DATE DUE

			PRINTED IN U.S.A.

Gynecologic Cancers

A Multidisciplinary Approach to
Diagnosis and Management

Current Multidisciplinary Oncology Series

Charles R. Thomas, Jr., MD
Series Editor

Current Multidisciplinary Oncology

Gynecologic Cancers
A Multidisciplinary Approach to Diagnosis and Management

Edited by

Kunle Odunsi, MD, PhD

The M. Steven Piver Professor and Chair
Department of Gynecologic Oncology
Director, Center for Immunotherapy
Roswell Park Cancer Institute
Buffalo, New York

Tanja Pejovic, MD, PhD

Associate Professor
Department of Obstetrics and Gynecology
The Knight Cancer Institute
Oregon Health & Science University
Portland, Oregon

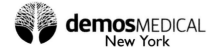
demosMEDICAL
New York

Acquisitions Editor: Rich Winters
Compositor: NewGen Imaging
Printer: Bradford & Bigelow

Visit our website at www.demosmedpub.com

Library of Congress Cataloging-in-Publication Data
Gynecologic cancers (2013)
 Gynecologic cancers : a multidisciplinary approach to diagnosis and management / [edited by] Kunle Odunsi, Tanja Pejovic.
    p. ; cm. — (Current multidisciplinary oncology)
 Includes bibliographical references and index.
 ISBN 978-1-936287-89-5
 I. Odunsi, Kunle, editor of compilation. II. Pejovic, Tanja, editor of compilation. III. Title. IV. Series: Current multidisciplinary oncology.
 [DNLM: 1. Genital Neoplasms, Female—diagnosis. 2. Genital Neoplasms, Female—therapy. WP 145]
 RC280.G4
 616.99'46—dc23   2013023405

Medicine is an ever-changing science. Research and clinical experience are continually expanding our knowledge, in particular our understanding of proper treatment and drug therapy. The authors, editors, and publisher have made every effort to ensure that all information in this book is in accordance with the state of knowledge at the time of production of the book. Nevertheless, the authors, editors, and publisher are not responsible for errors or omissions or for any consequences from application of the information in this book and make no warranty, expressed or implied, with respect to the contents of the publication. Every reader should examine carefully the package inserts accompanying each drug and should carefully check whether the dosage schedules mentioned therein or the contraindications stated by the manufacturer differ from the statements made in this book. Such examination is particularly important with drugs that are either rarely used or have been newly released on the market.

Special discounts on bulk quantities of Demos Medical Publishing books are available to corporations, professional associations, pharmaceutical companies, health care organizations, and other qualifying groups. For details, please contact:

Special Sales Department
Demos Medical Publishing
11 W. 42nd Street, 15th Floor
New York, NY 10036
Phone: 800-532-8663 or 212-683-0072
Fax: 212-941-7842
E-mail: special sales@demosmedpub.com

Made in the United States of America
13 14 15 16   5 4 3 2 1

Contents

Series Foreword

This volume in the series Current Multidisciplinary Oncology, devoted to gynecologic oncology, brings me great pleasure to introduce the practicing clinician to a valuable resource that will aid in the multidisciplinary approach of these common solid tumors.

Drs. Kunle Odunsi and Tanja Pejovic have put together a cadre of leading-edge investigators as contributors on the multidisciplinary approach to tumors of the female reproductive system.

Over the past decade, a myriad of advances in the diagnosis and treatment of gynecologic neoplasms have occurred. Some of the advances include, but are not limited to, diagnostic molecular tools that may aid in predicting a response to certain treatment approaches and/or in providing a guide of a prognostic outcomes for certain patients.

Thirty-three chapters have been compiled into well-defined sections by the volume co-editors.

Gynecologic neoplasms comprise some of the most common malignancies in the world and hence warrant intense efforts to find a cure. In recent years, investment of resources to help further understand the nature of this malignancy have increased.

Drs. Odunsi and Pejovic represent the current generation of academic, forward-thinking oncologists who have committed their careers to eradicating gynecologic cancer using multidisciplinary approaches. Their collective vision and ability to assemble an outstanding group of investigators in the field has provided a very high quality product that will be a useful resource to the busy clinician as well as those along various stages of the learning spectrum. I'm sure that you will enjoy this innovative and easy-to-read volume as you look for guidance in the multidisciplinary approach of your patients with gynecologic cancer.

Charles R. Thomas, Jr., MD
Series Editor
Department of Radiation Medicine
Oregon Health and Science University
Knight Cancer Institute
Portland, Oregon

Preface

The care of women with gynecologic cancer is best performed by multidisciplinary teams including gynecologic oncologists, radiation oncologists, medical oncologists, pathologists, geneticists, social workers, and palliative care specialists. Such multidisciplinary care has become imperative as a consequence of rapid advances in the understanding of the clinical, cellular, and molecular basis of cancer. These advances are leading to the development of novel strategies for screening, risk assessment, diagnosis, personalized treatments, supportive care, and survivorship. Ultimately, multidisciplinary care is critical for improving the quality of care of gynecologic cancer patients.

It is against this background that we have assembled an extraordinary team of leading experts from across different disciplines to distill the most current information in a succinct format, with sufficient depth and breadth.

While each chapter can stand alone, the final product is a unique textbook of gynecologic oncology with continuity of the multidisciplinary theme across chapters, covering the entire spectrum of gynecologic oncology topics. The book is designed to be a comprehensive text with up to date, relevant material for all providers of gynecologic cancer care including practicing physicians, nurse practitioners, physician assistants, residents, and fellows. It is our hope that we have accomplished our goal of providing a distinct reference text for the contemporary provider of gynecologic cancer care.

We are grateful to Dr. Charles Thomas for his scholarly vision and encouragement, and Mr. Rich Winters of Demos Medical Publishing for editorial guidance and timeliness. Finally we are indebted to our colleagues who contributed their time and knowledge toward this effort.

Contributors

Roshan Agarwal
Department of Oncology
Northampton General Hospital
Northampton, UK

Jay E. Allard, MD
Gynecologic Oncology
Naval Medical Center Portsmouth
Portsmouth, VA

Allison Ambrosio, BA
Gillette Center for Gynecologic Oncology
Massachusetts General Hospital Cancer Center
Boston, MA

Matthew L. Anderson, MD, PhD
Department of Obstetrics and Gynecology and
    Dan L. Duncan Cancer Center
Baylor College of Medicine
Houston, TX

Masoud Azodi, MD
Division of Gynecologic Oncology
Department of Obstetrics/Gynecology and Reproductive
    Sciences
Yale University School of Medicine
New Haven, CT

Paul B. Bascom, MD
Palliative Medicine Physician
Portland, OR

Jonathan S. Berek, MD, MMS
Laurie Kraus Lacob Professor
Stanford Women's Center
Stanford Clinic Institute
Department of Obstetrics and Gynecology
Stanford University School of Medicine
Stanford, CA

Michelle Berlin, MD, MPH
Departments of Obstetrics and Gynecology,
    Public Health and Preventive Medicine,
    Medical Informatics and Clinical Epidemiology
OHSU Center for Women's Health
Oregon Health & Science University
Portland, OR

Emily Berry, MD
Division of Gynecologic Oncology
Department of Obstetrics and Gynecology
Robert H. Lurie Comprehensive Cancer Center
Northwestern University Feinberg School of Medicine
Chicago, IL

Michael A. Bidus, MD
Division of Gynecologic Oncology
Department of Obstetrics and Gynecology
Naval Medical Center Portsmouth
Portsmouth, VA

Michael J. Birrer, MD, PhD
Professor
Department of Medicine
Harvard Medical School
Department of Hematology/Oncology
Massachusetts General Hospital
Boston, MA

Michelle M. Boisen, MD
Division of Gynecologic Oncology
Department of Obstetrics, Gynecology, and Reproductive
    Sciences
Magee-Womens Hospital of UPMC
Pittsburgh, PA

Leslie Bradford, MD
Gillette Center for Gynecologic Oncology
Massachusetts General Hospital Cancer Center
Boston, MA

Molly A. Brewer, DVM, MD, MS
Division of Gynecologic Oncology
Department of Obstetrics and Gynecology
University of Connecticut School of Medicine
Farmington, CT

Russell R. Broaddus, MD, PhD
Department of Pathology
University of Texas
MD Anderson Cancer Center
Houston, TX

Setsuko K. Chambers, MD
Division of Women's Cancers
University of Arizona Cancer Center
Division of Gynecologic Oncology
Department of Obstetrics and Gynecology
University of Arizona
Tucson, AZ

Dennis S. Chi, MD
Memorial Sloan-Kettering Cancer Center
New York, NY

Christina S. Chu, MD
Obstetrics and Gynecology
Division of Gynecologic Oncology
Hospital of the University of Pennsylvania
Jordan Center for Gynecologic Cancer
Philadelphia, PA

Sayeema Daudi, MD
Department of Gynecologic Oncology
Roswell Park Cancer Institute
Buffalo, NY

Ben Davidson, MD, PhD
Institute of Clinical Medicine
University of Oslo and Division of Pathology
Oslo University Hospital
The Norwegian Radium Hospital
Oslo, Norway

Elena Diaz, MD
Department of Obstetrics and Gynecology
David Geffen School of Medicine
University of California
Los Angeles, CA

Bojana Djordjevic, MD
Department of Pathology and Laboratory Medicine
University of Ottawa
The Ottawa Hospital
Ottawa, Ontario, Canada

Oliver Dorigo, MD, PhD
Manager
Gynecologic Endoscopy
Assistant Professor
Gynecologic Oncology Institute for Molecular Medicine
David Geffen School of Medicine
University of California
Los Angeles, CA

Shona Dougherty, MB, ChB, PhD
Department of Radiation Oncology
University of Arizona
University Medical Center
Tucson, AZ

Elizabeth A. Dubil, MD
Walter Reed National Military Medical Center
Bethesda, MD

Robert P. Edwards, MD
Division of Gynecologic Oncology
Department of Obstetrics, Gynecology and Reproductive Sciences
Magee-Womens Hospital of UPMC
Pittsburgh, PA

Ane Gerda Zahl Eriksson, MD
Department of Gynaecological Oncology
Oslo University Hospital
The Norwegian Radium Hospital
Oslo, Norway

Jim Fanning, DO
Division of Gynecologic Oncology
Department of Obstetrics and Gynecology
Pennsylvania State University
Milton S. Hershey Medical Center
Hershey, PA

Tamara Finger, MD
Division of Minimally Invasive Surgery
Department of Obstetrics and Gynecology
St. Luke's Roosevelt Hospital
New York, NY

Ashley Ford Haggerty, MD
Division of Gynecologic Oncology
Hospital of the University of Pennsylvania
Jordan Center for Gynecologic Cancer
Philadelphia, PA

Katherine C. Fuh, MD, PhD
Division of Gynecologic Oncology
Department of Obstetrics and Gynecology
Stanford University School of Medicine
Stanford Women's Cancer Center
Stanford, CA

Heidi Godoy, DO
Department of Gynecologic Oncology
Roswell Park Cancer Institute
Buffalo, NY

Keith A. Joiner, MD, MPH
Health Promotion and Sciences Division
Mel and Enid Zuckerman College of Public Health
University of Arizona
Tucson, AZ

Janne Kaern, MD, PhD
Department of Gynaecological Oncology
Oslo University Hospital
The Norwegian Radium Hospital
Oslo, Norway

Joshua P. Kesterson, MD
Division of Gynecologic Oncology
Department of Obstetrics and Gynecology
Pennsylvania State University
Milton S. Hershey Medical Center
Hershey, PA

Susan S. Khalil, MD
Division of Minimally Invasive Surgery
Department of Obstetrics and Gynecology
St. Luke's Roosevelt Hospital
New York, NY

Nonna Kolomeyevskaya, MD
Gynecologic Oncology Fellow
Roswell Park Cancer Center
Buffalo, NY

Colleen McCormick, MD, MPH
Compass Oncology
Portland, OR

Loren K. Mell MD
Division of Clinical and Translational Research
Department of Radiation Medicine and Applied Sciences
University of California San Diego
La Jolla, CA

Emily Meserve, MD, MPH
Brigham and Women's Hospital
Boston, MA

Terry Morgan, MD, PhD
Departments of Pathology and Obstetrics and Gynecology
Oregon Health and Science University
Portland, OR

Arno J. Mundt, MD
Department of Radiation Medicine and Applied Sciences
University of California San Diego
La Jolla, CA

Farr R. Nezhat, MD
Division of Minimally Invasive Surgery
Department of Obstetrics and Gynecology
St. Luke's Roosevelt Hospital
Columbia University Medical Center
New York, NY

Kunle Odunsi, MD, PhD
Department of Gynecologic Oncology
Center for Immunotherapy
Roswell Park Cancer Institute
Buffalo, NY

Tanja Pejovic, MD, PhD
Department of Obstetrics and Gynecology
The Knight Cancer Institute
Oregon Health & Science University
Portland, OR

Evgenia Polosina, MD
Division of Minimally Invasive Surgery
Department of Obstetrics and Gynecology
St. Luke's Roosevelt Hospital
New York, NY

Susan J. Ramus, MD
Department of Preventive Medicine
Keck School of Medicine
USC/Norris Comprehensive Cancer Center
University of Southern California
Los Angeles, CA

Elena Ratner, MD
Department of Obstetrics, Gynecology,
    and Reproductive Sciences
Division of Gynecologic Oncology
Yale University School of Medicine
New Haven, CT

Dana M. Roque, MD
Department of Obstetrics, Gynecology,
    and Reproductive Sciences
Division of Gynecologic Oncology
Yale University School of Medicine
New Haven, CT

Peter G. Rose, MD
Section of Gynecologic Oncology
The Cleveland Clinic Foundation
Cleveland, OH

Alessandro D. Santin, MD
Department of Obstetrics, Gynecology,
    and Reproductive Sciences
Division of Gynecologic Oncology
Yale University School of Medicine
New Haven, CT

John O. Schorge, MD
Vincent Department of Obstetrics and Gynecology
Division of Gynecologic Oncology
Massachusetts General Hospital
Harvard Medical School
Boston, MA

Peter E. Schwartz, MD
Department of Obstetrics, Gynecology,
    and Reproductive Sciences
Division of Gynecologic Oncology
Yale University School of Medicine
New Haven, CT

Neil J. Sebire
Department of Medical Oncology
Charing Cross Hospital Campus
Imperial College NHS Healthcare Trust and
    Imperial College London
London, UK

Michael J. Seckl
Department of Medical Oncology
Charing Cross Hospital Campus
Imperial College NHS Healthcare Trust and
    Imperial College London
London, UK

Tyler M. Seibert, MD, PhD
Department of Radiation Medicine and Applied Sciences
University of California San Diego
La Jolla, CA

Jay P. Shah, MD
Division of Gynecologic Oncology
Department of Obstetrics and Gynecology Orange County
Southern California Permanente Medical Group
Assistant Clinical Professor
University of California-Irvine
Irvine, CA

Daniel R. Simpson MD
Department of Radiation Medicine and Applied Sciences
University of California San Diego
La Jolla, CA

Tijana Skrepnik, MD
Department of Radiation Oncology
University of Arizona Medical Center
Tucson, AZ

Anil K. Sood, MD
Departments of Gynecologic Oncology and Cancer Biology
Blanton-Davis Ovarian Cancer Research Program
Center for RNA Interference and Non-Coding RNA
MD Anderson Cancer Center
Houston, TX

Amy Stenson, MD, MSc
Oregon Health & Science University
Department of Obstetrics and Gynecology
Portland, OR

Jason Sternchos, MD
Division of Minimally Invasive Surgery
Department of Obstetrics and Gynecology
North Shore University Hospital
Manhasset, NY

Devansu Tewari, MD
Division of Gynecologic Oncology
Department of Obstetrics and Gynecology Orange County
Southern California Permanente Medical Group
University of California-Irvine
Irvine, CA

Premal H. Thaker, MD
Division of Gynecologic Oncology
Department of Obstetrics and Gynecology
Washington University School of Medicine
St. Louis, MO

Eugene P. Toy, MD
Division of Gynecologic Oncology
Department of Obstetrics and Gynecology
The University of Rochester
Rochester, NY

Claes Göran Tropé, MD, PhD
Department of Gynaecological Oncology
Oslo University Hospital
The Norwegian Radium Hospital and
    Institute of Clinical Medicine
University of Oslo
Oslo, Norway

Joyce Varughese, MD
Department of Obstetrics, Gynecology,
    and Reproductive Sciences
Division of Gynecologic Oncology
Yale University School of Medicine
New Haven, CT

Lori E. Weinberg, MD
Section of Gynecologic Oncology
The Cleveland Clinic Foundation
Cleveland, OH

William E. Winter, III, MD
Division of Gynecologic Oncology/Pelvic Surgery
Compass Oncology: Rose Quarter/St. Vincent Cancer Centers
Portland, OR

Catheryn M. Yashar, MD
Division of Clinical Radiation Oncology
Department of Radiation Medicine and Applied Sciences
University of California San Diego
La Jolla, CA

Cervical Cancer and Precancerous Lesions

I

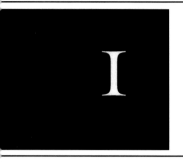

The Biology of Human Papillomavirus and the Etiology of Female Genital Tract Cancers

EUGENE P. TOY

The human papillomavirus (HPV) belongs to a family of papillomaviruses that have been discerned through the ages and studied in a variety of animal models. Genital warts portrayed by fig leaves have been the subject of classical art and sculpture dating back to ancient times. While equally as elegant and artful in terms of research, the bovine, canine, and cottontail rabbit (CTR) papillomavirus models are a few of the well-established animal systems employed over the years to study the virus (1–3). With difficulties in the propagation of papillomavirus presenting an obstacle to in vitro culture, reliance on these animal papillomavirus models has provided much information into mutagenesis of DNA sequence, overexpression of early and late gene products, and transcriptional regulation in order to better understand the viral replication cycle and design novel therapeutics for HPV-associated disease.

In spite of these models, little is known of the active phase of productive HPV replication following initial exposure and inoculation (4). The virus is highly epitheliotropic, entering through gaps or breeches in the cervix, vagina, and/or vulvar skin with great affinity, even to the extent of self-inoculation in directly opposed tissues such as the labia or with transmission via the "field effect," which is not readily deterred by barriers such as condoms. Once penetrating the surface epithelium, the virus begins to express its early proteins under the regulation of the host promoter.

■ VIRAL STRUCTURE AND GENOMIC ORGANIZATION

The infectious viral particle of HPV is known as a virion and is composed of one molecule of double-stranded circular DNA, 8 kb in length, contained within an icosahedral structure formed from the natural assembly of its L1 and L2 proteins forming a protein coat or capsid (Figure 1.1).

Sequence Homology

Based on genotyping, the *Papillomaviridae* family contains over 100 types that can be recognized and grouped into 18 genera by sequence homology. While the mucosal infecting types, such as those associated with lower genital tract disease, belong to the *Alpha papillomavirus* genus, there is crossover of species from types causing benign warts to those causing low- and high-grade dysplasia (Table 1.1) with their associated disease manifestations seen in Figure 1.2.

Regulatory Proteins

URR—The "upstream regulatory region" where, under the influence of both cellular and viral factors, the main control of viral genome transcription is exerted, which leads to the encoded messages responsible for viral replication. Downstream from the URR, well-conserved gene sequences of the HPV genome produce the necessary viral proteins, which leads to active viral production in an orchestrated manner.

Early Proteins

E2—The main transcriptional regulatory protein that has four binding sites on the URR (6) and exerts control over the two predominant early proteins, E6 and E7, which are synthesized early in viral replication. Interruption of this viral control is found after the integration of the HPV viral genome into the host genome and results in unregulated overexpression of E6 and E7.

E6—Part of the dicistronic message produced early after initial viral infection leading to the production of both E6 and E7 in the basal layers of the epithelium shortly after infection. In oncogenic HPV types causing cancer, E6 binds the tumor suppressor protein p53, targeting it for the ubiquitination pathway and subsequent degradation.

E7—The distal part of the dicistronic message produced under the regulation of E2 protein. E7 from oncogenic HPV types will bind to pRb (retinoblastoma) protein and cause its inhibition, which also leads to subsequent loss of cell-cycle control from G1 to S phase.

E1—A "late" early protein subsumed by its counterpart E4 protein. It is involved in viral replication and controls gene transcription. It also is involved in the maintenance of the viral episome.

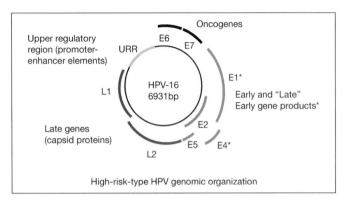

FIGURE 1.1 The exemplary viral genome of high-risk oncogenic HPV-16 is shown. Both the early and late genes are highly conserved amongst noncancer and cancer-causing types, respectively.

■ **Table 1.1** Clinical manifestations of specific HPV types are shown. Most commonly associated types are presented first with more inclusive listing provided in parentheses.

Biologic (Disease) Manifestation	Commonly Associated HPV Type
Condyloma (benign lower genital tract warts)	6, 11
Low-grade dysplasia (productive infection)	42, 43, 44 (as well as 6, 11)
High-grade dysplasia (neoplastic infection)	31, 33, 35, 52, 58 (as well as types below)
Invasive carcinoma	16, 18, 45, 56

E4—The other "late" early protein that marks the onset of viral genome amplification and comprises the E1^E4 gene product that has been found to localize and bind to intermediate filaments of the cytoskeleton. In oncogenic HPV types, the E1^E4 protein will cause the collapse of the cytoskeleton, thus suggesting a role for viral propagation in cancer-causing types.

Late Proteins

L1—Major capsid protein that is involved in the formation of the pentamer structure, which comprises the virion, and is highly immunogenic in the native conformation of the virion, providing a neutralizing epitope.

L2—Minor capsid protein involved with the assembly of the virion and the formation of the infectious particle to be released. Not detected by the neutralizing antibody elicited by commercial vaccine, but still may provide protection by more sensitive second-generation assays (7).

■ VIRAL LIFE CYCLE

Early Infection

In the basal layer of the epithelium, the early E6 and E7 gene products are expressed under the regulation of the host promoter. HPV viral DNA synthesis occurs early after infection as part of an initial amplification of viral genomic DNA in order to reach a baseline number of approximately 50 to 100 DNA copies per infected cell (4). Little is known about the factors that control these events. Viral gene expression following this maintenance level of viral amplification is highly regulated and occurs only in cells that have lost their ability

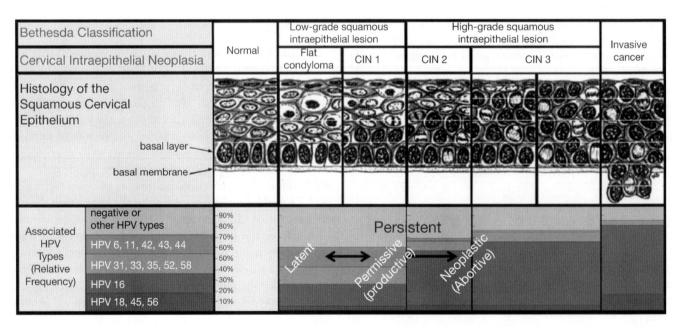

FIGURE 1.2 Transformation of normal epithelium through preinvasive change to invasive carcinoma is presented in schematic form. Associated HPV types and the frequency in which they are found are presented in parallel with histologic representations. (Modified with permission from [5].)

to divide. On histologic sections, cells that are found differentiating through the layers of the epithelium lose their ability to divide and become enucleated as seen in the superficial layer. Through these layers of cell maturation, there is production of early gene products necessary for virus production, with gene amplification occurring under the influence of E1, E2, and E4 with production on the order of 1000 copies of genome produced. Virion assembly occurs and cytopathic changes can be seen in the layer just below the surface epithelium. These classic cytopathic changes with pathognomonic wrinkled nuclei occur as a result of HPV infection. Release of infectious particles through the superficial epithelium may occur as a result of trauma or potentially as an effect of HPV E1^E4 protein in association with cytoskeletal elements leading to the collapse of the cell structure and subsequent release of viral particles (8).

Viral Gene Transcription and Regulation

The HPV genome exists in an extrachromosomal form known as an episome in low-grade lesions caused by HPV from both low- and high-risk types. The prevalence of high-risk HPV types in low-grade dysplasia of the cervix is quite evident from the ALTS (Atypical Squamous Cells of Undetermined Significance/Low-Grade Squamous Intraepithelial Lesion Triage Study) trial and had preempted the completion of the low-grade arm (9). This illustrates the importance of tight regulation of viral DNA transcription by E2 where its open reading frame (ORF) encodes the regulatory proteins controlling the transcription of E6 and E7 early proteins. E6 protein has many well-characterized roles that may function in a pleiotropic manner. It has the ability to cause heterologous viral infection as well as host-cell transcriptional transactivation (10). As it is part of a dicistronic message with the E7 gene, E6 acts in concert with E7 during the early "basal" and productive phases of a viral infection. Both E1 and E2 proteins are required for this extrachromosomal DNA replication. However, due to the occurrence of alternate splicing, E1 is subsumed by E4, and the two act during the "late" early phase of the replication process, with E4 resembling the late proteins. The E5 gene product enhances the growth effects seen in the same layers beneath the surface where koilocytes are found manifest from the cytopathic effects of HPV. The HPV early proteins E2 and E1^E4 have been shown to elicit G2 arrest prior to cell division or mitosis (11). This function of E1^E4 is conserved in spite of this alternate splicing with several subtypes of HPV including 11, 16, and 18 also exhibiting E1^E4-induced G2 arrest. This delay prior to cell division may represent yet another level of control that these early proteins exert over viral replication.

The highly ordered process of natural virus infection and productive replication must be distinguished from aberrant neoplastic infection that leads to precancer and

ultimate invasive cancer. This "abortive" type of infection represents a neoplastic process of viral replication that occurs with cancer-causing HPV types and leads to integration of the HPV genome into the host genome and loss of regulation by the host promoter (8). In addition, there is redundancy in the feedback loop of p53 that may also affect the G2 to M progression. On both levels from G1 to S and G2 to M, the deleterious effect of p53 degradation may enhance the pathogenesis process leading to HPV-induced dysplasia and neoplasia.

Persistent Infection

Persistence of high-risk HPV represents the one true risk factor associated in the development of invasive cancer. Although persistent infection occurs in 20% of women who have no overt evidence of disease on colposcopy, up to 30% will develop high-risk lesions within 2 years due to persistence of HPV infection (12). If clearance of the virus does not occur, as is the norm in over 90% of affected women, an alternating pattern of regression and progression may occur over the course of several years (13). Small lesions may be imperceptible on colposcopy, but with larger apparent lesions, there will be progression to invasive carcinoma about one-third of the time (14). Over time, with the E6 and E7 oncogenes becoming overexpressed after integration into the host genome combined with additional tissue differentiation due to hormonal effects, genetic instability due to epigenetic factors may lead to changes in the expression of host-cell genes and progression of these in situ lesions to become frankly invasive. An increase in telomerase activity by transactivation of hTERT by E6 protein and other chromosomal aberrations have both been cited as potential causes of this disease progression (15).

Natural or innate immunity to the HPV virus is responsible for 90% of clearance of initial viral infection in spite of the relative lack of detectable systemic humoral response and a blunted cellular immune response to the early proteins produced after infection (16). The innate immune response then kick-starts the adaptive immune response with Th1 (cell-mediated) and Th2 (humoral-mediated) responses. In the case of invasive cancer, an antibody response is generated against oncoproteins E6 and E7 and is clinically detectable (17). Otherwise, the L1 capsid protein is able to evoke a humoral response albeit slow in vivo (18), but has been found in vaccine trials to be highly protective for disease prevention based on serum transfer experiments in CTR, dog, and rhesus monkey models with currently available commercial vaccines produced from recombinant L1 protein providing vaccination levels 50–10,000× higher than natural infection. E6 downregulates toll-like receptors (TLR), while Langerhans cells are inactivated by E2. Such an immunosuppressed environment is commonplace in transformed cells (19). HIV patients are exemplary of the reduced clearance of the HPV virus with reactivation of latent infection despite abstinence of new exposures from new sexual encounters (20). The E5 protein has been shown to be responsible for the virus' ability to evade the immune system by interfering with antigen presentation. Ultimately, however, the resolution of active infection requires cellular immunity.

Transformation and Integration of HPV DNA

Once integration of the viral HPV genome takes place and/or E2 function is lost by mutation, there is a loss of E2-mediated control of E6 and E7 expression which then becomes unregulated (21). This corresponds with the transition of permissive HPV infection in its episomal form associated with low-grade dysplasia to an integrated form that results clinically in the neoplastic phenotype (Figure 1.2). E6 protein from these oncogenic-type HPV strains can bind to p53 causing its degradation and loss of checkpoint control in the cell cycle from G1 to S phase as the oncoprotein is overexpressed. This loss of cell-cycle regulation will allow damaged or transformed cells to progress through the cell cycle to cell division and produce daughter cells thereby perpetuating changes in DNA that have resulted from HPV infection.

HPV E7 protein acts in analogous fashion to bind to another tumor suppressor protein pRb, which is also involved in checkpoint control at G1 to S. When HPV E7 from oncogenic types binds pRb, it releases pRb inhibition of E2F, which is then free to act as a catalyst to cell-cycle progression from G1 to S.

Several years after these events are caused by "abortive" or nonproductive infection by HPV, there can be progression of dysplasia from moderate to severe disease, or even neoplasia. Just as permissive or productive infection can occur after chronic latent HPV infection over the course of many years, the time frame of neoplastic progression can take as long as a decade and is affected by multiple factors including age, immunocompromised status, histology, and tissue type (22). Intervention by ablative procedures, however, can usually abrogate this process of transformation but will not eliminate the viral cause of the pathogenesis.

■ TISSUE-SPECIFIC PATHOGENESIS

Cervix

Highly susceptible to the effects of HPV infection particularly in the adolescent cervix, the protuberance, known as the portio, provides a larger surface area for inoculation with HPV to occur. As puberty takes place, this expansive ectropion becomes exposed to the acid environment in the vagina and the process of squamous metaplasia takes place leading to creation of the transformation zone. This relatively thin, vulnerable region of epithelium represents the area at most risk for introduction of HPV and subsequent development of cervical dysplasia.

The endocervical canal is sequestered from the changes in vaginal pH. Glandular abnormalities occurring in this central portion of the canal most commonly are related to infection with types HPV-18 and HPV-16. The less common cancers with small cell and neuroendocrine-type histology are also found to contain HPV-18 but occur infrequently and have a very aggressive phenotype.

Vagina

While vaginal dysplasia is rare, it follows the same pattern of risk factors as with cervical dysplasia. Those with known history of treatment for cervical dysplasia or neoplasia are at significant risk for vaginal dysplasia with 30% of primary vaginal cancers having had a history of in situ or invasive cervical cancer within the prior 5 years, and the majority of these having undergone hysterectomy (23). Disease is most commonly found at the apex of the vagina, often following surgery. HPV infection with low-risk HPV-6 is associated with low-grade disease, while high-risk types, particularly HPV-16, place individuals at risk for high-grade squamous dysplasia and neoplasia as with its cervical counterpart, albeit at much lower frequency for progression of high-grade or severe dysplasia to invasive cancer (9%–10%).

Vulva

The bimodal distribution of disease illustrates the susceptibility of the vulvar skin to the effects of HPV infection after exposure, particularly in women of young reproductive age. Similar high-risk types such as HPV-16 responsible for cervical cancer are found in vulvar dysplasia and neoplasia. Smoking as a cofactor seems to be associated with this younger group at risk for high-grade dysplasia. While low-risk HPV types 6 and 11 are generally associated with vulvar condyloma, low-grade dysplasia can be found containing HPV-6 with the rare variant of verrucous carcinoma manifesting from malignant transformation of warty disease.

While high-grade cervical dysplasia portends approximately 30% of progression to invasive carcinoma from in situ disease and vaginal dysplasia even less, vulvar carcinoma in situ progresses to frank invasion in over 90% of cases if left untreated (24). Only 5% of treated high-grade dysplasia will progress to invasive disease. The high rate of progression may be related to difficulty in diagnosing invasive disease on preoperative biopsy prior to definitive resection in addition to noncompliance in the elderly population. Regardless, the relatively low incidence of this disease results in a lag in providing translational data as is now becoming available from cervical cancer studies using molecular markers of progression.

■ BIOLOGICAL MARKERS OF PROGRESSION

As surrogates for viral-induced carcinogenesis, markers of disease progression have been the subject of ongoing research in order to determine individuals most at risk for progression to invasive cancer. These markers reflect the sequelae of aberrant infection that does not necessarily result in productive viral infection but instead in the development of malignant transformation from preinvasive disease (Figure 1.2). These markers will become more crucial in triage of women in the era of HPV-vaccinated cohorts worldwide where the majority of HPV-16- and HPV-18-associated cancers will inevitably decline (25).

p16 INK4a

This protein normally functions as one of the cyclin-dependent kinase (cdk) inhibitors, which regulate cdk-4 and cdk-6 activity. When E7 oncoprotein interacts with pRB, p16 INK4a levels increase as negative feedback to the loss of pRb protein by the release of E2F. This increase in p16 can therefore represent a marker for loss of checkpoint control from G1 to S phase, which upregulates cell proliferation. The interaction of E7 and pRb is present in nearly all CIN2/CIN3 (88%–98%) and in invasive carcinoma and represents an important threshold for treatment intervention (26).

Ki-67

One of the markers of proliferation, it is found in all phases of the cell-cycle except for G0 or senescence. Thus, it reflects actively proliferating cells. It has been found to be overexpressed in a variety of cancers and is associated with malignant transformation. Dual staining with p16 has been used in triage of HPV+/normal PAP women (27).

Mini-Chromosome Maintenance (MCM)

The MCM proteins are a family of proteins that are involved in the initiation of the DNA replication complex. Among others in this family, MCM-5 expression in cervical dysplasia and neoplasia specimens has been shown to have the most potential clinical value with 100% sensitivity and 67% specificity. It is found expressed solely in the nucleus and reflects proliferating cells in the parabasal layer.

PCNA

Involved in the initiation of DNA synthesis, productive HPV virus replication requires host machinery, as the more superficial layers of the epithelium have lost their ability to divide. As another marker of proliferation, it has been used in conjunction with Ki-67.

Methylation Markers

The detection of methylation sites of promoters where tumor suppressor function has been lost is also being used in clinical practice to predict disease progression. Hypermethylation occurs early during the transformation events leading to cervical cancer. Examples include the CADM1 and MAL-m1 promoter sites in high-risk HPV types. Epigenetic models with methylation of E2-binding sites have supported this pathway of progression (28).

Cyclin D

Functioning as regulatory subunits of the cdk-4 and cdk-6, cyclin D1 and D3 have been explored as surrogate markers of disease progression. As they exert negative control over the cdks responsible for progression from G1 to S, decreases in cyclin D1 and D3 expression have been found associated with high-grade cervical dysplasia and invasive carcinoma (29).

Cyclins A and B

The regulatory subunits of cdk-2 and cdk-1, respectively, these cyclins, responsible for transition to M phase, have been studied particularly in invasive carcinoma of the cervix. Poor sensitivity using this test has limited its clinical utility although it has been found to have some correlation with the less common glandular adenocarcinomas.

■ CLINICAL MODELS FOR HPV-RELATED DISEASE

With the inability to clear the virus causing persistent infection, the events that are responsible for progression through the spectrum of disease (Figure 1.2) into invasive cancer become harder to delineate. The wealth of clinical data in young adolescent patients supports the finding that even with high-grade changes noted on cytology, the majority of these lesions will regress. Infection and/or reinfection with high-risk oncogenic-type HPV portends the highest risk found for high-grade disease vs low-grade change where 90% regression rate is noted. Only a nominal few cases of invasive cervical cancer were noted from SEER data from 2002 in the under 20 age group in a time where screening of adolescents was more commonplace (30). Current admonition is for HPV co-testing in women 30 years of age and older.

The alternative scenario in older women presents another challenge to effective screening. With about a quarter of cervical cancer patients being in their postmenopausal years, lack of screening becomes the fore-most reason for this increase in incident cases from this age group over 50. Again, the majority of women who had been exposed to HPV would have cleared their infection over the years. Guidelines for HPV testing in those women over age 65 have been established, and compliance with guidelines continues to be reinforced actively among primary care providers and gynecologic specialists (31).

■ REFERENCES

1. Brandsma JL. The cottontail rabbit papillomavirus model of high-risk HPV-induced disease. *Methods Mol Med.* 2005;119:217–235.

2. Venuti A, Paolini F, Nasir L, et al. Papillomavirus E5: the smallest oncoprotein with many functions. *Mol Cancer.* 2011;10:140.

3. Suprynowicz FA, Disbrow GL, Simic V, Schlegel R. Are transforming properties of the bovine papillomavirus E5 protein shared by E5 from high-risk human papillomavirus type 16? *Virology.* 2005;332(1):102–113.

4. Howley P, Lowy DR. Papillomaviruses and their replication. In: Knip DM, Howley PM, eds. *Fields Virology.* Vol. II, 4th ed., chapter 65. Philadelphia, PA: Lippincott Williams & Wilkins, 2001: 2210.

5. Rose RC, Stoler MH. Biology. In Bonnez W, ed. *Guide to Genital HPV Diseases and Prevention.* New York, NY: Informa Healthcare, 2009.

6. Hegde RS. The papillomavirus E2 proteins: structure, function, and biology. *Annu Rev Biophys Biomol Struct.* 2002;31:343–360.

7. Day PM, Pang YY, Kines RC, Thompson CD, Lowy DR, Schiller JT. A human papillomavirus (HPV) *in vitro* neutralization assay that recapitulates the *in vitro* process of infection provides a sensitive measure of HPV L2 infection-inhibiting antibodies. *Clin Vaccine Immunol.* 2012;19(7):1075–1082.

8. Doorbar J, Quint W, Banks L, et al. The biology and life-cycle of human papillomaviruses. *Vaccine.* 2012;30 Suppl 5:F55–F70.

9. ALTS Group. Human papillomavirus testing for triage of women with cytologic evidence of low-grade squamous intraepithelial lesions: baseline data from a randomized trial. *J Natl Cancer Inst.* 2000;92(5):397–402.

10. Myers G, Androphy E. The E6 protein In: Myers G, Delius H, Icenogel J, et al. eds. *Human Papillomaviruses.* Vol. III. Los Alamos, NM: Los Alamos National Laboratory.

11. Davy CE, Jackson DJ, Wang Q, et al. Identification of a G(2) arrest domain in the E1 wedge E4 protein of human papillomavirus type 16. *J Virol.* 2002;76(19):9806–9818.

12. Gage JC, Schiffman M, Solomon D, Wheeler CM, Castle PE. Comparison of measurements of human papillomavirus persistence for postcolposcopic surveillance for cervical precancerous lesions. *Cancer Epidemiol Biomarkers Prev.* 2010;19(7):1668–1674.

13. Moscicki AB, Ma Y, Wibbelsman C, et al. Rate of and risks for regression of cervical intraepithelial neoplasia 2 in adolescents and young women. *Obstet Gynecol.* 2010;116(6):1373–1380.

14. McCredie MR, Sharples KJ, Paul C, et al. Natural history of cervical neoplasia and risk of invasive cancer in women with cervical intraepithelial neoplasia 3: a retrospective cohort study. *Lancet Oncol.* 2008;9(5):425–434.

15. Van Doorslaer K, Burk RD. Association between hTERT activation by HPV E6 proteins and oncogenic risk. *Virology.* 2012;433(1):216–219.

16. Trimble CL, Clark RA, Thoburn C, et al. Human papillomavirus 16-associated cervical intraepithelial neoplasia in humans excludes CD8 T cells from dysplastic epithelium. *J Immunol.* 2010;185(11):7107–7114.

17. Woo YL, van den Hende M, Sterling JC, et al. A prospective study on the natural course of low-grade squamous intraepithelial lesions and the presence of HPV16 E2-, E6-, and E7-specific T-cell responses. *Int J Cancer.* 2010;126(1):133–141.

18. Stanley M. Immune responses to human papillomavirus. *Vaccine.* 2006;24 Suppl 1:S16–S22.

19. Stanley MA, Pett MR, Coleman N. HPV: from infection to cancer. *Biochem Soc Trans.* 2007;35(Pt 6):1456–1460.

20. Strickler HD, Burk RD, Fazzari M, et al. Natural history and possible reactivation of human papillomavirus in human immunodeficiency virus-positive women. *J Natl Cancer Inst.* 2005;97(8):577–586.

21. Park TW, Fujiwara H, Wright TC. Molecular biology of cervical cancer and its precursors. *Cancer.* 1995;76(10 Suppl):1902–1913.

22. Kelly JG, Cheung KT, Martin C, et al. A spectral phenotype of oncogenic human papillomavirus-infected exfoliative cervical cytology distinguishes women based on age. *Clin Chim Acta.* 2010;411(15–16):1027–1033.

23. Gurumurthy M, Cruickshank ME. Management of vaginal intraepithelial neoplasia. *J Low Genit Tract Dis.* 2012;16(3):306–312.

24. van Seters M, van Beurden M, de Craen AJ. Is the assumed natural history of vulvar intraepithelial neoplasia III based on enough evidence? A systematic review of 3322 published patients. *Gynecol Oncol.* 2005;97(2):645–651.

25. Franco EL, Bosch FX, Cuzick J, et al. Chapter 29: Knowledge gaps and priorities for research on prevention of HPV infection and cervical cancer. *Vaccine.* 2006;24 Suppl 3:S3/242–249.

26. Tsoumpou I, Arbyn M, Kyrgiou M, et al. p16(INK4a) immunostaining in cytological and histological specimens from the uterine cervix: a systematic review and meta-analysis. *Cancer Treat Rev.* 2009;35(3):210–220.

27. Petry KU, Schmidt D, Scherbring S, et al. Triaging Pap cytology negative, HPV positive cervical cancer screening results with p16/Ki-67 Dual-stained cytology. *Gynecol Oncol.* 2011;121(3):505–509.

28. Vinokurova S, von Knebel Doeberitz M. Differential methylation of the HPV 16 upstream regulatory region during epithelial differentiation and neoplastic transformation. *PLoS ONE.* 2011;6(9):e24451.

29. Malinowski DP. Molecular diagnostics for cervical neoplasia: emerging markers for the detection of high-grade cervical disease. *Biotechniques.* 2005;38:S17–S23.

30. Saslow D, Solomon D, Lawson HW, et al.; ACS-ASCCP-ASCP Cervical Cancer Guideline Committee. American Cancer Society, American Society for Colposcopy and Cervical Pathology, and American Society for Clinical Pathology screening guidelines for the prevention and early detection of cervical cancer. *CA Cancer J Clin.* 2012;62(3):147–172.

31. Berkowitz A, Saraiya M, Sawaya G. Cervical cancer screening intervals, 2006 to 2009: moving beyond annual testing. *JAMA Intern Med.* 2013;1–3. doi:10.1001/jamainternmed.

2 Cervical Cancer Prevention: HPV Vaccines

MICHELLE BERLIN

Cervical cancer remains the most common cancer in women worldwide. High-risk human papillomavirus (HPV) types are considered to be the etiology of the majority of cases of cervical cancer; the most common types are 16 and 18. HPV vaccine development focused on immunization against types 16 and 18 due to their predominance. This chapter describes the two HPV vaccines licensed in the United States and current challenges to immunization.

■ HPV VACCINE DEVELOPMENT

Once HPV was identified as the etiology of most types of cervical carcinoma, efforts began to develop a vaccine. Two key proteins required for HPV replication were targeted in vaccine development: E6 and E7. The main role of E6 is to bind the tumor suppressor protein p53, a DNA protein important to suppress viral replication (1). E7 alters pRb retinoblastoma gene product to facilitate cell-cycle progression and subsequent proliferation of HPV. While E6 and E7 can act alone to induce HPV production and elaboration, their combined efforts more efficiently lead to cell proliferation and subsequent release of HPV.

After working in mammalian models, Frazer (2) and others realized that virus-like particles (VLPs) could be constructed to induce cell-mediated and humoral immune responses to HPV in humans. The two vaccines currently approved by the U.S. Food and Drug Administration (FDA) utilize VLPs designed to express L1, the primary HPV capsid protein, using recombinant DNA. Antibodies are formed to the capsid through humoral and cellular antibody development, leading to immunity. The two vaccines licensed in the United States use VLP technology with a different adjuvant system to induce immunity to HPV.

The quadrivalent vaccine HPV4 (Gardasil, manufactured by Merck) was approved by the FDA in 2006. HPV4 has activity against high-risk HPV strains 16 and 18 and against low-risk HPV strains 11 and 16. Four coordinated studies were conducted to assess the efficacy of HPV4. As described by the investigators of the largest study (Females United to Unilaterally Reduce Endo/Ectocervical Disease [FUTURE] II Study Group [3]), these trials were designed to assess vaccine efficacy in the prevention of cervical intraepithelial neoplasia (CIN) grade 2 & 3, and adenocarcinoma in situ (AIS). These surrogate endpoints were chosen because prevention of cervical cancer per se was "neither feasible nor ethical" (3). In brief, 20,583 women worldwide primarily aged 16 to 23 participated in these randomized, double-blind, placebo-controlled trials (three trials used the HPV4 vaccine; one used only the HPV16 component of the vaccine). Enrollment criteria included no pregnancy at enrollment, no known history of an abnormal Pap test and a history of less than four or five sexual partners in her lifetime; all were requested to use contraception during study participation. Vaccine, or placebo, was administered on the first study day, with subsequent administration at 2 months and at 6 months. At enrollment and at specified intervals thereafter, Pap, cervicovaginal, and serum samples were tested for antibodies to HPV 16, 18, 6, and 11. Women found to have atypical squamous cells of undetermined significance (ASCUS) (with HPV positive results for three trials; ASCUS alone for one trial) or more were referred for colposcopy. Potential HPV-associated lesions identified at colposcopy were biopsied, with protocol-specified subsequent evaluation and clinical management. A final outcome ("endpoint determination") of HPV 16- or 18-associated CIN2, CIN3, or AIS was determined by consensus of a group of pathologists blinded to treatment allocation, HPV results, clinical assessment, and initial evaluation at the central laboratory (3,4).

Among women who were HPV-naïve (i.e., seronegative for HPV 16 or 18 at baseline), HPV4 showed efficacy of 99% (95% CI 93%–100%) in preventing CIN2, CIN 3, AIS, or cervical cancer associated with HPV 16 or 18. Using intention-to-treat analyses of all women randomized to vaccine (i.e., women seronegative for HPV 16 or 18 at baseline and women seropositive for HPV 16 or 18 on study day 1) was 44% (95% CI 31%–55%). A study conducted in Colombia showed similar results in 24- to

45-year-old seronegative women, with per-protocol efficacy of 90.5% (95% CI 73.7%–97.5%) and intention-to-treat efficacy of 30.9% (95% CI 11.1%–46.5%). The duration of efficacy is unclear, but appears to be at least 6 years (5). Recent results suggest efficacy for 8.5 years, based on testing of the HPV16 component (6).

The bivalent vaccine, HPV2 (Cervarix, manufactured by GlaxoSmithKline) was approved by the FDA in 2009 (7). This vaccine is designed to induce immunity to two high-risk HPV types, 16 and 18. Final results for the major HPV2 trial (PATRICIA—PApilloma TRIal against Cancer In young Adults) were published in 2009 (8). The primary outcomes were vaccine efficacy in prevention of infection with HPV16 and/or HPV18 among subjects initially seronegative for these HPV types. Similar to the HPV4 trials, PATRICIA was designed to evaluate the efficacy of HPV2 in the prevention of CIN 2 and 3, AIS, invasive carcinoma "associated with HPV16 or HPV18," and persistent infection with 14 high-risk HPV types (16,18,31,33,35,39,45, 51,52,56,58,59,66,68). Worldwide, 18,644 women aged 15 to 25 participated in this randomized, double-blind trial. Enrollment criteria included not being pregnant (or breastfeeding) at enrollment, no history of colposcopy or chronic condition (including immunodeficiency), an intact cervix, agreement to use contraception, and no more than six lifetime partners (except in some countries where the latter was not applied to minors). Enrollees received HPV2 or hepatitis A vaccine at 0, 1, and 6 months. Women who tested positive twice for HPV DNA, or were found to have ASCUS or more, were referred for colposcopy with biopsy of any suspicious lesions. Cone biopsy was recommended if CIN 2 or higher was detected. All histopathologic outcomes were verified by experts blinded to vaccine administration, HPV DNA findings prior to biopsies, and cytologic results.

Several sets of analyses were performed. In the per-protocol analysis, the overall efficacy of HPV2 for the prevention of HPV 16- or 18-associated CIN 2 or 3 or AIS was 92.9% (95% CI 79.9%–98.3%; 7,8). This finding is garnered from the "according to protocol for efficacy" (ATP-E) group, who received three HPV2 doses, had sufficient evaluable laboratory data, and had normal or low-grade cytology at study onset. Among the "total vaccination cohort-naïve" (TVC-naïve) group (meaning enrollees with negative cytology, seronegative for HPV 16 and 18, HPV DNA negative for the 14 high-risk HPV types tested, and who received at least one HPV2 dose), vaccine efficacy against CIN2+ was 98.4% (95% CI 90.4%–100%). The TVC-naïve group is intended to represent adolescents who have not been exposed to HPV. Thus, the findings in this group suggest maximal HPV2 efficacy achievable before the onset of sexual activity (7).

Both vaccines appear to offer some cross-immunity to other types of high-risk HPV (7,8), which may be helpful for the 30% of cervical cancer not attributable to HPV 16 and 18 (9) (e.g., HPV 16 may help confer immunity to HPV31, while HPV18 may do so for HPV45) (10). In addition, immunization against high-risk HPV may help prevent HPV-mediated vulvar and vaginal carcinoma in addition to cervical carcinoma (11).

Challenges to Immunization

Despite the efficacy of the HPV vaccines, immunization rates in the United States are low. For females, current recommendations by the Advisory Committee on Immunization Practices (ACIP), a group of experts who counsel the U.S. Department of Health and Human Services on optimal immunization types and schedules, are (a) routine vaccination of all females ages 11 to 12, with (b) vaccination of 13- to 26-year-olds if not previously vaccinated. Vaccination can begin at age 9 (7). The three-dose series, with either HPV4 or HPV2, is scheduled at 0, 1–2 months, and 6 months. However, results from the 2010 National Immunization Survey-Teen indicate that only 32% of girls aged 13 to 17 received all three doses while 48.7% received at least one dose (12).

Several sets of reasons have been suggested for the lack of sufficient vaccination. While the magnitude of each effect is difficult to determine, several key issues are described below. These range from difficulties in administering vaccines in this age group to beliefs among the public about vaccine safety and other societal factors.

Before release of HPV4, considerable discussion occurred about how best to distribute and administer HPV vaccine. Given the expected age range for vaccination (ages 11–26), distribution through usual "well child" visits would not be sufficient. Administration of vaccine to adolescents is problematic. Only about 9% of health care visits are preventive among 11- to 21-year-old females and males (13). One suggestion for HPV vaccine and other vaccines administered during adolescence is to increase vaccination at acute care visits (13,14). Specialty-specific visit rates have a bearing on vaccine distribution as well: younger adolescents (less than age 15) tend to visit pediatricians or family medicine physicians, older female adolescents are likely to see an obstetrician–gynecologist, and older male adolescents are more likely to visit family medicine physicians (13). Familiarity and facility of vaccine storage and administration, as well as comfort with discussing risks and benefits of vaccination, can vary by specific practice, let alone by specialty type.

Public perception of vaccine safety and duration of efficacy impacts vaccination rates. The best source of data concerning safety of HPV vaccine (HPV4) is the Vaccine Safety Datalink (VSD). The VSD is conducted by seven large U.S. managed care organizations, representing visits by over 9 million patients yearly; by providing both the number of cases and the number of individuals at risk, rates of adverse events can be calculated. A key component is its Rapid Cycle Analysis (RCA), which provides surveillance, almost in real time, of adverse events associated with vaccine administration. Using 3+ years of data, no statistically significant risk of prespecified outcomes (Guillain–Barré syndrome, stroke, venous thromboembolism, appendicitis, seizures, syncope, allergic reactions, anaphylaxis) were found with HPV vaccine use (15). These outcomes were chosen based on the evaluation of adverse events reported in studies submitted for vaccine approval (i.e., the FDA approval process) as well as the Vaccine Adverse Event Report System (VAERS). The VAERS, administered by the U.S. Centers for Disease Control and Prevention (CDC) and the FDA, provides important information concerning possible adverse effects of vaccination. Unfortunately, because the VAERS is a passive surveillance system, neither an accurate number nor rate of adverse events can be determined (due to likely under reporting and lack of at-risk population size needed for the denominator in rate calculations, respectively). Thus, data from VSD are more reliable than VAERS in estimating rates of adverse outcomes.

In addition to HPV safety, some parents have other concerns about HPV vaccine. Parents who did not intend to immunize their 8- to 17-year-old daughters were asked why, as part of the 2008 National Health Interview Survey. The most common reasons were that the daughter did not need the vaccine, that the parent did not have enough information about the vaccine, and that the daughter was not sexually active (16). Some have voiced concerns that, once immunized, adolescents will be more inclined to engage in sexual activity; no evidence of increased sexual activity among vaccinated teens has been documented (17). Parents may underestimate the risk of HPV acquisition with the onset of sexual activity: one study suggests 28.5% of young women acquired HPV within 1 year of beginning sexual activity with a male partner, with nearly half acquiring HPV within 3 years with the same partner (18). Cost should not be a barrier to vaccination for most adolescents: most private insurers cover HPV vaccination, with public funding (including the CDC's Vaccines for Children Program) covering the cost for virtually all others. Nevertheless, insured girls and women are more likely to receive HPV vaccination (17).

Sexual contact between males and females (as well as male–male and female–female) is a key factor in transmission of HPV. Routine vaccination of boys and young men with HPV4 was approved in 2009. While the indication for approval was for prevention of genital condyloma by immunization against HPV 6 and 11, immunization against HPV 16 and 18 is a side benefit. The recommended schedule for males, like for females, is routine vaccination at ages 11 to 12. Catch-up vaccination in males is recommended for ages 13 to 21, and males aged 22 to 26 may be vaccinated (19). While routine vaccination of males was not initially found to be cost-effective for the prevention of cervical cancer (20), in scenarios with low rates of female vaccination (as we currently face in the United States) and with consideration of prevention of other serious HPV-associated conditions (anal cancer, oropharyngeal cancer, and perhaps recurrent respiratory papillomatosis) the overall cost-effectiveness ratio may improve (21).

Future activity in HPV vaccine research is likely on several fronts (22,23). How best to increase uptake of existing HPV2 and HPV4 vaccines will continue to be of interest. The next generation of vaccines is under development: similar vaccines for additional HPV types are anticipated, and other vaccine mechanisms are being evaluated as well (24,25).

■ REFERENCES

1. Boulet G, Horvath C, Vanden Broeck D, Sahebali S, Bogers J. Human papillomavirus: E6 and E7 oncogenes. *Int J Biochem Cell Biol.* 2007;39(11):2006–2011.
2. Frazer I. God's gift to women: the human papillomavirus vaccine. *Immunity.* 2006;25(2):179–184.
3. Ault KA; Future II Study Group. Effect of prophylactic human papillomavirus L1 virus-like-particle vaccine on risk of cervical intraepithelial neoplasia grade 2, grade 3, and adenocarcinoma in situ: a combined analysis of four randomised clinical trials. *Lancet.* 2007;369(9576):1861–1868.
4. Koutsky LA, Harper DM. Chapter 13: Current findings from prophylactic HPV vaccine trials. *Vaccine* 2006;24 Suppl 3:S3/114–121.
5. CDC. HPV Vaccine Information for Clinicians - Fact Sheet. http://www.cdc.gov/std/HPV/STDFact-HPV-vaccine-hcp.htm accessed 18 Nov 2012.
6. Rowhani-Rahbar A, Alvarez FB, Bryan JT, et al. Evidence of immune memory 8.5 years following administration of a prophylactic human papillomavirus type 16 vaccine. *J Clin Virol.* 2012;53(3):239–243.
7. Centers for Disease Control and Prevention. FDA licensure of bivalent human papillomavirus vaccine (HPV2, Cervarix) for use in females and updated HPV vaccination recommendations from the Advisory Committee on Immunization Practices (ACIP). *MMWR Morb Mortal Wkly Rep.* 2010;59:626–629.
8. Paavonen J, Naud P, Salmerón J, et al.; HPV PATRICIA Study Group. Efficacy of human papillomavirus (HPV)-16/18 AS04-adjuvanted vaccine against cervical infection and precancer caused by oncogenic HPV types (PATRICIA): final analysis of a double-blind, randomised study in young women. *Lancet.* 2009;374(9686):301–314.
9. Schiffman M, Wentzensen N. From human papillomavirus to cervical cancer. *Obstet Gynecol.* 2010;116(1):177–185.
10. Frazer I. HPV vaccines. International journal of gynaecology and obstetrics: the official organ of the International Federation of Gynaecology and Obstetrics 2006;94:S81–S88.
11. Hampl M, Sarajuuri H, Wentzensen N, Bender HG, Kueppers V. Effect of human papillomavirus vaccines on vulvar, vaginal, and anal intraepithelial lesions and vulvar cancer. *Obstet Gynecol.* 2006;108(6):1361–1368.
12. Centers for Disease Control and Prevention. National and state vaccination coverage among adolescents aged 13 through 17 years—United States, 2010. MMWR morbidity and mortality weekly report 2011;60:1117–1123.
13. Rand CM, Shone LP, Albertin C, Auinger P, Klein JD, Szilagyi PG. National health care visit patterns of adolescents: implications for

delivery of new adolescent vaccines. *Arch Pediatr Adolesc Med.* 2007;161(3):252–259.

14. Rand CM, Szilagyi PG, Albertin C, Auinger P. Additional health care visits needed among adolescents for human papillomavirus vaccine delivery within medical homes: a national study. *Pediatrics.* 2007;120(3):461–466.

15. Gee J, Naleway A, Shui I, et al. Monitoring the safety of quadrivalent human papillomavirus vaccine: findings from the Vaccine Safety Datalink. *Vaccine.* 2011;29(46):8279–8284.

16. Wong CA, Berkowitz Z, Dorell CG, Anhang Price R, Lee J, Saraiya M. Human papillomavirus vaccine uptake among 9- to 17-year-old girls: National Health Interview Survey, 2008. *Cancer.* 2011;117(24):5612–5620.

17. Liddon NC, Leichliter JS, Markowitz LE. Human papillomavirus vaccine and sexual behavior among adolescent and young women. *Am J Prev Med.* 2012;42(1):44–52.

18. Winer RL, Feng Q, Hughes JP, O'Reilly S, Kiviat NB, Koutsky LA. Risk of female human papillomavirus acquisition associated with first male sex partner. *J Infect Dis.* 2008;197(2):279–282.

19. Centers for Disease Control and Prevention. FDA licensure of quadrivalent human papillomavirus vaccine (HPV4, Gardasil) for use in males and guidance from the Advisory Committee on Immunization Practices (ACIP). MMWR Morbidity and mortality weekly report 2010;59:630–632.

20. Kim JJ, Goldie SJ. Cost effectiveness analysis of including boys in a human papillomavirus vaccination programme in the United States. *BMJ.* 2009;339:b3884.

21. Chesson HW, Ekwueme DU, Saraiya M, Dunne EF, Markowitz LE. The cost-effectiveness of male HPV vaccination in the United States. *Vaccine.* 2011;29(46):8443–8450.

22. Schiller JT, Nardelli-Haefliger D. Chapter 17: Second generation HPV vaccines to prevent cervical cancer. Vaccine 2006;24 Suppl 3:S3/147–153.

23. zur Hausen H. Perspectives of contemporary papillomavirus research. *Vaccine.* 2006;24 Suppl 3:S3/iii–S3/iiv.

24. Hildesheim A, Markowitz L, Avila MH, Franceschi S. Chapter 27: Research needs following initial licensure of virus-like particle HPV vaccines. Vaccine 2006;24 Suppl 3:S3/227–232.

25. Palmer KE, Jenson AB, Kouokam JC, Lasnik AB, Ghim SJ. Recombinant vaccines for the prevention of human papillomavirus infection and cervical cancer. *Exp Mol Pathol.* 2009;86(3):224–233.

3 Cervical Cancer Prevention: Screening and Diagnostic Accuracy

TERRY MORGAN

EMILY MESERVE

MICHELLE BERLIN

Cervical carcinoma is the second most common cancer in women worldwide, leading to nearly 300,000 deaths each year (1). In the United States, there are about 12,000 new cases of invasive cervical cancer each year with a mortality rate of approximately 33% (2). The incidence of cervical cancer has decreased more than 50% in the past 40 years, largely because of cost-effective screening methods, but more than *half of the patients who die from this disease have never had a screening test.* Screening is especially important for cervical cancer, because even limited superficial invasion (3.0 mm of invasion or more) has metastatic potential (3). In this chapter, we will discuss cervical cancer screening and diagnostic accuracy.

■ CERVICAL CANCER SCREENING AND THE PAPANICOLAOU (PAP) SMEAR

Dr. Georgios Papanicolaou published a 2-page manuscript in 1925 with no figures, tables, or references, describing the diagnosis of early human pregnancy by the vaginal smear method (4). He made what are now called conventional cytologic smears on glass slides from various mammals, including women, to determine whether the animal was pregnant. After reviewing human smears from "normal cases as well as from cases of pregnancy, and from several pathologic conditions," he reported that "...different pathologic conditions of the ovaries and genital tract might be diagnosed *more or less* (emphasis added) accurately by such smears." In 1928, he reported cancer cells in cervical smears, but this breakthrough was not widely appreciated until 1941 (5), and Pap smears did not become common until the 1960s (6).

In countries where the Pap smear is now routine, it is recommended that screening begin after age 21 (7–9). The recommended screening frequency depends on the methods used due to differing sensitivities and specificities as well as the patient's comorbidities (i.e., history of immunosuppression) and history of any prior abnormal Pap smears (8). For example, Pap smear alone has a sensitivity of 45%–80% (7–12) to detect precancerous high-grade dysplasia (high-grade squamous intraepithelial lesion [HSIL]). Prevalence and the predictive value of Pap smears are dependent on the diagnostic category (Table 3.1). Because the Pap smear has only moderate sensitivity, it is recommended to have a Pap smear every 3 years for women between ages 21 and 29 years (8, 9). Women older than 29 years may be screened every 5 years if they have negative co-testing by cytology and are negative for high risk HPV (9). Screening may be discontinued after age 65 to 70 in low-risk women who had at least three consecutive negative Pap smears within the preceding decade. Of course there are exceptions such as immunosuppression and a previous history of high-grade cervical dysplasia or cervical cancer (8). This schedule is effective because although 20% of HSIL diagnoses may be missed in a given year, nearly all of these cases should be detected in a 3-year period. Screening failures occur if women miss their scheduled Pap smear, or if rare HSIL cells are missed by cytopathologists reviewing the Pap smear slide.

Most Pap smears are normal, but 10%–20% are abnormal (8,9). Abnormal Pap smears are classified into various diagnostic categories that imply the likelihood of the patient having precancerous high-grade cervical dysplasia (cervical intraepithelial neoplasia [CIN] grade 2 and grade 3), or invasive cancer, in follow-up surgical biopsies (8–13) (Table 3.1). In brief, most of these *abnormal Pap smears* are diagnosed as "atypical squamous cells of undetermined significance" (ASCUS, 6% of all Pap smears). An ASCUS diagnosis indicates mild changes in nuclear size, color, texture, and nuclear:cytoplasmic ratio. The differential diagnosis includes reactive changes or low-grade dysplasia (low-grade squamous intraepithelial lesion [LSIL]). However, cervical dysplasia classified as moderate (CIN2) or worse (CIN2+) is discovered in only about 10%–15% of women with an ASCUS Pap. LSIL (3% of Pap smears) is characterized by squamous cells with nuclear enlargement with dark coarse chromatin and clearing of the cytoplasm around the nucleus (koilocyte). The positive predictive value (PPV) of a LSIL

■ Table 3.1 Prevalence and predictive values for Pap smear diagnostic categories

Diagnostic Category (%)	Pap Smear NPV	Pap Smear PPV	Pap and HPV NPV	Pap and HPV PPV	High Risk HPV Prevalence
Negative (90%)	80%	—	99%	—	10%
ASCUS (6%)	—	10%	98%	15%[a]	60%[a]
LSIL (3%)	—	20%	90%	25%	85%
ASC-H (0.25%)	—	40%	80%	50%	75%
HSIL (0.5%)	—	75%	—	81%	99%

High-risk HPV genotypes are common in abnormal Pap smears and do not significantly improve positive predictive value (PPV).
[a]The exception is in women older than 30 years of age, who despite having a reduced HPV positive prevalence (from 60% to 10%), have an improved PPV (approximately 40%). HPV testing is also useful to improve negative predictive value (NPV) in negative Pap smears (from 80% to >99%) (11,17).
ASCUS, atypical squamous cells of undetermined significance; ASC-H, atypical squamous cells, cannot exclude HSIL; HSIL, high-grade squamous intraepithelial lesion; LSIL, low-grade squamous intraepithelial lesion; PAP, papanicolaou.

diagnosis for CIN2+ on biopsy is about 20%, and consequently, guidelines recommend colposcopy to visualize the cervix with directed biopsies of gross lesions to exclude high-grade dysplasia (Figure 3.1). HSIL (0.5% of Paps) is characterized by squamous cells with dark, coarse irregular nuclei, and high nuclear:cytoplasmic ratios. It implies high-grade dysplasia is present, but surprisingly, the PPV for CIN2+ in follow-up surgical biopsies is only 75%–80%. This means the Pap smear HSIL diagnosis is incorrect in at least 20% of cases. There are also less common diagnostic categories, such as "atypical squamous cells, cannot exclude HSIL" (ASC-H, 0.25% of Paps with PPV of CIN2+ on biopsy of 40%) and "atypical glandular cells" (AGC [or AGUS], 0.2% of Paps with PPV for carcinoma of 50%). An AGC diagnosis is important to recognize because it implies a 50% chance of carcinoma, including adenocarcinoma of the endocervix, endometrium, or ovaries. *It should not be mistaken either clinically or morphologically as ASCUS.* An AGC diagnosis should prompt both colposcopy with endocervical curettage and endometrial biopsy to exclude malignancy (7).

■ HIGH-RISK HUMAN PAPILLOMAVIRUS (HPV) TESTING

The story of Eva Perón (Evita), the First Lady of Argentina (1946–1952), evokes images of her social life and tragic end. Despite having a hysterectomy for cervical cancer in 1952 she died at the age of 33 (14). She was dictator Juan Perón's second wife to die of cervical cancer. His first wife (Aurelia Tizon) died when she was only 28 years old. Notably, Evita's mother also died of cervical cancer. Cervical cancer is a sexually transmitted disease, and HPV is ubiquitous.

It is well accepted that HPV causes cervical cancer, but it has also been shown to be a common cause of anal cancer (15) and many tonsillar cancers (16). Although there are

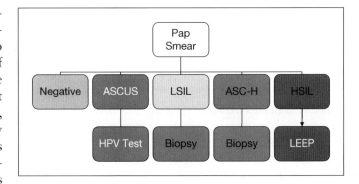

FIGURE 3.1 Pap smear management guidelines (2012). Clinicians may "see and treat" or "leap to LEEP" women with HSIL Pap. However, most clinicians remain cautious and prefer colposcopic biopsies to confirm high-grade cervical dysplasia (7,8,27,28). LEEP, loop electrosurgical excisional procedure.

about 40 varieties of HPV, only 14 genotypes are known to cause cancer. Among these, HPV16 and HPV18 account for 70% of cases. Most of the remaining subtypes cause warts, including genital warts (i.e., HPV genotypes 6 and 11).

Currently, there are a number of U.S. Food and Drug Administration-approved kits for cervical HPV testing in clinical practice (i.e., Digene Hybrid Capture 2 [Qiagen] and Cervista [Hologic Inc.]), which may be performed on the residual cell pellet of liquid-based cytology (LBC) preparations (18) (i.e., ThinPrep [Hologic], or SurePath [BD Diagnostics]). This is one advantage of LBC; the other may be improved Pap smear sensitivity compared with conventional cytology (18). Nonetheless, when conventional smears are used, additional collection for HPV testing may also be performed using a separate cervical cytology specimen, which may be submitted directly for HPV DNA analysis (11).

The advantage of HPV testing is excellent negative predictive value (NPV). The disadvantage is less than moderate PPV (50%) for precancerous CIN2+ lesions (11). That is to say, many sexually active men and women are positive for high-risk HPV, but the infection is likely transient and the large majority of these people do not have a precancerous lesion (11). Because the prevalence of high-risk HPV is common in all abnormal Pap smears (Table 3.1) HPV testing is only recommended as a reflex test for women with an ASCUS diagnosis, in postmenopausal women with a LSIL diagnosis, or Pap/HPV cotesting in women after 30 years of age to increase the NPV of the combined test to 99% (8).

Ironically, this problem may be magnified if HPV vaccinations fulfill their promise. Vaccination reduces the prevalence of some types of HPV (19,20), but not all. Decreased prevalence will improve the already excellent NPV of HPV screening assays. But in turn, decreased prevalence is also likely to *decrease PPV*. This will be significant because false-positive test results lead to unnecessary treatment of women without disease. Fortunately, a nationwide postvaccination surveillance program is underway to better understand the issue.

Even if patients have easy access to health care with excellent compliance, the poor PPV of HPV testing poses a problem. Consider Kaiser Northwest in Portland, Oregon. It was a leading center validating the use of HPV testing in cases of abnormal Pap smears (11). However, the reflex HPV test (8) has led to a significant increase in the number of colposcopic cervical biopsies despite the frequency of high-grade dysplasia being less than 0.5% (1/200 women). Therefore, it may not be cost-effective to biopsy all of these cases.

■ THE ROLE OF COLPOSCOPIC BIOPSIES

Visual examination of the cervix by colposcopy with directed biopsies is the standard of care to confirm precancerous lesions after an atypical Pap smear (8,9). Pap smears are a sensitive test to screen for disease, while colposcopic examination and biopsies are specific to confirm the presence of high-grade dysplasia (CIN2+). If the biopsy is positive for CIN2+, the patient may have definitive loop electrosurgical excisional procedure (LEEP), or cold knife cone surgical therapy (7). The sensitivity of a colposcopic examination to visualize and biopsy a CIN2+ lesion is less than 66% (21–23). In turn, studies suggest it may require two to three colposcopic examinations before biopsies provide tissue confirmation of CIN2+ when present (22). This problem is further compounded by low-to-moderate diagnostic reproducibility by the surgical pathologists evaluating these biopsies (24–29). Although histologic criteria for grading cervical dysplasia are based on widely accepted features (24), there is significant variability in interobserver reproducibility (kappa statistic) (25–26). This is especially true when diagnosing moderate dysplasia (CIN2), which is essentially not reproducible (Table 3.2). This is significant because a CIN2 colposcopic diagnosis prompts follow-up surgery in some women, but not others (7–9).

Current management guidelines have recognized these problems and allow clinicians to progress directly to surgical treatment, so-called "leap to LEEP" when patients have an HSIL Pap diagnosis (30,31). If the HSIL Pap smear diagnosis is a false-positive, the consequence may be excision of nonneoplastic cervical tissue (32). This unnecessary treatment is undesirable, especially provided the 6%–10% risk of cervical incompetence during pregnancy (33,34), and/or scarring cervical stenosis (35) associated with LEEP/cone. False-positive HSIL diagnoses and inaccurate colposcopic biopsy diagnoses need to be minimized for more effective patient management. The problem should not be a surprise. Pap-stained cervical cytology is nearly 100 years old. A pathologic diagnosis based on hematoxylin and eosin (H&E)-stained histologic sections is 19th-century technology.

■ **Table 3.2** Diagnostic reproducibility and accuracy in cervical biopsies evaluated by surgical pathologists using routine histology or aided by p16 immunohistochemistry

Kappa Statistic (95% CI)	CIN1	CIN2	CIN3	CIN2+
H&E only	0.64 (0.58–0.70)	0.40 (0.34–0.47)	0.68 (0.61–0.74)	0.67 (0.60–0.73)
H&E + p16	0.69 (0.63–0.75)	0.48 (0.42–0.54)	0.67 (0.61–0.73)	0.69 (0.63–0.75)
H&E + p16/Ki67	0.75 (0.68–0.81)	0.52 (0.46–0.58)	0.60 (0.54–0.66)	0.75 (0.69–0.81)

CIN2+	Accuracy	Sensitivity (95% CI)	Specificity (95% CI)
H&E only	82%	81% (76%–87%)	87% (82%–91%)
H&E + p16	95%	94% (91%–97%)	100%

Reproducibility of CIN2 diagnoses are significantly improved by p16 staining compared with H&E alone ($p < .05$). A kappa statistic of 1.0 implies perfect agreement. Scores above 0.81 are considered near-perfect agreement in tissue-based diagnoses, 0.61–0.8 excellent, 0.41–0.6 moderate, and less than 0.4 poor. Most studies show a CIN2 kappa of less than 0.40 (25–29). P16-assisted diagnoses also provide significantly improved accuracy, sensitivity, and specificity compared with H&E and long-term clinical outcomes (29).
CI, confidence interval; CIN, cervical intraepithelial neoplasia; H&E, hematoxylin and eosin.

■ MOLECULAR MARKERS OF HPV-MEDIATED NEOPLASTIC TRANSFORMATION

During the past decade, molecular biologists, pathologists, and clinicians have identified and validated a number of "neoplastic markers" to assist pathologists with cervical biopsy and Pap smear diagnoses (36–48). To understand how these neoplastic markers work requires a basic understanding of the effect HPV infection has on cell-cycle regulation (Figure 3.2). First, the virus is most likely to infect immature cells at the transformation zone between the squamous ectocervix and glandular endocervical mucosa. Interestingly, these immature cells may have a specific immunophenotype (50), which is also seen in the anal transformation zone and perhaps the tonsil. Proliferating virus within these infected cells leads to koilocytic changes characteristic of low-grade dysplasia in a Pap smear (LSIL) and cervical biopsy (CIN1)

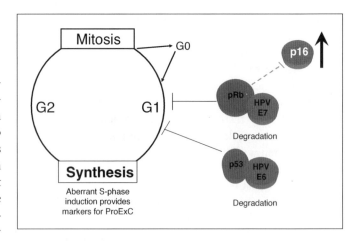

FIGURE 3.2 Persistent high-risk HPV infection leads to cell-cycle deregulation, aberrant S-phase induction, and upregulation of E6 and E7, which lead to degradation of p54 and pRb [49]. This process increases expression of potential "neoplastic immunohistochemical markers" such as p16 and ProExC (46). HPV, human papillomavirus.

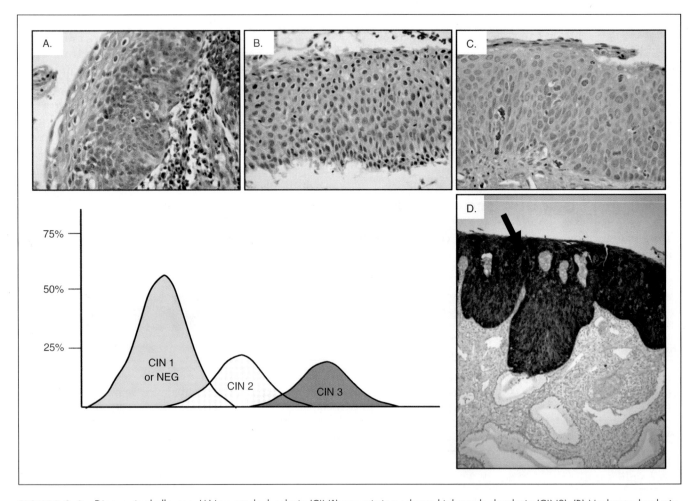

FIGURE 3.3 Diagnostic challenges. (A) Low-grade dysplasia (CIN1) may mimic moderate high-grade dysplasia (CIN2). (B) Moderate dysplasia, CIN2, and reactive metaplasia have similar features. (C) Severe dysplasia (CIN3) is a more reproducible diagnosis because of nuclear:cytoplasmic ratios and mitotic activity. The consequence of diagnostic overlap and incorrect classification is inappropriate LEEP. (D) Immunostaining for p16 (arrow) can reliably distinguish CIN2 and CIN3 from CIN1 when it shows diffuse full thickness signal (brown). CIN, cervical intraepithelial neoplasia; LEEP, loop electrosurgical excisional procedure.

(Figure 3.3). Most of these transient infections are cleared within 6 to 12 months by the patient's immune system (11,49), but when infection persists, or if there are other risk factors (i.e., immunosuppression, smoking), the virus may intercalate into the host DNA and induce neoplastic transformation (49).

Precancerous squamous dysplasia (HSIL) and endocervical adenocarcinoma (AIS) begin with persistent high-risk HPV infections (often cited as at least 2 years) (11,49). The molecular switch from an infected cell into a neoplastic cell begins with upregulation of the HPV E6 and E7 genes (Figure 3.2). These genes promote downregulation of the tumor suppressor genes p53 and pRB, respectively. The consequence of pRB inactivation is upregulation of the p16INK4 protein, which may be detected by immunohistochemistry (CINtec; Roche/mtm Laboratories) showing p16 protein in the nucleus

and cytoplasm of neoplastic cells (Figure 3.3D). This marker is now routinely used to evaluate histologic tissue sections (44) and in many practices is becoming the standard of care to distinguish CIN2 from CIN1 and reactive changes (Figure 3.3A–C). The loss of p53 and pRB also leads to aberrant S-phase induction and associated upregulation of topoisomerase II-a (TOP2A) and minichromosome maintenance protein-2 (MCM2). These markers are detected with the ProEx™ C antibody cocktail (BD Diagnostics, Women's Health Research) and have utility distinguishing CIN1 from CIN2 from CIN3 (Figure 3.4). Finally, since dysplastic cells are proliferating, the Ki-67 nuclear maker is sometimes used in conjunction with p16. Although commonplace in routine surgical pathology, the use of these molecular markers to assist with Pap smear diagnoses is only in the early stages of clinical validation (46–48).

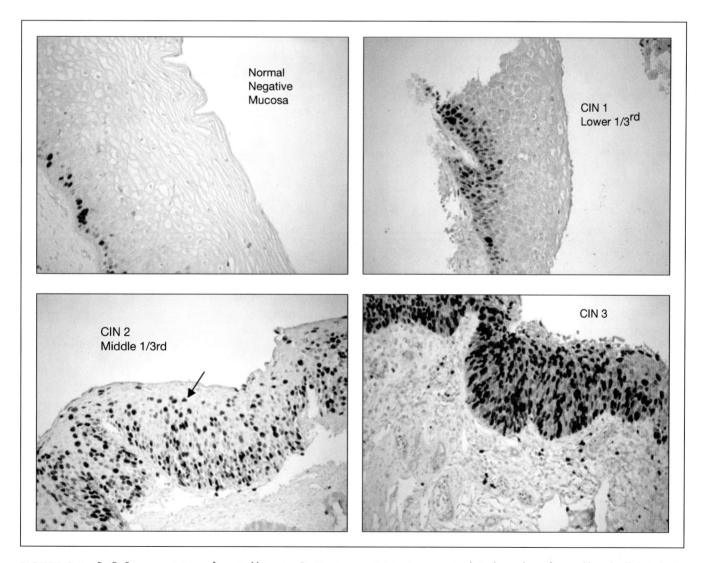

FIGURE 3.4 ProExC immunostaining of cervical biopsies. Positive immunostaining is seen not only in the nucleus of normal basal cells but also in neoplastically transformed dysplastic cells above the basal layer (arrow). The added value of ProExC is the ability to more reliably distinguish CIN2 from CIN3. CIN, cervical intraepithelial neoplasia.

■ IMPROVED DIAGNOSTIC ACCURACY USING NEOPLASTIC MARKERS

Numerous studies have now shown that marker-assisted diagnoses improve a pathologist's reproducibility and accuracy for both cervical biopsies (25–29) and Pap smears (46–48). Our group (29) and others (26–28) have shown using p16-assisted diagnoses that approximately 30% of the original H&E histology-based cervical biopsy diagnoses were misclassified compared with the gold standard consensus diagnosis and 5-year clinical outcome. P16 improves diagnostic reproducibility and accuracy (Table 3.2).

Similar results are anticipated for marker-assisted Pap smears. A problem with p16 *immunocytochemistry*

in early studies was false-positive highlighting of benign endometrial cells and metaplastic cells (tubal or squamous metaplasia). Dual staining with Ki-67 seems to reduce this problem (46,47) because metaplastic cells are usually not proliferating. Similar promising results have been obtained using ProExC (Figure 3.5) alone (41,48), or in combination with p16 (45). In turn, marker-assisted Pap smear diagnoses in all diagnostic categories (negative, ASCUS, ASC-H, LSIL, HSIL, AGC) seem to show significantly improved predictive value compared with routine cytology (41,46–48). *Although molecular Pap smears are not yet approved for routine clinical use,* it is likely that they will become more commonplace in the near future (Figure 3.6).

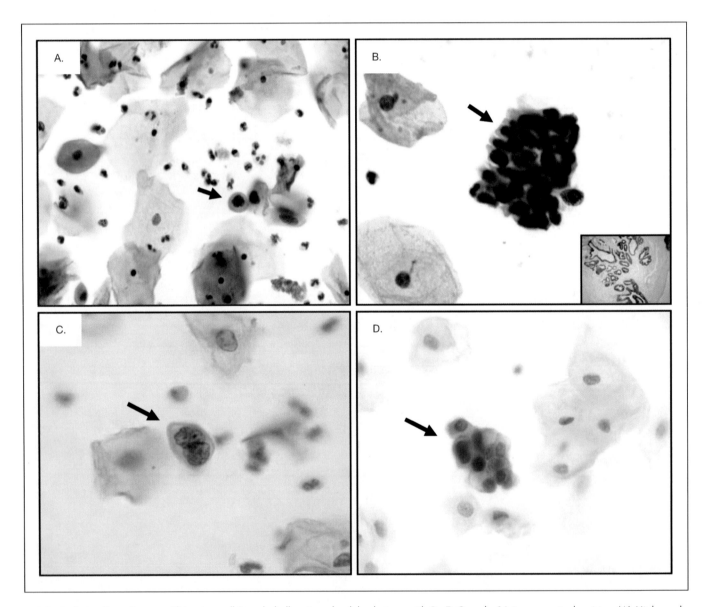

FIGURE 3.5 Detecting rare "litigation cells" and challenging glandular lesions with ProExC and p16 immunocytochemistry. (A) High-grade dysplasia (HSIL) is easily missed, especially when only rare atypical cells are present (arrow). (B) Similarly, endocervical glandular lesions are notoriously challenging to diagnose in cervical Pap smears (arrow), but are highlighted by p16 immunostaining (inset: endocervical adenocarcinoma labeled with p16). Immunocytochemistry for (C) ProExC and/or (D) p16 may improve both diagnostic sensitivity and specificity compared with cytology alone. Chromogen is brown. HSIL, high-grade cervical squamous intraepithelial lesion.

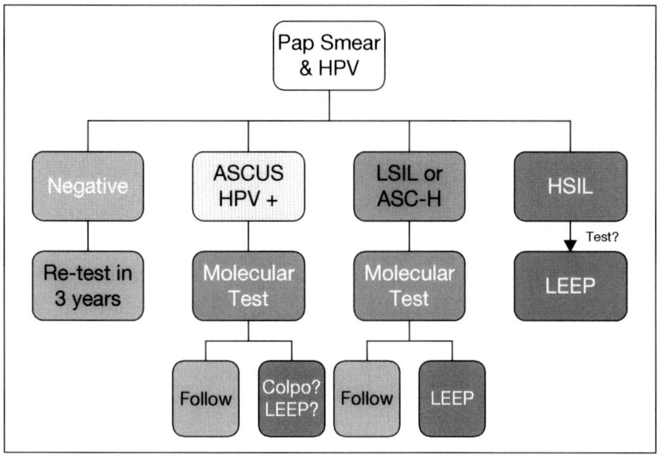

FIGURE 3.6 Potential future algorithm to manage cervical Pap smears with HPV and molecular testing. HPV, human papillomavirus.

■ FUTURE SCREENING

Future changes to screening algorithms are likely. These changes will likely reflect the superior sensitivity of HPV testing and specificity of the molecular Pap smear. Improved specificity may even replace traditional colposcopic biopsies in many cases, allowing clinicians to see and treat their patients (leap to LEEP), similar to what is currently allowed for a HSIL Pap smear diagnosis. Molecular testing is more expensive than a conventional Pap smear, but we suspect the improved PPV and potential to eliminate colposcopic biopsies may provide a favorable cost-benefit analysis [48].

In addition, we anticipate that the molecular Pap is only an intermediate step toward a more optimal evaluation of the entire Pap smear sample. LBC Pap slides actually represent only a subset of all the cells collected in a Pap smear specimen. The remaining cells may be used for HPV testing, but the vast majority of the collected cells are usually not visualized in the Pap slide. Future methods will make use of these cells. For example, whole sample multiplex analyses like flow cytometry are capable of testing millions of cells and are routinely employed to screen blood and tissue specimens for lymphoma and leukemia. Although there are substantial technical difficulties to overcome, if applied to cervical cytology specimens, methods like these would provide automated *objective quantitative data* rather than subjective qualitative diagnoses. In this light, it is interesting to recognize that one of the earliest applications of flow cytometry was an attempt to screen Pap smears (51). It failed in the 1960s, before immunocytochemistry, but methods like this (52) may come to dominate cervical cancer screening in the 21st century.

■ REFERENCES

1. Walboomers J, Jacobs M, Manos M, et al. Human papillomavirus is a necessary cause of invasive cervical cancer worldwide. *J Pathol.* 1999;189(1):12–19.
2. U.S. Cancer Statistics Working Group. *United States Cancer Statistics: 1999–2008 Incidence and Mortality Web-based Report.* Atlanta, GA: Department of Health and Human Services, Centers for Disease Control and Prevention, and National Cancer Institute; 2012. Available at: http://www.cdc.gov/uscs.
3. Morris M. Management of stage IA cervical carcinoma. *J Natl Cancer Inst Monographs.* 1996;(21):47–52.
4. Papanicolaou GN. The diagnosis of early human pregnancy by the vaginal smear method. *Scientific Proceedings.* 1925;207:436–437.
5. Vilos GA. The history of the Papanicolaou smear and the odyssey of George and Andromache Papanicolaou. *Obstet Gynecol.* 1998;91(3):479–483.
6. Albrow R, Kitchener H, Gupta N, Desai M. Cervical screening in England: the past, present, and future. *Cancer Cytopathol.* 2012;120(2):87–96.
7. Wright TC Jr, Massad LS, Dunton CJ, Spitzer M, Wilkinson EJ, Solomon D; 2006 American Society for Colposcopy and Cervical Pathology-sponsored Consensus Conference. 2006 consensus guidelines for the management of women with cervical intraepithelial neoplasia or adenocarcinoma in situ. *Am J Obstet Gynecol.* 2007;197(4):340–345.
8. ACOG Practice Bulletin. *Cervical Cytology Screening.* 2009;109:1–12.
9. Saslow D, Solomon D, Lawson HW, et al.; American Cancer Society; American Society for Colposcopy and Cervical Pathology; American Society for Clinical Pathology. American Cancer Society, American Society for Colposcopy and Cervical Pathology, and American Society for Clinical Pathology screening guidelines for the prevention and early detection of cervical cancer. *Am J Clin Pathol.* 2012;137(4):516–542.
10. Nanda K, McCrory DC, Myers ER, et al. Accuracy of the Papanicolaou test in screening for and follow-up of cervical cytologic abnormalities: a systematic review. *Ann Intern Med.* 2000;132(10):810–819.
11. Sherman ME, Lorincz AT, Scott DR, et al. Baseline cytology, human papillomavirus testing, and risk for cervical neoplasia: a 10-year cohort analysis. *J Natl Cancer Inst.* 2003;95(1):46–52.
12. Whitlock EP, Vesco KK, Eder M, Lin JS, Senger CA, Burda BU. Liquid-based cytology and human papillomavirus testing to screen for cervical cancer: a systematic review for the U.S. Preventive Services Task Force. *Ann Intern Med.* 2011;155(10):687–697, W214.
13. Solomon D, Davey D, Kurman R, et al.; Forum Group Members; Bethesda 2001 Workshop. The 2001 Bethesda System: terminology for reporting results of cervical cytology. *JAMA.* 2002;287(16):2114–2119.
14. Lerner BH. The illness and death of Eva Perón: cancer, politics, and secrecy. *Lancet.* 2000;355(9219):1988–1991.
15. Pirog EC, Quint KD, Yantiss RK. P16/CDKN2A and Ki-67 enhance the detection of anal intraepithelial neoplasia and condyloma and correlate with human papillomavirus detection by polymerase chain reaction. *Am J Surg Pathol.* 2010;34(10):1449–1455.
16. Fakhry C, Rosenthal BT, Clark DP, Gillison ML. Associations between oral HPV16 infection and cytopathology: evaluation of an oropharyngeal "pap-test equivalent" in high-risk populations. *Cancer Prev Res (Phila).* 2011;4(9):1378–1384.
17. Muñoz N, Bosch FX, de Sanjosé S, et al.; International Agency for Research on Cancer Multicenter Cervical Cancer Study Group. Epidemiologic classification of human papillomavirus types associated with cervical cancer. *N Engl J Med.* 2003;348(6):518–527.
18. Hardie A, Moore C, Patnick J, et al. High-risk HPV detection in specimens collected in SurePath preservative fluid:

comparison of ambient and refrigerated storage. *Cytopathology.* 2009;20(4):235–241.

19. Kollar LM, Kahn JA. Education about human papillomavirus and human papillomavirus vaccines in adolescents. *Curr Opin Obstet Gynecol.* 2008;20(5):479–483.

20. Giuliano AR. Human papillomavirus vaccination in males. *Gynecol Oncol.* 2007;107(2 Suppl 1):S24–S26.

21. Pretorius RG, Zhang WH, Belinson JL, et al. Colposcopically directed biopsy, random cervical biopsy, and endocervical curettage in the diagnosis of cervical intraepithelial neoplasia II or worse. *Am J Obstet Gynecol.* 2004;191(2):430–434.

22. Gage JC, Hanson VW, Abbey K, et al.; ASCUS LSIL Triage Study (ALTS) Group. Number of cervical biopsies and sensitivity of colposcopy. *Obstet Gynecol.* 2006;108(2):264–272.

23. Pretorius RG, Belinson JL, Burchette RJ, Hu S, Zhang X, Qiao YL. Regardless of skill, performing more biopsies increases the sensitivity of colposcopy. *J Low Genit Tract Dis.* 2011;15(3):180–188.

24. Tavassoli FA, Devilee P, eds. *WHO Classification of Tumors of the Breast & Female Genital Tract.* Lyon: IARC Press; 2003.

25. Stoler MH, Schiffman M; Atypical Squamous Cells of Undetermined Significance-Low-grade Squamous Intraepithelial Lesion Triage Study (ALTS) Group. Interobserver reproducibility of cervical cytologic and histologic interpretations: realistic estimates from the ASCUS-LSIL Triage Study. *JAMA.* 2001;285(11):1500–1505.

26. Klaes R, Benner A, Friedrich T, et al. p16INK4a immunohistochemistry improves interobserver agreement in the diagnosis of cervical intraepithelial neoplasia. *Am J Surg Pathol.* 2002;26(11):1389–1399.

27. Horn LC, Reichert A, Oster A, et al. Immunostaining for p16INK4a used as a conjunctive tool improves interobserver agreement of the histologic diagnosis of cervical intraepithelial neoplasia. *Am J Surg Pathol.* 2008;32(4):502–512.

28. Galgano MT, Castle PE, Atkins KA, Brix WK, Nassau SR, Stoler MH. Using biomarkers as objective standards in the diagnosis of cervical biopsies. *Am J Surg Pathol.* 2010;34(8):1077–1087.

29. Meserve E, Berlin M, Mori T, Krum R, Morgan T. Reducing misclassification bias in cervical dysplasia risk factor analysis with p16-based diagnoses. *JLGTD* (submitted)

30. Szurkus DC, Harrison TA. Loop excision for high-grade squamous intraepithelial lesion on cytology: correlation with colposcopic and histologic findings. *Am J Obstet Gynecol.* 2003;188(5):1180–1182.

31. Berdichevsky L, Karmin R, Chuang L. Treatment of high-grade squamous intraepithelial lesions: a 2- versus 3-step approach. *Am J Obstet Gynecol.* 2004;190(5):1424–1426.

32. Sarian LO, Derchain SF, Andrade LA, Tambascia J, Morais SS, Syrjänen KJ. HPV DNA test and Pap smear in detection of residual and recurrent disease following loop electrosurgical excision procedure of high-grade cervical intraepithelial neoplasia. *Gynecol Oncol.* 2004;94(1):181–186.

33. Moinian M, Andersch B. Does cervix conization increase the risk of complications in subsequent pregnancies? *Acta Obstet Gynecol Scand.* 1982;61(2):101–103.

34. Acharya G, Kjeldberg I, Hansen SM, Sørheim N, Jacobsen BK, Maltau JM. Pregnancy outcome after loop electrosurgical excision procedure for the management of cervical intraepithelial neoplasia. *Arch Gynecol Obstet.* 2005;272(2):109–112.

35. Suh-Burgmann EJ, Whall-Strojwas D, Chang Y, Hundley D, Goodman A. Risk factors for cervical stenosis after loop electrocautery excision procedure. *Obstet Gynecol.* 2000;96(5 Pt 1):657–660.

36. Sano T, Oyama T, Kashiwabara K, Fukuda T, Nakajima T. Expression status of p16 protein is associated with human papillomavirus oncogenic potential in cervical and genital lesions. *Am J Pathol.* 1998;153(6):1741–1748.

37. Keating JT, Cviko A, Riethdorf S, et al. Ki-67, cyclin E, and p16INK4 are complimentary surrogate biomarkers for human papilloma virus-related cervical neoplasia. *Am J Surg Pathol.* 2001;25(7):884–891.

38. Kruse AJ, Baak JP, de Bruin PC, et al. Ki-67 immunoquantitation in cervical intraepithelial neoplasia (CIN): a sensitive marker for grading. *J Pathol.* 2001;193(1):48–54.

39. Ishimi Y, Okayasu I, Kato C, et al. Enhanced expression of Mcm proteins in cancer cells derived from uterine cervix. *Eur J Biochem.* 2003;270(6):1089–1101.

40. Santin AD, Zhan F, Bignotti E, et al. Gene expression profiles of primary HPV16- and HPV18-infected early stage cervical cancers and normal cervical epithelium: identification of novel candidate molecular markers for cervical cancer diagnosis and therapy. *Virology.* 2005;331(2):269–291.

41. Shroyer KR, Homer P, Heinz D, Singh M. Validation of a novel immunocytochemical assay for topoisomerase II-alpha and minichromosome maintenance protein 2 expression in cervical cytology. *Cancer.* 2006;108(5):324–330.

42. Shi J, Liu H, Wilkerson M, et al. Evaluation of p16INK4a, minichromosome maintenance protein 2, DNA topoisomerase II alpha, ProEX C, and p16INK4a/ProEX C in cervical squamous intraepithelial lesions. *Hum Pathol.* 2007;38(9):1335–1344.

43. Pinto AP, Schlecht NF, Woo TY, Crum CP, Cibas ES. Biomarker (ProEx C, p16(INK4A), and MiB-1) distinction of high-grade squamous intraepithelial lesion from its mimics. *Mod Pathol.* 2008;21(9):1067–1074.

44. CINtec p16 Cervical Histology Compendium & Staining Atlas by K. Shroyer, M. Chivukula, B. Ronnett, and T. Morgan by Roche/mtm labs. 2011.

45. Guo M, Baruch AC, Silva EG, et al. Efficacy of p16 and ProExC immunostaining in the detection of high-grade cervical intraepithelial neoplasia and cervical carcinoma. *Am J Clin Pathol.* 2011;135(2):212–220.

46. Schmidt D, Bergeron C, Denton KJ, Ridder R; European CINtec Cytology Study Group. p16/ki-67 dual-stain cytology in the triage of ASCUS and LSIL papanicolaou cytology: results from the European equivocal or mildly abnormal Papanicolaou cytology study. *Cancer Cytopathol.* 2011;119(3):158–166.

47. Singh M, Mockler D, Akalin A, Burke S, Shroyer A, Shroyer KR. Immunocytochemical colocalization of P16(INK4a) and Ki-67 predicts CIN2/3 and AIS/adenocarcinoma. *Cancer Cytopathol.* 2012;120(1):26–34.

48. Morgan T, Rozelle C, Schreiner A, et al. Cost-benefit analysis of immunostaining SurePath Pap smears for p16 or ProEx C. Cancer Cytopathology (in submitted).

49. zur Hausen H. Papillomaviruses and cancer: from basic studies to clinical application. *Nat Rev Cancer.* 2002;2(5):342–350.

50. Herfs M, Yamamoto Y, Laury A, et al. A discrete population of squamocolumnar junction cells implicated in the pathogenesis of cervical cancer. *Proc Natl Acad Sci USA.* 2012;109(26):10516–10521.

51. Koenig SH, Brown RD, Kamentsky LA, Sedlis A, Melamed MR. Efficacy of a rapid cell spectrophotometer in screening for cervical cancer. *Cancer.* 1968;21(5):1019–1026.

52. Narimatsu R, Patterson BK. High-throughput cervical cancer screening using intracellular human papillomavirus E6 and E7 mRNA quantification by flow cytometry. *Am J Clin Pathol.* 2005;123(5):716–723.

4 Management of Cervical Dysplasia and Precancerous Lesions

JOYCE VARUGHESE

ELENA RATNER

MASOUD AZODI

Up to 4 million women per year in the United States have an abnormal Papanicolaou (Pap) smear. Of these women, approximately 1 million are diagnosed with low-grade cervical intraepithelial lesions and approximately 500,000 are diagnosed with high-grade cervical cancer precursor lesions, referred to as *cervical intraepithelial neoplasia* (CIN) 2,3 (1). The reduction in incidence and mortality of cervical cancer in developed countries is related to the fact that the cervix is accessible to direct visualization and sampling. Therefore, the diagnosis of cervical dysplasia has increased.

The management of cervical dysplasia has changed several times over the past decade. While the standard of care for moderate dysplasia used to be aggressive management, given the potential obstetric complications in young women after cervical conization, the trend has shifted toward surveillance and less surgical interventions, especially in women who have not yet completed childbearing.

CIN3 progresses to cancer over 15% of the time, whereas CIN1 progresses only 1% of the time. Patients with CIN3 or carcinoma in situ can often be treated with conservative excisional procedures as discussed below, although simple hysterectomy can also be considered in patients with persistent dysplasia and no desire for future fertility. Local therapies such as cold-knife conization, laser ablation, and cryotherapy have comparable efficacy in patients with intact immune systems (2). All procedures in which women retain their uterus carry the risks of cervical stenosis and persistent vaginal discharge. In reproductive-age women, possible infertility and preterm labor in subsequent pregnancies are also considerations (3).

All cytologic findings should be reported using the standard terminology set forth by the Bethesda system in 1998 with revisions in 2001. Terminology included in this system describes the adequacy of the specimen, a general categorization of whether the specimen is within normal limits or not, and a description of cytologic dysplasia. Epithelial cell abnormalities are reported as atypical squamous cells of undetermined significance (ASCUS), atypical squamous cells—cannot rule out high-grade squamous intraepithelial lesion (ASC-H), low-grade squamous intraepithelial lesion (LSIL), high-grade squamous intraepithelial lesion (HSIL), or squamous cell carcinoma. Glandular lesions are reported as atypical glandular cells (AGC), with the origin noted if possible (endocervix, endometrial, or not otherwise specified), AGC favor neoplastic, adenocarcinoma in situ (AIS), or frank adenocarcinoma (4).

■ COLPOSCOPIC TERMINOLOGY

Colposcopy is the mainstay of diagnostic evaluation of cervical dysplasia and precancerous lesions. A complete colposcopic examination involves inspection of the lower genital tract, including the vulva, vagina, cervical epithelium, and endocervix. Acetic acid and Lugol's solution are used to aid in identifying areas of dysplasia.

As most patients with cervical dysplasia and precancerous lesions are ultimately referred for colposcopy, it is important to review the terminology used to describe and interpret colposcopic findings. Current recommendations are that the 2011 International Federation of Cervical Pathology and Colposcopy Colposcopic Terminology of the Cervix be used for diagnosis, treatment, and research (Table 4.1; 5).

Excision treatment types and specimen dimensions are also classified in this terminology schema. This addition is for the purposes of standardizing the description of excisions of the transformation zone, as previously undefined terminologies, such as *cone biopsy* or *big loop excision*, were subject to interpretation. Type 1 excision is the most conservative type of excision and denotes complete resection of ectocervical or Type 1 transformation zone. Type 2 excision indicates resection of a small amount of endocervical epithelium visible with a colposcope. Finally, Type 3 excision resects the most amount of tissue including a significant amount of endocervical epithelium. A Type 3

■ Table 4.1   2011 International Federation of Cervical Pathology and Colposcopy colposcopic terminology of the cervix

Section	Pattern
General assessment	Adequate or inadequate for the reason (e.g., cervix obscured by inflammation, bleeding, scar) Squamocolumnar junction visibility: completely visible, partially visible, not visible Transformation zone types 1,2,3
Normal colposcopic findings	Original squamous epithelium: mature, atrophic Columnar epithelium: ectopy/ectropion Metaplastic squamous epithelium, nabothian cysts, crypt (gland) openings Deciduosis in pregnancy
Abnormal colposcopic findings	Location of the lesion: inside or outside of the transformation zone, location by clock position Size of the lesion: number of cervical quadrants the lesion covers Size of the lesion: as percentage of the cervix Grade 1 (minor): Fine mosaic; fine punctation; thin acetowhite epithelium; irregular, geographic border Grade 2 (major): Sharp border; inner-border sign; ridge sign; dense acetowhite epithelium; coarse mosaic; coarse punctation; rapid appearance of acetowhitening; cuffed crypt (gland) openings Nonspecific: Leukoplakia (keratosis, hyperkeratosis), erosion Lugol's staining (Schiller's test): stained or nonstained
Suspicious for invasion	Atypical vessels Additional signs: fragile vessels, irregular surface, exophytic lesion, necrosis, ulceration (necrotic), tumor, or gross neoplasm
Miscellaneous findings	Congenital transformation zone, condyloma, polyp (ectocervical or endocervical), inflammation, stenosis, congenital anomaly, posttreatment consequence, endometriosis

excision may also be used in previously treated women with glandular disease or microinvasive disease (5).

The excision specimen dimensions that are to be used are: "length," defined as the distance from the distal (external) margin to the proximal (internal) margin; "thickness," defined as the distance from the stromal margin to the surface of the specimen; and "circumference," defined as the perimeter of the excised specimen. It is optional to include the dimension of circumference when describing the excision specimen. Given that several studies have shown that cervical conization effects on future pregnancy outcomes are related to the size of the excised cervical specimen, this terminology is an attempt to standardize the description (5).

■ HUMAN PAPILLOMAVIRUS (HPV) POSITIVE, CYTOLOGY NEGATIVE

The risk of patients who test HPV positive with negative cytology of developing CIN3 in the short term is much lower than the risk threshold of HPV positive patients with ASCUS and LSIL lesions. Therefore, management of such patients involves two options. These patients can either have repeat cotesting in 12 months or immediate HPV genotype-specific testing for HPV16 alone or HPV 16 and 18. If the first option of repeat cotesting is done, then patients who either test positive for HPV or have a PAP showing LSIL or greater should be referred to colposcopy. Women who test negative for both tests should be referred for routine screening (6).

■ HPV NEGATIVE, ASCUS CYTOLOGY

Given the great variation in inter- and intraobserver reproducibility of an ASCUS PAP test, as well as the fact that ASCUS cytology represents a category of morphologic uncertainty, the current recommendation is to continue routine screening with 3-year interval for cytology screening and 5-year interval for cotesting for women aged 30 to 65 years (6). This recommendation is based on data showing that the risk of precancerous lesions is very low in patients who have ASCUS cytology but are HPV negative.

■ HPV POSITIVE, ASCUS CYTOLOGY OR LSIL OR MORE SEVERE CYTOLOGY REGARDLESS OF HPV STATUS

Given the risk of progressing to CIN3 and cancer, women with LSIL or more severe cytology should be referred for colposcopy, irrespective of HPV status. Similarly, women who are found to have ASCUS cytology and are high-risk HPV positive should also undergo colposcopic evaluation (7).

■ CIN1 WITH ASCUS, ASC-H, OR LSIL CYTOLOGY

Given the low rate of progression of CIN1 to cervical cancer, these patients can be followed without treatment. Two management options are available. Cytology can be repeated at 6 and 12 months from the time of initial abnormal cytology, or patients can have oncogenic HPV testing at 12 months. If the cytology is negative at both subsequent screenings or HPV testing is negative, the patient can return to routine cytological screening (7).

If either cytology shows ASCUS or more severe cytology or the patient is found to be high-risk HPV positive at 12 months, the patient should again be referred for colposcopy. If colposcopically directed biopsies show no CIN or CIN2,3, management is per appropriate American Society for Colposcopy and Cervical Pathology (ASCCP) guidelines. If the biopsy shows CIN1 again, and it persists for at least 2 years, clinicians may discuss continued follow-up vs ablative or excisional treatment, depending on specific patient circumstances, including age and parity (7).

■ CIN1 WITH HSIL OR AGC CYTOLOGY

There are three acceptable management options in patients whose colposcopically directed biopsies for HSIL or AGC cytology show CIN1. One can proceed directly to a diagnostic excisional procedure. Another option is to correlate all findings (cytology, colposcopic findings, and all biopsies). If no change in diagnosis of CIN1, can proceed with either observation or a diagnostic excisional procedure after discussion with the patient. If there is a change in the diagnosis, one should manage per ASCCP guidelines for the new diagnosis (7).

■ CIN2,3

Women with a diagnosis of CIN2,3 who have had a satisfactory colposcopy should have excision or ablation of the transformation zone performed. Those with an unsatisfactory colposcopy or recurrent CIN2,3 should undergo a diagnostic excisional procedure.

Once the appropriate management for the above two scenarios has been performed, there are two options for follow-up. Patients may undergo oncogenic HPV DNA testing 6 to 12 months after treatment for the CIN2,3. If HPV testing returns positive, patients should again be referred for colposcopy with endocervical sampling. If HPV testing is negative, patients should return to routine screening for at least 20 years. The other option after treatment for CIN2,3 is for patients to have cytologic

sampling at 6-month intervals or cytology and colposcopy at 6-month intervals. If these yield two consecutive negative results, the patient may return to routine screening for at least 20 years. If any repeat cytology shows ASC or more severe cytology, colposcopy with endocervical sampling should be performed (7).

■ CIN2,3 IN ADOLESCENT AND YOUNG WOMEN

Given the risks of cervical insufficiency and preterm delivery in women of reproductive age, either treatment using excision or ablation of the transformation zone or observation is acceptable in young women with CIN2,3, provided they have undergone a satisfactory colposcopy. If observation is chosen, colposcopy and cytology should be performed every 6 months for up to 2 years. If cytology is negative × 2 and the patient has normal colposcopic examinations, she can return to routine screening. If the colposcopic findings worsen or the patient has high-grade cytology, a repeat biopsy is recommended. If that shows CIN2,3 that persists for 2 years since initial diagnosis or CIN3, treatment is recommended (7).

■ AIS

The preferred management of women with AIS is simple hysterectomy as up to 33% of patients with AIS who have a cone biopsy already have invasive disease (8). However, in patients desiring future fertility, conservative management is acceptable (3). If the excisional biopsy has negative margins, the patient should continue with long-term follow-up. If the excisional procedure specimen has positive margins or a positive ECC, reexcision is recommended although a reevaluation using cytology, HPV testing, and colposcopy with endocervical sampling at 6 months is also acceptable (7).

■ PREGNANCY

The overall incidence of abnormal cytology in pregnancy is approximately 5%. Colposcopy and biopsies are safe in pregnancy, while endocervical sampling is not recommended as it can lead to bleeding and rupture of membranes. Any abnormal cervical lesions seen in pregnancy should be biopsied. If cervical dysplasia is identified during pregnancy using colposcopy and directed biopsies, serial colposcopy should be performed every 8 weeks or at least every trimester and managed definitively per ASCCP guidelines postpartum (9).

■ HIV-POSITIVE WOMEN

The HPV prevalence in HIV-positive women has been estimated to be as high as 60%, which is double the prevalence identified in HIV-negative women. Although the rate of clearance of HPV is directly correlated with CD4 count in HIV-positive women, HIV-negative women still have a twofold greater rate of clearance than HIV-positive women with adequate CD4 counts and low or undetectable HIV viral loads.

The treatment of low-grade cervical dysplasia in HIV-positive women follows the same algorithms as above for HIV-negative women, as the rate of progression of CIN1 to high-grade CIN is very low. However, follow-up in HIV-positive women with dysplasia tends to be even more conservative with cytology or colposcopy recommended every 4 months, as opposed to 6-month intervals. Highly active antiretroviral therapy is also recommended to help in the regression of CIN (10).

For CIN2,3, an excisional procedure is preferred in the setting of adequate colposcopy that has ruled out invasive disease. The rate of recurrence of dysplasia, however, is higher in HIV-positive women, therefore close follow-up is recommended posttreatment (1).

■ REFERENCES

1. Creasman WT. Preinvasive disease of the cervix. In: Disaia PJ, Creasman WT, eds. *Clinical Gynecologic Oncology*. Philadelphia, PA: Elsevier, 2007:1–37.

2. Randall ME, Michael H, Long H, et al. Uterine cervix. In: Barakat RR, Markman M, Randall ME, eds. *Principles and Practice of Gynecologic Oncology*. Philadelphia, PA: Lippincott Williams & Wilkins, 2009:623–681.

3. Campion MJ. Preinvasive disease. In: Berek JS, Hacker NF, eds. *Gynecologic Oncology*. Philadelphia, PA: Lippincott Williams & Wilkins, 2005:268–340.

4. Solomon D, Davey D, Kurman R, et al.; Forum Group Members; Bethesda 2001 Workshop. The 2001 Bethesda System: terminology for reporting results of cervical cytology. *JAMA*. 2002;287(16):2114–2119.

5. Bornstein J, Bentley J, Bösze P, et al. 2011 colposcopic terminology of the International Federation for Cervical Pathology and Colposcopy. *Obstet Gynecol*. 2012;120(1):166–172.

6. Saslow D, Solomon D, Lawson HW, et al.; ACS-ASCCP-ASCP Cervical Cancer Guideline Committee. American Cancer Society, American Society for Colposcopy and Cervical Pathology, and American Society for Clinical Pathology screening guidelines for the prevention and early detection of cervical cancer. *CA Cancer J Clin*. 2012;62(3):147–172.

7. Wright TC Jr, Massad LS, Dunton CJ, Spitzer M, Wilkinson EJ, Solomon D; 2006 American Society for Colposcopy and Cervical Pathology-sponsored Consensus Conference. 2006 consensus guidelines for the management of women with cervical intraepithelial neoplasia or adenocarcinoma in situ. *J Low Genit Tract Dis*. 2007;11(4):223–239.

8. Azodi M, Chambers SK, Rutherford TJ, Kohorn EI, Schwartz PE, Chambers JT. Adenocarcinoma in situ of the cervix: management and outcome. *Gynecol Oncol*. 1999;73(3):348–353.

9. Campion MJ, Sedlacek TV. Colposcopy in pregnancy. *Obstet Gynecol Clin North Am*. 1993;20(1):153–163.

10. Ahdieh L, Klein RS, Burk R, et al. Prevalence, incidence, and type-specific persistence of human papillomavirus in human immunodeficiency virus (HIV)-positive and HIV-negative women. *J Infect Dis*. 2001;184(6):682–690.

5 Management of Recurrent Cervical Cancer

LORI E. WEINBERG

PETER G. ROSE

■ BACKGROUND

Cervical cancer is the third most common cancer among women worldwide. In 2008, there were approximately 530,000 cases reported with 275,000 deaths (1). In the United States, there were approximately 11,000 cases reported with 3869 deaths in 2012 (2). Although the incidence of cervical cancer has decreased dramatically in developed countries compared with developing countries, cervical cancer is still a large public health burden worldwide. Fortunately, in the United States, 50% of cervical cancers are Stage I (2), but 10%–20% of these patients will recur, and in one series where 11% of the patients with Stage IB cervical cancer recurred, 56% died after 2 years despite adjuvant treatments (3,4).

The likelihood of recurring is dependent on a patient's initial stage and other risk factors. The risk of recurrence by stage is as follows: Stage IB 15%, Stage IIA 30%, Stage IIB 28%, Stage III 48%, and among 20 patients with Stage IVA disease all recurred by 5 years after primary radiotherapy (5). Recurrence rates are also increased among patients with larger tumors (greater than 2 cm), close surgical margins (less than 5 mm), parametrial spread, lymphatic space invasion, outer-third cervical stromal invasion, and lymph node involvement (6–10). For example, among patients with Stage IB to IIA disease with no evidence of lymph node spread, recurrence rate is 10%–20%, whereas among patients with lymph node spread, recurrence rate is up to 70% (11–14).

Cervical cancer may recur locally—in the vagina, cervix, parametria, or in the pelvis—or at distant sites. The majority of patients who succumb to their cervical cancer do so because of uncontrollable disease in the pelvis. However, a subset of patients with local recurrences can be cured with either surgery and/or radiotherapy. The success of salvage therapy is often determined by the primary treatment received, the extent and location of the recurrence, the disease-free interval (DFS), the patients' performance status and comorbidities, as well as the toxicities/complications of the salvage therapy. Unfortunately, distant recurrences are often fatal, and palliative chemotherapy is often utilized to control disease with no likelihood of cure.

■ SURVEILLANCE

Typically, the majority of cervical cancers will recur in the first 2 to 3 years after diagnosis. A large retrospective study of 564 patients treated for cervical cancer reported an overall 31% recurrence rate with 58% of the recurrences occurring within 1 year and 76% occurring within 2 years (15). Therefore, the National Comprehensive Cancer Networks (NCCN) and the Society of Gynecologic Oncology (SGO) recommend follow-up every 3 to 6 months for the first 2 years and then every 6 months to annually for years 2 to 5 and annually thereafter. The NCCN recommends cervical/vaginal cytology at each visit and annual chest X-rays for the first 5 years with positron emission tomography-computed tomography (PET-CT) scans as clinically indicated. The SGO recommends yearly cytology but notes that there is insufficient evidence in its detection of cancer recurrence. The SGO also does not recommend routine radiographic imaging (chest X-ray, PET-CT, MRI), again because there is insufficient evidence to support its detection of recurrence. In fact, few recurrences, 26% to 36%, are actually detected during follow-up examination. This is likely due to the fact that there is a high incidence of poor follow-up among cervical cancer patients and because recurrences are usually symptomatic—provoking unscheduled visits in approximately 40% of patients (16,17). In fact, 46%–95% of patients diagnosed with a recurrence present with symptoms (16–22). Symptoms often include weight loss, lower extremity edema or pain, pelvic pain, vaginal bleeding or discharge, urinary symptoms, shortness of breath, or cough. Therefore, patients need to be counseled about signs and symptoms of recurrence.

Surveillance with routine imaging is still unclear. Whereas older modalities such as chest X-rays detect only 20%–47% of pulmonary recurrences with limited ability to affect survival outcomes, newer modalities such as CT scans and especially PET-CT scans have improved sensitivity and specificity and have the ability to detect asymptomatic local recurrences that may be amenable to treatment with a potential for cure. In fact, recent studies have reported PET-CT scans to have a high sensitivity (87%–100%) and specificity (73%–87%) for detection of recurrent disease (16,23). Furthermore, a recent study reported on the utility of PET-CT in surveillance and found that PET-CT detected local recurrences in 8 of the 9 asymptomatic patients compared with 4 of the 21 patients who presented with symptoms that were being evaluated (17). Additionally, asymptomatic patients are potentially more treatable than those who present with symptoms. For example, a multicenter retrospective series from Italy reviewed 327 cases of recurrent cervical cancer and found that the median overall survival for symptomatic patients was 37 months compared with 109 months for asymptomatic patients ($p = 0.00001$) (22).

The treatment of recurrent cervical cancer is highly dependent on the site of recurrence and the type of primary therapy (surgery vs radiation). Additionally, the size of the recurrence, proximity to other vital structures/organs, and the nature of the recurrence (isolated vs multifocal) will significantly alter treatment planning. Thus, we will address the scenarios separately and discuss the evidence to support adjuvant therapies.

■ LOCAL RECURRENCES AFTER PRIMARY SURGICAL MANAGEMENT

The prognosis for patients with local recurrences is highly dependent on tumor size and location. Approximately 60% of recurrences after radical hysterectomy are local without extrapelvic disease at the time of diagnosis (4). These patients typically have 5-year survival rates of 20%–50% (24–27). However, patients with recurrences in the pelvis, typically on the sidewall, often are poorly controlled with patients with central-type recurrences (4,15,24,25,28).

Central Recurrences

Approximately 30%–45% of recurrences after a radical hysterectomy are central—situated atop the vaginal cuff between the bladder and rectum (29). However, in a series of 564 patients that underwent a radical hysterectomy at Mayo Clinic, among 20 patients with central-type recurrences, 11 had other sites of recurrence (15). Therefore, it is imperative that imaging such as a PET-CT be done to evaluate possible areas of distant metastasis before planning treatments. In cases where there is multifocal and

especially distant disease, overall survival is significantly diminished.

Once it has been determined that the recurrence is an isolated central-type tumor, there are several other factors that can dramatically alter survival. In a retrospective series of 90 patients, Ito et al found that among patients with central recurrences at the vaginal cuff treated with external radiation and/or high-dose-rate brachytherapy, size was highly predictive of survival. Among patients with nonpalpable tumors, the 10-year survival was 72% compared with 48% among patients with tumors less than 3 cm and 0% among patients with tumors greater than 3 cm. In fact, all the patients with tumors greater than 3 cm died within 5 years. They also found that patients with nonpalpable tumors had equal outcomes when treated with brachytherapy alone or brachytherapy and external radiation. Therefore, they recommended using brachytherapy only among patients with central nonpalpable recurrences. Additionally, the response to radiotherapy for recurrent disease was predictive of long-term survival. The 10-year overall survival among patients with a complete response (no evidence of disease on physical examination within 2 months after completion of radiotherapy) was 63% compared with 10% for patients with residual disease (25). Additionally, the DFS is also predictive of survival outcomes. For example, Krebs et al found that 80% of their patients that recurred within 6 months of surgery died within the first year whereas patients who recurred more than 6 months after surgery had a 50% survival 1 year later (30).

The traditional approach to patients with central recurrences after surgery with no prior radiotherapy is brachytherapy with or without external radiotherapy. In radiotherapy-naïve patients, doses of 40 to 50 Gy are often given to the pelvis to cover the primary tumor and regional lymphatics. Inguinofemoral nodal basins should be covered in the fields if the recurrence involves the distal third of the vagina. Furthermore, any recurrence involving the vagina or the vaginal cuff should be treated to a dose of 60 to 65 Gy to the vagina from external beams with additional doses of 15 to 30 Gy via brachytherapy or intensity-modulated radiotherapy (IMRT) (31). Additionally, interstitial brachytherapy may be considered for recurrences involving deeper tissues such as the parametria.

In light of five randomized studies that show an approximate 30%–50% improvement in survival with the addition of radiosensitizing chemotherapy to radiotherapy for Stage IB2 to IVA cervical cancer, it is reasonable to consider giving concomitant chemotherapy to radiotherapy in the recurrent setting. There are no randomized trials supporting this practice, but several Phase I/II trials show good response and tolerability (32–37). Grigsby studied 22 patients with recurrent disease after primary surgery who received concurrent 5-fluorouracil (5-FU) and cisplatin with radiation at the time of their recurrence. He showed a 35% 5- and 10-year survival rate with few acute toxicities, but significant late toxicities in a few patients (34). Smaniotto et al studied 33 patients with locoregional recurrences of which 64% were with central-type recurrences after surgery. They were treated with 5-FU and mitomycin for two cycles with radiation. Smaniotto et al reported a clinical response rate of 45% and a 3-year overall survival of 56% among patients with central recurrences (35). Subsequently, Bazhenov et al published a series on 285 patients with recurrences and showed a better response rate with combination chemotherapy and radiation (69%) compared with radiation alone (26%) and chemotherapy alone (20%) (37).

Radiation therapy is indicated for patients with central-type recurrences after surgery, and concurrent chemotherapy (usually cisplatin) should be considered. Pelvic exenteration should be considered in cases where either there is still residual disease after completion of radiotherapy or if fistulas are present when the recurrence is diagnosed. However, there are several contraindications to pelvic exenteration that need to be considered.

Pelvic Sidewall Recurrences

As mentioned earlier, patients with pelvic sidewall recurrences often do worse than patients with central recurrences. For example, the clinical response rate to chemoradiation after a central recurrence was 45% compared with only 18% among patients with a pelvic recurrence in a prospective Phase II trial of 33 patients (35). Nonetheless, in radiation-naïve patients, there is still a chance to be salvaged with pelvic radiation and pelvic sidewall boost directed at the tumor. Again, it is reasonable to consider concomitant chemotherapy with radiation.

Thomas et al reviewed 40 cases of pelvic recurrences after surgical management of cervical cancer. These patients were treated with tumor-directed radiotherapy with concurrent 5-FU—and mitomycin C in 10 patients. Thirty-one of the 40 patients had a pelvic sidewall recurrence. Twenty-three of the 40 patients (58%) had a complete response, but 5 of these patients eventually relapsed, with 18 patients (45%) still free of disease at a median follow-up of 57 months (range 3–113 months). Of the five patients that recurred, three were distant recurrences and only two recurred in the treated area. In multivariate analysis, location of recurrence (central vs sidewall) was not predictive of a complete response, but these results are limited by the small number of patients in the study. Interestingly, the only significant predictor of complete response was the number of 5-FU cycles administered (32).

Cerrotta et al subsequently published a series of 20 patients treated with radiotherapy and concurrent paclitaxel, 6 of these patients had a local recurrence (5 with sidewall recurrences and 1 with bulky parametrial disease). A complete response was seen in four of the six

(60%) patients with local recurrence after completion of chemoradiation (36). As mentioned earlier, Smaniotto et al reviewed 33 cases of local recurrences after surgery treated with radiation and concurrent 5-FU. The majority of patients had central recurrences, but 36% had pelvic recurrences. They reported a clinical response rate of 18% and a 3-year overall survival of 48% among these patients with pelvic recurrences (35).

More recently, Miglietta et al published a Phase II trial of radiation with cisplatin and paclitaxel for locally advanced or recurrent cervical cancer. Five of the 27 patients had pelvic recurrences and they reported a complete response in all 5 patients, but 1 patient had local progression 6 months after completion of radiotherapy (38).

These studies provide evidence for the use of chemoradiation as the treatment of choice for patients with local recurrences, central and pelvic. However, unlike patients with central recurrences, if patients with pelvic sidewall recurrences fail adjuvant radiotherapy, with or without chemotherapy, they typically are not candidates for surgical resection.

■ LOCAL RECURRENCES AFTER RADIOTHERAPY

Central Recurrences

Unfortunately, most patients who recur locally after radiotherapy are not candidates for further radiation due to dose-limiting toxicities. The only option for cure remains pelvic exenteration. However, in select cases with small central recurrences or persistent disease at the cervix, one may consider radical hysterectomy as long as adequate margins free of disease can be accomplished and patients understand the elevated risk of fistula formation.

Rutledge et al in 1994 published a series of 42 patients that underwent radical surgeries, less than exenterations, for recurrent or persistent cervical cancer after radiotherapy. They divided the patients into three groups based upon original stage/size of recurrence. Thirteen of the patients had recurrent or persistent disease localized to the vagina and/or cervix with Stage IB to IIA disease whereas 20 patients had more extensive disease (Stage IIB to III tumors) and/or tumor extending into the parametria at the time of recurrence. The remaining eight patients in this series had even more extensive disease that required either resection of the bladder base and/or ureteral transections with reanastamosis or partial bowel resections. None of the patients had pelvic sidewall disease as this was an exclusion criterion. The 5-year disease-free survival (DFS) rates for the three subsets of patients with small-, medium-, and large-volume disease were 84%, 49%, and 25%, respectively, with a mean follow-up of 6.6 years. However, major complication rates increased as the volume of recurrent/persistent disease increased with rates of 31%, 50%, and 75%, respectively. The most common complication was fistula formation, which occurred in 11 patients (26%). In the group with small central tumors at the time of salvage surgery, there were two vesicovaginal fistulas and two rectovaginal fistulas. However, the rectovaginal fistulas occurred only in the two patients that had vaginectomy performed (39). There were two deaths related to surgical complications, but deaths were limited to the group with large-volume disease. They concluded that among patients with early Stage IB to IIA disease that have central recurrences limited to the cervix with limited vaginal extension radical hysterectomy should be considered if not recommended in lieu of a pelvic exenteration.

That same year, Coleman et al published a series of 50 patients again with central recurrent or persistent disease after primary radiotherapy that underwent radical hysterectomy for salvage. The reported overall survival rates at 5 and 10 years were 72% and 60%, respectively. However, among a subset of patients with lesions less than 2 cm their 5-year survival was 90% compared with 64% in patients with lesions greater than 2 cm ($p < .01$). They reported a 42% rate of severe complications with one death and a 28% fistula rate. However, among a subset of patients with small tumors (less than 2 cm) and normal intravenous pyelograms preoperatively, the rate of fistula was only 10%. They also concluded that patients with small central recurrences may be salvaged with radical hysterectomy rather than exenterative procedures (40).

Maneo et al in 1999 published a similar series of 34 patients with central recurrent or persistent disease after primary radiotherapy treated with radical hysterectomy to salvage disease. They reported a 5-year survival rate of 49% with a 44% rate of major complications and 15% fistula rate. Again, they identified a subset of patients with a better prognosis. Patients with Stage IB to IIA disease, no clinical parametrial involvement, and tumors less than or equal to 4 cm had a 35% subsequent recurrence rate, whereas the remaining subset of patients that had at least one of the aforementioned features had a 76% recurrence rate. Similar to the prior studies, they concluded that radical hysterectomy can be an alternative option to pelvic exenteration in a highly selected group of patients with small central recurrences (41).

Nonetheless, among patients with larger central recurrence or involvement of lateral parametria and/or vagina after primary or adjuvant radiotherapy (with or without chemotherapy), pelvic exenteration remains the only option for cure in highly selected cases. The 5-year survival rates after pelvic exenteration range from 20% to 66%, with a cumulative average of 34% (42). Overall morbidity of the procedure approaches 70% (43,44) and the rate of intraoperative death averages 10%, but estimates of rates over the last 20 years are closer to 5% (42).

Surgical complications typically involve excessive blood loss, wound infections and dehiscences, sepsis, veno-occlusive events, and pulmonary complications. In addition, in previously irradiated patients, there is an increased risk of fistula, bowel perforations or anastamotic leaks, and obstructions. Long-term complications include urinary tract infections, renal insufficiency, obstruction, and loss of sexual function, as well as the typical complications of stomas. Thus, when selecting patients for pelvic exenteration, one must consider the likelihood of cure or risk of severe complications and even death.

Prognostic factors that predict improved survival after pelvic exenteration include DFSs greater than 6 months, recurrences less than 3 cm in size, and lack of pelvic sidewall involvement (45–50). The clinical signs of pelvic sidewall involvement include the triad of unilateral lymphatic leg edema, sciatic pain, and hydronephrosis. However, nowadays, imaging typically detects sidewall involvement prior to the presentation of the clinical triad. Many consider pelvic sidewall disease an absolute contraindication to pelvic exenteration due to its unresectability. Jurado et al published resectability rates of 48 patients who had been previously irradiated and underwent pelvic exenteration. Among patients with central recurrence, 65% were resectable (negative margins) compared with 29% of the patients with pelvic sidewall disease (51). Evidence of metastasis outside the pelvis is also considered an absolute contraindication to pelvic exenteration (46,52). Morley et al in 1989 reported a series of 100 carefully selected patients for pelvic exenteration. Thirteen of these patients had positive lymph nodes (seven with only microscopic involvement) and none of these patients were alive after 5 years, compared with a 70% 5-year survival among the patients with negative nodes (52). Thus, a patient should have a PET-CT scan to assess for distant metastasis and an MRI to assess for tumor size/invasion and resectability. Of course, there are some individuals who may still consider exenteration if there is an isolated distant metastasis that is resectable such as a para-aortic lymph node. This of course will diminish their overall prognosis, but may still afford them a chance of cure (53). Despite all the preoperative workup, approximately one-third of cases will be found to be inappropriate for exenteration at the time of surgery due to peritoneal disease, para-aortic node involvement, or pelvic sidewall disease (50).

Regardless of the resectability of the tumor, the patient's overall performance status and psychosocial well-being need to be considered. Pelvic exenterations are life-altering surgeries often requiring caring for two ostomies, a loss of sexual functioning, and a myriad of potential short- and long-term surgical complications. Thus, all women who are candidates for exenteration need to undergo extensive counseling regarding the potential complications and changes in lifestyle and daily functioning (54).

Pelvic Sidewall Recurrences

As mentioned earlier, if extension to the pelvic sidewall occurs, these patients typically are not candidates for exenteration. However, as mentioned earlier, Jurado et al reported a 28% resectability rate among 28 patients with previously irradiated sidewall disease with a 10-year local control rate of 32% compared with 43% among patients with central recurrences only; this was not significant. The group with sidewall disease also had higher rates of 10-year distant failure, 83% compared with 57% among patients with central recurrences only; this also was not significant. More importantly, the location of the recurrence (central vs lateral) was not predictive of disease-specific survival among the patients with completely resected disease and the morbidity of the exenteration was not different between patients with central versus sidewall disease (65% vs 73%) (51). Thus, if a patient has sidewall disease but it is felt to be surgically resectable it may be reasonable to consider pelvic exenteration.

In Germany, Hockel published a series of 36 patients with sidewall disease from locally advanced or recurrent cervical cancer where two-thirds had been previously irradiated. These patients underwent a laterally extended endopelvic resection (LEER), which, in addition to the standard procedures of exenteration, includes exposing the entire internal iliac vessel system and ligating the internal iliac vessels at the bifurcation. The vessels are mobilized medially to expose the sacral plexus. The lesser pelvic sidewall and pelvic floor muscles are then resected by incising the obturator internus muscle and detaching it from the acetabulum and the lesser sciatic foramen in order to resect the tumor en bloc with the adjacent pelvic floor muscles. In this first series, he reported a 5-year survival rate of 49% with one treatment-related death and a 39% rate of severe complications (55).

Hockel later published a series of 102 patients that underwent LEER where 63 of the patients had cervical cancer, the majority being recurrent tumors. Seventy-six patients had tumor fixed to the sidewall. Despite the heterogeneous nature of this series, after a median follow-up of 30 months (range 1–136 months), he reported 5-year recurrence rates and disease-specific survival rates of 52% and 55%, respectively. In this series, 97% of the patients had resectable disease and there were two treatment-related deaths with a 70% severe complication rate. Eighty-four percent of recurrences involved distant sites, while only six patients had isolated local pelvic recurrences. However, patients with tumors greater than 5 cm, a DFS of less than 5 months after completing radiotherapy, or tumor involvement of the sciatic nerve were not eligible for LEER (56). Thus, again, patients must be highly selected based on the probability of resectability and potential for cure. Preoperative determination of resectability can be difficult. However, clinical exam and radiographic imaging are highly predictive of resectability. Jurado et al reported odds ratios for clinical exam and imaging in predicting negative margins of 4.70 (95% confidence interval [CI] 1.29–17.69) and 5.80 (95% CI 1.06–33.38), respectively. In addition, positive lymph node status portends a worse prognosis with 5-year survival rates of 23% vs 47% for patients with negative lymph nodes (51). Thus, at the time of exploratory laparotomy, a surgeon must fully evaluate the potential for resectability and lymph node status to help determine if it is warranted to proceed with exenterative surgery.

When exenterative surgery is performed and there is a concern for gross positive margins or positive microscopic margins, some have utilized intraoperative radiotherapy (IORT) to sterilize residual disease. The benefit of IORT is that the treatment area can be directly visualized and critical structures can be mobilized away or shielded. Recommended doses vary from 10 to 12 Gy for microscopic disease and 15 to 20 Gy for gross residual disease; however, optimal doses must take into account previous radiation doses to the region being treated. Several studies have shown that IORT is beneficial only in scenarios where there is no gross residual disease (57–59). Haddock et al reported 5-year survival rates of approximately 42% for patients with microscopic residual disease compared with only 11% for patients with gross residual disease, and 3-year local control rates of 83% for patients with microscopic residual compared with 25% with gross residual disease (58). Therefore, ideal situations where IORT may be beneficial include cases where tumor is resectable but the patient has poor prognostic factors for local recurrence or residual microscopic disease such as close positive margins and lymphatic-space or perineural invasion (60).

If a patient is felt to have nonresectable disease and still no other evidence of distant disease, one may consider neoadjuvant chemotherapy in attempts to decrease the tumor volume to render it resectable in order to perform a pelvic exenteration. Lopez-Graniel et al recently published on a series of 17 patients with recurrent or persistent cervical cancer deemed to not be candidates for exenteration due to the extent of their local disease. The patients received an average of four cycles of platinum-based chemotherapy. Nine (53%) of the patients had a clinical and/or radiographic response to chemotherapy and underwent exenteration. Of these nine patients, four had a complete pathological response and eight of the nine patients had completely resectable disease with negative margins, 1 patient died during surgery due to complications. At a median follow-up of 11 months, the median survival among the operable patients was 32 months compared with only 3 months in the nonoperable group (61). Maggioni et al also recently reported a 73% response rate on 44 patients that received neoadjuvant chemotherapy prior to pelvic exenteration. Tumor size was reduced in 65% of the patients (62). Thus, preoperative neoadjuvant chemotherapy may render certain patients amenable to pelvic exenteration that otherwise would not have been operable.

Some authors have also investigated the utility of intra-arterial chemotherapy directed at the tumor for isolated pelvic recurrences. In 1988, Rettenmaier et al reported on a small series of seven patients with untreated locally advanced cervical cancer and five patients with isolated pelvic recurrences from cervical cancer. These patients received a continuous infusion of cisplatin via an implantable device infusing directly into the internal iliac artery. Unfortunately, only two of the five patients with recurrent disease were evaluable and they died at 32 and 60 months after initiating treatment (63). In 1987, a group from Italy reported more success with intermittent intra-arterial infusion of peptichemio, doxorubicin, and cisplatin. In fact, 9 of the 13 patients (69%) with recurrent disease experienced a response. However, among this series of 25 patients, there was one treatment-related death due to sepsis and two femoral thromboses, one of which requiring an arterial bypass (64). Subsequent studies from Japan and in the United States have only evaluated intra-arterial chemotherapy in the setting of primary therapy for locally advanced cervical cancer in combination with radiotherapy, and have reported excellent response rates up to 98% with acceptable toxicities and side effects (65–69). However, in one randomized trial in the treatment of Stage III and IV disease, the addition of concurrent intra-arterial chemotherapy to primary radiotherapy did not provide any additional benefit at the expense of more complications (70). However, it may be beneficial to administer intra-arterial chemotherapy to patients with unresectable local recurrences. In the event of a complete response, no further therapy may be needed, but in the event of a partial response, patients may then be considered for exenterative procedures. Such treatment(s) should be given in the setting of clinical trials.

■ DISTANT RECURRENCES OR NONOPERABLE LOCAL RECURRENCES

Unfortunately, many patients will recur in extrapelvic sites or else have locally advanced disease that is unresectable despite radiotherapy. In these cases, chemotherapy is given in an attempt to control disease progression, but rarely do patients get a complete response. However, in cases of isolated lung metastasis, chemotherapy may result in a complete response. In fact, surgical resection of isolated lung metastasis (1–3 metastases) followed by adjuvant chemotherapy showed a 5-year survival of 46% (71). However, in most cases, chemotherapy is used as a palliative measure to decrease symptoms and possibly increase survival. No randomized trials have been done that have compared

chemotherapy to best supportive care to assess the impact of chemotherapy on survival and quality of life.

There are many chemotherapeutic agents that are active in cervical cancer. However, cisplatin is the single most active agent used to treat cervical cancer (72,73). Several Gynecologic Oncology Group (GOG) trials including approximately 800 patients have shown response rates of 20%–30% with median survivals of approximately 7 months (72–74). GOG 43 evaluated different dose regimens of cisplatin and reported a 21% response rate with 50 mg/m^2 every 3 weeks compared with a 31% response rate with 100 mg/m^2 every 3 weeks. However, the 100 mg/m^2 regimen was more toxic with no improvement in progression-free survival (PFS) or overall survival. Therefore, they recommended using 50 mg/m^2 every 3 weeks (73). Also, in GOG 26C, patients who were chemotherapy-naïve have a much greater response rate of 50% compared with patients that received prior chemotherapy, response rate 17% (72). These rates are similar to subsequent rates reported in other studies (75,76). In another small study of single-agent cisplatin, 30% of patients had an objective response to treatment, but 67% had palliation of their pain (77).

Many trials have subsequently looked at cisplatin-based combination therapy. However, very few of the trials have proven any survival benefit in doublet therapy, with obvious increases in toxicity. Furthermore, initial high response rates in Phase II trials have not been confirmed in larger Phase III studies. In 1997, GOG 110 reported evaluation of cisplatin 50 mg/m^2 with or without ifosfamide 5 g/m^2 over 24 hours with mesna in patients with advanced or recurrent disease. They reported a higher response rate and PFS with the addition of ifosfamide, –31% vs 18% response rate and 4.6 vs 3.2 months PFS. However, this benefit was at the expense of significantly higher toxicities with no difference in overall survival (78). In 2002, GOG 149 reported that evaluated cisplatin 50 mg/m^2 and ifosfamide 5 g/m^2 over 24 hours with or without bleomycin 30 units over 24 hours in patients with recurrent or persistent disease. However, the addition of bleomycin had no difference in response rates (31% vs 32%), PFS, or overall survival (79). In 2004, GOG 169 was reported which evaluated cisplatin compared with cisplatin and paclitaxel in 260 patients with recurrent or advanced disease. The overall response rates were 36% vs 19% for the doublet vs singlet therapy, respectively, and the median PFS was 4.8 vs 2.8 months for doublet and singlet therapy, respectively. These differences were significantly different at the expense of increased toxicity with the doublet, but overall survival was not different (9.7 vs 8.8 months) nor was quality of life (80). In 2005, GOG 179 was reported which evaluated cisplatin at 50 mg/m^2 every 3 weeks compared with cisplatin at a similar dose and frequency in combination with topotecan 0.75 mg/m^2 on days 1 to 3 every 3 weeks in 294 patients with recurrent or advanced disease. A third arm in this trial receiving methotrexate, vinblastine, doxorubicin, and cisplatin (MVAC) was closed early due to four treatment-related deaths. A significantly improved response rate *and* survival were reported with the administration of cisplatin and topotecan compared with cisplatin alone (27% vs 13% response rates and 9.4 vs 6.5 months overall survival). The quality of life between the two arms was no different despite more toxicity with cisplatin and topotecan (81). This was the first and only trial to show a survival benefit with a doublet regimen compared with cisplatin alone.

Since combination chemotherapy was beneficial in GOG 179, the GOG performed another trial, GOG 204, that compared cisplatin with one of four different agents: paclitaxel at 135 mg/m^2 every 3 weeks, vinorelbine 30 mg/m^2 every 3 weeks, gemcitabine 1 g/m^2 on days 1 and 8 every 3 weeks, and again topotecan at 0.75 mg/m^2 on days 1 to 3 every 3 weeks. The response rates between the four arms were not significantly different ranging from 22% to 29% and the trial was closed early for futility as there was no probability that the three combinations with vinorelbine, topotecan, or gemcitabine would be superior to paclitaxel (82). Nor was there a difference in quality of life between the four arms (83).

Despite the apparent equivalency between the chemotherapeutic regimens, there are several prognostic factors that are important in predicting individual patient responses. Moore et al reviewed 428 patients from GOG 110, 169, and 179 and with multivariate analysis identified five significant independent poor prognostic factors: African-American race, performance status greater than 0, pelvic disease, prior radiosensitizing chemotherapy, and time interval from diagnosis to recurrence less than 1 year. In fact, patients with four to five of these risk factors were estimated to have a response rate of only 13% and a median PFS of 2.8 months and overall survival of 5.5 months (84). Thus, each patient should be assessed individually with respect to their likelihood of response to chemotherapy when considering the benefits and risks of treatment.

Carboplatin has also been studied in advanced or recurrent disease but initial studies by the GOG were not as promising as cisplatin (85,86). GOG 77 showed a response rate of 28% among chemotherapy-naïve patients receiving single-agent carboplatin (85), but a subsequent GOG trial comparing carboplatin with iproplatin reported a response rate of only 15% among 175 patients (86). However, several more recent Phase II trials of carboplatin and paclitaxel (CT) have shown promising responses (87,88). In Australia, a series of 25 patients with recurrent or advanced cervical cancer was reported. The patients were treated with CT and had a response rate of 40% with a median overall survival of 21 months and a median PFS of 3 months (87). A multicentered Phase II trial in the United States reported on

48 patients treated with CT for advanced or recurrent disease and found a response rate of 53% with a median overall survival of 11 months. These results were not significantly different from a similar group of 14 patients treated with the traditional regimen of cisplatin and paclitaxel (PT; 88).

Recently, the Japan Clinical Oncology Group (JCOG) reported results from their randomized controlled Phase III trial comparing CT with PT in patients with advanced or recurrent disease (89). This was an equivalency trial powered to detect a difference of at least 30% between the two arms. Among the 253 patients, they reported similar median overall survivals (18.3 vs 17.5 months) and similar median PFSs (6.9 vs 6.2 months) in the PT arms compared with the CT arms. However, a subset analysis revealed that patients previously treated with platinum (typically cisplatin) had worse survival outcomes when given PT compared with CT, hazard ratio (HR) 0.69 (95% CI 0.47–1.02); whereas, patients who were chemotherapy-naïve had better survival outcomes when treated with PT compared with CT, overall survival HR 1.57 (95% CI 1.06–2.32). Thus, cisplatin appears to remain the best choice among chemotherapy-naïve patients, but carboplatin may be a better second-line treatment after previous cisplatin exposure (89). In addition, carboplatin is easier to administer and is less nephrotoxic—a common concern among patients with ureteral obstruction from their cervical cancer.

Many other chemotherapy regimens have also been studied as first- and second-line treatments, but perhaps one of the most promising new drugs is gemcitabine (90). Gemcitabine is a fluorine-substituted pyrimidine antimetabolite with increased membrane permeability, greater enzyme affinity, more prolonged intracellular retention, and a broader spectrum of activity. It also has a proposed synergistic role when given with cisplatin (90). Initial studies of single-agent gemcitabine revealed response rates of only 8% (91), but subsequent Phase I/II trials of gemcitabine in combination with cisplatin have shown promising response rates of 41%–75% (92–94). In fact, the addition of gemcitabine to cisplatin in the setting of primary treatment for locally advanced disease in conjunction with radiotherapy has recently been shown to significantly decrease overall survival by 32% in a randomized controlled trial (95).

The GOG has also studied irinotecan with and without cisplatin but reported response rates of only 18% and 13%, respectively (96,97). Oral capecitabine has been studied as a single agent in a Phase II trial, but showed a response rate of only 15% among 26 patients with recurrent or metastatic disease (98). Ifosfamide as a single agent has shown response rates of 15%–33% (99,100). Thus, cisplatin and paclitaxel remain the most commonly used regimen for metastatic or recurrent cervical cancer not amenable to radiotherapy or surgical resection.

Despite the aforementioned response rates, improvements are usually temporary and the vast majority of the patients will succumb to their disease in less than a year. Newer drugs are desperately needed among this group of patients with unresectable and/or metastatic disease who generally have a grim prognosis and poor quality of life. Antiangiogenesis and endothelial growth factor receptor (EGFR) inhibitors are under investigation (101,102). In fact, HPV E6 has been shown to upregulate hypoxia inducible factor 1 (HIF-1) alpha, which then upregulates vascular EGF (VEGF) (102). Therefore, bevacizumab, a humanized monoclonal antibody directed against VEGF-A, seems to be an appropriate targeted therapy against HPV-induced cervical cancer. A recent Phase II multicenter clinical trial, GOG 227C, studied single-agent bevacizumab among 46 patients with recurrent or persistent cervical cancer who may have received up to two prior chemotherapy regimens. The response rate was 11% and the median overall survival was 7.3 months and median PFS 3.4 months (103). According to the investigators, these results favored comparably to historical controls in other similar GOG trials. Because cisplatin is so commonly used during primary treatment with chemoradiation a recent trial (GOG 240) evaluated cisplatin and paclitaxel to paclitaxel and topotecan, with a secondary randomization adding bevacizumab (102). This trial demonstrated superiority of cisplatin and paclitaxel over paclitaxel and topotecan in response rate (38.4% vs 24.7% $P = .03$) and PFS (HR = 1.39, $P = .008$), but not survival (15 vs 12.5 months, $P = .88$). The addition of bevacizumab to cisplatin and paclitaxel further improved response rate (48% vs 36%, $P = .0081$), median PFS (8.2 vs 5.9 months, $P = .0002$), and overall survival 17.5 vs 14.3 months ($P = .035$).

Studies of EGFR inhibitors, cetuximab and erlotinib, have not shown to have any benefit in treating patients with recurrent or persistent cervical cancer in recent GOG trials (104,105). Another Phase II trial studied newer EGFR inhibitors, pazopanib and lapatinib, as monotherapy or in combination. The study showed a benefit with pazopanib in terms of PFS with a response rate of 9% (106). However, a randomized Phase III trial would be needed to determine if there is any benefit to these drugs over standard therapies. In light of the small response rate, such a trial may not be feasible.

The first ever Phase I trial of a live-attenuated *Listeria monocytogenes* therapeutic vaccine delivering the HPV-16 E7 antigen was recently tested in 15 patients for dose tolerability and safety. Although there was only one partial responder among the group of patients with advanced or recurrent disease, the vaccine was safe and tolerable (107). Additionally, new therapies using nanotechnology and nanoparticles are currently being studied in the laboratory to offer more directed treatments for cancer and potentially could be applied to treating recurrent cervical cancer in the future (108,109).

■ CONCLUSION

The treatment of recurrent cervical cancer is highly dependent on the location of the recurrence (central, regional, or distant), the primary therapy given (surgery and/or radiotherapy), the size of the recurrence, the time to recurrence, and the patients' symptoms. Also, the overall well-being of the patient and their ability to endure treatment(s) and their side effects weighed against the projected benefit of such treatment(s) needs to be carefully considered. In situations where patients have metastatic disease or unresectable pelvic disease not amenable to further radiotherapy, chemotherapy is given as a palliative measure to control disease progression and hopefully relieve symptoms. Rarely, in cases with isolated pulmonary disease, chemotherapy may be curative. Therefore, when the side effects of chemotherapy are too burdensome and the chemotherapy is no longer controlling the disease or alleviating symptoms, patients and their physicians need to consider transitioning to providing symptom management alone. Unfortunately, the symptoms related to progressive cervical cancer are often very debilitating and painful requiring high doses of pain medications and at time palliative radiation for bone pain. Hopefully, with the development of new systemic therapies, we may improve survival and quality of life among patients with incurable recurrent disease. In the meantime, we need to be judicious about which patients with recurrences have the potential for cure with aggressive treatments including but not limited to: salvage radiotherapy and concurrent chemotherapy after surgery, radical resection of tumor often involving pelvic exenteration with or without intraoperative radiotherapy, and possibly neoadjuvant chemotherapy prior to surgical resection.

■ REFERENCES

1. Ferlay JSH, Bray F, Forman D, Mathers C, Parkin DM. GLOBOCAN 2008, *Cancer Incidence and Mortality Worldwide: IARC CancerBase No. 10*. Internet. Lyon, France. International Agency for Research on Cancer, 2010. http://globocan.iarc.fr.
2. Siegel R, Naishadham D, Jemal A. *Cancer Statistics, 2012*.
3. Elit L, Fyles AW, Oliver TK, Devries-Aboud MC, Fung-Kee-Fung M; members of the Gynecology Cancer Disease Site Group of Cancer Care Ontario's Program in Evidence-Based Care. Follow-up for women after treatment for cervical cancer. *Curr Oncol*. 2010;17(3):65–69.
4. Larson DM, Copeland LJ, Stringer CA, Gershenson DM, Malone JM Jr, Edwards CL. Recurrent cervical carcinoma after radical hysterectomy. *Gynecol Oncol*. 1988;30(3):381–387.
5. Perez CA, Grigsby PW, Camel HM, Galakatos AE, Mutch D, Lockett MA. Irradiation alone or combined with surgery in stage IB, IIA, and IIB carcinoma of uterine cervix: update of a nonrandomized comparison. *Int J Radiat Oncol Biol Phys*. 1995;31(4):703–716.
6. Marchiolé P, Buénerd A, Benchaib M, Nezhat K, Dargent D, Mathevet P. Clinical significance of lympho vascular space involvement and lymph node micrometastases in early-stage cervical cancer: a retrospective case-control surgico-pathological study. *Gynecol Oncol*. 2005;97(3):727–732.

7. Grisaru DA, Covens A, Franssen E, et al. Histopathologic score predicts recurrence free survival after radical surgery in patients with stage IA2-IB1-2 cervical carcinoma. *Cancer.* 2003;97(8):1904–1908.

8. Sedlis A, Bundy BN, Rotman MZ, Lentz SS, Muderspach LI, Zaino RJ. A randomized trial of pelvic radiation therapy versus no further therapy in selected patients with stage IB carcinoma of the cervix after radical hysterectomy and pelvic lymphadenectomy: A Gynecologic Oncology Group Study. *Gynecol Oncol.* 1999;73(2):177–183.

9. Estape RE, Angioli R, Madrigal M, et al. Close vaginal margins as a prognostic factor after radical hysterectomy. *Gynecol Oncol.* 1998;68(3):229–232.

10. Hopkins MP, Morley GW. Radical hysterectomy versus radiation therapy for stage IB squamous cell cancer of the cervix. *Cancer.* 1991;68(2):272–277.

11. Delgado G, Bundy B, Zaino R, Sevin BU, Creasman WT, Major F. Prospective surgical-pathological study of disease-free interval in patients with stage IB squamous cell carcinoma of the cervix: a Gynecologic Oncology Group study. *Gynecol Oncol.* 1990;38(3):352–357.

12. Zaino RJ, Ward S, Delgado G, et al. Histopathologic predictors of the behavior of surgically treated stage IB squamous cell carcinoma of the cervix. A Gynecologic Oncology Group study. *Cancer.* 1992;69(7):1750–1758.

13. Burghardt E, Baltzer J, Tulusan AH, Haas J. Results of surgical treatment of 1028 cervical cancers studied with volumetry. *Cancer.* 1992;70(3):648–655.

14. Stehman FB, Bundy BN, DiSaia PJ, Keys HM, Larson JE, Fowler WC. Carcinoma of the cervix treated with radiation therapy. I. A multi-variate analysis of prognostic variables in the Gynecologic Oncology Group. *Cancer.* 1991;67(11):2776–2785.

15. Webb MJ, Symmonds RE. Site of recurrence of cervical cancer after radical hysterectomy. *Am J Obstet Gynecol.* 1980;138(7 Pt 1):813–817.

16. Havrilesky LJ, Wong TZ, Secord AA, Berchuck A, Clarke-Pearson DL, Jones EL. The role of PET scanning in the detection of recurrent cervical cancer. *Gynecol Oncol.* 2003;90(1):186–190.

17. Brooks RA, Rader JS, Dehdashti F, et al. Surveillance FDG-PET detection of asymptomatic recurrences in patients with cervical cancer. *Gynecol Oncol.* 2009;112(1):104–109.

18. Soisson AP, Geszler G, Soper JT, Berchuck A, Clarke-Pearson DL. A comparison of symptomatology, physical examination, and vaginal cytology in the detection of recurrent cervical carcinoma after radical hysterectomy. *Obstet Gynecol.* 1990;76(1):106–109.

19. Bodurka-Bevers D, Morris M, Eifel PJ, et al. Posttherapy surveillance of women with cervical cancer: an outcomes analysis. *Gynecol Oncol.* 2000;78(2):187–193.

20. Zanagnolo V, Minig LA, Gadducci A, et al. Surveillance procedures for patients for cervical carcinoma: a review of the literature. *Int J Gynecol Cancer.* 2009;19(3):306–313.

21. Morice P, Deyrolle C, Rey A, et al. Value of routine follow-up procedures for patients with stage I/II cervical cancer treated with combined surgery-radiation therapy. *Ann Oncol.* 2004;15(2):218–223.

22. Zola P, Fuso L, Mazzola S, et al. Could follow-up different modalities play a role in asymptomatic cervical cancer relapses diagnosis? An Italian multicenter retrospective analysis. *Gynecol Oncol.* 2007;107(1 Suppl 1):S150–S154.

23. Husain A, Akhurst T, Larson S, Alektiar K, Barakat RR, Chi DS. A prospective study of the accuracy of 18Fluorodeoxyglucose positron emission tomography (18FDG PET) in identifying sites of metastasis prior to pelvic exenteration. *Gynecol Oncol.* 2007;106(1):177–180.

24. Jobsen JJ, Leer JW, Cleton FJ, Hermans J. Treatment of locoregional recurrence of carcinoma of the cervix by radiotherapy after primary surgery. *Gynecol Oncol.* 1989;33(3):368–371.

25. Ito H, Shigematsu N, Kawada T, et al. Radiotherapy for centrally recurrent cervical cancer of the vaginal stump following hysterectomy. *Gynecol Oncol.* 1997;67(2):154–161.

26. Tan R, Chung CH, Liu MT, Lai YL, Chang KH. Radiotherapy for postoperative recurrent uterine cervical carcinoma. *Acta Oncol.* 1991;30(3):353–356.

27. Ijaz T, Eifel PJ, Burke T, Oswald MJ. Radiation therapy of pelvic recurrence after radical hysterectomy for cervical carcinoma. *Gynecol Oncol.* 1998;70(2):241–246.

28. Deutsch M, Parsons JA. Radiotherapy for carcinoma of the cervix recurrent after surgery. *Cancer.* 1974;34(6):2051–2055.

29. Friedlander M, Grogan M; U.S. Preventative Services Task Force. Guidelines for the treatment of recurrent and metastatic cervical cancer. *Oncologist.* 2002;7(4):342–347.

30. Krebs HB, Helmkamp BF, Sevin BU, Poliakoff SR, Nadji M, Averette HE. Recurrent cancer of the cervix following radical hysterectomy and pelvic node dissection. *Obstet Gynecol.* 1982;59(4):422–427.

31. Randall M, M.H., Long III H, Tedjarati S., in *Principles and Practice of Gynecologic Oncology.*, M.M. Barakat R, Randall M., Editor 2009, Lippincott Williams & Wilkins: Baltimore, MD. p. 667.

32. Thomas GM, Dembo AJ, Myhr T, Black B, Pringle JF, Rawlings G. Long-term results of concurrent radiation and chemotherapy for carcinoma of the cervix recurrent after surgery. *Int J Gynecol Cancer.* 1993;3(4):193–198.

33. Maneo A, Landoni F, Cormio G, et al. Concurrent carboplatin/5-fluorouracil and radiotherapy for recurrent cervical carcinoma. *Ann Oncol.* 1999;10(7):803–807.

34. Grigsby PW. Prospective phase I/II study of irradiation and concurrent chemotherapy for recurrent cervical cancer after radical hysterectomy. *Int J Gynecol Cancer.* 2004;14(5):860–864.

35. Smaniotto D, D'Agostino G, Luzi S, et al. Concurrent 5-fluorouracil, mitomycin C and radiation with or without brachytherapy in recurrent cervical cancer: a scoring system to predict clinical response and outcome. *Tumori.* 2005;91(4):295–301.

36. Cerrotta A, Gardan G, Cavina R, et al. Concurrent radiotherapy and weekly paclitaxel for locally advanced or recurrent squamous cell carcinoma of the uterine cervix. A pilot study with intensification of dose. *Eur J Gynaecol Oncol.* 2002;23(2):115–119.

37. Bazhenov AG, Guseinov KD, Khadzhimba AV, Baranov SB, Il'iashenko SA, Maksimov SIa. [Results of treatment for recurrent cancer of the uterine cervix]. *Vopr Onkol.* 2009;55(3):319–326.

38. Miglietta L, Franzone P, Centurioni MG, et al. A phase II trial with cisplatin-paclitaxel cytotoxic treatment and concurrent external and endocavitary radiation therapy in locally advanced or recurrent cervical cancer. *Oncology.* 2006;70(1):19–24.

39. Rutledge S, Carey MS, Prichard H, Allen HH, Kocha W, Kirk ME. Conservative surgery for recurrent or persistent carcinoma of the cervix following irradiation: is exenteration always necessary? *Gynecol Oncol.* 1994;52(3):353–359.

40. Coleman RL, Keeney ED, Freedman RS, Burke TW, Eifel PJ, Rutledge FN. Radical hysterectomy for recurrent carcinoma of the uterine cervix after radiotherapy. *Gynecol Oncol.* 1994;55(1):29–35.

41. Maneo A, Landoni F, Cormio G, Colombo A, Mangioni C. Radical hysterectomy for recurrent or persistent cervical cancer following radiation therapy. *Int J Gynecol Cancer.* 1999;9(4):295–301.

42. Peiretti M, Zapardiel I, Zanagnolo V, Landoni F, Morrow CP, Maggioni A. Management of recurrent cervical cancer: a review of the literature. *Surg Oncol.* 2012;21(2):e59–e66.

43. Fotopoulou C, Neumann U, Kraetschell R, et al. Long-term clinical outcome of pelvic exenteration in patients with advanced gynecological malignancies. *J Surg Oncol.* 2010;101(6):507–512.

44. Maggioni A, Roviglione G, Landoni F, et al. Pelvic exenteration: ten-year experience at the European Institute of Oncology in Milan. *Gynecol Oncol.* 2009;114(1):64–68.

45. Shingleton HM, Soong SJ, Gelder MS, Hatch KD, Baker VV, Austin JM Jr. Clinical and histopathologic factors predicting recurrence and survival after pelvic exenteration for cancer of the cervix. *Obstet Gynecol.* 1989;73(6):1027–1034.

46. Rutledge FN, Smith JP, Wharton JT, O'Quinn AG. Pelvic exenteration: analysis of 296 patients. *Am J Obstet Gynecol.* 1977;129(8):881–892.

47. Symmonds RE, Pratt JH, Webb MJ. Exenterative operations: experience with 198 patients. *Am J Obstet Gynecol.* 1975; 121(7):907–918.

48. Stanhope CR, Symmonds RE. Palliative exenteration–what, when, and why? *Am J Obstet Gynecol.* 1985;152(1):12–16.

49. Matthews CM, Morris M, Burke TW, Gershenson DM, Wharton JT, Rutledge FN. Pelvic exenteration in the elderly patient. *Obstet Gynecol.* 1992;79(5 (Pt 1)):773–777.

50. Estape R, Angioli R. Surgical management of advanced and recurrent cervical cancer. *Semin Surg Oncol.* 1999;16(3):236–241.

51. Jurado M, Alcázar JL, Martinez-Monge R. Resectability rates of previously irradiated recurrent cervical cancer (PIRCC) treated with pelvic exenteration: is still the clinical involvement of the pelvis wall a real contraindication? a twenty-year experience. *Gynecol Oncol.* 2010;116(1):38–43.

52. Morley GW, Hopkins MP, Lindenauer SM, Roberts JA. Pelvic exenteration, University of Michigan: 100 patients at 5 years. *Obstet Gynecol.* 1989;74(6):934–943.

53. Höckel M, Dornhöfer N. Pelvic exenteration for gynaecological tumours: achievements and unanswered questions. *Lancet Oncol.* 2006;7(10):837–847.

54. Ruth-Sahd LA, Zulkosky KD. Cervical cancer: caring for patients undergoing total pelvic exenteration. *Crit Care Nurse.* 1999;19(1):46–57.

55. Höckel M. Laterally extended endopelvic resection. Novel surgical treatment of locally recurrent cervical carcinoma involving the pelvic side wall. *Gynecol Oncol.* 2003;91(2):369–377.

56. Höckel M. Laterally extended endopelvic resection (LEER)–principles and practice. *Gynecol Oncol.* 2008;111(2 Suppl): S13–S17.

57. Gemignani ML, Alektiar KM, Leitao M, et al. Radical surgical resection and high-dose intraoperative radiation therapy (HDR-IORT) in patients with recurrent gynecologic cancers. *Int J Radiat Oncol Biol Phys.* 2001;50(3):687–694.

58. Haddock MG, Petersen IA, Webb MJ, Wilson TO, Podratz KC, Gunderson LL. IORT for locally advanced gynecological malignancies. *Front Radiat Ther Oncol.* 1997;31:256–259.

59. del Carmen MG, McIntyre JF, Fuller AF, Nikrui N, Goodman A. Intraoperative radiation therapy in the treatment of pelvic gynecologic malignancies: a review of fifteen cases. *Gynecol Oncol.* 2000;79(3):457–462.

60. Beitler JJ, Anderson PS, Wadler S, et al. Pelvic exenteration for cervix cancer: would additional intraoperative interstitial brachytherapy improve survival? *Int J Radiat Oncol Biol Phys.* 1997;38(1):143–148.

61. Lopez-Graniel C, Dolores R, Cetina L, et al. Pre-exenterative chemotherapy, a novel therapeutic approach for patients with persistent or recurrent cervical cancer. *BMC Cancer.* 2005;5:118.

62. Maggioni A, L.F., Sanguineti F, Lopes A, Zanagnolo V, Aletti G, et al., *Neoadjuvant Chemotherapy Prior to Pelvic Exenteration in Patients With Recurrent or Advanced Cervical Cancer.* Presented at the ICGS Meeting 2010, Prague, Czech Republic, October 23–26 (Abstract #2010–150).

63. Rettenmaier MA, Moran MF, Ramsinghani NF, et al. Treatment of advanced and recurrent squamous carcinoma of the uterine cervix with constant intraarterial infusion of cisplatin. *Cancer.* 1988;61(7):1301–1303.

64. Scarabelli C, Tumolo S, De Paoli A, et al. Intermittent pelvic arterial infusion with peptichemio, doxorubicin, and cisplatin for locally advanced and recurrent carcinoma of the uterine cervix. *Cancer.* 1987;60(1):25–30.

65. Kaku S, Takahashi K, Murakami Y, et al. Neoadjuvant intraarterial chemotherapy for stage IIB-IIIB cervical cancer in Japanese women. *Exp Ther Med.* 2010;1(4):651–655.

66. Motoyama S, Hamana S, Ku Y, et al. Neoadjuvant high-dose intraarterial infusion chemotherapy under percutaneous pelvic perfusion with extracorporeal chemofiltration in patients with stages IIIa-IVa cervical cancer. *Gynecol Oncol.* 2004;95(3):576–582.

67. Kawase S, Okuda T, Ikeda M, et al. Intraarterial cisplatin/nedaplatin and intravenous 5-fluorouracil with concurrent radiation therapy for patients with high-risk uterine cervical cancer. *Gynecol Oncol.* 2006;102(3):493–499.

68. Patton TJ Jr, Kavanagh JJ, Delclos L, et al. Five-year survival in patients given intra-arterial chemotherapy prior to radiotherapy for advanced squamous carcinoma of the cervix and vagina. *Gynecol Oncol.* 1991;42(1):54–59.

69. Chaney AW, Eifel PJ, Logsdon MD, Morris M, Wharton JT. Mature results of a pilot study of pelvic radiotherapy with concurrent continuous infusion intra-arterial 5-FU for stage IIIB-IVA squamous cell carcinoma of the cervix. *Int J Radiat Oncol Biol Phys.* 1999;45(1):113–118.

70. Onishi H, Yamaguchi M, Kuriyama K, et al. Effect of concurrent intra-arterial infusion of platinum drugs for patients with stage III or IV uterine cervical cancer treated with radical radiation therapy. *Cancer J Sci Am.* 2000;6(1):40–45.

71. Shiromizu K, Kasamatsu T, Honma T, Matsumoto K, Shirai T, Takahashi M. clinicopathological study of recurrent uterine cervical squamous-cell carcinoma. *J Obstet Gynaecol Res.* 1999;25(6):395–399.

72. Thigpen T, Shingleton H, Homesley H, Lagasse L, Blessing J. Cis-platinum in treatment of advanced or recurrent squamous cell carcinoma of the cervix: a phase II study of the Gynecologic Oncology Group. *Cancer.* 1981;48(4):899–903.

73. Bonomi P, Blessing JA, Stehman FB, DiSaia PJ, Walton L, Major FJ. Randomized trial of three cisplatin dose schedules in squamous-cell carcinoma of the cervix: a Gynecologic Oncology Group study. *J Clin Oncol.* 1985;3(8):1079–1085.

74. Thigpen JT, Blessing JA, DiSaia PJ, Fowler WC Jr, Hatch KD. A randomized comparison of a rapid versus prolonged (24 hr) infusion of cisplatin in therapy of squamous cell carcinoma of the uterine cervix: a Gynecologic Oncology Group study. *Gynecol Oncol.* 1989;32(2):198–202.

75. Potter ME, Hatch KD, Potter MY, Shingleton HM, Baker VV. Factors affecting the response of recurrent squamous cell carcinoma of the cervix to cisplatin. *Cancer.* 1989;63(7): 1283–1286.

76. Brader KR, Morris M, Levenback C, Levy L, Lucas KR, Gershenson DM. Chemotherapy for cervical carcinoma: factors determining response and implications for clinical trial design. *J Clin Oncol.* 1998;16(5):1879–1884.

77. Chambers SK, Lamb L, Kohorn EI, Schwartz PE, Chambers JT. Chemotherapy of recurrent/advanced cervical cancer: results of the Yale University PBM-PFU protocol. *Gynecol Oncol.* 1994;53(2):161–169.

78. Omura GA, Blessing JA, Vaccarello L, et al. Randomized trial of cisplatin versus cisplatin plus mitolactol versus cisplatin plus ifosfamide in advanced squamous carcinoma of the cervix: a Gynecologic Oncology Group study. *J Clin Oncol.* 1997; 15(1):165–171.

79. Bloss JD, Blessing JA, Behrens BC, et al. Randomized trial of cisplatin and ifosfamide with or without bleomycin in squamous carcinoma of the cervix: a Gynecologic Oncology Group study. *J Clin Oncol.* 2002;20(7):1832–1837.

80. Moore DH, Blessing JA, McQuellon RP, et al. Phase III study of cisplatin with or without paclitaxel in stage IVB, recurrent, or persistent squamous cell carcinoma of the cervix: a Gynecologic Oncology Group. *J Clin Oncol.* 2004;22(15):3113–3119.

81. Long HJ 3rd, Bundy BN, Grendys EC Jr, et al.; Gynecologic Oncology Group Study. Randomized phase III trial of

cisplatin with or without topotecan in carcinoma of the uterine cervix: a Gynecologic Oncology Group Study. *J Clin Oncol.* 2005;23(21):4626–4633.

82. Monk BJ, Sill MW, McMeekin DS, et al. Phase III trial of four cisplatin-containing doublet combinations in stage IVB, recurrent, or persistent cervical carcinoma: a Gynecologic Oncology Group study. *J Clin Oncol.* 2009;27(28):4649–4655.

83. Cella D, Huang HQ, Monk BJ, et al. Health-related quality of life outcomes associated with four cisplatin-based doublet chemotherapy regimens for stage IVB recurrent or persistent cervical cancer: a Gynecologic Oncology Group study. *Gynecol Oncol.* 2010;119(3):531–537.

84. Moore DH, Tian C, Monk BJ, Long HJ, Omura GA, Bloss JD. Prognostic factors for response to cisplatin-based chemotherapy in advanced cervical carcinoma: a Gynecologic Oncology Group Study. *Gynecol Oncol.* 2010;116(1):44–49.

85. Arseneau J, Blessing JA, Stehman FB, McGehee R. A phase II study of carboplatin in advanced squamous cell carcinoma of the cervix (a Gynecologic Oncology Group Study). *Invest New Drugs.* 1986;4(2):187–191.

86. McGuire WP 3rd, Arseneau J, Blessing JA, et al. A randomized comparative trial of carboplatin and iproplatin in advanced squamous carcinoma of the uterine cervix: a Gynecologic Oncology Group study. *J Clin Oncol.* 1989;7(10):1462–1468.

87. Tinker AV, Bhagat K, Swenerton KD, Hoskins PJ. Carboplatin and paclitaxel for advanced and recurrent cervical carcinoma: the British Columbia Cancer Agency experience. *Gynecol Oncol.* 2005;98(1):54–58.

88. Moore KN, Herzog TJ, Lewin S, et al. A comparison of cisplatin/paclitaxel and carboplatin/paclitaxel in stage IVB, recurrent or persistent cervical cancer. *Gynecol Oncol.* 2007;105(2):299–303.

89. Kitagawa, R., *A randomized, phase III trial of paclitaxel and carboplatin (TC) versus paclitaxel plus cisplatin (TP) in stage IVb, persistent or recurrent cervical cancer: Japan Clinical Oncology Group study (JCOG0505). 2012 ASCO Annual Meeting.* J Clin Oncol 30, 2012 (suppl; abstr 5006).

90. Mutch DG, Bloss JD. Gemcitabine in cervical cancer. *Gynecol Oncol.* 2003;90(2 Pt 2):S8–15.

91. Schilder RJ, Blessing JA, Morgan M, Mangan CE, Rader JS. Evaluation of gemcitabine in patients with squamous cell carcinoma of the cervix: a Phase II study of the Gynecologic Oncology Group. *Gynecol Oncol.* 2000;76(2):204–207.

92. Burnett AF, Roman LD, Garcia AA, Muderspach LI, Brader KR, Morrow CP. A phase II study of gemcitabine and cisplatin in patients with advanced, persistent, or recurrent squamous cell carcinoma of the cervix. *Gynecol Oncol.* 2000;76(1):63–66.

93. Matulonis UA, Campos S, Duska L, et al.; Gynecologic Cancer Program of Dana Farber-Harvard Cancer Center. Phase I/II dose finding study of combination cisplatin and gemcitabine in patients with recurrent cervix cancer. *Gynecol Oncol.* 2006;103(1):160–164.

94. Lorvidhaya V, Kamnerdsupaphon P, Chitapanarux I, Sukthomya V, Tonusin A. Cisplatin and gemcitabine in patients with metastatic cervical cancer. *Gan To Kagaku Ryoho.* 2004;31(7):1057–1062.

95. Dueñas-González A, Zarbá JJ, Patel F, et al. Phase III, open-label, randomized study comparing concurrent gemcitabine plus cisplatin and radiation followed by adjuvant gemcitabine and cisplatin versus concurrent cisplatin and radiation in patients with stage IIB to IVA carcinoma of the cervix. *J Clin Oncol.* 2011;29(13):1678–1685.

96. Muggia FM, Blessing JA, McGehee R, Monk BJ. Cisplatin and irinotecan in squamous cell carcinoma of the cervix: a phase II study of the Gynecologic Oncology Group. *Gynecol Oncol.* 2004;94(2):483–487.

97. Look KY, Blessing JA, Levenback C, Kohler M, Chafe W, Roman LD. A phase II trial of CPT-11 in recurrent squamous carcinoma of the cervix: a Gynecologic Oncology Group study. *Gynecol Oncol.* 1998;70(3):334–338.

98. Garcia AA, Blessing JA, Darcy KM, et al. Phase II clinical trial of capecitabine in the treatment of advanced, persistent or recurrent squamous cell carcinoma of the cervix with translational research: a Gynecologic Oncology Group study. *Gynecol Oncol.* 2007;104(3):572–579.

99. Sutton GP, Blessing JA, Manetta A, Homesley H, McGuire W. Gynecologic Oncology Group studies with ifosfamide. *Semin Oncol.* 1992;19(6 Suppl 12):31–34.

100. Meanwell CA, Mould JJ, Blackledge G, et al. Phase II study of ifosfamide in cervical cancer. *Cancer Treat Rep.* 1986;70(6):727–730.

101. Willmott LJ, Monk BJ. Cervical cancer therapy: current, future and anti-angiogensis targeted treatment. *Expert Rev Anticancer Ther.* 2009;9(7):895–903.

102. Tewari KS, Sill M, Long HJ, et al. Incorporation of bevacizumab in the treatment of recurrent and metastatic cervical cancer: a phase III randomized trial of the Gynecologic Oncology Group. *J Clin Oncol.* 2013;31(suppl; abstr 3).

103. Monk BJ, Sill MW, Burger RA, Gray HJ, Buekers TE, Roman LD. Phase II trial of bevacizumab in the treatment of persistent or recurrent squamous cell carcinoma of the cervix: a Gynecologic Oncology Group study. *J Clin Oncol.* 2009;27(7):1069–1074.

104. Schilder RJ, Sill MW, Lee YC, Mannel R. A phase II trial of erlotinib in recurrent squamous cell carcinoma of the cervix: a Gynecologic Oncology Group Study. *Int J Gynecol Cancer.* 2009;19(5):929–933.

105. Santin AD, Sill MW, McMeekin DS, et al. Phase II trial of cetuximab in the treatment of persistent or recurrent squamous or nonsquamous cell carcinoma of the cervix: a Gynecologic Oncology Group study. *Gynecol Oncol.* 2011;122(3):495–500.

106. Monk BJ, Mas Lopez L, Zarba JJ, et al. Phase II, open-label study of pazopanib or lapatinib monotherapy compared with pazopanib plus lapatinib combination therapy in patients with advanced and recurrent cervical cancer. *J Clin Oncol.* 2010;28(22):3562–3569.

107. Maciag PC, Radulovic S, Rothman J. The first clinical use of a live-attenuated Listeria monocytogenes vaccine: a Phase I safety study of Lm-LLO-E7 in patients with advanced carcinoma of the cervix. *Vaccine.* 2009;27(30):3975–3983.

108. Shanker M, Jin J, Branch CD, et al. Tumor suppressor gene-based nanotherapy: from test tube to the clinic. *J Drug Deliv.* 2011;2011:465845.

109. Liu L, Ni F, Zhang J, et al. Silver nanocrystals sensitize magnetic-nanoparticle-mediated thermo-induced killing of cancer cells. *Acta Biochim Biophys Sin (Shanghai).* 2011;43(4):316–323.

6 Multimodality Treatment of Rare Cervical Cancer

MOLLY A. BREWER

The most common malignancies of the uterine cervix are squamous cell carcinoma (SCC) and adenocarcinoma (AC) which comprise about 90% of all cervical carcinomas. Rarer cervical cancers include neuroendocrine cancer (2%), glassy cell carcinoma (GCC) (1%–5%), adenoma malignum (1%–3%), sarcomas (including rhabdomyosarcoma, alveolar soft part sarcoma (ASPS) [very rare], and embryonal rhabdomyosarcoma), primitive neuroectodermal tumor (PNET) (very rare), and lymphoma (extremely rare). Due to the rarity of these tumors, they are typically treated with multimodality treatment including neoadjuvant chemotherapy (NACT), +/– surgery and +/– radiation. The majority of these rare cervical cancers are reported in case reports or small case series with heterogeneous treatments, which limits data available on the most efficacious treatments with even large cancer centers having limited experience.

■ RARE AC

Clear cell AC of the cervix (CCAC) accounts for 4%–9% of all cervical ACs. There is a bimodal age distribution with two distinct peaks: one at a mean age of 26 years and a later peak at a mean age of 71 years. Prognosis for patients with early-stage CCAC is similar to patients with early-stage SCC and non-CCAC. However, the standard treatment results in infertility, a concern for the younger age group. Development of fertility-conserving alternatives such as radical trachelectomy can be performed by either a vaginal or abdominal route and can preserve fertility (1). This case report described a patient who received NACT with Taxol Carboplatin (TC), followed by radical trachelectomy and nodal dissection with residual disease in the cervix. To preserve fertility, she received three additional cycles of TC and remains free of disease. Clear cell carcinoma of the cervix is an even more rare disease in the pediatric population, with less than 50 patients reported (2). In this case report, a 14-year-old was treated with ovarian transposition and pelvic and brachy chemoradiation and remains free of disease. Although the literature consists of case reports, this appears to be amenable to conservative multimodal treatment with preservation of fertility.

Papillary-serous AC (PSCC) is one of the rarest subtypes of cervical cancer. It is of Mullerian origin, similar to the other gynecologic papillary serous cancers. Based on a small case series of reported cases, the prognosis for early-stage PSCC is probably similar to that for other cervical ACs. The literature consists of several case reports (3) and one case series of 17 patients (4). Multimodality treatment with surgery followed by radiotherapy (RT) or chemotherapy showed poor survival in the case series with 9/17 dead of disease at 5 years. However, this publication was in 1998 before there had been the transition from RT as the main adjuvant treatment for uterine papillary serous carcinoma (UPSC) which has now changed to chemotherapy as adjuvant treatment with improved survival and this is often extrapolated to PSCC. Thus, these data may not be relevant to the current standard of care with surgery and adjuvant chemotherapy.

Signet-ring cell carcinoma presenting in the uterine cervix is usually a metastasis from a primary gastric tumor; only rarely, cervical involvement is the first manifestation of the disease (5). Primary signet-ring carcinoma of the cervix is extremely unusual, and it is always necessary to rule out a metastatic neoplasm. There are only a few case reports and case series in the literature and these have been typically treated with surgery alone (5–7) with surprisingly good results, probably attributable to the early stage in most of these cancers.

Mesonephric ACs are rare neoplasms that most commonly arise in the uterine cervix and rarely in the uterine corpus. They are assumed to arise from benign mesonephric remnants located in the lateral walls of the cervix (8). There are limited case reports and case series, and patients have been treated with surgery followed by radiation in a few cases with few recurrences. The majority of patients (4/7) were alive following treatment. Two patients received postoperative pelvic RT and one patient received postoperative chemotherapy. The majority of these patients had Stage I disease (9).

Adenoma Malignum (AM)

AM is a rare variant of AC of the uterine cervix and has been associated with Peutz-Jeghers syndrome (10). AM comprises 1%–3% of all cervical ACs (11). In a case series of 18 patients, there was a better survival than with AC, suggesting this is a less aggressive variant. All patients had radical surgery and eight patients underwent adjuvant treatment with chemotherapy, radiation, or chemoradiation. All patients with local disease survived and the two with metastatic disease died. In a smaller series in which all patients received adjuvant treatment after surgery (chemotherapy, radiation, or both), 3/4 patients died of disease (12), which was contradictory to the prior report.

■ GCC

GCC of the uterine cervix is a rare form of cervical cancer, accounting for only 1%–5% of all cervical cancer cases. It has traditionally been classified as the most poorly differentiated form of adenosquamous carcinoma of the uterine cervix. The clinical behavior is characterized by a poor prognosis due to its rapid growth, its frequent distant metastases, and its relative resistance to conventional treatment modalities including surgery, RT, and chemotherapy, in the majority of cases. Radical surgery for GCC followed by aggressive chemoradiation has been proposed in an attempt to improve patient survival (13). A recent case report described a young woman with Stage IIB disease who was treated with radical surgery, followed by whole pelvic radiation therapy (XRT) and concurrent every 3-week TC with an excellent response. A second case report described a patient diagnosed during pregnancy who was successfully treated with NACT carboplatin, etoposide, and epirubicin followed by delivery and radical surgery (14), with an excellent response and who delivered a viable infant. Although the role of NACT has not been studied extensively, Mikami et al (15) reported that NACT with cisplatin, etoposide, and mitomycin-C (PEM) regimen was effective for the treatment of Stage IIIb GCC of the uterine cervix.

Lymphoma

Approximately one-fourth of the malignant lymphomas arise in extranodal organs. The most common locations are gastrointestinal tract and skin, and primary non-Hodgkin's lymphoma (NHL) of the female genital tract is extremely rare. Treatment for gynecologic lymphoma has not been standardized (16–18). In a review of 74 cases, which included 43 patients with primary cervical lymphoma, different modalities of treatment were used: surgery only (25%); surgery and chemotherapy (25%); chemotherapy and RT (19%); chemotherapy only (19%); chemotherapy, RT, and surgery (8%); surgery with RT (3%). CHOP is the most preferred chemotherapy regimen and is considered the current standard of care for intermediate grade lymphomas. Rituximab, the first anti-CD20 antibody registered for B-cell lymphoma, is now an accepted part of this regimen. Lymphoma of the cervix has been treated with surgery, chemotherapy, and/or radiation, and there is no consensus of the optimal treatment. Two patients with B-cell lymphoma were treated with rituximab-CHOP and showed excellent responses with no evidence of disease at 20 and 19 months posttreatment, suggesting this may be a reasonable approach (16). Another case report described a young woman with diffuse B-cell lymphoma who was treated with CHOP and pelvic RT with an excellent response (17).

Melanoma

There is no standard treatment for melanoma of the cervix, and although the majority of case reports describe radical hysterectomy as the mainstay of treatment, survival is poor (18–22). The 5-year survival after radical hysterectomy is less than 40% in Stage I and only 14% in Stage II. One case report suggests that pelvic exenteration is the optimal surgery (19–26). The majority of patients have Stage I or II disease at diagnosis, suggesting that surgery may be appropriate in this population (20).

RT may reduce tumor size (18–20) or treat inadequate margins despite the low level of radiosensitivity typically exhibited by melanoma. RT has not yet been evaluated in the palliative setting for cervical melanoma. While it does not eradicate the melanoma, it often causes tumor shrinkage and symptomatic relief and may therefore be useful for palliation.

No chemotherapy regimens have been reported that substantially reduce the possibility of recurrence. Dacarbazine has been used in advanced disease and up to 20% of patients may have a response. Cisplatin, bleomycin, and vinblastine may have a better response than the use of dacarbazine, while in other cases, combining dacarbazine with vincristine and carmustine has been reported as well as immunotherapy utilizing local Bacillus Calmette Guérin (BCG) or the transfusion of activated lymphocytes. Patients who received chemotherapy or immunotherapy did not have a significantly different survival compared with those who did not receive treatment (26). With the data emerging on the use of *BRAF* inhibitors in the treatment of melanoma, there may be treatment options in the future for treatment of these rare cancers arising in the cervix.

Neuroendocrine Tumors

Neuroendocrine cervical carcinomas are a rare subtype of cervical carcinomas first recognized in 1972. The College of American Pathologists and the National Cancer Institute have described four types of cervical neuroendocrine tumors: classical carcinoid, atypical carcinoid, large-cell and small-cell neuroendocrine carcinomas (NECs). These are typically aggressive tumors treated with chemotherapy and radiation.

Small-cell carcinoma is the most common of the neuroendocrine tumors but are still quite rare. Primary small-cell cervical cancers are the most common gynecologic small-cell carcinomas and, as in other cervical cancers, are associated with HPV, primarily HPV18 infections. They are more likely to be diagnosed at advanced stages and have a poorer prognosis, with a higher risk of lymph node involvement and distant metastases, often to the liver, lung, brain, bone, and bone marrow. For all stages, combined 5-year survival rates ranging from 11% to 54% have been reported (27–30). Most of the current therapeutic regimens for small-cell cervical carcinoma have been derived from larger trials in the treatment of small-cell lung cancer. The treatment of early-stage cervical cancers has historically involved surgery; however, a multimodality approach is needed even in early-stage cervical small-cell carcinoma because of the risk of recurrence and distant metastasis. If surgery is performed in early stage of the disease, a multimodality approach including adjuvant chemotherapy with cisplatin and etoposide with or without local-regional radiation is recommended. Another case series included surgical resection (radical hysterectomy), chemotherapy, RT, and combinations of these treatments. If the tumor was Stage Ib1 or IIa and smaller than 4 cm, a radical hysterectomy was the first choice. If not, patients received NACT using VP-16, bleomycin, and cisplatin as the first-line followed by surgery (28). The mean survival time of the six patients who underwent multimodality treatment of surgery, chemotherapy, and RT was 23.7 months, the longest of any other series, suggesting that multimodality treatment is optimal in this type of cancer. A third series from Memorial Sloan-Kettering Cancer Center (MSKCC) (29) evaluated 17 patients whose treatment consisted of primary surgery with or without individualized adjuvant treatment, definitive RT, chemoradiation with cisplatin/etoposide, or chemotherapy with carboplatin/etoposide alone. Distant recurrence was significantly reduced in patients receiving chemotherapy, and 100% of the patients with early disease who did not receive chemotherapy as part of their initial treatment plan developed recurrent disease. In a fourth case series, the 3-year survival for early-stage patients who received postoperative adjuvant chemotherapy was 57.1% compared with 56.4% for those who underwent adjuvant chemoradiotherapy, and their median survival periods were 84.7 and 89.1 months, respectively (30). Most studies report long-term survival only for those patients that have undergone surgical resection when performed in the context of a multimodality treatment approach with adjuvant chemotherapy (31). There are no prospective data to compare

surgery with primary chemoradiation for small resectable cervical NECs. For advanced disease or nonsurgical candidates, chemoradiation is a reasonable option. Patients with evidence of lymphadenopathy or fluorodeoxyglucose (FDG)-avid nodal basins may also be candidates for primary chemoradiation. To extrapolate from lung cancer regimens, chemoradiation with etoposide/cisplatin (EP) concurrent with pelvic radiation may be appropriate (31).

Large-cell NEC (LCNEC) of the uterine cervix is a very rare malignancy that is highly aggressive and usually results in unfavorable outcomes. It is considerably less common than the well-recognized small-cell NEC of the cervix. The treatment of LCNEC of the cervix remains controversial due to the rarity of the disease. In one case series, three cycles of adjuvant chemotherapy and concurrent radiation was offered to patients with positive para-aortic lymph nodes. However, there is no solid evidence to support or oppose this treatment regimen. Aggressive initial multimodality treatment with radical hysterectomy and adjuvant chemoradiation is recommended (31–33).

Although atypical carcinoid tumors are exceedingly rare, with about 14 reported cases in the literature, their recognition is important because they are regarded as highly aggressive tumors that frequently show subclinical hematogenous and lymphatic metastases, even in early disease. There is only one case report of successful treatment in a patient for whom the tumor recurred in the liver after radical surgery and was treated with hepatic arterial chemoembolization with streptozotocin (STZ) and 5-fluorouracil (5-FU; 34).

There are limited publications about cervical carcinoid (35). One case report concluded that even in patients with early-stage (FIGO I or II) carcinoid of the cervix, systemic metastases are common, and a cause of death. Despite the moderate response rate, adjuvant chemotherapy should be considered (34).

In a large series of 26 patients with neuroendocrine cervical neoplasms, multimodality treatment was evaluated (35). Eleven patients in total (42%) and 9/11 patients (82%) with Stage I disease were no evidence of disease (NED) at the last reported follow-up. The two patients with Stage I who died of disease either declined adjuvant therapy or had peritoneal metastasis at the time of surgery (36). Thus, there is reasonable consensus that neuroendocrine tumors of the cervix are best treated with multimodality treatment to include systemic chemotherapy.

Sarcoma

There are multiple subgroups within sarcoma, the most common is rhabdomyosarcoma, which is divided into three subgroups: embryonal, alveolar, and undifferentiated. Although approximately 20% of rhabdomyosarcomas in children arise in the genitourinary tract, only 0.5% of primary rhabdomyosarcomas in girls are found on the cervix. Primary cervical rhabdomyosarcoma in adults is even rarer (37). Ferguson et al (38) found only eight cases of adult cervical rhabdomyosarcoma diagnosed over 40 years at MSKCC. Kriseman et al (37) found that at the end of primary surgical therapy, all 11 patients were free of disease but 3 patients (27%) had local recurrence. Some groups recommend chemotherapy with vincristine, dactinomycin, and cyclophosphamide (39) and others recommend conservative surgery (40). Case reports of four patients with embyronal rhabdomyosarcoma reported that two had surgical treatment only and died of their disease, with one having recurrence at 4 months, and the other having three recurrences and surgical excisions during a period of 6 years. Of the two surviving patients, one was treated with surgical excision followed by chemotherapy alone, and is disease-free and the other underwent complete surgical excision and chemotherapy, recurred 2 months after completion of chemotherapy, received radiation, and has been disease-free for 22 years (41). ASPS is an exceedingly rare mesenchymal cancer that typically presents as a painless mass in the buttocks or thighs of young adults. ASPS also occurs in the female reproductive tract, where less than 1% of all cervical sarcomas can be classified as ASPSs. Given that so few cases have been described, optimal clinical management of ASPS arising in the female reproductive tract remains uncertain (42). Carcinosarcomas most commonly occur in the uterus and rarely occur in the uterine cervix, with only 40 cases documented in the literature and no consensus on treatment (43).

Peripheral PNET of the cervix is extremely rare. A recent case report reviewed the available literature and developed a multimodal approach based on the literature in Ewing's sarcoma (44). PNETs belong to the family of Ewing's sarcoma, which are tumors with a 90% mortality without systemic treatment from secondary hematogeneous metastases, occurring mainly in the lungs. Based on these data, they treated with NACT with doxorubicin, ifosfamide, mesna, and etoposide, followed by hysterectomy and RT. This was then followed with consolidation chemotherapy by means of 6 to 8 courses of vincristine, ifosfamide, and dactinoycin with a complete response.

CONCLUSION

Rare cervical cancers encompass many different cell types and are not only a challenge to accurately diagnose but also a challenge to determine the best treatment. The data in the literature are in the form of case reports and case series, and treatments in the larger case series are heterogeneous, making it difficult to determine the most effective treatment. The majority of patients diagnosed with these rare cancers appear to be best treated with a multidisciplinary approach using multimodality treatment regimens.

■ REFERENCES

1. Singh P, Nicklin J, Hassall T. Neoadjuvant chemotherapy followed by radical vaginal trachelectomy and adjuvant chemotherapy for clear cell cancer of the cervix: a feasible approach and review. *Int J Gynecol Cancer*. 2011;21(1):137–140.

2. Ansari DO, Horowitz IR, Katzenstein HM, Durham MM, Esiashvili N. Successful treatment of an adolescent with locally advanced cervicovaginal clear cell adenocarcinoma using definitive chemotherapy and radiotherapy. *J Pediatr Hematol Oncol*. 2012;34(5):e174–e176.

3. Watrowski R, Striepecke E, Jäger C, Bauknecht T, Horst C. Papillary-serous adenocarcinoma of the uterine cervix during tamoxifen therapy after bilateral breast cancer. *Anticancer Res*. 2012;32(11):5075–5078.

4. Zhou C, Gilks CB, Hayes M, Clement PB. Papillary serous carcinoma of the uterine cervix: a clinicopathologic study of 17 cases. *Am J Surg Pathol*. 1998;22(1):113–120.

5. Balcı S, Saglam A, Usubutun A. Primary signet-ring cell carcinoma of the cervix: Case report and review of the literature. *Am J Surg Pathol*. 1998;29:181–184.

6. Suárez-Peñaranda JM, Abdulkader I, Barón-Duarte FJ, González Patiño E, Novo-Domínguez A, Varela-Durán J. Signet-ring cell carcinoma presenting in the uterine cervix: report of a primary and 2 metastatic cases. *Int J Gynecol Pathol*. 2007;26(3):254–258.

7. Insabato L, Simonetti S, De Cecio R, Di Tuoro S, Bifulco G, Di Spiezio Sardo A. Primary signet-ring cell carcinoma of the uterine cervix with long term follow-up: case report. *Eur J Gynaecol Oncol*. 2007;28(5):411–414.

8. Kenny SL, McBride HA, Jamison J, McCluggage WG. Mesonephric adenocarcinomas of the uterine cervix and corpus: HPV-negative neoplasms that are commonly PAX8, CA125, and HMGA2 positive and that may be immunoreactive with TTF1 and hepatocyte nuclear factor 1-ß. *Am J Surg Pathol*. 2012;36(6):799–807.

9. Bagué S, Rodríguez IM, Prat J. Malignant mesonephric tumors of the female genital tract: a clinicopathologic study of 9 cases. *Am J Surg Pathol*. 2004;28(5):601–607.

10. Lim KT, Lee IH, Kim TJ, Kwon YS, Jeong JG, Shin SJ. Adenoma malignum of the uterine cervix: Clinicopathologic analysis of 18 cases. *Kaohsiung J Med Sci*. 2012;28(3):161–164.

11. Fujiwaki R, Takahashi K, Kitao M. Adenoma malignum of the uterine cervix associated with Peutz-Jeghers syndrome. *Int J Gynaecol Obstet*. 1996;53(2):171–172.

12. Kudo R, Sagae S, Kusanagi T, Mizuuchi H, Hayakawa O, Hashimoto M. Minimal-deviation adenocarcinoma (adenoma malignum) of the uterine cervix; four case reports. *Eur J Obstet Gynecol Reprod Biol*. 1990;34(1–2):179–188.

13. Hirai Y, Takeshima N, Haga A, Arai Y, Akiyama F, Hasumi K. A clinicocytopathologic study of adenoma malignum of the uterine cervix. *Gynecol Oncol*. 1998;70(2):219–223.

14. Hirai Y, Takeshima N, Haga A, Arai Y, Akiyama F, Hasumi K. Multimodal treatment for glassy cell carcinoma of the uterine cervix. *J Obstet Gynaecol Res*. 2009;35(3):584–587.

15. Mikami M, Ezawa S, Sakaiya N, et al. Response of glassy-cell carcinoma of the cervix to cisplatin, epirubicin, and mitomycin C. *Lancet*. 2000;355(9210):1159–1160.

16. Upanal N, Enjeti A. Primary lymphoma of the uterus and cervix: two case reports and review of the literature. *Aust N Z J Obstet Gynaecol*. 2011;51(6):559–562.

17. Baijal G, Vadiraja BM, Fernandes DJ, Vidyasagar MS. Diffuse large B-cell lymphoma of the uterine cervix: a rare case managed novelly. *J Cancer Res Ther*. 2009;5(2):140–142.

18. Novotny S, Ellis T, Stephens J. Cervical lymphoma with hydronephrosis. *Obstet Gynecol.* 2011;117(2):444–446.

19. Calderón-Salazar L, Cantú de Leon D, Perez Montiel D, Almogabar-Villagrán E, Villavicencio V, Cetina L. Primary malignant melanoma of the uterine cervix treated with ultraradical surgery: a case report. *ISRN Obstet Gynecol.* 2011;2011:683020.

20. Zhang J, Cao Y, Xiao L, Tang J, Tang L. A peculiar site: melanoma of the cervix. *Am J Obstet Gynecol.* 2011;205(5):508.e1–508.e3.

21. Mousavi AS, Fakor F, Nazari Z, Ghaemmaghami F, Hashemi FA, Jamali M. Primary malignant melanoma of the uterine cervix: case report and review of the literature. *J Low Genit Tract Dis.* 2006;10(4):258–263.

22. Baruah J, Roy KK, Kumar S, Kumar L. A rare case of primary malignant melanoma of cervix. *Arch Gynecol Obstet.* 2009;280(3):453–456.

23. Yücesoy G, Kus E, Cakiroglu Y, Muezzinoglu B, Yildiz K, Yucesoy I. Primary malignant melanoma of the cervix: report of a case. *Arch Gynecol Obstet.* 2009;279(4):573–575.

24. Sonja BK, Ralph A, Donald MC. Primary malignant melanoma of the cervix and review of literature (a case report). *Gynecol Oncol.* 1992;47:398–403.

25. Ma SQ, Bai CM, Zhong S, Yu XH, Lang JH. Clinical analysis of primary malignant melanoma of the cervix. *Chin Med Sci J.* 2005;20(4):257–260.

26. Tcheung WJ, Selim MA, Herndon JE 2nd, Abernethy AP, Nelson KC. Clinicopathologic study of 85 cases of melanoma of the female genitalia. *J Am Acad Dermatol.* 2012;67(4):598–605.

27. Cohen JG, Chan JK, Kapp DS. The management of small-cell carcinomas of the gynecologic tract. *Curr Opin Oncol.* 2012;24(5):572–579.

28. Li JD, Zhuang Y, Li YF, et al. A clinicopathological aspect of primary small-cell carcinoma of the uterine cervix: a single-centre study of 25 cases. *J Clin Pathol.* 2011;64(12):1102–1107.

29. Zivanovic O, Leitao MM Jr, Park KJ, et al. Small cell neuroendocrine carcinoma of the cervix: Analysis of outcome, recurrence pattern and the impact of platinum-based combination chemotherapy. *Gynecol Oncol.* 2009;112(3):590–593.

30. Lan-Fang L, Hai-Yan S, Zuo-Ming Y, Jian-Qing Z, Ya-Qing C. Small cell neuroendocrine carcinoma of the cervix: analysis of the prognosis and role of radiation therapy for 43 cases. *Eur J Gynaecol Oncol.* 2012;33(1):68–73.

31. Gardner GJ, Reidy-Lagunes D, Gehrig PA. Neuroendocrine tumors of the gynecologic tract: A Society of Gynecologic Oncology (SGO) clinical document. *Gynecol Oncol.* 2011;122(1):190–198.

32. Embry JR, Kelly MG, Post MD, Spillman MA. Large cell neuroendocrine carcinoma of the cervix: prognostic factors and survival advantage with platinum chemotherapy. *Gynecol Oncol.* 2011;120(3):444–448.

33. Ko ML, Jeng CJ, Huang SH, Shen J, Chen SC, Tzeng CR. Large cell neuroendocrine carcinoma of the uterine cervix associated with adenocarcinoma. *Taiwan J Obstet Gynecol.* 2007;46(1):68–70.

34. Yoshida Y, Sato K, Katayama K, Yamaguchi A, Imamura Y, Kotsuji F. Atypical metastatic carcinoid of the uterine cervix and review of the literature. *J Obstet Gynaecol Res.* 2011;37(6):636–640.

35. Seidel R Jr, Steinfeld A. Carcinoid of the cervix: natural history and implications for therapy. *Gynecol Oncol.* 1988;30(1):114–119.

36. McCann GA, Boutsicaris CE, Preston MM, et al. Neuroendocrine carcinoma of the uterine cervix: the role of multimodality therapy in early-stage disease. *Gynecol Oncol.* 2013;129(1):135–139.

37. Kriseman ML, Wang WL, Sullinger J, et al. Rhabdomyosarcoma of the cervix in adult women and younger patients. *Gynecol Oncol.* 2012;126(3):351–356.

38. Ferguson SE, Gerald W, Barakat RR, Chi DS, Soslow RA. Clinicopathologic features of rhabdomyosarcoma of gynecologic origin in adults. *Am J Surg Pathol.* 2007;31(3):382–389.

39. Adams BN, Brandt JS, Loukeris K, Holcomb K. Embryonal rhabdomyosarcoma of the cervix and appendiceal carcinoid tumor. *Obstet Gynecol.* 2011;117(2 Pt 2):482–484.

40. Karaman E, Akbayir O, Kocatürk Y, Cekic S, Filiz FB, Gulkilik A. Successful treatment of a very rare case: locally treated cervical rhabdomyosarcoma. *Arch Gynecol Obstet.* 2011;284:1019–1022.

41. Sanders MA, Gordinier M, Talwalkar SS, Moore GD. Embryonal rhabdomyosarcoma of the uterine cervix in a 41-year-old woman treated with radical hysterectomy and adjuvant chemotherapy. *Gynecol Oncol.* 2008;111(3):561–563.

42. Guntupalli S, Anderson ML, Bodurka DC. Alveolar soft part sarcoma of the cervix: case report and literature review. *Arch Gynecol Obstet.* 2009;279(2):263–265.

43. Kadota K, Haba R, Ishikawa M, et al. Uterine cervical carcinosarcoma with heterologous mesenchymal component: a case report and review of the literature. *Arch Gynecol Obstet.* 2009;280:839–843.

44. Snijders-Keilholz A, Ewing P, Seynaeve C, Burger CW. Primitive neuroectodermal tumor of the cervix uteri: a case report – changing concepts in therapy. *Gynecol Oncol.* 2005;98(3):516–519.

7 Principles of Radiation Therapy for Cervical Cancer

DANIEL R. SIMPSON

CATHERYN M. YASHAR

LOREN K. MELL

ARNO J. MUNDT

■ INTRODUCTION

Radiation therapy (RT) has long occupied an important role in the treatment of cervical cancer, dating back over 100 years to its first reported use in 1902 (1). Over the years, RT techniques have advanced considerably, not only in terms of the equipment used but also in terms of how radiation is planned and delivered. Today, RT is commonly used in the treatment of patients with nearly all stages of cervical cancer, either as definitive or adjuvant therapy. RT also plays an important role in the palliation of patients when cure is no longer possible.

This chapter focuses on the principles of conventional RT in cervical cancer and provides an overview of both external beam RT (EBRT) and brachytherapy approaches. The application of newer, more novel RT approaches, including intensity-modulated RT (IMRT), image-guided RT (IGRT), and stereotactic body RT (SBRT), is presented in Chapter 27.

■ EBRT

EBRT (also known as teletherapy) is at the heart of the radiotherapeutic treatment of patients with cervical cancer and is delivered using a linear accelerator (linac) capable of producing high-energy X-ray (photon) beams, with energies ranging from 4 to 24 megavolts (MV) (Figure 7.1). Previously, EBRT was delivered with Cobalt-60 machines using low-energy beams, a practice that remains commonplace throughout the developing world. Low-energy beams are not desirable since they are less penetrating and deposit considerable dose in superficial tissues resulting in increased risk of side effects.

EBRT fields are designed to treat the primary tumor and surrounding involved tissues as well as potential disease spread to the regional lymph nodes. Fields used in an individual patient depend on multiple factors, including disease extent and stage. Most cervical cancer patients are treated using whole pelvic RT (WPRT) fields, which encompass the cervix, uterus, parametria, and proximal vagina, as well as the pelvic lymph nodes (internal, external, and common iliac and presacral lymph nodes). Patients with para-aortic lymph node involvement undergo extended-field RT (EFRT) treating both the pelvis and para-aortic regions. In women with disease extension to the lower vagina and those with inguinal node involvement, pelvic-inguinal fields are used to treat the pelvis and inguinal regions.

EBRT in cervical cancer patients has traditionally been delivered using either two (opposed anterior–posterior) or four (opposed anterior–posterior and opposed lateral) fields. In patients receiving WPRT, four field techniques are currently favored since this approach allows considerably more normal tissue sparing, including the anterior small bowel and posterior rectum (2). EFRT and pelvic-inguinal RT are typically delivered using opposed anterior–posterior beams although more sophisticated approaches may be used (3).

Treatment planning for EBRT begins with a "simulation" at which patients are positioned in the treatment position and a customized immobilization device is fabricated to reproduce daily setup and minimize their movement during treatment. Patients are typically immobilized in the supine position; however, at select centers, prone positioning with a "belly board" is favored, particularly in women undergoing WPRT, to reduce the volume of small bowel irradiated. Field borders have been traditionally selected based on bony landmarks. In women undergoing WPRT, the superior and inferior borders are typically placed at the L4–5 interspace and the inferior obturator foramen, respectively. The lateral borders of the anterior–posterior fields are set 1 to 1.5 cm beyond the pelvic brim. The anterior border of the lateral fields is at (or 1 cm anterior) to the pubic symphysis to ensure coverage of the external iliac lymph nodes; the posterior border

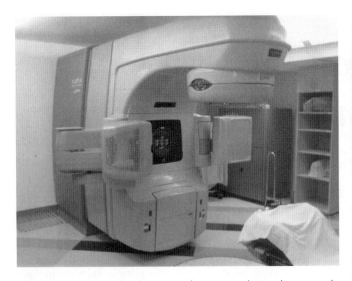

FIGURE 7.1 A modern linear accelerator in radiation therapy vault.

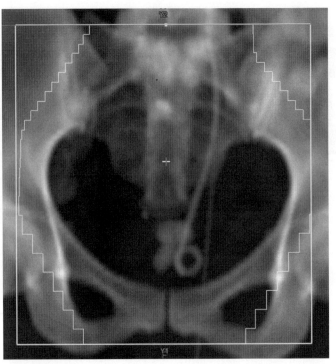

is at the S2–3 interspace. In patients undergoing EFRT, the superior field extent is typically placed at the T12–L1 interspace; in those treated with pelvic-inguinal RT, the inferior border is placed 5 cm inferior to the perineum to ensure coverage of the inguinal nodes. However, these standard field borders are often modified. For example, the upper and lower borders may be extended in patients with involved common iliac nodes and significant vaginal involvement, respectively. In women with bulky primary tumors, the posterior border may be moved posteriorly to include the entire sacrum.

Customized blocking is added to the various treatment fields to help shield surrounding normal tissues. An example of the fields and blocking used in a patient undergoing WPRT is shown in Figure 7.2. Oral and rectal contrast may be used at simulation in the design of these blocks. At many centers today, computed tomography (CT) simulators have replaced conventional fluoroscopic simulators allowing the field design to be based on patient anatomy instead of bony landmarks. Multiple investigators have shown that reliance on bony landmarks may inadvertently underdose target tissues and/or inadequately shield normal tissues (4,5).

EBRT is delivered at most centers using conventional daily fraction sizes (1.8–2 Gy) to total doses ranging from 39.4 to 50.4 Gy. In select high-risk women, that is, patients with documented involved lymph nodes and/or gross residual disease following surgery, higher doses (greater than or equal to 60 Gy) may be delivered using reduced fields; however, careful attention is needed to minimize the dose to normal tissues, particularly the small bowel. In the past, considerable interest focused on altered fractionation schedules in an attempt to deliver higher than conventional EBRT doses. However, several studies (6,7), including a prospective Radiation Therapy Oncology Group (RTOG) trial (8), have failed to show a benefit to this approach.

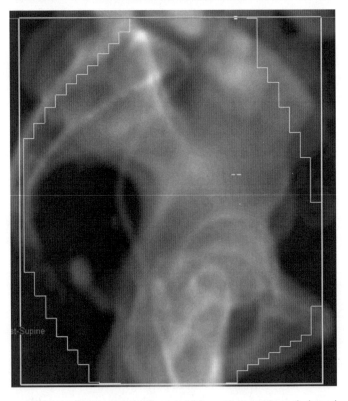

FIGURE 7.2 Conventional anterior/posterior (top) and lateral (bottom) pelvic radiation therapy fields.

In addition to blocks used to shape the EBRT treatment fields, some investigators recommend the placement of a midline block (typically after 20 Gy) in cervical cancer patients undergoing both EBRT and brachytherapy, allowing a higher proportion of dose to be delivered via brachytherapy (9). A midline block may also be placed *following* brachytherapy with parametrial and/or lymph node involvement, allowing the delivery of an additional EBRT boost, typically 10 to 12 Gy in 5 to 6 fractions. Such blocks are not standardized; however, at some centers they are customized based on the brachytherapy isodose distributions (10).

Considerable interest is currently focused on IMRT planning and delivery in cervical cancer patients. Interested readers are referred to Chapter 27 for a review of IMRT as well as for a discussion of other novel techniques including IGRT and SBRT.

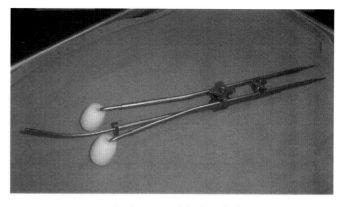

FIGURE 7.3 A Fletcher-Suit-Delclos brachytherapy applicator.

■ BRACHYTHERAPY

Brachytherapy (also known as internal RT) involves the delivery of radiation using radioactive sources (Cesium-137, Iridium-192) placed in close proximity to (intracavitary) or within (interstitial) the tumor. Brachytherapy takes advantage of the rapid dose fall-off from a radioactive source and allows for delivery of high doses to tumor while sparing nearby critical structures. It is typically given in conjunction with EBRT, but may be delivered as the sole treatment or as a boost following EBRT in patients treated adjuvantly.

Traditionally, brachytherapy was performed by placing radioactive sources directly within the vagina and/or uterus. By the 1960s, after-loading approaches were introduced whereby an applicator was first positioned with the sources placed at a later time, typically after the patient had been transferred to a shielded hospital room. Using this approach, radioactive sources were initially inserted manually but, more recently, remote after-loading techniques have been developed, reducing the exposure of the radiation and nursing staff.

There are currently a wide range of commercial intracavitary, interstitial, and combined applicators available. In intact cervical cancer patients treated with intracavitary brachytherapy (ICB), applicators typically include a central strut or tandem, which is inserted into the uterine cavity in combination with some form of a vaginal source holder. The most widely utilized ICB device is the Fletcher-Suit-Delclos applicator comprised of ovoids (colpostats) and a tandem (Figure 7.3). Other applicators include the Henschke applicator, the modified Stockholm tandem and ring, and the Vienna combined intracavitary and interstitial devices (11). Applicators used for interstitial brachytherapy include the Syed–Neblett template and the Martinez universal perineal interstitial template (MUPIT) (12), comprised of templates with an array of equally spaced holes through which hollow needles are inserted. Postoperative cervical cancer patients undergoing ICB are treated using either colpostats or a vaginal cylinder.

Whether a patient undergoes ICB or interstitial brachytherapy depends on several factors including disease extent and physician preference. While the majority of patients undergoing brachytherapy today are treated with ICB (13), interstitial brachytherapy is recommended in women in whom ICB would result in suboptimal dose distributions. Interstitial brachytherapy should also be considered in patients with extensive parametrial involvement, bulky primary tumors, narrow vagina cavities precluding optimal applicator placement, distal vaginal involvement, a posthysterectomy recurrence or a history of prior RT. Unlike intact cervical cancer patients who can be treated with either ICB or interstitial approaches, ICB is the sole approach utilized in the adjuvant setting.

Brachytherapy is delivered utilizing either low-dose-rate (LDR) or high-dose-rate (HDR) techniques. Historically, LDR techniques using initially Radium-226 and later Cesium-137 have been standard practice. In contrast, interstitial LDR brachytherapy has been delivered primarily using Iridium-192. Both ICB and interstitial LDR treatments are delivered over multiple hours to days. Today, HDR techniques (both ICB and interstitial) are commonly performed using high-activity Iridium-192, reducing treatment times to several minutes.

Controversy remains as to which brachytherapy method is best, with various proposed advantages and disadvantages of each technique. LDR has a long reported treatment history with high local control and low toxicity rates. However, due to the length of treatment, LDR brachytherapy requires inpatient administration and can be burdensome for both the patients and providers and is not ideal in the elderly, particularly those with multiple comorbidities. In contrast, HDR offers the advantage of comparatively fast treatment performed in an outpatient setting. Proponents of LDR brachytherapy argue that HDR has a higher potential for toxicity. However, a meta-analysis (14) and multiple prospective randomized trials (15,16) comparing LDR and HDR have demonstrated that the two techniques are similar in terms of both tumor control and toxicity. Moreover, national cooperative groups including the RTOG have deemed both LDR and HDR techniques as acceptable forms of therapy when done properly. An alternative technique, pulsed-dose-rate (PDR) brachytherapy has also been proposed. This strategy replicates the dose rate of LDR using an Iridium-192 source delivered at intervals with a stepping after-loader device in an attempt to lower normal tissue complications and improve target coverage (17). However, outcome data using this approach remain limited (18).

Various prescription points have been used for patients undergoing brachytherapy. In intact cervical cancer patients undergoing ICB, reference points are used based on the original Manchester formulation developed in the 1930s (19). This system specifies two prescription points, A and B. Point A is defined as 2 cm superior to the external cervical os and 2 cm lateral to the intrauterine canal, presumably at the medial edge of the broad ligament where the uterine artery crosses the ureter. Point B is defined as 3 cm lateral to Point A and is felt to represent the location of the obturator lymph nodes, although CT-based studies reveal that this is rarely the case (20). In patients undergoing adjuvant therapy, ICB is prescribed either to the vaginal surface or to 0.5 cm depth. Additional planning points include bladder and rectal reference points. In intact cervical cancer patients treated with intersitital brachytherapy, the treatment volume is typically defined by the peripheral needles with or without an additional 5 mm margin, with the dose prescribed to an isodose line (IDL) encompassing this volume.

The number of brachytherapy treatments depends on the technique used (intracavitary vs interstitial), the dose rate (HDR vs LDR), and the overall treatment approach (definitive or adjuvant). Cervical cancer patients undergoing definitive treatment with LDR ICB typically receive two separate treatments (also referred to as *insertions*), although comparable tumor control and complication rates have been reported with a single insertion, particularly in early-stage patients (21). Intact cervical cancer patients undergoing definitive treatment with HDR ICB typically receive 4 to 6 insertions. Since multiple investigators have demonstrated that treatment courses more than 8 weeks are associated with poorer outcomes (22), care needs to be taken to avoid unnecessary treatment protraction by performing the first insertion as soon as pelvic geometry allows. For postoperative patients, ICB is delivered with either 1 to 2 LDR or 3 to 5 HDR treatments. Most patients undergoing LDR interstitial brachytherapy are treated with a single treatment. Women undergoing HDR interstitial brachytherapy undergo 1 to 3 implants, often with multiple fractions delivered during each implant.

Brachytherapy treatment planning has traditionally been based on two-dimensional (2-D) radiographs. More recently, however, CT-based planning with computerized dosimetry has come into wider use. In intact cervical cancer patients undergoing LDR ICB, given the limited overall number of source activities and positions, planning is performed manually by varying the various source activities and positions focusing on the doses to Point A as well as normal tissues. The goal is to deliver a total Point A dose (including the EBRT dose) of 80 to 85 Gy for small tumors and 85 to 90 Gy for bulky disease, while limiting the rectal and bladder doses to less than 80% of the Point A dose. Different investigators recommend different maximum acceptable rectal and bladder doses, typically less than 75 to 80 Gy for the bladder and less than 70 to 75 Gy for the rectum. Patients treated postoperatively with LDR ICB receive surface dose rates of 80 to 100 cGy/hour or 50 to 80 cGy/hour to 0.5 cm. Given the increased number of potential dwell positions and times, HDR ICB optimization lends itself to more sophisticated optimization approaches. The American Brachytherapy Society (ABS) has provided detailed guidelines using multiple points along the tandem and vaginal surface (23). Consensus guidelines have also been published by the ABS on the optimal dose-fractionation regimens in patients undergoing HDR (23), LDR (24,25), and PDR (25) ICB.

Treatment planning in patients undergoing interstitial brachytherapy is more complex. Preplanning using CT and/ or MRI is typically used to help determine source number and placement, particularly in patients treated with LDR interstitial brachytherapy which required ordering of radioactive seeds and/or wires. Computerized dosimetry is important to ensure dose homogeneity. Maximum doses to adjacent normal tissues should be calculated and efforts made to spare the surrounding bladder and rectum. No consensus exists regarding maximum allowable doses to these organs in patients undergoing interstitial brachytherapy. Total rectal doses of more than 76 Gy were noted in one study to be highly correlated with the development of severe gastrointestinal (GI) toxicity (26). Unlike ICB, no consensus exists regarding the optimal schedule for cervical cancer patients receiving interstitial brachytherapy. The ABS has endorsed the dose-fractionation regimens employed at the California Endocurietherapy Center (CEC) (23).

In recent years, increasing attention has been focused on the use of volume-directed IGRT treatment planning in intact cervical cancer patients undergoing definitive treatment (27,28). This approach utilizes MRI- and CT-compatible applicators allowing imaging to be performed prior to each brachytherapy treatment allowing the dose prescribed to the tumor volume (instead of Point A). Promising results using this approach have been reported and are presented in Chapter 27.

■ INDICATIONS AND TREATMENT OUTCOMES

Early-Stage Disease

RT is commonly used in early-stage cervical cancer patients. The one exception is in women with very early (microscopic) Stage IA tumors, which are primarily treated with definitive surgery. However, RT consisting of ICB alone is associated with excellent outcomes (5-year disease-free survivals [DFS] greater than 95%) in these patients (29) and is thus an appealing approach in women unfit for surgery due to advanced age and/or multiple comorbidities. EBRT is not indicated given their low risk of pelvic lymph node involvement.

In early-stage patients with gross disease (Stages IB-IIA), RT is also commonly delivered, consisting of both EBRT and brachytherapy, with results comparable to radical surgery. In fact, in a large prospective randomized trial performed by Landoni et al comparing radical surgery with definitive RT in Stage IB-IIA disease, there were no differences between the two arms in terms of 5-year overall survival (OS) (83%) and DFS (74%) (30). However, the rate of severe treatment morbidity was considerably *higher* in the surgery arm (28% vs 12%, p = .004), possibly due to the need for adjuvant RT in 63% of the patients randomized to surgery.

The choice of surgery vs RT in early-stage patients depends on a number of factors, including patient age, comorbidities, and various tumor characteristics. Older women, particularly those with multiple comorbidities, are generally treated with RT, whereas younger women receive surgery. A common reason for favoring surgery in young women is the ability to preserve their ovarian function. However, it may be possible to preserve ovarian function in premenopausal patients by performing an ovarian transposition prior to RT (31). An oft-stated reason for favoring surgery in young women is the commonly held belief that sexual function would be less adversely affected. However, prospective quality-of-life analyses have found equivalent sexual function following surgery compared to RT (32). Moreover, new approaches have been developed to address sexual dysfunction in irradiated women (33).

When RT is delivered in Stage IB-IIA patients, it is commonly administered alone. The exception, however, is in women with bulky (greater than 4 cm) tumors who also receive chemotherapy. The Gynecologic Oncology Group (GOG) performed a randomized trial comparing RT vs chemoradiation in bulky Stage IB (greater than or equal to 4 cm) tumors (34). All patients underwent both EBRT and LDR ICB with a cumulative Point A dose of 75 Gy, followed by adjuvant hysterectomy. Chemotherapy consisted of cisplatin 40 mg/m²/week. Patients receiving both chemotherapy and RT had a superior 4-year DFS (p < .001) and OS (p = .008) than patients treated with RT alone. However, chemoradiation patients also had a higher rate of severe hematologic (21% vs 2%) and GI toxicities (14% vs 5%). Such patients today are typically treated with chemoradiation alone without adjuvant hysterectomy (35).

Locally Advanced Disease

In patients with locally advanced disease (Stage IIB-IVA), RT consisting of both EBRT and brachytherapy is the cornerstone of treatment. As in bulky early-stage patients, such women are treated with combined chemoradiation. Multiple randomized trials in the United States have demonstrated improvements in DFS and OS with the addition of concurrent platinum-based chemotherapy in these patients, with only one randomized trial showing no benefit (Table 7.1; 36–40).

Although platinum-based therapy is the standard of care, more recent studies have examined the role of multiagent chemotherapy. Dueñas-González et al conducted a multinational randomized Phase III study comparing standard concurrent cisplatin with concurrent and adjuvant gemcitabine and cisplatin in locally advanced patients (41). Patients receiving cisplatin–gemcitabine had a better 3-year DFS (p = .029) and OS (p = .0224) than those treated

			DFS (%)		OS (%)	
Study	Patients	Design	+ CDDP	–CDDP	+CDDP	–CDDP
RTOG 90–01 (36)	386 pts; Stage IIB-IVA, IB-IIA ≥ 5 cm, PLN+	EFRT + BT vs WPRT + BT + CDDP/5FU	61	46	67	41
GOG 120 (37)	526 pts; Stage IIB-IVA	WPRT + BT + CDDP vs CDDP/5FU/HU vs HU	43–46	26	53	34
GOG 85 (38)	368 pts; Stage IIB-IVA	WPRT + BT + CDDP/5FU vs HU	57	47	55	43
NCIC (39)	259 pts; Stage IB-IVA >5 cm or PLN+	WPRT + BT ± CDDP	NR	NR	62	58

■ **Table 7.1** Randomized trials of concurrent chemotherapy and radiation therapy in locally advanced cervical cancer

5FU, 5-fluorouracil; BT, brachytherapy; CDDP, cisplatin; DFS, disease-free survival; EFRT, extended-field radiotherapy; GOG, Gynecologic Oncology Group; HU, hydroxyurea; NCIC, National Cancer Institute of Canada; NR, not reported; OS, overall survival; RTOG, Radiation Therapy Oncology Group; WPRT, whole pelvic radiation therapy.

with cisplatin alone. However, the addition of gemcitabine resulted in higher severe hematologic and GI toxicities as well as two possible treatment-related deaths.

Following surgery, patients with high-risk features have been shown to benefit from adjuvant RT with or without chemotherapy. Delgado et al performed a prospective surgical-pathological study designed to identify the pathologic features of disease recurrence in women following radical hysterectomy and pelvic lymphadenectomy (42). They found that nodal involvement, tumor size, lymphovascular space invasion (LVI), and depth of invasion were all independent predictors of recurrence.

Sedlis et al performed a randomized trial of adjuvant RT in 277 women who had undergone radical hysterectomy, and while they were found to have no lymph node involvement, they had two or more high-risk features (lymphovascular invasion [LVI], deep stromal invasion, and/or tumor size greater than 4 cm) (43). Following surgery, patients were randomized to pelvic EBRT or no further therapy. At 10-year follow-up, adjuvant RT reduced the risk of recurrence by 46%, with reductions seen in both local and distant failures. A nonsignificant trend to a superior OS was also noted with the addition of RT (19.7% vs 28.6%, $p = .07$). A modest increase in the rate of severe treatment-related toxicity in the RT arm (6% vs 2.1%) was also noted. The ongoing GOG 263 is evaluating whether women with intermediate risk factors (LVI plus deep stromal invasion, middle-third invasion with tumors greater than or equal to 2 cm, superficial stromal invasion with tumors greater than or equal to 5 cm, or middle or deep third invasion with tumors greater than or equal to 4 cm and no LVI) benefit from chemotherapy in addition to RT.

Adjuvant chemoradiation is the standard of care in cervical cancer patients undergoing radical surgery and found to have positive pelvic nodes, positive surgical margins, and/or parametrial invasion. GOG 109 compared adjuvant pelvic EBRT with pelvic RT plus chemotherapy in these patients (44). Chemotherapy consisted of two cycles of 5-fluorouracil (5-FU) and cisplatin delivered concurrently, followed by two additional cycles after RT. The addition of chemotherapy improved both 4-year OS (71% vs 81%, $p = .007$) and DFS (63% vs 80%, $p = .003$) compared with RT alone. Not surprisingly, there were more serious toxicities reported in the chemotherapy arm (17% vs 4%), predominantly hematologic and GI toxicities.

While most cervical cancer patients undergoing RT (definitive or adjuvant) receive pelvic RT, considerable attention was previously focused on the use of EFRT, particularly in patients with bulky early or locally advanced disease (45,46). The European Organization for Research and Treatment of Cancer (EORTC) performed a trial of prophylactic EFRT in women with high-risk features including radiographic or pathologic evidence of pelvic nodal involvement, distal vaginal involvement, or Stage III disease but without demonstrable para-aortic involvement (47). Patients were randomized to pelvic vs EFRT irradiation. While there was a decrease in para-aortic nodal failure, no differences were seen in OS, local control, or distant metastases. EFRT was associated with a higher rate of small-bowel injury (2.3% vs 0.9%) and severe complications (9% vs 4.8%).

Although prophylactic EFRT is rarely performed today, EFRT is commonly used in patients with documented para-aortic lymph node involvement. Given their poor outcomes with EFRT alone (48), the GOG conducted a Phase II study to assess the feasibility and outcomes of EFRT plus concominant chemotherapy in these patients (49). Three-year OS and DFS rates were 39% and 34%, respectively. However, significant rates of severe GI (19%) and hematologic toxicity (15%) were noted. Grigsby et al evaluated combining concomitant cisplatin with EFRT in patients with involved para-aortic nodes by using a hyperfractionated approach (48 Gy delivered in fractions of 1.2 Gy given twice per day, followed by a boost of 54–60 Gy to involved nodes) (50). The results were disappointing with a 4-year OS rate of 29% and a 3-year locoregional failure rate of 50%. Acute Grade 3 (21%) and 4 (28%) sequelae were unacceptably high. It is hoped that newer approaches including IMRT will allow EFRT to be combined with chemotherapy with less toxicity (see Chapter 27).

Palliative Radiotherapy

RT can also serve as an effective palliative tool for women experiencing pain and bleeding from advanced cervical cancer. A variety of fractionation regimens ranging from a single fraction to twice-daily split-course treatment have been employed. Halle et al prospectively evaluated the efficacy and safety of a single fraction of 10 Gy to the pelvis in 42 patients with painful or bleeding cervical or endometrial tumors (51). Forty percent of women required retreatment either a second or even a third time for recurrent or persistent symptoms. Complete or partial pain relief was achieved in 44% of women, and complete or partial resolution of bleeding was observed in 90% of cases. Of note, five patients (12%) suffered serious treatment complications including fistula, small bowel obstruction, and skin ulceration.

Spanos and coworkers performed two prospective trials evaluating the use of different palliative regimens. RTOG 79–05 was a Phase I/II trial that included various pelvic malignancies (43% gynecologic) and treated to a total of 30 Gy delivered in three fractions with 4-week intervals (52). Overall, 44% of patients experienced either partial or complete palliation. However, there were unacceptably high rates of late severe (30%) GI toxicities. In RTOG 85–02, patients with pelvic tumors (40% gynecologic) were randomized to two regimens consisting of 12 twice-daily fractions of 3.7 Gy given over three courses spaced by either 2- or 4-week intervals (53,54). Forty-five percent of patients experienced either complete or partial palliation, with no differences in the proportion receiving either partial or complete response seen between the two arms. However, more patients in the 2-week rest arm completed treatment (72% vs 63%), and the rates of overall response rates were higher among patients who received all three arms (42% vs 5%). Of note, the rate of severe late toxicity was 6%, which was much lower than that observed in the previous RTOG trial (48).

■ REFERENCES

1. Cleaves M. Radium: with a preliminary note on radium rays in the treatment of cancer. *Med Rec.* 1903;64:1719–1723.
2. Eifel PJ, Moughan J, Erickson B, Iarocci T, Grant D, Owen J. Patterns of radiotherapy practice for patients with carcinoma of the uterine cervix: a patterns of care study. *Int J Radiat Oncol Biol Phys.* 2004;60(4):1144–1153.
3. Moran MS, Castrucci WA, Ahmad M, et al. Clinical utility of the modified segmental boost technique for treatment of the pelvis and inguinal nodes. *Int J Radiat Oncol Biol Phys.* 2010;76(4):1026–1036.
4. Finlay MH, Ackerman I, Tirona RG, Hamilton P, Barbera L, Thomas G. Use of CT simulation for treatment of cervical cancer to assess the adequacy of lymph node coverage of conventional pelvic fields based on bony landmarks. *Int J Radiat Oncol Biol Phys.* 2006;64(1):205–209.
5. Zunino S, Rosato O, Lucino S, Jauregui E, Rossi L, Venencia D. Anatomic study of the pelvis in carcinoma of the uterine cervix as related to the box technique. *Int J Radiat Oncol Biol Phys.* 1999;44(1):53–59.
6. MacLeod C, Bernshaw D, Leung S, Narayan K, Firth I. Accelerated hyperfractionated radiotherapy for locally advanced cervix cancer. *Int J Radiat Oncol Biol Phys.* 1999;44(3):519–524.
7. Kavanagh BD, Gieschen HL, Schmidt-Ullrich RK, et al. A pilot study of concomitant boost accelerated superfractionated radiotherapy for stage III cancer of the uterine cervix. *Int J Radiat Oncol Biol Phys.* 1997;38(3):561–568.
8. Grigsby P, Winter K, Komaki R, et al. Long-term follow-up of RTOG 88–05: twice-daily external irradiation with brachytherapy for carcinoma of the cervix. *Int J Radiat Oncol Biol Phys.* 2002;54(1):51–57.
9. Perez CA, Grigsby PW, Chao KS, Mutch DG, Lockett MA. Tumor size, irradiation dose, and long-term outcome of carcinoma of uterine cervix. *Int J Radiat Oncol Biol Phys.* 1998;41(2):307–317.
10. Wolfson AH, Abdel-Wahab M, Markoe AM, et al. A quantitative assessment of standard vs. customized midline shield construction for invasive cervical carcinoma. *Int J Radiat Oncol Biol Phys.* 1997;37(1):237–242.
11. Dimopoulos JC, Kirisits C, Petric P, et al. The Vienna applicator for combined intracavitary and interstitial brachytherapy of cervical cancer: clinical feasibility and preliminary results. *Int J Radiat Oncol Biol Phys.* 2006;66(1):83–90.
12. Martinez A, Cox RS, Edmundson GK. A multiple-site perineal applicator (MUPIT) for treatment of prostatic, anorectal, and gynecologic malignancies. *Int J Radiat Oncol Biol Phys.* 1984;10(2):297–305.
13. Erickson B, Eifel P, Moughan J, Rownd J, Iarocci T, Owen J. Patterns of brachytherapy practice for patients with carcinoma of the cervix (1996–1999): a patterns of care study. *Int J Radiat Oncol Biol Phys.* 2005;63(4):1083–1092.
14. Wang X, Liu R, Ma B, et al. High dose rate versus low dose rate intracavity brachytherapy for locally advanced uterine cervix cancer. *Cochrane Database Syst Rev.* 2010;(7):CD007563.
15. Hareyama M, Sakata K, Oouchi A, et al. High-dose-rate versus low-dose-rate intracavitary therapy for carcinoma of the uterine cervix: a randomized trial. *Cancer.* 2002;94(1):117–124.
16. Lertsanguansinchai P, Lertbutsayanukul C, Shotelersuk K, et al. Phase III randomized trial comparing LDR and HDR brachytherapy in treatment of cervical carcinoma. *Int J Radiat Oncol Biol Phys.* 2004;59(5):1424–1431.
17. Davidson SE, Hendry JH, West CM. Point: why choose pulsed-dose-rate brachytherapy for treating gynecologic cancers? *Brachytherapy.* 2009;8(3):269–272.
18. Rath GK, Sharma DN, Julka PK, Subramani V, Bahl A, Haresh KP. Pulsed-dose-rate intracavitary brachytherapy for cervical carcinoma: the AIIMS experience. *Am J Clin Oncol.* 2010;33(3):238–241.
19. Tod M, Meredith WJ. Treatment of cancer of the cervix uteri, a revised Manchester method. *Br J Radiol.* 1953;26(305):252–257.
20. Lee LJ, Sadow CA, Russell A, Viswanathan AN. Correlation of point B and lymph node dose in 3D-planned high-dose-rate cervical cancer brachytherapy. *Int J Radiat Oncol Biol Phys.* 2009;75(3):803–809.
21. Rotmensch J, Connell PP, Yamada D, Waggoner SE, Mundt AJ. One versus two intracavitary brachytherapy applications in early-stage cervical cancer patients undergoing definitive radiation therapy. *Gynecol Oncol.* 2000;78(1):32–38.
22. Pereit DG, Sarkaria JN, Chappell R, et al. The adverse effect of treatment prolongation in cervical carcinoma. *Int J Radiat Oncol Biol Phys.* 1995;32(5):1301–1307.
23. Nag S, Erickson B, Thomadsen B, Orton C, Demanes JD, Pereit D. The American Brachytherapy Society recommendations for high-dose-rate brachytherapy for carcinoma of the cervix. *Int J Radiat Oncol Biol Phys.* 2000;48(1):201–211.
24. Nag S, Chao C, Erickson B, et al.; American Brachytherapy Society. The American Brachytherapy Society recommendations for low-dose-rate brachytherapy for carcinoma of the cervix. *Int J Radiat Oncol Biol Phys.* 2002;52(1):33–48.
25. Lee LJ, Das IJ, Higgins SA, et al.; American Brachytherapy Society. American Brachytherapy Society consensus guidelines for locally advanced carcinoma of the cervix. Part III: low-dose-rate and pulsed-dose-rate brachytherapy. *Brachytherapy.* 2012;11(1):53–57.
26. Kasibhatla M, Clough RW, Montana GS, et al. Predictors of severe gastrointestinal toxicity after external beam radiotherapy and interstitial brachytherapy for advanced or recurrent gynecologic malignancies. *Int J Radiat Oncol Biol Phys.* 2006;65(2):398–403.
27. Haie-Meder C, Pötter R, Van Limbergen E, et al.; Gynaecological (GYN) GEC-ESTRO Working Group. Recommendations from Gynaecological (GYN) GEC-ESTRO Working Group (I): concepts and terms in 3D image based 3D treatment planning in cervix cancer brachytherapy with emphasis on MRI assessment of GTV and CTV. *Radiother Oncol.* 2005;74(3):235–245.
28. Dimopoulos JC, Pötter R, Lang S, et al. Dose-effect relationship for local control of cervical cancer by magnetic resonance image-guided brachytherapy. *Radiother Oncol.* 2009;93(2):311–315.
29. Grigsby PW, Perez CA. Radiotherapy alone for medically inoperable carcinoma of the cervix: stage IA and carcinoma in situ. *Int J Radiat Oncol Biol Phys.* 1991;21(2):375–378.
30. Landoni F, Maneo A, Colombo A, et al. Randomised study of radical surgery versus radiotherapy for stage Ib-IIa cervical cancer. *Lancet.* 1997;350(9077):535–540.
31. Bloemers MC, Portelance L, Legler C, Renaud MC, Tan SL. Preservation of ovarian function by ovarian transposition prior to concurrent chemotherapy and pelvic radiation for cervical cancer. A case report and review of the literature. *Eur J Gynaecol Oncol.* 2010;31(2):194–197.

32. Bergmark K, Avall-Lundqvist E, Dickman PW, Henningsohn L, Steineck G. Vaginal changes and sexuality in women with a history of cervical cancer. *N Engl J Med.* 1999;340(18):1383–1389.

33. Schroder M, Mell LK, Hurteau JA, et al. Clitoral therapy device for treatment of sexual dysfunction in irradiated cervical cancer patients. *Int J Radiat Oncol Biol Phys.* 2005;61(4):1078–1086.

34. Keys HM, Bundy BN, Stehman FB, et al. Cisplatin, radiation, and adjuvant hysterectomy compared with radiation and adjuvant hysterectomy for bulky stage IB cervical carcinoma. *N Engl J Med.* 1999;340(15):1154–1161.

35. Keys HM, Bundy BN, Stehman FB, et al.; Gynecologic Oncology Group. Radiation therapy with and without extrafascial hysterectomy for bulky stage IB cervical carcinoma: a randomized trial of the Gynecologic Oncology Group. *Gynecol Oncol.* 2003;89(3):343–353.

36. Morris M, Eifel PJ, Lu J, et al. Pelvic radiation with concurrent chemotherapy compared with pelvic and para-aortic radiation for high-risk cervical cancer. *N Engl J Med.* 1999;340(15): 1137–1143.

37. Rose PG, Ali S, Watkins E, et al.; Gynecologic Oncology Group. Long-term follow-up of a randomized trial comparing concurrent single agent cisplatin, cisplatin-based combination chemotherapy, or hydroxyurea during pelvic irradiation for locally advanced cervical cancer: a Gynecologic Oncology Group Study. *J Clin Oncol.* 2007;25(19):2804–2810.

38. Whitney CW, Sause W, Bundy BN, et al. Randomized comparison of fluorouracil plus cisplatin versus hydroxyurea as an adjunct to radiation therapy in stage IIB-IVA carcinoma of the cervix with negative para-aortic lymph nodes: a Gynecologic Oncology Group and Southwest Oncology Group study. *J Clin Oncol.* 1999;17(5):1339–1348.

39. Pearcey R, Brundage M, Drouin P, et al. Phase III trial comparing radical radiotherapy with and without cisplatin chemotherapy in patients with advanced squamous cell cancer of the cervix. *J Clin Oncol.* 2002;20(4):966–972.

40. Eifel PJ, Winter K, Morris M, et al. Pelvic irradiation with concurrent chemotherapy versus pelvic and para-aortic irradiation for high-risk cervical cancer: an update of radiation therapy oncology group trial (RTOG) 90–01. *J Clin Oncol.* 2004;22(5):872–880.

41. Dueñas-González A, Zarba JJ, Patel F, et al. Phase III, open-label, randomized study comparing concurrent gemcitabine plus cisplatin and radiation followed by adjuvant gemcitabine and cisplatin versus concurrent cisplatin and radiation in patients with stage IIB to IVA carcinoma of the cervix. *J Clin Oncol.* 2011;1; 29(13):1678–1685.

42. Delgado G, Bundy B, Zaino R, Sevin BU, Creasman WT, Major F. Prospective surgical-pathological study of disease-free interval in patients with stage IB squamous cell carcinoma of the cervix: a Gynecologic Oncology Group study. *Gynecol Oncol.* 1990;38(3):352–357.

43. Sedlis A, Bundy BN, Rotman MZ, Lentz SS, Muderspach LI, Zaino RJ. A randomized trial of pelvic radiation therapy versus no further therapy in selected patients with stage IB carcinoma of the cervix after radical hysterectomy and pelvic lymphadenectomy: A Gynecologic Oncology Group study. *Gynecol Oncol.* 1999; 73(2):177–183.

44. Peters WA 3rd, Liu PY, Barrett RJ 2nd, et al. Concurrent chemotherapy and pelvic radiation therapy compared with pelvic radiation therapy alone as adjuvant therapy after radical surgery in high-risk early-stage cancer of the cervix. *J Clin Oncol.* 2000;18(8):1606–1613.

45. Rotman M, Pajak TF, Choi K, et al. Prophylactic extended-field irradiation of para-aortic lymph nodes in stages IIB and bulky IB and IIA cervical carcinomas. Ten-year treatment results of RTOG 79–20. *JAMA.* 1995;274(5):387–393.

46. Rotman M, Sedlis A, Piedmonte MR, et al. A phase III randomized trial of postoperative pelvic irradiation in Stage IB cervical carcinoma with poor prognostic features: follow-up of a Gynecologic Oncology Group study. *Int J Radiat Oncol Biol Phys.* 2006;65(1):169–176.

47. Haie C, Pejovic MH, Gerbaulet A, et al. Is prophylactic para-aortic irradiation worthwhile in the treatment of advanced cervical carcinoma? Results of a controlled clinical trial of the EORTC radiotherapy group. *Radiother Oncol.* 1988;11(2):101–112.

48. Grigsby PW, Perez CA, Chao KS, Herzog T, Mutch DG, Rader J. Radiation therapy for carcinoma of the cervix with biopsy-proven positive para-aortic lymph nodes. *Int J Radiat Oncol Biol Phys.* 2001;49(3):733–738.

49. Varia MA, Bundy BN, Deppe G, et al. Cervical carcinoma metastatic to para-aortic nodes: extended field radiation therapy with concomitant 5-fluorouracil and cisplatin chemotherapy: a Gynecologic Oncology Group study. *Int J Radiat Oncol Biol Phys.* 1998;42(5):1015–1023.

50. Grigsby PW, Lu JD, Mutch DG, Kim RY, Eifel PJ. Twice-daily fractionation of external irradiation with brachytherapy and chemotherapy in carcinoma of the cervix with positive para-aortic lymph nodes: Phase II study of the Radiation Therapy Oncology Group 92–10. *Int J Radiat Oncol Biol Phys.* 1998;41(4):817–822.

51. Halle JS, Rosenman JG, Varia MA, Fowler WC, Walton LA, Currie JL. 1000 cGy single dose palliation for advanced carcinoma of the cervix or endometrium. *Int J Radiat Oncol Biol Phys.* 1986;12(11):1947–1950.

52. Spanos WJ Jr, Wasserman T, Meoz R, Sala J, Kong J, Stetz J. Palliation of advanced pelvic malignant disease with large fraction pelvic radiation and misonidazole: final report of RTOG phase I/II study. *Int J Radiat Oncol Biol Phys.* 1987;13(10): 1479–1482.

53. Spanos W Jr, Guse C, Perez C, Grigsby P, Doggett RL, Poulter C. Phase II study of multiple daily fractionations in the palliation of advanced pelvic malignancies: preliminary report of RTOG 8502. *Int J Radiat Oncol Biol Phys.* 1989;17(3):659–661.

54. Spanos WJ Jr, Perez CA, Marcus S, et al. Effect of rest interval on tumor and normal tissue response–a report of phase III study of accelerated split course palliative radiation for advanced pelvic malignancies (RTOG-8502). *Int J Radiat Oncol Biol Phys.* 1993;25(3):399–403.

Multidisciplinary Approach to Cancer of the Uterine Corpus

8 Surgical-Pathologic Features of Uterine Cancers

BOJANA DJORDJEVIC

RUSSELL R. BROADDUS

The central goal of this chapter is to provide a practical guide to key topics in surgical pathology of endometrial cancer. This includes the classification of endometrial adenocarcinoma and its precursor lesions and a discussion of interpretation and reporting of endometrial biopsies. Emphasis has been placed on everyday issues commonly encountered in clinical practice and problems commonly discussed between pathologists, oncologists, and surgeons in tumor board conferences.

■ ENDOMETRIAL CARCINOMA

Endometrial carcinoma is a heterogeneous disease characterized by a number of different histological subtypes. It is important to recognize these different subtypes, as they have distinct clinical behaviors. Endometrial carcinoma can broadly be divided into endometrioid and nonendometrioid types. Endometrioid tumors can arise from endometrial hyperplasia in pre- and postmenopausal patients, often in the setting of estrogen excess or obesity. Nonendometrioid tumors, on the other hand, have a hormone-independent pathogenesis and no known precursor lesions. They typically occur in older postmenopausal patients.

Endometrioid adenocarcinoma is the most common histological subtype and accounts for 80%–90% of all endometrial cancers (1,2). Microscopically, endometrioid carcinoma is composed of crowded, back-to-back and fused glands as well as of solid nests of tumor. The nuclei are pseudostratified and atypical, but generally maintain intraepithelial polarity. Morular, squamous, or mucinous metaplasia is often present. For a diagnosis of endometrial endometrioid adenocarcinoma, particularly on biopsy, one of the following diagnostic criteria must be met: (a) back-to-back proliferation of endometrial glands occupying an area of at least 2 × 2 mm; (b) an extensive papillary pattern; (c) a desmoplastic or fibroblastic stroma infiltrated by irregular glands (3,4). Endometrioid carcinomas are graded by the International Federation of Gynecology and Obstetrics (FIGO) system on a scale of 1 to 3, based on the amount of solid tumor component (5). Grade 1, 2, and 3 tumors have less than 6%, between 6% and 50%, and more than 50% of a solid tumor component, respectively (Figure 8.1) (6). Grade 1 and 2 tumors are considered low grade, and are generally associated with good prognosis, while grade 3 tumors have an intermediate to poor prognosis. Endometrioid endometrial carcinoma has several microscopic morphological variants including the variant with squamous differentiation, villoglandular variant, and secretory or ciliated variant; currently, these variants have no known clinical significance.

Mucinous endometrial adenocarcinoma represents approximately 1% of endometrial tumors and is composed predominantly of mucinous glands (Figure 8.2) (7). While endometrioid tumors commonly have focal areas of mucinous metaplasia, the World Health Organization (WHO) criteria define mucinous adenocarcinoma as having greater than 90% of such cells with intracytoplasmic mucin (6). However, some investigators have used cutoffs of greater than 50% (8,9) or greater than 70% (10) in their studies. Mucinous endometrial adenocarcinoma is graded in the same manner as endometrioid adenocarcinoma. Although mucinous carcinoma has a comparable prognosis to endometrioid adenocarcinoma (8–10), one group has recently shown that mucinous endometrial carcinomas have a slightly higher association with lymph node metastasis (8). The key differential diagnosis, particularly in biopsy specimens, is to distinguish this histotype from an endocervical primary or metastasis from the GI tract (see the section Practical Considerations on Endometrial Biopsy).

Nonendometrioid endometrial carcinomas include serous carcinoma, clear-cell carcinoma, and carcinosarcoma. These histotypes are associated with high-grade cytological features, and are not otherwise graded. Uterine serous carcinoma accounts for 5%–13% of endometrial carcinomas (2,7,11). The hallmark of this histotype is loss of intraepithelial polarity in combination with pronounced cytological atypia, including prominent nucleoli and a

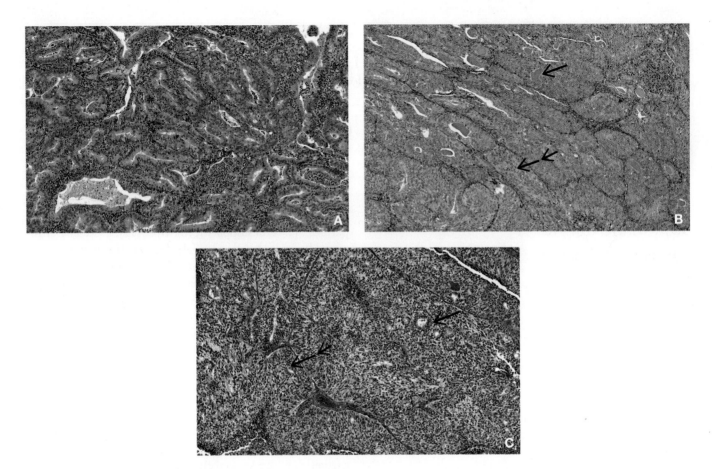

FIGURE 8.1   Endometrioid endometrial adenocarcinoma. (A) FIGO Grade 1 tumor consists of back-to-back and fused glands with no intervening stroma. (B) FIGO Grade 2 tumor contains a mixture of glands (arrow) and solid tumor nests (double arrow). (C) FIGO Grade 3 tumor consists of predominantly solid nests and sheets of cells (double arrow), with only focal glandular formations (arrow). FIGO, International Federation of Gynecology and Obstetrics.

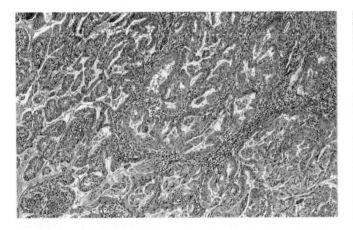

FIGURE 8.2   Mucinous endometrial adenocarcinoma, FIGO Grade 1. The tumor consists predominantly of glands with abundant blue-tinged intracytoplasmic mucin. The nuclei are small and show only mild cytological atypia. FIGO, International Federation of Gynecology and Obstetrics.

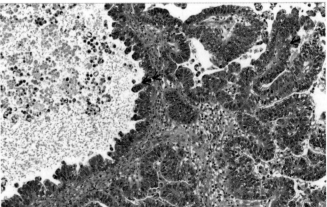

FIGURE 8.3   Serous endometrial adenocarcinoma. The tumor contains papillae with (arrow) and without (double arrow) fibrovascular cores. Tumor cells show loss of intraepithelial polarity and high-grade nuclear atypia with prominent nucleoli and large variation in nuclear size.

large variation in nuclear size and shape (Figure 8.3). The tumors may assume a variety of architectural configurations microscopically, ranging from intraepithelial carcinoma to invasive forms with glandular, papillary, or solid patterns. Uterine serous tumors have a poor prognosis,

with presence of extrauterine disease in as many as 37% of patients with no evidence of endometrial stromal or myometrial invasion (12).

Clear-cell carcinoma represents 1%–7% of endometrial adenocarcinomas (2,7,11). The tumor cells are typically polygonal with clear to eosinophilic cytoplasm and eccentrically placed atypical nuclei. They may be arranged in solid sheets, papillae, or glands. Papillae exhibit hyalinized cores, while glands are typically lined by a single layer of cells with hobnail nuclei. The tumor may contain hyaline globules (Figure 8.4). Overall, clear-cell carcinoma has a comparably poor prognosis to uterine serous carcinoma (2), although some studies have suggested that stage I tumors are associated with improved survival (13).

Carcinosarcomas (or malignant mixed müllerian tumors) contain distinct malignant epithelial (carcinomatous) and malignant mesenchymal (sarcomatous) components (Figure 8.5). Although carcinosarcoma is categorized as a sarcoma, rather than a carcinoma, in the current WHO classification of endometrial carcinoma (6), it is increasingly being regarded as a high-grade metaplastic carcinoma by pathologists. Its pattern of recurrence and metastasis mirrors that of carcinoma rather than of sarcoma (14), while clonality and mutational studies have shown that the carcinomatous and the sarcomatous components derive from the same precursor (15–18).

Carcinosarcomas typically have a worse outcome than endometrioid, clear-cell, and serous carcinomas (19,20). In a recent study, it has been shown that tumors with a polypoid shape are associated with lower rates of myometrial and lymphovascular invasion as well as with longer patient survival compared with their nonpolypoid counterparts (21).

Undifferentiated carcinoma is a recently described entity, which may represent up to 9% of endometrial carcinomas (11). This tumor does not exhibit any gland or solid tumor nest formation, but instead consists of monotonous discohesive cells arranged in solid sheets (Figure 8.6). It shows only focal evidence of epithelial differentiation, with only 5%–10% of cells expressing keratin markers by immunohistochemistry, and very minimal expression of the hormone receptors estrogen receptor (ER) and progesterone receptor (PR). Undifferentiated carcinoma is commonly underrecognized due to diagnostic confusion with FIGO Grade 3 endometrioid adenocarcinoma, which has a significantly better prognosis (22). Undifferentiated carcinoma may appear as a mixed carcinoma (see discussion below), commonly in combination with endometrioid adenocarcinoma. It has been hypothesized that the two entities may be biologically related and that undifferentiated carcinoma arises due to dedifferentiation of endometrioid adenocarcinoma (23), but definitive molecular evidence of this has not yet been uncovered. Thus far, it is only known that these tumors may focally express neuroendocrine markers (22,24) and may have DNA mismatch repair abnormalities (25,26). It is currently uncertain whether these undifferentiated tumors should be classified as endometrioid or nonendometrioid.

The WHO tumor classification states that mixed endometrial carcinomas are tumors composed of one endometrioid or mucinous carcinoma component and

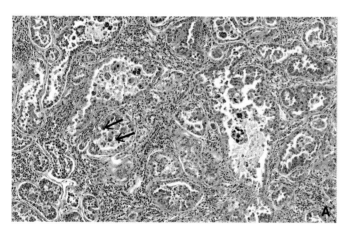

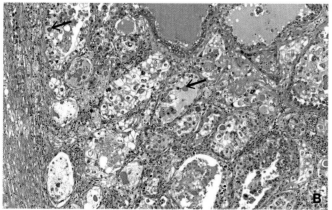

FIGURE 8.4 Clear-cell endometrial adenocarcinoma. (A) Glands comprising the tumor are lined by a single layer of cells with large atypical hobnail nuclei (arrows) and clear to eosinophilic cytoplasm. (B) Abundant hyaline globules are present (arrows).

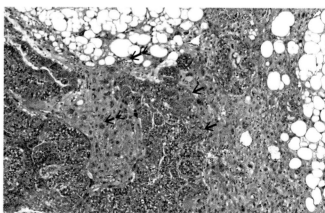

FIGURE 8.5 Carcinosarcoma of the endometrium. Two sharply demarcated malignant components are present. The carcinomatous component (arrows) is a high-grade endometrioid carcinoma. The sarcomatous component (double arrows) is a high-grade sarcoma with liposarcomatous differentiation.

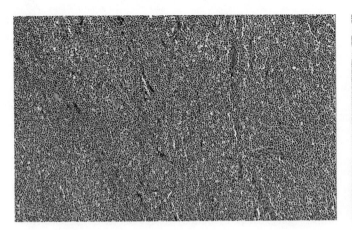

FIGURE 8.6 Undifferentiated endometrial carcinoma. The tumor consists of sheets of discohesive atypical cells. There is no gland or nest formation.

another nonendometrioid carcinoma component, with each representing at least 10% of the overall tumor (6). However, experience with mixed carcinoma is somewhat limited, and in practice, some pathologists tend to report any amount of nonendometrioid or nonmucinous endometrial component. In mixed endometrioid–serous tumors, it can be quite difficult to pinpoint the exact percentage of endometrioid and serous subtypes present, as the microscopic features of these subtypes can blend together. The most studied mixed carcinoma has been the endometrioid–serous type, with the percentage cutoffs for the relative amount of serous carcinoma ranging from greater than or equal to 50% (27), greater than or equal to 25% (28,29), to less than 10% (30,31) among various studies, which have shown these tumors to have a behavior comparable to that of pure serous carcinoma. Similarly, a few studies have reported that clear-cell carcinoma in combination with endometrioid carcinoma confers a poor outcome (31,32).

Other endometrial carcinoma histotypes include pure squamous cell carcinoma, transitional-cell carcinoma, and small-cell carcinoma. Squamous cell carcinomas likely represent endometrioid-type endometrial carcinomas that have undergone extensive squamous metaplastic changes. These three histotypes are exceedingly rare and are beyond the scope of this chapter.

■ ENDOMETRIAL HYPERPLASIA

Endometrial hyperplasia, especially complex hyperplasia with atypia, is a precursor to endometrioid-type endometrial carcinoma. Endometrial hyperplasia is a proliferation of endometrial glands causing an increased gland-to-stroma ratio within the endometrium. The WHO recognizes several different types of hyperplasia, including simple hyperplasia with or without atypia and complex hyperplasia with or without atypia (6; Figure 8.7). In simple

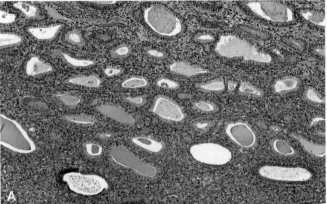

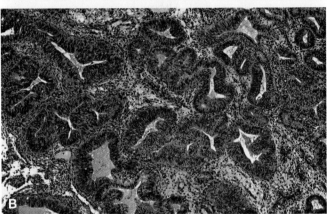

FIGURE 8.7 (A) Simple endometrial hyperplasia without atypia. The glands are crowded and have tubular outlines. The nuclei are small and have a smooth chromatin pattern. (B) Complex endometrial hyperplasia with atypia. The glands are crowded with irregular and branched outlines, but remain distinct from one another within endometrial stroma. The cells show pseudostratification and crowding within the epithelium. The nuclei are hyperchromatic and have a coarse chromatin pattern.

hyperplasia, the glands retain their tubular outlines, similar to the glands of proliferative endometrium. In complex hyperplasia, the glands exhibit branched and complex outlines. Glands with cytological atypia show an increased amount of cellular pseudostratification, enlarged nuclei, coarse chromatin, and prominent nucleoli. Complex atypical hyperplasia is the subtype associated with the highest risk of developing endometrioid endometrial adenocarcinoma, with progression to carcinoma occurring in 29% of cases (3). In addition, complex atypical hyperplasia and endometrioid carcinoma frequently coexist in the endometrium, and up to 42.6% of endometrial biopsies with complex atypical endometrial hyperplasia will result in a diagnosis of carcinoma in the subsequent hysterectomy specimen (33). Although the WHO classification system is widely used, some studies have suggested that it is not highly reproducible (34–36), which may be attributable to the lack of precisely defined diagnostic criteria and the morphologic continuum that exists between complex atypical hyperplasia and well-differentiated endometrioid carcinoma. Other classification systems including endometrial intraepithelial neoplasia (EIN) with D-score have been proposed (37–39), but have not gained wide acceptance.

■ PRACTICAL CONSIDERATIONS ON ENDOMETRIAL BIOPSY

Endometrial Versus Endocervical Adenocarcinoma

A common diagnostic scenario in gynecologic pathology involves the distinction of endometrial vs endocervical origin of adenocarcinoma obtained during endometrial or endocervical sampling. The presence of concurrent cervical squamous dysplasia or adenocarcinoma-in-situ favors the endocervical origin of the adenocarcinoma, while postmenopausal patient age and endometrial hyperplasia and/or squamous morules favor the endometrial tumor origin. However, morphological clues are not always present, and patient age may sometimes be misleading, particularly given the rising incidence of obesity and endometrial carcinoma in premenopausal women. For this reason, immunohistochemical testing may be useful in establishing the correct diagnosis.

A panel of four immunohistochemical markers is commonly used to distinguish endometrial from endocervical primaries and includes estrogen receptor (ER), vimentin, monoclonal carcinoembryonic antigen (mCEA) and p16 (40–43). Endometrial adenocarcinoma typically shows diffuse immunohistochemical expression of ER and vimentin, patchy p16 staining, and negative expression for mCEA. Endocervical adenocarcinoma is typically diffusely positive for p16 and shows diffuse membranous and/or cytoplasmic staining for mCEA, while it is negative for ER and vimentin. It is important to note, however, that up to 50% of endocervical and as many as 70% endometrial adenocarcinomas (44) may have aberrant positive or negative patterns of expression for at least one of the four markers in the panel. This underscores the need for judicious interpretation and correlation with tumor morphology by the pathologist. It should also be emphasized that this panel is only valid for tumors of endometrioid and mucinous differentiation. For example, serous or clear-cell carcinomas of endometrium and endocervix cannot be distinguished from one another by immunohistochemistry. Therefore, in some cases, the pathologist may not be able to specifically designate the origin (endocervical vs endometrial) of the tumor.

Uncommonly, independent primary endometrial and endocervical adenocarcinomas will coexist in the same patient. Such tumors will typically have a different histological appearance and discordant immunohistochemical profiles (45). Carcinomas arising in the lower uterine segment are generally thought to be endometrial carcinomas. They have been shown in one study to have the same immunohistochemical profile as conventional endometrioid adenocarcinomas arising in the uterine fundus (46).

Metastases to the Endometrium

Metastases to the endometrium are rare and typically originate either from breast or from colon (47). Breast carcinoma typically involves the lymphatics and does not form a mass lesion, thus making the diagnosis particularly challenging on endometrial biopsy. Gross cystic disease fluid protein-15 is the preferred marker to identify breast from an endometrial primary, as mammaglobin is expressed in the majority of endometrial tumors (48). Colorectal carcinoma metastases to the endometrium may mimic an endometrial primary with areas of mucinous differentiation. These two entities may be distinguished from ER, vimentin, and cytokeratin 7 (positive in endometrial carcinoma), and CDX2 and cytokeratin 20 (positive in colorectal carcinoma) immunostains. Pax 8 is a novel marker that will stain endometrial carcinoma, but not breast or colon carcinoma (49).

Endometrial Sampling Issues

Endometrial biopsies may be insufficient for histological evaluation in up to 15% of cases (50), leading to a recommendation for repeat sampling by the pathologist. For example, a biopsy may only contain endocervical tissue or lower uterine segment endometrium, without any endometrium from the corpus. Alternatively, the specimen may be fragmented, showing only glands with proliferative activity, with or without atypia, but with no underlying endometrial stroma that would permit assessment of the glandular to stromal ratio. 1.9%–6% of women with initially insufficient biopsies will be diagnosed with endometrial carcinoma on subsequent endometrial sampling (51,52).

Among adequately sampled endometrial biopsies, a positive biopsy result increases the pretest probability of endometrial carcinoma from 6.3% to 81.7%, while a negative result decreases the pretest probability to 0.9% (50). In the latter group of patients, repeat endometrial sampling, particularly if the endovaginal ultrasound shows an endometrial mass or an endometrial thickness of 5 mm or greater, is recommended (53).

When the endometrial biopsy uncovers premalignant or malignant entities, it is important to keep in mind that it may still not be a representative sample, leading to some discrepancies between the biopsy and the hysterectomy pathology. As noted earlier, complex atypical hyperplasia and endometrial endometrioid adenocarcinoma frequently coexist, leading to a situation in which only one of the two may be represented in the endometrial biopsy. Similarly, the biopsy may only capture one histological component of a mixed endometrial adenocarcinoma. On occasion, the hysterectomy specimen will grossly show no evidence of tumor that was detected on the biopsy, particularly if the tumor was confined to an endometrial polyp. In such instances, the pathologist will submit the endometrium in its entirety for histological examination.

■ REFERENCES

1. Clement PB, Young RH. Endometrioid carcinoma of the uterine corpus: a review of its pathology with emphasis on recent advances and problematic aspects. *Adv Anat Pathol.* 2002;9(3): 145–184.

2. Cirisano FD Jr, Robboy SJ, Dodge RK, et al. Epidemiologic and surgicopathologic findings of papillary serous and clear cell endometrial cancers when compared to endometrioid carcinoma. *Gynecol Oncol.* 1999;74(3):385–394.

3. Kurman RJ, Kaminski PF, Norris HJ. The behavior of endometrial hyperplasia. A long-term study of "untreated" hyperplasia in 170 patients. *Cancer.* 1985;56(2):403–412.

4. Malpica A, Deavers MT, Euscher ED. Biopsy interpretation of uterine cervix and corpus. In: Epstein JI, ed. *Biopsy Interpretation Series*. Philadelphia, PA: Lippincott Williams and Wilkins; 2009: 177.

5. Zaino RJ, Kurman RJ, Diana KL, Morrow CP. The utility of the revised International Federation of Gynecology and Obstetrics histologic grading of endometrial adenocarcinoma using a defined nuclear grading system. A Gynecologic Oncology Group study. *Cancer.* 1995;75(1):81–86.

6. Silverberg SG, Kurman RJ, Nogales F, Mutter GL, Kubik-Huch RA, Tavassoli FA. In: Tavassoli FA, Devillee P, eds. *World Health Organization Classification of Tumours: Tumours of the Breast and Female Genital Organs*. Lyon: IARC Press; 2003: 221–232.

7. Clement PB, Young RH. Non-endometrioid carcinomas of the uterine corpus: a review of their pathology with emphasis on recent advances and problematic aspects. *Adv Anat Pathol.* 2004;11(3):117–142.

8. Musa F, Huang M, Adams B, Pirog E, Holcomb K. Mucinous histology is a risk factor for nodal metastases in endometrial cancer. *Gynecol Oncol.* 2012;125(3):541–545.

9. Ross JC, Eifel PJ, Cox RS, Kempson RL, Hendrickson MR. Primary mucinous adenocarcinoma of the endometrium. A clinicopathologic and histochemical study. *Am J Surg Pathol.* 1983;7(8):715–729.

10. Melhem MF, Tobon H. Mucinous adenocarcinoma of the endometrium: a clinico-pathological review of 18 cases. *Int J Gynecol Pathol.* 1987;6(4):347–355.

11. Silva EG, Deavers MT, Malpica A. Undifferentiated carcinoma of the endometrium: a review. *Pathology.* 2007;39(1):134–138.

12. Slomovitz BM, Burke TW, Eifel PJ, et al. Uterine papillary serous carcinoma (UPSC): a single institution review of 129 cases. *Gynecol Oncol.* 2003;91(3):463–469.

13. Malpica A, Tornos C, Burke TW, Silva EG. Low-stage clear-cell carcinoma of the endometrium. *Am J Surg Pathol.* 1995; 19(7):769–774.

14. Sreenan JJ, Hart WR. Carcinosarcomas of the female genital tract. A pathologic study of 29 metastatic tumors: further evidence for the dominant role of the epithelial component and the conversion theory of histogenesis. *Am J Surg Pathol.* 1995;19(6):666–674.

15. Thompson L, Chang B, Barsky SH. Monoclonal origins of malignant mixed tumors (carcinosarcomas). Evidence for a divergent histogenesis. *Am J Surg Pathol.* 1996;20(3):277–285.

16. Costa MJ, Vogelsan J, Young LJ. p53 gene mutation in female genital tract carcinosarcomas (malignant mixed müllerian

17. Abeln EC, Smit VT, Wessels JW, de Leeuw WJ, Cornelisse CJ, Fleuren GJ. Molecular genetic evidence for the conversion hypothesis of the origin of malignant mixed müllerian tumours. *J Pathol.* 1997;183(4):424–431.

18. Kounelis S, Jones MW, Papadaki H, Bakker A, Swalsky P, Finkelstein SD. Carcinosarcomas (malignant mixed mullerian tumors) of the female genital tract: comparative molecular analysis of epithelial and mesenchymal components. *Hum Pathol.* 1998;29(1):82–87.

19. George E, Lillemoe TJ, Twiggs LB, Perrone T. Malignant mixed müllerian tumor versus high-grade endometrial carcinoma and aggressive variants of endometrial carcinoma: a comparative analysis of survival. *Int J Gynecol Pathol.* 1995;14(1):39–44.

20. Vaidya AP, Horowitz NS, Oliva E, Halpern EF, Duska LR. Uterine malignant mixed mullerian tumors should not be included in studies of endometrial carcinoma. *Gynecol Oncol.* 2006;103(2):684–687.

21. Djordjevic B, Gien LT, Covens A, Malpica A, Khalifa MA. Polypoid or non-polypoid? A novel dichotomous approach to uterine carcinosarcoma. *Gynecol Oncol.* 2009;115(1):32–36.

22. Altrabulsi B, Malpica A, Deavers MT, Bodurka DC, Broaddus R, Silva EG. Undifferentiated carcinoma of the endometrium. *Am J Surg Pathol.* 2005;29(10):1316–1321.

23. Silva EG, Deavers MT, Bodurka DC, Malpica A. Association of low-grade endometrioid carcinoma of the uterus and ovary with undifferentiated carcinoma: a new type of dedifferentiated carcinoma? *Int J Gynecol Pathol.* 2006;25(1):52–58.

24. Taraif SH, Deavers MT, Malpica A, Silva EG. The significance of neuroendocrine expression in undifferentiated carcinoma of the endometrium. *Int J Gynecol Pathol.* 2009;28(2):142–147.

25. Tafe LJ, Garg K, Chew I, Tornos C, Soslow RA. Endometrial and ovarian carcinomas with undifferentiated components: clinically aggressive and frequently underrecognized neoplasms. *Mod Pathol.* 2010;23(6):781–789.

26. Broaddus RR, Lynch HT, Chen LM, et al. Pathologic features of endometrial carcinoma associated with HNPCC: a comparison with sporadic endometrial carcinoma. *Cancer.* 2006;106(1):87–94.

27. Williams KE, Waters ED, Woolas RP, Hammond IG, McCartney AJ. Mixed serous-endometrioid carcinoma of the uterus: pathologic and cytopathologic analysis of a high-risk endometrial carcinoma. *Int J Gynecol Cancer.* 1994;4(1):7–18.

28. Sherman ME, Bitterman P, Rosenshein NB, Delgado G, Kurman RJ. Uterine serous carcinoma. A morphologically diverse neoplasm with unifying clinicopathologic features. *Am J Surg Pathol.* 1992;16(6):600–610.

29. Carcangiu ML, Chambers JT. Uterine papillary serous carcinoma: a study on 108 cases with emphasis on the prognostic significance of associated endometrioid carcinoma, absence of invasion, and concomitant ovarian carcinoma. *Gynecol Oncol.* 1992;47(3):298–305.

30. Lim P, Al Kushi A, Gilks B, Wong F, Aquino-Parsons C. Early stage uterine papillary serous carcinoma of the endometrium: effect of adjuvant whole abdominal radiotherapy and pathologic parameters on outcome. *Cancer.* 2001;91(4):752–757.

31. Quddus MR, Sung CJ, Zhang C, Lawrence WD. Minor serous and clear cell components adversely affect prognosis in "mixed-type" endometrial carcinomas: a clinicopathologic study of 36 stage-I cases. *Reprod Sci.* 2010;17(7):673–678.

32. Carcangiu ML, Chambers JT. Early pathologic stage clear cell carcinoma and uterine papillary serous carcinoma of the endometrium: comparison of clinicopathologic features and survival. *Int J Gynecol Pathol.* 1995;14(1):30–38.

33. Trimble CL, Kauderer J, Zaino R, et al. Concurrent endometrial carcinoma in women with a biopsy diagnosis of atypical endometrial hyperplasia: a Gynecologic Oncology Group study. *Cancer.* 2006;106(4):812–819.

tumors): a clinicopathologic study of 74 cases. *Mod Pathol.* 1994; 7(6):619–627.

34. Bergeron C, Nogales FF, Masseroli M, et al. A multicentric European study testing the reproducibility of the WHO classification of endometrial hyperplasia with a proposal of a simplified working classification for biopsy and curettage specimens. *Am J Surg Pathol.* 1999;23(9):1102–1108.

35. Zaino RJ, Kauderer J, Trimble CL, et al. Reproducibility of the diagnosis of atypical endometrial hyperplasia: a Gynecologic Oncology Group study. *Cancer.* 2006;106(4):804–811.

36. Kendall BS, Ronnett BM, Isacson C, et al. Reproducibility of the diagnosis of endometrial hyperplasia, atypical hyperplasia, and well-differentiated carcinoma. *Am J Surg Pathol.* 1998;22(8):1012–1019.

37. Mutter GL. Histopathology of genetically defined endometrial precancers. *Int J Gynecol Pathol.* 2000;19(4):301–309.

38. Baak JP, Mutter GL, Robboy S, et al. The molecular genetics and morphometry-based endometrial intraepithelial neoplasia classification system predicts disease progression in endometrial hyperplasia more accurately than the 1994 World Health Organization classification system. *Cancer.* 2005;103(11):2304–2312.

39. Baak JP, Ørbo A, van Diest PJ, et al. Prospective multicenter evaluation of the morphometric D-score for prediction of the outcome of endometrial hyperplasias. *Am J Surg Pathol.* 2001;25(7):930–935.

40. McCluggage WG, Sumathi VP, McBride HA, Patterson A. A panel of immunohistochemical stains, including carcinoembryonic antigen, vimentin, and estrogen receptor, aids the distinction between primary endometrial and endocervical adenocarcinomas. *Int J Gynecol Pathol.* 2002;21(1):11–15.

41. Dabbs DJ, Sturtz K, Zaino RJ. The immunohistochemical discrimination of endometrioid adenocarcinomas. *Hum Pathol.* 1996;27(2):172–177.

42. Castrillon DH, Lee KR, Nucci MR. Distinction between endometrial and endocervical adenocarcinoma: an immunohistochemical study. *Int J Gynecol Pathol.* 2002;21(1):4–10.

43. Staebler A, Sherman ME, Zaino RJ, Ronnett BM. Hormone receptor immunohistochemistry and human papillomavirus in situ hybridization are useful for distinguishing endocervical and endometrial adenocarcinomas. *Am J Surg Pathol.* 2002;26(8):998–1006.

44. Han CP, Lee MY, Kok LF, et al. Adding the p16(INK4a) marker to the traditional 3-marker (ER/Vim/CEA) panel engenders no supplemental benefit in distinguishing between primary endocervical and endometrial adenocarcinomas in a tissue microarray study. *Int J Gynecol Pathol.* 2009;28(5):489–496.

45. Jiang L, Malpica A, Deavers MT, et al. Endometrial endometrioid adenocarcinoma of the uterine corpus involving the cervix: some cases probably represent independent primaries. *Int J Gynecol Pathol.* 2010;29(2):146–156.

46. Westin SN, Lacour RA, Urbauer DL, et al. Carcinoma of the lower uterine segment: a newly described association with Lynch syndrome. *J Clin Oncol.* 2008;26(36):5965–5971.

47. Kumar NB, Hart WR. Metastases to the uterine corpus from extragenital cancers. A clinicopathologic study of 63 cases. *Cancer.* 1982;50(10):2163–2169.

48. Onuma K, Dabbs DJ, Bhargava R. Mammaglobin expression in the female genital tract: immunohistochemical analysis in benign and neoplastic endocervix and endometrium. *Int J Gynecol Pathol.* 2008;27(3):418–425.

49. Ozcan A, Shen SS, Hamilton C, et al. PAX 8 expression in non-neoplastic tissues, primary tumors, and metastatic tumors: a comprehensive immunohistochemical study. *Mod Pathol.* 2011;24(6):751–764.

50. Clark TJ, Mann CH, Shah N, Khan KS, Song F, Gupta JK. Accuracy of outpatient endometrial biopsy in the diagnosis of endometrial cancer: a systematic quantitative review. *BJOG.* 2002;109(3):313–321.

51. van Doorn HC, Opmeer BC, Burger CW, Duk MJ, Kooi GS, Mol BW; Dutch Study in Postmenopausal Bleeding (DUPOMEB). Inadequate office endometrial sample requires further evaluation in women with postmenopausal bleeding and abnormal ultrasound results. *Int J Gynaecol Obstet.* 2007;99(2):100–104.

52. Feldman S, Shapter A, Welch WR, Berkowitz RS. Two-year follow-up of 263 patients with post/perimenopausal vaginal bleeding and negative initial biopsy. *Gynecol Oncol.* 1994;55(1):56–59.

53. Smith-Bindman R, Kerlikowske K, Feldstein VA, et al. Endovaginal ultrasound to exclude endometrial cancer and other endometrial abnormalities. *JAMA.* 1998;280(17):1510–1517.

9 Multidisciplinary Approach to Treatment of Endometrioid Uterine Carcinoma

JIM FANNING

JOSHUA P. KESTERSON

The treatment of endometrial cancer has evolved significantly over the last 20 years. Surgical staging is the standard for early endometrial cancer and should be performed minimally invasively. The potential therapeutic role of resection of macroscopic lymphadenopathy (Stage IIIC) and cytoreductive surgery (Stage IV) is being investigated. Postoperative teletherapy for early endometrial cancer is no longer recommended. For advanced stage and recurrent disease, there has been a shift toward first-line chemotherapy. A "sandwich" approach for advanced and recurrent endometrial cancer consisting of chemotherapy and radiation has been described. For younger women interested in childbearing, conservative progestin hormonal therapy is an option for properly counseled patients.

■ SURGERY FOR EARLY ENDOMETRIAL CANCER

In 2005, the American College of Obstetricians and Gynecologists recommended that women with endometrial cancer should undergo surgical staging, which includes hysterectomy, oophorectomy, and lymphadenectomy (1). There are five main reasons for surgical staging:

1. Lymph node status is the most important prognosticator in endometrial cancer. In the prospective Gynecologic Oncology Group (GOG) trial, 50% of all recurrence occurred in patients with nodal metastasis (2).
2. Surgical staging allows tailoring of postoperative therapy by eliminating adjuvant teletherapy in patients with disease limited to the uterus. The GOG performed a prospective randomized trial comparing teletherapy versus observation in 448 patients with early endometrial cancer (3). There was no statistically significant survival difference between patients receiving no treatment versus those receiving teletherapy.
3. There appears to be a small survival advantage by performing lymphadenectomy. Kilgore et al reported an increased survival from approximately 72% to 88% in patients undergoing lymphadenectomy (4).
4. In experienced hands, lymphadenectomy can be performed with minimal morbidity. In prospective evaluation, we have shown that lymphadenectomy can be performed in a median of 25 min with a 1% complication rate (5).
5. This treatment strategy is cost-effective. Using a cost-effectiveness analysis, we have shown that this treatment strategy is 12% less expensive than selected lymphadenectomy and postoperative teletherapy (6,7). In a 2005 survey of the Society of Gynecologic Oncology (SGO), the vast majority of gynecologic oncologists recommend surgical staging in all cases of endometrial cancer (8).

Whenever feasible, surgery for endometrial cancer should be performed minimally invasive—laparoscopically or robotically. The GOG performed a prospective randomized trial (LAP2) comparing laparoscopic vs laparotomy surgical staging on 2181 patients (9,10). Five-year survival was identical, but complications were significantly reduced with laparoscopy (14% vs 21%). Although there was a 26% conversion to laparotomy in the laparoscopic group of LAP2, more recent trails have reported only a 3% conversion rate (11).

Complex atypical hyperplasia (CAH) is the precursor of endometrial cancer. The pathologic reproducibility of CAH is poor. The GOG reviewed 306 biopsy specimens of CAH and diagnosed 29% as cancer (12). Also, coexisting cancer can be present in the hysterectomy specimen in patients with biopsy specimens of CAH. The GOG prospectively reviewed 289 hysterectomy specimens and found coexisting cancer in 43% (13). Because of the poor pathologic reproducibility of CAH (29% are cancer), the significant likelihood of coexisting cancer (43%), and the benefits of surgical staging, it is reasonable to offer surgical staging at the time of hysterectomy in patients with CAH.

■ SURGERY FOR ADVANCED ENDOMETRIAL CANCER (STAGE III-IV)

Resection of Macroscopic Lymphadenopathy (Stage IIIC)

Unfortunately, there are no prospective randomized trials to guide evidence-based surgical treatment of advanced or recurrent endometrial cancer. The potential therapeutic role of resection of macroscopic lymphadenopathy (Stage IIIC) has been investigated. Studies have shown a significantly longer disease-specific survival (DSS) in patients who had a complete resection of macroscopic lymphadenopathy (38 months) compared with patients left with gross residual nodal disease (9 months) (14). We reported a DSS of 40 months for 22 patients who had complete resection of macroscopic lymphadenopathy (15). Similarly, investigators at Duke University reported a lower DSS for women who had gross nodal disease not debulked (16). Using the Surveillance, Epidemiology, and End Results (SEER) database, 2113 women were identified with Stage III and IV disease who underwent surgical staging with lymph node assessment (17). There was an improved 5-year survival for patients with Stage III and IV endometrial cancer who underwent a more extensive lymph node dissection (85.3% and 86.8%; $p < .001$), respectively. Furthermore, for Stage III and IV patients with nodal disease, the extent of nodal dissection was associated with an improved survival. Because of the limitations of these studies (small retrospective reports and SEER database), future studies need to assess the benefit of resection of macroscopic lymphadenopathy in patients with advanced-stage endometrial cancer.

Cytoreduction (Stage IV)

Cytoreductive surgery is the resection of advanced cancer to improve the response to chemotherapy. Although cytoreductive surgery is the standard in advanced-stage ovarian cancer, its role in advanced-stage endometrial cancer is less clear. In patients with Stage IV endometrial cancer (18), investigators reported improved outcomes for those with no gross residual (NGR) disease after surgery compared with those with residual disease. The overall survival (OS) for those with NGR was 42 versus 19 months for those with any residual disease and only 2 months for those who had no attempted cytoreduction. Similarly, Bristow et al noted a statistically significant improvement in survival for patients with Stage IVB endometrial cancer who were optimally cytoreduced (less than or equal to 1 cm residual tumor nodules) compared with those with greater than 1 cm residual tumor (34 vs 11 months, respectively) (19). In a review of 14 retrospective studies, there was an association between complete cytoreduction to NGR and improved OS (20). Because of the limitations of these studies (small retrospective reports), prospective studies are warranted to determine the benefits of cytoreductive surgery for advanced or recurrent endometrial cancer.

Adjuvant Radiation Therapy for Early Endometrial Cancer (Stage I-II)

Traditionally, postoperative teletherapy had been recommended to decrease recurrence in early endometrial cancer. However, with surgical staging, there has been a marked decrease in postoperative radiation therapy. No adjuvant radiation therapy is recommended for low-risk early endometrial cancer (Stage I, Grade 1 or 2). For intermediate-risk early endometrial cancer (Stage IC, Grade 3 or Stage II), brachytherapy, instead of teletherapy, has been shown to be as effective with less cost and morbidity (21). However, recently, multiple prospective randomized trials have failed to demonstrate a survival advantage with postoperative radiation therapy. The GOG performed a prospective randomized trial comparing teletherapy vs observation in 448 patients with early endometrial cancer (3). There was no statistically significant survival difference: no treatment (86%) vs teletherapy (92%). The radiation group experienced more frequent and severe toxicity. The Post-Operative Radiation Therapy in Endometrial Cancer (PORTEC) trial compared teletherapy vs observation in 714 patients and also failed to demonstrate a survival advantage: no treatment (85%) vs teletherapy (81%) (22). The radiation group experienced more toxicity, 25% vs 6%. In a Cochrane Database review of eight trials (4273 patients), postoperative teletherapy failed to demonstrate a survival advantage and was associated with significant morbidity and reduction in quality of life (23). Thus, there has been a significant decrease in the recommendation for postoperative radiation therapy for early-stage endometrial cancer. The majority of gynecologic oncologists do not recommend postoperative teletherapy for intermediate-risk early endometrial cancer (8).

Chemotherapy for Advanced and Recurrent Endometrial Cancer

For advanced-stage disease, there has been a shift toward first-line chemotherapy. The shift from radiation therapy to chemotherapy is based on the results of GOG trial 122 that randomized nearly 400 patients with Stage III/IV endometrial cancer after hysterectomy to whole abdominal radiation or combination chemotherapy with doxorubicin and cisplatin (24). At a median follow-up of greater than 6 years, chemotherapy resulted in a significantly improved progression-free survival (PFS) and OS. There has subsequently been a paradigm shift whereby women with advanced-stage endometrial cancer are treated first-line with chemotherapy.

Effective chemotherapy agents for the treatment of advanced and recurrent endometrial cancer have been elucidated through a series of prospective randomized trials. The most active regimen is a triplet combination of doxorubicin, cisplatin, and paclitaxel (25). When compared with a doxorubicin and cisplatin doublet, the addition of paclitaxel resulted in an improvement in PFS (8.3 vs 5.3 months) and OS (15.3 vs 12.3 months). However, this modest improvement in survival with the triplet regimen came at the expense of greater neuropathy and gastrointestinal toxicity, as well as several treatment-related deaths, and thus widespread acceptance of the regimen of doxorubicin, cisplatin, and paclitaxel has been limited. The doublet combination of carboplatin and paclitaxel has demonstrated efficacy and acceptable tolerability. We reported a 63% response rate in 18 patients treated with carboplatin and paclitaxel (26). Recently, interim results from GOG trial 209, comparing the triplet regimen of doxorubicin, cisplatin, and paclitaxel with carboplatin and paclitaxel in patients with metastatic or recurrent endometrial cancer, were published in abstract form (27). The doublet of carboplatin and paclitaxel was not inferior to the triplet regimen with regard to PFS and OS. The toxicity profile favored the doublet regimen as fewer patients experienced neurologic and hematologic toxicity. More patients randomized to the carboplatin and paclitaxel arm were able to complete all planned cycles (69% vs 62%). Considering these findings, the authors concluded that the doublet of carboplatin and paclitaxel should serve as the backbone for further trials in combination with targeted therapies.

"Sandwich" Chemotherapy and Radiotherapy

A "sandwich" approach for the treatment of advanced and recurrent endometrial cancer consisting of initial chemotherapy (~3 cycles), radiation, and consolidation chemotherapy (~3 cycles) has been described. Two small (43 and 41 patients) prospective nonrandomized trials have reported a 53% and 71% 3-year DSS (28,29). Additional trials are warranted.

Hormonal Therapy for Advanced and Recurrent Endometrial Cancer

Progestin therapy for the treatment of advanced and recurrent endometrial cancer has limited success, because the majority of advanced and recurrent tumors are estrogen/progesterone receptor negative. In a prospective GOG trial of 299 patients, there was only a 15% response rate (30). In another GOG trial, combining tamoxifen with progestin increased the response rate to 33% (31). Women with late recurrence of a well-differentiated cancer respond the best.

Treatment of Isolated Vaginal Recurrences

A majority of regional endometrial cancer recurrences will be in the vaginal vault. Patients who have not had prior radiation therapy are candidates for radiation of their pelvic recurrence, with an expected excellent outcome. In a series of radiation-naïve patients with isolated vaginal recurrences treated with radiation therapy, 81% of women were salvaged with a 5-year OS of 75% (32). Other studies have also shown that a majority of isolated pelvic recurrences can be cured with radiation therapy (33).

Patients with vaginal recurrences in the setting of prior radiation therapy have a worse OS than their nonradiated counterparts (34). Treatment options are limited in previously radiated patients, because radiating previously radiated tissue is generally contraindicated due to the toxicity incurred to adjacent tissues. However, there are limited series reporting on attempts to radiate in a more site-specific manner using stereotactic radiotherapy (35). Considering the limited feasibility of reirradiation, patients with isolated vaginal recurrences may be candidates for surgical resection. Surgical resection with adequate margins may necessitate a pelvic exenteration, and appropriate candidate selection is of paramount importance.

Fertility-Sparing Treatment of Endometrial Cancer

While the majority of cases of endometrial cancer are diagnosed in postmenopausal women, a portion occurs in younger women (usually with polycystic ovarian disease) interested in childbearing, and thus fertility-sparing treatment options. Fortunately, the majority of cases in younger women are low-grade and early-stage. Although there are no prospective randomized trials, conservative progestin hormonal therapy is an option for properly counseled patients (36). The greatest risk associated with conservative management of endometrial cancer is an unrecognized metastatic endometrial cancer or synchronous ovarian cancer. Various oral progestin agents have been used, including medroxyprogesterone acetate (MPA) and megestrol acetate as well as the levonorgestrel-releasing intrauterine system (Mirena). Usual treatment lasts for 6 months and resampling is required. Those who have a documented histologic response should pursue childbearing immediately. Preferably, fertility counseling should begin during progestin therapy.

In a prospective trial of 28 women with endometrial cancer, 55% responded, 60% obtained a pregnancy, and 57% recurred (37). In a meta-analysis of 27 articles, including 81 patients, 76% of patients responded to treatment (38).

Estrogen Replacement Therapy for Menopausal Symptoms

Estrogen replacement therapy (ERT) for the treatment of menopausal symptoms in patients with early-stage endometrial cancer does not appear to affect survival. The GOG performed a prospective randomized double-blind trial comparing ERT with placebo in 1236 women with early-stage endometrial cancer and found no difference in cancer recurrence, 2% in both arms (39).

■ REFERENCES

1. ACOG Practice Bulletin. Clinical management guidelines for obstetrician-gynecologists. *Management of Endometrial Cancer.* 2005;65:1–14.

2. Morrow CP, Bundy BN, Kurman RJ, et al. Relationship between surgical-pathological risk factors and outcome in clinical stage I and II carcinoma of the endometrium: a Gynecologic Oncology Group study. *Gynecol Oncol.* 1991;40(1):55–65.

3. Keys HM, Roberts JA, Brunetto VL, et al.; Gynecologic Oncology Group. A phase III trial of surgery with or without adjunctive external pelvic radiation therapy in intermediate risk endometrial adenocarcinoma: a Gynecologic Oncology Group study. *Gynecol Oncol.* 2004;92(3):744–751.

4. Kilgore LC, Partridge EE, Alvarez RD, et al. Adenocarcinoma of the endometrium: survival comparisons of patients with and without pelvic node sampling. *Gynecol Oncol.* 1995;56(1):29–33.

5. Fanning J, Firestein S. Prospective evaluation of the morbidity of complete lymphadenectomy in endometrial cancer. *Int J Gynecol Cancer.* 1998;8:270–273.

6. Fanning J. Treatment for early endometrial cancer. Cost-effectiveness analysis. *J Reprod Med.* 1999;44(8):719–723.

7. Fanning J, Hoffman ML, Andrews SJ, Harrah AW, Feldmeier JJ. Cost-effectiveness analysis of the treatment for intermediate risk endometrial cancer: postoperative brachytherapy vs. observation. *Gynecol Oncol.* 2004;93(3):632–636.

8. Naumann RW, Coleman RL. The use of adjuvant radiation therapy in early endometrial cancer by members of the Society of Gynecologic Oncologists in 2005. *Gynecol Oncol.* 2007;105(1):7–12.

9. Walker JL, Piedmonte MR, Spirtos NM, et al. Laparoscopy compared with laparotomy for comprehensive surgical staging of uterine cancer: Gynecologic Oncology Group Study LAP2. *J Clin Oncol.* 2009;27(32):5331–5336.

10. Walker JL, Piedmonte MR, Spirtos NM, et al. Recurrence and survival after random assignment to laparoscopy versus laparotomy for comprehensive surgical staging of uterine cancer: Gynecologic Oncology Group LAP2 Study. *J Clin Oncol.* 2012;30(7):695–700.

11. Fanning J, Hossler C. Laparoscopic conversion rate for uterine cancer surgical staging. *Obstet Gynecol.* 2010;116(6):1354–1357.

12. Zaino RJ, Kauderer J, Trimble CL, et al. Reproducibility of the diagnosis of atypical endometrial hyperplasia: a Gynecologic Oncology Group study. *Cancer.* 2006;106(4):804–811.

13. Trimble CL, Kauderer J, Zaino R, et al. Concurrent endometrial carcinoma in women with a biopsy diagnosis of atypical endometrial hyperplasia: a Gynecologic Oncology Group study. *Cancer.* 2006;106(4):812–819.

14. Bristow RE, Zahurak ML, Alexander CJ, Zellars RC, Montz FJ. FIGO stage IIIC endometrial carcinoma: resection of macroscopic nodal disease and other determinants of survival. *Int J Gynecol Cancer.* 2003;13(5):664–672.

15. Katz LA, Andrews SJ, Fanning J. Survival after multimodality treatment for stage IIIC endometrial cancer. *Am J Obstet Gynecol.* 2001;184(6):1071–1073.

16. Havrilesky LJ, Cragun JM, Calingaert B, et al. Resection of lymph node metastases influences survival in stage IIIC endometrial cancer. *Gynecol Oncol.* 2005;99(3):689–695.

17. Chan JK, Cheung MK, Huh WK, et al. Therapeutic role of lymph node resection in endometrioid corpus cancer: a study of 12,333 patients. *Cancer.* 2006;107(8):1823–1830.

18. Shih KK, Yun E, Gardner GJ, Barakat RR, Chi DS, Leitao MM Jr. Surgical cytoreduction in stage IV endometrioid endometrial carcinoma. *Gynecol Oncol.* 2011;122(3):608–611.

19. Bristow RE, Zerbe MJ, Rosenshein NB, Grumbine FC, Montz FJ. Stage IVB endometrial carcinoma: the role of cytoreductive surgery and determinants of survival. *Gynecol Oncol.* 2000;78(2):85–91.

20. Barlin JN, Puri I, Bristow RE. Cytoreductive surgery for advanced or recurrent endometrial cancer: a meta-analysis. *Gynecol Oncol.* 2010;118(1):14–18.

21. Fanning J, Nanavati PJ, Hilgers RD. Surgical staging and high dose rate brachytherapy for endometrial cancer: limiting external radiotherapy to node-positive tumors. *Obstet Gynecol.* 1996;87(6):1041–1044.

22. Creutzberg CL, van Putten WL, Koper PC, et al. Surgery and postoperative radiotherapy versus surgery alone for patients with stage-1 endometrial carcinoma: multicentre randomised trial. PORTEC Study Group. Post Operative Radiation Therapy in Endometrial Carcinoma. *Lancet.* 2000;355(9213):1404–1411.

23. Kong A, Johnson N, Kitchener HC, Lawrie TA. Adjuvant radiotherapy for stage I endometrial cancer. *Cochrane Database Syst Rev.* 2012;Mar 14;3:CD003916.

24. Randall ME, Filiaci VL, Muss H, et al.; Gynecologic Oncology Group Study. Randomized phase III trial of whole-abdominal irradiation versus doxorubicin and cisplatin chemotherapy in advanced endometrial carcinoma: a Gynecologic Oncology Group study. *J Clin Oncol.* 2006;24(1):36–44.

25. Fleming GF, Brunetto VL, Cella D, et al. Phase III trial of doxorubicin plus cisplatin with or without paclitaxel plus filgrastim in advanced endometrial carcinoma: a Gynecologic Oncology Group study. *J Clin Oncol.* 2004;22(11):2159–2166.

26. Akram T, Maseelall P, Fanning J. Carboplatin and paclitaxel for the treatment of advanced or recurrent endometrial cancer. *Am J Obstet Gynecol.* 2005;192(5):1365–1367.

27. Miller D, Filiaci V, Gleming G, et al. Late-Breaking Abstract 1: Randomized phase III non-inferiority trial of first line chemotherapy for metastatic or recurrent endometrial carcinoma: A Gynecologic Oncology Group study. *Gynecol Oncol.* 2012;125:771–773.

28. Geller MA, Ivy JJ, Ghebre R, et al. A phase II trial of carboplatin and docetaxel followed by radiotherapy given in a "Sandwich" method for stage III, IV, and recurrent endometrial cancer. *Gynecol Oncol.* 2011;121(1):112–117.

29. Lupe K, D'Souza DP, Kwon JS, et al. Adjuvant carboplatin and paclitaxel chemotherapy interposed with involved field radiation for advanced endometrial cancer. *Gynecol Oncol.* 2009;114(1):94–98.

30. Thigpen JT, Brady MF, Alvarez RD, et al. Oral medroxyprogesterone acetate in the treatment of advanced or recurrent endometrial carcinoma: a dose-response study by the Gynecologic Oncology Group. *J Clin Oncol.* 1999;17(6):1736–1744.

31. Whitney CW, Brunetto VL, Zaino RJ, et al.; Gynecologic Oncology Group study. Phase II study of medroxyprogesterone acetate plus tamoxifen in advanced endometrial carcinoma: a Gynecologic Oncology Group study. *Gynecol Oncol.* 2004;92(1):4–9.

32. Huh WK, Straughn JM, Jr, Mariani A, et al. Salvage of isolated vaginal recurrences in women with surgical stage I endometrial cancer: A multi-institutional experience. *Int J Gyn Cancer.* 2007;17(4):886–889.

33. Lin LL, Grigsby PW, Powell MA, Mutch DG. Definitive radiotherapy in the management of isolated vaginal recurrences of endometrial cancer. *Int J Radiat Oncol Biol Phys.* 2005;63(2):500–504.

34. Creutzberg CL, van Putten WL, Koper PC, et al.; PORTEC Study Group. Survival after relapse in patients with endometrial cancer: results from a randomized trial. *Gynecol Oncol.* 2003;89(2):201–209.

35. Deodato F, Macchia G, Grimaldi L, et al. Stereotactic radiotherapy in recurrent gynecological cancer: a case series. *Oncol Rep.* 2009;22(2):415–419.

36. Kesterson JP, Fanning J. Fertility-sparing treatment of endometrial cancer: options, outcomes and pitfalls. *J Gynecol Oncol.* 2012;23(2):120–124.

37. Ushijima K, Yahata H, Yoshikawa H, et al. Multicenter phase II study of fertility-sparing treatment with medroxyprogesterone acetate for endometrial carcinoma and atypical hyperplasia in young women. *J Clin Oncol.* 2007;25(19):2798–2803.

38. Ramirez PT, Frumovitz M, Bodurka DC, Sun CC, Levenback C. Hormonal therapy for the management of grade 1 endometrial adenocarcinoma: a literature review. *Gynecol Oncol.* 2004;95(1):133–138.

39. Barakat RR, Bundy BN, Spirtos NM, Bell J, Mannel RS; Gynecologic Oncology Group Study. Randomized double-blind trial of estrogen replacement therapy versus placebo in stage I or II endometrial cancer: a Gynecologic Oncology Group study. *J Clin Oncol.* 2006;24(4):587–592.

10 Principles of Radiation Therapy for Uterine Cancers

TIJANA SKREPNIK

SHONA DOUGHERTY

Endometrial cancer is primarily a surgical disease with more than 75% of women presenting with organ-confined tumors (1,2). The standard surgical treatment remains a total hysterectomy and bilateral salpingo-oophorectomy (TH/BSO) with or without full pelvic and para-aortic lymph node dissection (LND). Recommendations for adjuvant therapy are based on the findings of the pathological staging and risk status, and may include observation, pelvic radiation therapy (RT), vaginal cuff brachytherapy (VBT), and systemic therapy such as chemotherapy or hormone-blocking agents. Radiation therapy also has a role in the management of recurrent disease and in the treatment of patients who are deemed medically inoperable.

■ ADJUVANT RADIATION

Adjuvant therapy may be offered to decrease the risk of local, locoregional, or systemic recurrence utilizing RT or systemic drug therapy. Adjuvant RT may be delivered to the tissues of the vaginal cuff using brachytherapy and/or external beam RT (EBRT) directed to pelvic tissues and lymph nodes (LNs).

EBRT

EBRT includes both 3D-conformal RT (3D-CRT) and intensity-modulated RT (IMRT) techniques. The target tissues are the pelvic LNs and the vaginal cuff. Para-aortic LNs can also be addressed with more extensive fields. Limiting the radiation dose to the normal tissues in order to reduce the risk of short- and long-term complications is of high priority. The small bowel frequently falls into the true pelvis postoperatively and can become fixed, leading to higher exposure when compared with the undisturbed mobile organ. Also, the daily movement of central pelvic target tissue needs to be accounted for to avoid underdosing.

EBRT may be used alone or supplemented by a vaginal cuff boost using brachytherapy. Typical EBRT prescriptions deliver 1.8 to 2 Gy fractions daily to total doses of 45 to 50.4 Gy. Additional pelvic sidewall boosts with EBRT may be necessary for residual disease or enlarged LNs.

3D-CRT may more reliably encompass all target tissue within a high-dose volume or four-field box and so pelvic organ motion may occur with less risk of underdosing but at the price of higher radiation doses to normal tissues such as the rectum, bladder, femoral heads, and small bowel (Figure 10.1).

The use of IMRT is growing due to the considerable advantages in normal tissue sparing, but care must be taken to avoid underdosing mobile central pelvic structures (i.e., the vaginal cuff) which are influenced by the filling of the rectum and bladder. IMRT provides the opportunity to limit the total dose to the small bowel and other normal tissue within the pelvis and so reduces the risk of both short- and long-term toxicities (3–11). In addition, marrow within the pelvic bones can also be spared, preserving it for sequential or salvage chemotherapy.

A 2012 multi-institutional Radiation Therapy Oncology Group (RTOG) study, RTOG 0418, analyzed pelvic IMRT for patients with endometrial cancer to determine its influence on short-term bowel adverse events compared with standard pelvic RT. It found a nonsignificant reduction of 12% in short-term events in comparison to historic controls (12). Data on long-term toxicities are awaited and may influence recommendations on the routine use and dose constraints of IMRT.

Strategies to avoid underdosing of mobile organs include the use of appropriate margins to account for this motion and can be achieved by simple expansion of the margins on the target or undertaking simulation with the full and empty bladder after clearing the rectum with a presimulation enema. Generally, expansions of 1.0 to 1.5 cm around the vaginal cuff tissue are commonly used and details of IMRT contouring guidelines are well documented in the RTOG consensus guidelines (13).

VBT

VBT utilizes high-dose-rate (HDR) and low-dose-rate (LDR) radioactive sources placed within delivery devices such as ovoids or cylinders to deliver high doses of radiation

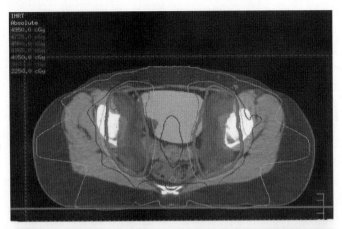

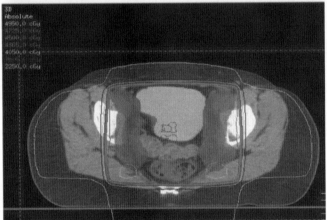

FIGURE 10.1   3D-CRT versus IMRT plan for endometrial cancer.

to well-circumscribed areas at the vaginal cuff and upper vagina to prevent local recurrences. As stated above, this technique can be a sole adjuvant therapy or be used as a boost to the vaginal cuff after external beam. Results from the Postoperative Radiation Therapy in Endometrial Cancer #2 (PORTEC-2) trial suggested that VBT is equivalent to EBRT in preventing local vaginal recurrences and distant metastases, and may avoid some of the toxicities associated with pelvic RT (14). VBT has its limits as to the extent of tissues that it can sterilize and is generally used to address the risk of microscopic disease in the rich lymphatics of the vaginal cuff and the top one- to two-thirds of the vagina to a depth of 5 mm of tissue beyond the surface of the vagina.

Usually, the vaginal cuff will heal 4 weeks after surgery and permit the placement of a suitable device to hold the radioactive source in proximity to the target tissue. Such devices include vaginal cylinders (smooth tubes with hollow centers) or ovoids or rings. Only cylinders allow the length of the vagina treated to be individualized. Ovoids and rings will treat the cuff with only a limited amount of upper vagina included to a therapeutic dose. Both the cylinder (diameters of 2.0–3.5 cm) and ovoids (mini, small, medium, and large) used should be the maximum size that can be comfortably accommodated to ensure an even dose

over the target tissues, avoiding redundant mucosal folds and air gaps which will affect optimal tissue dosimetry.

Various dosing schemes are well accepted for both sole and boost regimens and are documented in the ABS guidelines paper (15). Clear documentation of the prescription point is required as institutional standards vary with respect to dosing at a depth of 5 mm beyond the mucosa or on the vaginal surface. Errors can lead to gross overdosing of the vaginal tissue with risk of injury. Typical LDR dose is 60 Gy to the vaginal surface, and HDR dose is 7 Gy in three fractions prescribed to 0.5 cm as used in PORTEC-2, or 6 Gy in five fractions (MD Anderson) or 4 Gy in six fractions (Dana Farber/Brigham and Women's) prescribed to the surface (16). The use of computed tomography (CT) planning is becoming more widely used and allows for consideration of bowel and bladder dosimetry.

Recommendations for Adjuvant Radiation

Pathological staging permits patients to be stratified according to their risk of recurrence, either local or systemic. Factors known to predict for recurrence include stage, tumor grade and size, lymphovascular space invasion (LVSI), LN status, age, and comorbidities, which allow patients to be assigned to low- (LR), intermediate- (IR), or high-risk (HR) categories (17) (Table 10.1).

PORTEC-1 is a prospective trial of 714 postoperative L-IR patients randomized to EBRT vs no additional therapy with follow-up over 15 years, and found that there was no significant survival difference between the two arms (18). GOG99 studied 448 patients with early-stage disease and all risk categories randomized to EBRT or observation for the risk of recurrence and death (19). This study found that two-thirds of recurrences occurred in the H-IR subset, and that the risk of recurrence in the observation group at 48 months was 27%. It showed that local recurrence was reduced from 13% to 5% with the addition of EBRT and distant recurrence was reduced from 19% to 10%. Although PORTEC-1 and GOG-99 showed that whole pelvic RT (WPRT) reduced vaginal and pelvic recurrences, survival differences were not statistically significant, perhaps related to the high proportion of LR patients studied.

In general, low-risk (Grade 1 or 2) patients are adequately treated with surgery alone. IR patients who are in Stage I-II most commonly are offered RT due to the decreased risk of local and pelvic recurrence. While local control is improved, there is yet no convincing evidence of survival benefit in this group. For example, PORTEC-2 was a prospective study of 427 patients with IR-HR features randomized to WPRT and VBT to determine vaginal recurrence rates (20). Vaginal and local recurrence rates were equivalent between the two modalities, and no difference was seen in survival. However, on final pathology, again a higher proportion of LR patients were included, more than originally intended, which may account for these findings.

■ Table 10.1 Definition of high-risk groups

Study	Definition of High Risk Based on 1988 FIGO Staging
PORTEC-1	60 years old and older and those with Grade 3 lesions or early-stage uterine papillary serous or clear-cell tumors.
PORTEC-2	60 years old and older and Stage 1C, Grades 1 and 2; or Stage IB, Grade 3; or Stage IIA.
GOG-99	70 years old and older with one of the following factors or at least 50 years old with two factors or any age with all three factors. The factors are: Grade 2–3 tumors; positive lymphovascular space involvement (LVSI); outer 1/3 myometrial invasion.

■ Table 10.2 SEPAL definitions of risk

Low Risk	Intermediate Risk	High Risk
Ia, Ib, AND Grade 1–2 AND (–) LVSI	Ia, Grade 3 or serous/clear cell, and any LVSI OR Ib, Grade 3 or serous/clear cell, and (+) LVSI OR Ic or II, any grade, any LVSI	III or IV AND Any grade AND any LVSI

LVSI, lymphovascular space invasion; SEPAL, survival effect of para-aortic lymphadenectomy in endometrial cancer.

Complete pathological staging should, by definition, include a full LND, but doubt has been raised as to the benefit of extensive LND given its potential for morbidity, particularly for patients with low-risk disease. Generally, adjuvant therapy is not recommended for women with biopsy-proven Grade 1–2 tumors that are confined to the endometrium. However, it is estimated that full surgical staging will result in a change of grade assignment in 30% of patients thought to be Grade 1, and 61% of clinical Stage I patients were found to have deeper invasion, resulting in a change of adjuvant therapy recommendations (21–25).

While this controversy continues, the National Comprehensive Cancer Network (NCCN) recommends full surgical staging including peritoneal lavage for cytology for all patients (26). The ASTEC and Panici studies reported no benefit for LND with regard to survival or relapse-free survival (RFS) in early-stage disease (27,28). Once again, however, these large randomized studies were performed on predominantly low-risk patients. ASTEC had 74%–77% Grade 1–2, 51%–60% FIGO Stage IA-IB, and 59%–63% with no LVSI. Further study is much needed for early-stage high-grade patients to determine a survival benefit (29).

Tailoring the extent of LND to risk status may achieve the balance of benefit vs morbidity. Recent studies have shown that LND improves survival, specifically in patients with intermediate and high risk of nodal metastasis but not in LR patients (30–36). The SEPAL study in particular showed benefit of pelvic and para-aortic LND in IR and HR patients, and a recent meta-analysis yielded similar results for systematic LND (greater than 10 nodes removed) (37,38).

In 2009, FIGO updated the surgical staging, and the interpretation of risk categories changed compared with PORTEC and GOG99 definitions; for example, the SEPAL definitions are summarized in Table 10.2.

A recent study prospectively assessed survival, site of recurrence, morbidity, and cost in an LR cohort of 385 patients (39). The authors found that LND dramatically increased morbidity and cost of care without discernible benefits in LR patients. Furthermore, the Korean Gynecologic Oncology Group (KGOG) recently published a retrospective study proposing a preoperative LN metastasis risk assessment model based on MRI and CA-125 that accurately predicted an LR group for LN metastasis (40). This and future models may allow selection of patients for LND, reducing the cost and morbidity of unnecessary procedures.

Studies with concurrent VBT and LND show benefit with added LND. A recent study from Korea analyzing the survival of 156 patients concludes that a comprehensive staging surgery with LND followed by adjuvant VBT improves survival rates for IR endometrial cancer, and these results are comparable to those of LR patients (41).

A large SEER database analysis reported in 2011 looked at 56,000 patients for the influence of RT and LND on overall survival (OS; 42). This study determined risk category based on modified GOG99 and PORTEC criteria and 70% were LR, 26% were IR, and 3.4% were HR. This study found that, in LR patients, LND alone was associated with higher survival while RT alone was not. Results from the IR group showed that both WPRT and VBT alone were associated with an increased survival in this group. In the HR group, LND showed significant 5-year OS improvement, as expected. In those HR patients that underwent LND, all types of RT showed superior survival results with insignificant difference between modality, although WPRT and WPRT+VBT were superior to VBT alone. In fact, in this group, RT was associated with improved survival regardless of LND ($p < .001$), offering a retrospective answer to the question of the benefit of LND in HR patients.

GOG0099 found that two-thirds of recurrences occurred in the H-IR subset, and that the risk of recurrence in this group at 48 months without therapy was 27%. GOG0099 showed that local recurrence was reduced from 13% to 5% with the addition of RT and distant recurrence was reduced from 19% to 10%. Although PORTEC-1 and GOG0099 showed that whole pelvic radiation reduced vaginal and pelvic recurrences, survival differences were not statistically significant, possibly related to the high numbers of LR patients.

ADVANCED DISEASE

Previously, patients with advanced-stage disease received adjuvant WPRT. However, GOG-0107, 0163, 0177 Phase I trials showed that cisplatin and doxorubicin had a survival advantage over WPRT. GOG-0122 showed that nearly 20% of patients receiving chemotherapy alone had disease recur in the pelvis, vagina, and/or para-aortic regions (43). Other studies have shown similar results with 3-year pelvic recurrence rates as high as 46.5% in the chemotherapy-alone arms (44). Furthermore, overall survival is improved with chemotherapy compared with radiation alone as seen in the Japanese Gynecologic Oncology Group (JGOG) trial for Stage II-IIIA patients with 5-year OS 97% compared with 80% for cover atypical pathogens (CAP) regimen vs radiation, respectively (45). Therefore, currently the optimum combination therapy involving chemotherapeutic agents and the ideal sequencing with radiation is evolving.

RECURRENT DISEASE

While most Stage I endometrial cancers are cured by surgery alone, 12%–27% will recur with higher rates in patients with more advanced-stage disease (46). Salvage therapies need to be tailored to the site of the recurrence, and in general, recurrences at the vaginal cuff receive EBRT usually with some form of brachytherapy (vaginal cuff or interstitial) (47). Salvage therapy can be very effective with 2-year survival after an isolated recurrence at vaginal cuff as high as 75% (48–52). If pelvic EBRT has previously been used, then local control may be achieved with surgical resection and limited EBRT or intraoperative RT (IORT) or interstitial brachytherapy.

MEDICALLY INOPERABLE PATIENTS

Patients with severe comorbidities who develop endometrial cancer require alternative management strategies with RT becoming the mainstay of treatment, and the results are encouraging.

Early-stage disease with low-grade histology can be treated with intracavity brachytherapy alone, or after EBRT, using devices such as the Martinez-Y applicator, or Tandem and cylinder, placed in the endometrial and vaginal cavities and used to deliver HDR therapy. Disease free survival (DFS) of 85% has been documented (53) for brachytherapy alone

and EBRT followed with LDR brachytherapy has shown similar 2-year survival of 81.5% (54). For more advanced-stage or higher grade disease, intracavity brachytherapy after EBRT should be considered, and a recent study of 74 inoperable patients treated with either EBRT alone, brachytherapy alone, or EBRT followed by brachytherapy showed a 17.6% recurrence rate with a mean follow-up of 31 months (55). The median progression free survival (PFS) and OS were 43.5 and 47.2 months, respectively, and among the 31 surviving women after 3 years, recurrence rates were less than 16%. A recent study of 32 inoperable patients has shown no significant difference in OS, disease-specific survival (DSS), local control (LC) and toxicity between EBRT with HDR boost and EBRT with IMRT boost. Also, stereotactic body radiotherapy (SBRT) has been explored in a recent retrospective review of 11 women with medically inoperable Stage I-III endometrial cancer who were treated with EBRT followed by 30 Gy SBRT to the endometrium (56). This study found that in patients with Stage IA disease, freedom from progression (FFP) was 100% at 18 months, compared with 33% for IB disease.

FUTURE STUDIES

Studies are still needed to define the role of LND, extent of radiation, and optimal chemotherapeutic or other drugs, particularly for H-IR patients. Several organizations are actively addressing these issues, and three ongoing studies are:

GOG-0249: Prospective study of H-IR patients with early-stage disease receiving chemotherapy with three cycles of paclitaxel and carboplatinum and randomized to VBT vs WPRT to assess the impact of RT on RFS.

JGOG-2041: Prospective study looking at the most feasible chemotherapy regimen without radiotherapy for women with IR endometrial cancer (57).

PORTEC-3: prospective trial comparing WPRT and WPRT plus chemotherapy for women with H-IR and HR disease to determine the impact on overall and failure-free survival.

SUMMARY

- Recommendations for adjuvant therapy are based on full pathological staging
- Radiation is an effective adjuvant therapy for local control but does not affect overall survival
- Low-risk patients usually do not require adjuvant therapy
- Optimal combinations of surgery (+/–LND), radiation extent (VBT vs EBRT), and systemic therapy (chemotherapy or other agents) still require clinical study, particularly in high-risk patients

■ REFERENCES

1. Creasman WT, Morrow CP, Bundy BN, Homesley HD, Graham JE, Heller PB. Surgical pathologic spread patterns of endometrial cancer. A Gynecologic Oncology Group study. *Cancer.* 1987;60(8 Suppl):2035–2041.

2. Morrow CP, Bundy BN, Kurman RJ, et al. Relationship between surgical-pathological risk factors and outcome in clinical stage I and II carcinoma of the endometrium: a Gynecologic Oncology Group study. *Gynecol Oncol.* 1991;40(1):55–65.

3. Roeske JC, Lujan A, Rotmensch J, Waggoner SE, Yamada D, Mundt AJ. Intensity-modulated whole pelvic radiation therapy in patients with gynecologic malignancies. *Int J Radiat Oncol Biol Phys.* 2000;48(5):1613–1621.

4. Lujan AE, Mundt AJ, Yamada SD, Rotmensch J, Roeske JC. Intensity-modulated radiotherapy as a means of reducing dose to bone marrow in gynecologic patients receiving whole pelvic radiotherapy. *Int J Radiat Oncol Biol Phys.* 2003;57(2):516–521.

5. Ahamad A, D'Souza W, Salehpour M, et al. Intensity-modulated radiation therapy after hysterectomy: comparison with conventional treatment and sensitivity of the normal-tissue-sparing effect to margin size. *Int J Radiat Oncol Biol Phys.* 2005;62(4):1117–1124.

6. Portelance L, Chao KS, Grigsby PW, Bennet H, Low D. Intensity-modulated radiation therapy (IMRT) reduces small bowel, rectum, and bladder doses in patients with cervical cancer receiving pelvic and para-aortic irradiation. *Int J Radiat Oncol Biol Phys.* 2001;51(1):261–266.

7. Wong E, D'Souza DP, Chen JZ, et al. Intensity-modulated arc therapy for treatment of high-risk endometrial malignances. *Int J Radiat Oncol Biol Phys.* 2005;61(3):830–841.

8. Heron DE, Gerszten K, Selvaraj RN, et al. Conventional 3D conformal versus intensity-modulated radiotherapy for the adjuvant treatment of gynecologic malignancies: a comparative dosimetric study of dose-volume histograms small star, filled. *Gynecol Oncol.* 2003;91(1):39–45.

9. Mundt AJ, Lujan AE, Rotmensch J, et al. Intensity-modulated whole pelvic radiotherapy in women with gynecologic malignancies. *Int J Radiat Oncol Biol Phys.* 2002;52(5):1330–1337.

10. Brixey CJ, Roeske JC, Lujan AE, Yamada SD, Rotmensch J, Mundt AJ. Impact of intensity-modulated radiotherapy on acute hematologic toxicity in women with gynecologic malignancies. *Int J Radiat Oncol Biol Phys.* 2002;54(5):1388–1396.

11. Mundt AJ, Mell LK, Roeske JC. Preliminary analysis of chronic gastrointestinal toxicity in gynecology patients treated with intensity-modulated whole pelvic radiation therapy. *Int J Radiat Oncol Biol Phys.* 2003;56(5):1354–1360.

12. Jhingran A, Winter K, Portelance L, et al. Phase II study of IMRT to the pelvic for postoperative patients with endometrial carcinoma: Radiation Therapy Oncology Group Trial 0418. *Int J Radiat Oncol Biol Phys.* 2012;84(1):23–28.

13. Small W Jr, Mell LK, Mundt AJ et al. Consensus Guidelines for delineation of clinical target volume for intensity-modulated pelvic radiotherapy in postoperative treatment of endometrial and cervical cancer. *Int J Radiat Oncol Biol Phys.* 2008;71(2):428–434.

14. Nout RA, Smit VT, Putter H, et al.; PORTEC Study Group. Vaginal brachytherapy versus pelvic external beam radiotherapy for patients with endometrial cancer of high-intermediate risk (PORTEC-2): an open-label, non-inferiority, randomised trial. *Lancet.* 2010;375(9717):816–823.

15. Small W Jr, Beriwal S, Demanes DJ, et al.; American Brachytherapy Society. American Brachytherapy Society consensus guidelines for adjuvant vaginal cuff brachytherapy after hysterectomy. *Brachytherapy.* 2012;11(1):58–67.

16. Small W Jr, Beriwal S, Demanes DJ, et al.; American Brachytherapy Society. American Brachytherapy Society consensus guidelines for adjuvant vaginal cuff brachytherapy after hysterectomy. *Brachytherapy.* 2012;11(1):58–67.

17. NCCN Guidelines. *Uterine Neoplasms.* Version 3.2012.

18. Creutzberg CL, Nout RA, Lybeert MLM. Fifteen-year radiotherapy outcomes of the randomized PORTEC-1 trial for endometrial cancer. *Int J Radiat Oncol Biol Phys.* 2011;91(4):631–638.

19. Keys HM, Roberts JA, Brunetto VL, et al.; Gynecologic Oncology Group. A phase III trial of surgery with or without adjunctive external pelvic radiation therapy in intermediate risk endometrial adenocarcinoma: a Gynecologic Oncology Group study. *Gynecol Oncol.* 2004;92(3):744–751.

20. Nout RA, Smit VT, Putter H, et al.; PORTEC Study Group. Vaginal brachytherapy versus pelvic external beam radiotherapy for patients with endometrial cancer of high-intermediate risk (PORTEC-2): an open-label, non-inferiority, randomised trial. *Lancet.* 2010;375(9717):816–823.

21. Ben-Shachar I, Pavelka J, Cohn DE, et al. Surgical staging for patients presenting with grade 1 endometrial carcinoma. *Obstet Gynecol.* 2005;105(3):487–493.

22. Huang GS, Gebb JS, Einstein MH, Shahabi S, Novetsky AP, Goldberg GL. Accuracy of preoperative endometrial sampling for the detection of high-grade endometrial tumors. *Am J Obstet Gynecol.* 2007;196(3):243.e1–243.e5.

23. Case AS, Rocconi RP, Straughn JM Jr, et al. A prospective blinded evaluation of the accuracy of frozen section for the surgical management of endometrial cancer. *Obstet Gynecol.* 2006;108(6):1375–1379.

24. Vorgias G, Lekka J, Katsoulis M, Varhalama E, Kalinoglou N, Akrivos T. Diagnostic accuracy of prehysterectomy curettage in determining tumor type and grade in patients with endometrial cancer. *MedGenMed.* 2003;5(4):7.

25. Mitchard J, Hirschowitz L. Concordance of FIGO grade of endometrial adenocarcinomas in biopsy and hysterectomy specimens. *Histopathology.* 2003;42(4):372–378.

26. NCCN *Clinical Practice Guidelines in Oncology,* Uterine Neoplasms. Version 3.2012.

27. The ASTEC Writing Group. Efficacy of systematic pelvic lymphadenectomy in endometrial cancer (MRC ASTEC trial): a randomized study. *The Lancet.* 2009;373:125–136.

28. Benedetti Panici P, Basile S, Maneschi F, et al. Systematic pelvic lymphadenectomy vs. no lymphadenectomy in early-stage endometrial carcinoma: randomized clinical trial. *J Natl Cancer Inst.* 2008;100(23):1707–1716.

29. Naumann RW. The role of lymphadenectomy in endometrial cancer: was the ASTEC trial doomed by design and are we destined to repeat that mistake? *Gynecol Oncol.* 2012;126(1):5–11.

30. Kitchener H, Swart AM, Qian Q, Amos C, Parmar MK. Efficacy of systematic pelvic lymphadenectomy in endometrial cancer (MRC ASTEC trial): A randomised study. *Lancet.* 2009;373(9658):125–136.

31. Panici PB, Maggioni A, Hacker N, et al. Systematic aortic and pelvic lymphadenectomy versus resection of bulky nodes only in optimally debulked advanced ovarian cancer: a randomized clinical trial. *J Natl Cancer Inst.* 2005;97(8):560–566.

32. Benedetti Panici P, Basile S, Maneschi F, et al. Systematic pelvic lymphadenectomy vs. no lymphadenectomy in early-stage endometrial carcinoma: randomized clinical trial. *J Natl Cancer Inst.* 2008;100(23):1707–1716.

33. Bassarak N, Blankenstein T, Brüning A, et al. Is lymphadenectomy a prognostic marker in endometrioid adenocarcinoma of the human endometrium? *BMC Cancer.* 2010;10:224.

34. Chan JK, Cheung MK, Huh WK, et al. Therapeutic role of lymph node resection in endometrioid corpus cancer: a study of 12,333 patients. *Cancer.* 2006;107(8):1823–1830.

35. Cragun JM, Havrilesky LJ, Calingaert B, et al. Retrospective analysis of selective lymphadenectomy in apparent early-stage endometrial cancer. *J Clin Oncol.* 2005;23(16):3668–3675.

36. Jeong NH, Lee JM, Lee JK, et al. Role of systematic lymphadenectomy and adjuvant radiation in early-stage endometrioid uterine cancer. *Ann Surg Oncol.* 2010;17(11):2951–2957.

37. Todo Y, Kato H, Kaneuchi M, Watari H, Takeda M, Sakuragi N. Survival effect of para-aortic lymphadenectomy in endometrial cancer (SEPAL study): a retrospective cohort analysis. *Lancet.* 2010;375(9721):1165–1172.

38. Kim HS, Suh DH, Kim MK, Chung HH, Park NH, Song YS. Systematic lymphadenectomy for survival in patients with endometrial cancer: a meta-analysis. *Jpn J Clin Oncol.* 2012;42(5):405–412.

39. Dowdy SC, Borah BJ, Bakkum-Gamez JN, et al. Prospective assessment of survival, morbidity, and cost associated with lymphadenectomy in low-risk endometrial cancer. *Gynecol Oncol.* 2012;127(1):5–10.

40. Kang S, Kang WD, Chung HH, et al. Preoperative identification of a low-risk group for lymph node metastasis in endometrial cancer: a Korean Gynecologic Oncology Group study. *J Clin Oncol.* 2012;30(12):1329–1334.

41. Kong TW, Paek J, Chang SJ, Chun M, Chang KH, Ryu HS. Comprehensive staging surgery including complete pelvic and para-aortic lymphadenectomy followed by adjuvant vaginal brachytherapy improves survival rates for intermediate-risk endometrial cancer patients. *Gynecol Obstet Invest.* 2012;74(1):68–75.

42. Chino JP, Jones E, Berchuck A, Secord AA, Havrilesky LJ. The influence of radiation modality and lymph node dissection on survival in early-stage endometrial cancer. *Int J Radiat Oncol Biol Phys.* 2012;82(5):1872–1879.

43. Randall ME, Filiaci VL, Muss H, et al. Randomized phase III trial of whole-abdominal irradiation versus doxorubicin and cisplatin chemotherapy in advanced endometrial carcinoma: A Gynecologic Oncology Group study. *J Clin Oncol.* 2006;24:11.

44. Mundt AJ, McBride R, Rotmensch J, Waggoner SE, Yamada SD, Connell PP. Significant pelvic recurrence in high-risk pathologic stage I–IV endometrial carcinoma patients after adjuvant chemotherapy alone: implications for adjuvant radiation therapy. *Int J Radiat Oncol Biol Phys.* 2001;50(5):1145–1153.

45. Susumu N, Sagae S, Kudo R et al. Randomized phase III trial of pelvic radiotherapy versus cisplatin-based combined chemotherapy in patients with intermediate- and high-risk endometrial cancer: a Japanese Gynecologic Oncology Group study. *Gynecol Oncol.* 2008;108(1):226–233.

46. McMeekin SD, Randall ME. A phase III trial of pelvic radiation therapy versus vaginal cuff brachytherapy followed by paclitaxel/carboplatin chemotherapy in patients with high risk, early stage encometrial carcinoma (GOG-0249). Ongoing Trial.

47. Wright JD, Barrena Medel NI, Sehouli J, Fujiwara K, Herzog TJ. Contemporary management of endometrial cancer. *Lancet.* 2012;379(9823):1352–1360.

48. Wright JD, Barrena Medel NI, Sehouli J, Fujiwara K, Herzog TJ. Contemporary management of endometrial cancer. *Lancet.* 2012;379(9823):1352–1360.

49. Huh WK, Straughn JM Jr, Mariani A, et al. Salvage of isolated vaginal recurrences in women with surgical stage I endometrial cancer: a multiinstitutional experience. *Int J Gynecol Cancer.* 2007;17(4):886–889.

50. Creutzberg CL, van Putten WL, Koper PC, et al.; PORTEC Study Group. Survival after relapse in patients with endometrial cancer: results from a randomized trial. *Gynecol Oncol.* 2003;89(2):201–209.

51. Bristow RE, Santillan A, Zahurak ML, Gardner GJ, Giuntoli RL 2nd, Armstrong DK. Salvage cytoreductive surgery for recurrent endometrial cancer. *Gynecol Oncol.* 2006;103(1):281–287.

52. Keys HM, Roberts JA, Brunetto VL, et al.; Gynecologic Oncology Group. A phase III trial of surgery with or without adjunctive external pelvic radiation therapy in intermediate risk endometrial adenocarcinoma: a Gynecologic Oncology Group study. *Gynecol Oncol.* 2004;92(3):744–751.

53. Nguyen TV, Petereit DG. High-dose-rate brachytherapy for medically inoperable stage I endometrial cancer. *Gynecol Oncol.* 1998;71(2):196–203.

54. Rose PG, Baker S, Kern M, et al. Primary radiation therapy for endometrial carcinoma: a case controlled study. *Int J Radiat Oncol Biol Phys.* 1993;27(3):585–590.

55. Podzielinski I, Randall ME, Breheny PJ, et al. Primary radiation therapy for medically inoperable patients with clinical stage I and II endometrial carcinoma. *Gynecol Oncol.* 2012;124:36–41.

56. Kemmerer E, Hernandez E, Ferriss JS, Valakh V, Miyamoto C, Li S. Use of image-guided stereotactic body radiation therapy in lieu of intracavitary brachytherapy for the treatment of inoperable endometrial neoplasia. *Int J Radiat Oncol Biol Phys.* 2013;85(1):129–135.

57. Nomura H, Aoki D, Takahashi F, et al. Randomized phase II study comparing docetaxel plus cisplatin, docetaxel plus carboplatin, and paclitaxel plus carboplatin in patients with advanced or recurrent endometrial carcinoma: a Japanese Gynecologic Oncology Group study (JGOG2041). *Ann Oncol.* 2011;22(3):636–642.

II Multidisciplinary Management of Serous Carcinoma of the Endometrium

DANA M. ROQUE

ALESSANDRO D. SANTIN

PETER E. SCHWARTZ

■ EPIDEMIOLOGY, MOLECULAR PATHOGENESIS, AND BIOLOGIC BEHAVIOR

Pathogenesis of Type I and Type II Disease

Endometrial cancer is the most common gynecologic malignancy in developed countries, with 49,560 new cases and 8190 deaths projected in the United States alone for 2013 (1). Ninety percent of endometrial cancers arise purely from epithelial glands (2) and may be broadly dichotomized into two classes with distinct underlying pathogenetic mechanisms, histopathology, and clinical behavior (3).

Type I endometrial cancers comprise 80% of cases and are associated with endometrioid histology (grade 1 or 2; 4,5), a history of exposure to unopposed estrogen with retention of estrogen (ER)/progestin (PR) receptor status (6), and younger age at onset (mean 63 years; 7). Deleterious mutations in k-Ras, PTEN, or mismatch repair mechanisms predominate (8,9). Hyperplasia is a common precursor.

Type II endometrial cancers constitute a minority of cases and are characterized by serous, clear cell, or grade 3 endometrioid histology (10,11). Uterine serous carcinoma (USC) was first reported in 1972 (12) and is the most biologically aggressive Type II variant. USC is typified by a higher prevalence in black patients, as well as more advanced stage and age at presentation (13). An antecedent history of unopposed estrogen is often absent. Endometrial intraepithelial carcinoma (EIC) is a recognized precursor that frequently exhibits dysregulated p53 expression. Loss of heterozygosity in chromosome 17p on which p53 is located can be demonstrated in 100% of USCs and 43% of serous EIC, suggesting an important role in the pathogenesis of USC (14). Loss of ER/PR (15) as well as e-cadherin (16), aneuploidy, and HER2/Neu overexpression are common (6,17–19). Recently, altered expression of BAF250a, the protein encoded by the chromatin remodeling tumor suppressor gene *ARID1A*, has been implicated in 18% of serous cancers of the endometrium as examined by immunohistochemistry (IHC; 20). PPP2R1A, the scaffolding subunit of the serine/threonine protein phosphatase 2A (PP2A) holoenzyme, is also frequently mutated (21).

Uterine Serous Carcinoma in Association With Breast Cancer and Tamoxifen Use

USC has been described in association with breast cancer. In a Surveillance Epidemiology and End Results (SEER)–based study of 52,109 women with endometrial cancer, 1922 had a history of breast cancer; compared to women without breast cancer, the rate of USC was 9.4% vs 6.3% (22). BRCA mutation status has been implicated in some (23) but not other (24) reports, and the contribution of tamoxifen is controversial (25–29). Magriples and colleagues (1993) studied 53 patients diagnosed with breast cancer who subsequently developed a uterine malignancy and found that 67% of tamoxifen users harbored a cancer of high-risk histologic type as compared to 24% of tamoxifen non-users (P = .03) and were subsequently more likely to die of endometrial disease (P = .005; 27). In a separate analysis, breast cancer survivors with Type II histology were found to have a longer median duration of prior tamoxifen use compared to those with Type I histology (60 vs 46 months, P = .034; 28). Nevertheless, among 6681 women treated with tamoxifen for 5 years in the National Surgical Adjuvant Breast and Bowel Project (NSABP-P1), none of the resultant endometrial cancers were serous in nature (29).

Prior Radiation and Development of Uterine Serous Carcinoma

In patients who have received radiation for gynecologic disorders, the risk of subsequent development of high-risk endometrial cancers is increased. The risk of sarcoma may be raised by as much as 4-fold (30), and several reports have also described the tendency for development of USC (31,32), sometimes at intervals that exceed a decade (33,34). Gallion and colleagues (1987) found that 37.5% of endometrial cancers diagnosed after radiation therapy for cervical cancer were serous in nature (31).

Clinical Behavior and the Role of the Serous Component in Mixed Endometrial Cancers

USC is characterized by a relatively poor prognosis. While USC constitutes only 10% of cases, it accounts for as many as 40% of deaths (35). The 5-year disease-specific survival rate for USC is only 55% (36), which compares unfavorably to the rate of 89% for grade 1 or 2 endometrioid cancers (7). As many as 46% of patients have extrauterine spread at time of diagnosis, compared to only 26% of patients with Type I disease. Five-year overall survival for Stage I, II, III, and IV disease is 50%–80%, 50%, 20%, and 5%–10%, respectively (37).

By World Health Organization (WHO) guidelines for epithelial tumors, only those who contain less than 10% of a second malignant component are considered "pure" USC (38). The Gynecologic Oncology Group (GOG) Pathology Committee requires that the serous component comprise more than 50% of a mixed component tumor to be classified as USC in protocols. Presence of a serous component as small as 10% confers poorer prognosis (39). Boruta and colleagues (2004) described clinical outcomes for 87 patients with mixed serous histologies in comparison to grade 3 endometrioid disease; for patients with early stage disease, a significant trend existed for worse overall survival with increasing percentage of serous component (40).

Synchronous Serous Uterine and Ovarian Cancers

Synchronous primaries of the ovary and endometrium exist in 5%–8% of uterine cancers (41). In one study of 108 cases of USC identified retrospectively at a single institution, 10 were associated with synchronous ovarian primaries (39). In all instances, the endometrial cancer was confined to a polyp or demonstrated only scant superficial invasion without evidence of lymphovascular space invasion. Though treatments rendered were not reported in detail, overall survival in these patients with synchronous primaries was equivalent to survival outcome for Stage IV USC.

DNA flow cytometry, loss of heterozygosity, X chromosome inactivation, PTEN/MMAC1, beta-catenin, p53, and microsatellite instability have been proposed as methods to distinguish dual primaries, but there is no consensus regarding their use (42,43). Distinguishing concomitant uterine and ovarian primaries from Stage IV USC is often difficult and may not yield much relevance for purposes of protocols or management.

■ DIAGNOSIS, MANAGEMENT, AND PROGNOSIS

Diagnostic Utility of Preoperative Ultrasound, Endometrial Sampling, and Serum Biomarkers

As the surgical management of Type I and II cancers differs, preoperative identification is helpful. Given rates of cervical stenosis that may approach 17% in patients over 70 years (43) and a 5%–15% rate of insufficient specimen on office biopsy (44), clinicians increasingly turn to ultrasound for guidance. As USC is generally not preceded by endometrial hyperplasia, an ultrasonographic double endometrial stripe thickness less than 5 mm does not reliably exclude Type II as it does Type I disease (45). In a study of 52 women with Type II cancers, including 46% with USC, only 65% had endometrial thickening on transvaginal ultrasound assessment (46).

USC may also be misdiagnosed on tissue specimens. In a series of 67 patients with USC treated over a 10-year period from 1994 to 2003 at a teaching institution, the diagnostic accuracy of endometrial biopsy by pipelle was only 63%, though upon re-review of pathology specimens this rate approached 98.5% (47). In another series that examined dilatation and curettage specimens from 154 patients for which the prevalence of USC was 11%, sensitivity, specificity, positive predictive value, and negative predictive value were 59%, 97%, 71%, and 95%, respectively (48).

CA-125 is the most commonly used clinical biomarker for serous cancers including those of the endometrium (49) as elevations often reflect disease status by means of advanced stage, omental metastases, and lymphatic spread, though preoperative levels do not serve as an independent predictor for recurrence (50). Nevertheless, it is an imperfect marker and sensitivity for advanced USC may be as low as 57% (51). The acute phase reactant serum amyloid A (52) as well as human kallikreins 6 and 10 (53,54) have been proposed as novel biomarkers for USC.

Importance of Comprehensive Surgical Staging and the Role of Laparoscopy

Treatment for USC begins with complete surgical staging with intent for cytoreduction to no residual disease (37,55). Staging should consist of total hysterectomy, bilateral salpingo-oophorectomy, bilateral pelvic/para-aortic lymphadenectomy, omentectomy, and peritoneal washings with biopsies (37,49) given the unpredictable pattern of extrauterine spread (56,57), which may be as high as 60% even with a noninvasive disease (58). Gross inspection of the omentum has a reported sensitivity of 89% (59), but in some series upstaging by microscopic inspection of an otherwise disease-free omentum occurred in as many as 25% of cases (60,61).

No data currently exist to suggest that a laparoscopic approach is contraindicated for management of early-stage

USC. GOG-LAP2 (62) randomized 2181 patients with clinical Stage I to IIA disease to laparoscopy vs laparotomy (2:1), including 289 (13%) with USC. Among all patients, the 3-year recurrence rates differed by only 1.14% (11.4% vs 10.2%, 90% CI, –1.28%, 4.0%) with identical estimated 5-year overall survival rates (89.8%). In patients with USC, there were 82 recurrences (30.8%), but the relative hazard ratio among those randomized to laparoscopy vs laparotomy was 1.087. Overall, port site metastases were observed in only 0.24% of cases, the strongest risk factor for which appeared to be extrauterine disease at the time of staging but not necessarily having serous histology.

Treatment of Advanced Stage Disease: Adjuvant, Neoadjuvant, and Sandwich Therapy

Chemotherapeutic strategies for advanced disease draw largely upon the cumulative experience from six large phase III studies conducted by the GOG, each of which enrolled patients with both Type I and II disease (63–68). Historically, GOG 177 (64) established doxorubicin/cisplatin/paclitaxel (TAP) as standard of care for advanced or recurrent endometrial cancers. GOG 184 (67) subsequently demonstrated equivalent hazard ratios for recurrence or death in patients who received postoperative radiation followed by TAP vs doxorubicin/cisplatin (0.90, 95% CI, 0.69–1.17, P = .21), though there was a 50% reduction in risk of relapse or death with the former regimen in patients with residual disease after debulking at the expense of increased hematologic toxicity. Preliminary analyses of GOG 209 now suggest the noninferiority and favorable side effect profile of six cycles of carboplatin (AUC 6)/paclitaxel (175 mg/m^2) over cisplatin (50 mg/m^2)/doxorubicin (45 mg/m^2)/paclitaxel (160 mg/m^2; 68); this regimen appears to have utility in high-risk disease (69) and is regarded by most as standard of care in conjunction with or without tumor-directed radiation therapy (70).

Although the experience is much more limited compared to women with serous ovarian cancers, neoadjuvant chemotherapy has been employed successfully in patients with medical comorbidities that prevent immediate operative management or those at risk of suboptimal debulking. Patients with USC who undergo optimal cytoreduction (less than or equal to 1 cm residual disease) exhibit a trend toward longer median overall survival (71). Complete responses have been observed after three (72) to six (73) cycles of carboplatin/paclitaxel in women with Stage IV cancers, even in instances with bulky disease burden (74).

Recently, there has been growing interest in exploring sandwich techniques with the intention of reducing the individual toxicities of each modality (75). In one such scheme, carboplatin/paclitaxel was administered for three cycles, followed by external beam radiation therapy with extended fields in the event of positive nodes, and in most instances vaginal brachytherapy, prior to completion of the last three cycles of chemotherapy. Though the number of patients treated in this report was small, 3-year survival probability for patients with advanced USC was 50% (76).

Treatment of Early Stage Disease With Invasion

More controversy exists surrounding the treatment of early-stage USC. Whole-abdominal radiation is of little benefit (GOG-94; 77,78). Adjuvant carboplatin/paclitaxel administration clearly improves recurrence rates, overall survival, and progression-free survival in this population (79–82). There is also evidence to support the use of vaginal cuff brachytherapy in conjunction with platinum-based chemotherapy for Stage I disease. In a retrospective review of 74 patients with Stage I uterine serous cancers, no local recurrences occurred in patients who received vaginal cuff brachytherapy, but were diagnosed in 6 of 31 (19%) of patients who did not. As anticipated, recurrences were far more common in the absence of adjuvant chemotherapy: 6/14 vs 0/7 in FIGO (Fédération Internationale de Gynécologie et d'Obstétrique 1988) IA, 10/13 vs 0/15 in IB, 4/5 vs 1/7 in IC disease (83). In a similar single-institution review of Stage I/II serous cancers, a regimen consisting of six cycles of carboplatin/paclitaxel with vaginal cuff brachytherapy was very well tolerated and resulted in 5-year progression-free and overall survival rates of 88% (84).

Treatment of Uterine Serous Carcinoma Arising From Polyps and Minimal Serous Carcinoma

The natural history of serous carcinoma arising from endometrial polyps was first described in 1990 by Silva and Jenkins, who also noted a high rate of concurrent hyperplasia of ovarian surface and fallopian tube epithelium suggestive of a multicentric disease (85). In the original series, 37.5% of patients had extrauterine disease at the time of presentation, though lymphadenectomy was not performed, and therefore this rate might have been underestimated. In some instances, the serous component constituted only 5% of the polyp. Of the 10 without extrauterine extension, 6 had an abdominal recurrence and 4 out of 6 died of disease within 19 months; only 1 of these 6 patients had received adjuvant therapy in the form of radiation. Of the 4 patients without recurrence at the time of last follow-up, 2 had undergone radiation and 1 had received chemotherapy. Trahan and colleagues (2005) similarly described a 5-year overall survival rate of only 67% in patients with Stage IA USC arising from a polyp (86). Approximately 66% of these patients received adjuvant radiation therapy; none were treated with chemotherapy until recurrence. Overall these patients appear to experience outcomes equivalent to patients with early stage disease and myometrial invasion (39).

The term "minimal serous carcinoma" has since been put forth to describe both the disease confined to the endometrium (superficial serous carcinoma [SSC]) and that without any stromal invasion (EIC, serous EIC; 87). In a series of 8 patients with serous EIC and 13 patients with SSC first described by Wheeler and colleagues (2000), extrauterine disease was the single most important factor in outcome. At 52 months, 100% of patients with disease confined to the uterus were alive. In contrast, all patients with extrauterine spread were dead of disease or alive with recurrences despite disposition to adjuvant platinum-based chemotherapy or, in one instance, Megace and whole pelvic radiation. In nearly 60% of patients, extrauterine disease was solely microscopic (87). Hui and colleagues (2005) described a series of 40 minimal serous carcinomas including 23% EIC and 77% SSC. A total of 5/9 SSC and 16/31 EIC represented disease arising from an endometrial polyp alone (88). A total of 38% had extrauterine spread, consistent with rates reported by others (89); this included one instance of isolated positive peritoneal cytology. Five-year overall survival in patients with and without evidence of extrauterine disease was 94% and 44%, respectively.

Due to the strong association of minimal serous carcinoma with extrauterine disease that may approach 89% in some series (90), full surgical staging is recommended (91). Giuntoli and colleagues (2012) described the outcome of 41 patients with comprehensively staged (total hysterectomy, bilateral salpingo-oophorectomy, pelvic/para-aortic lymph node dissection, omentectomy, peritoneal biopsies) and noncomprehensively staged noninvasive or minimally invasive USC. Only 7% received adjuvant carboplatin/ paclitaxel, all of whom were noncomprehensively staged. Five-year disease-specific survival rates were 100% vs 61%, respectively (P = .039; 92).

Significance of Peritoneal Cytology

Though the 2009 revised FIGO staging criteria no longer incorporate peritoneal cytology, guidelines put forth by the National Comprehensive Cancer Network (NCCN) recommend collection as status may add to risk assessment within treatment algorithms (70). Publications that refute the upstaging of endometrial cancers based on cytology alone and led to the 2009 FIGO staging amendments include predominantly endometrioid histologies (93–95). These series include too few USC to draw definitive conclusions regarding the exact role of peritoneal cytology for this entity, and data are often conflicting. Preyer (2002) studied patients with FIGO 1988 Stage III disease (96 low-risk and 40 high-risk histologic subtypes); while only 15.4% of the entire population received adjuvant chemotherapy, positive peritoneal washings did not influence survival in either group (95). In contrast, Havrilesky and colleagues (2007) reported that positive peritoneal cytology alone conferred a similar prognosis to adnexal/serosal involvement among 57 patients with FIGO 1988 Stage IIIA disease, including 9% with USC (96).

Attempts have been made to stratify patients with positive peritoneal cytology at risk of poor outcome based on molecular characteristics as disseminated cells may have varying malignant potential. For example, a meta-analysis of 19 studies (one randomized trial, one prospective study, and 17 retrospective analyses) showed that while preoperative hysteroscopy may increase the probability of positive peritoneal cytology, there was no evidence to suggest that these patients had compromised outcomes (97). Benevolo and colleagues (2007) examined the role of HER2 overexpression and loss of PR expression in identification of those at risk of reduced overall survival in the setting positive peritoneal cytology (98). Some authors have suggested a role for concentration of cells in prediction of clinical outcome in Stage I disease (99). Among 12 of 54 patients with positive peritoneal cytology and disease otherwise confined to the uterus not restricted to endometrioid histology, 100% of those with greater than 1000 cells/ 100 mL were dead of disease within 2 years whereas those with less than 1000 cells/100 mL the majority had no evidence of disease after 37 to 64 months of follow-up. Others have attempted to identify specific morphologic cellular characteristics indicative of high-risk; in endometrioid cancers, "scalloped edges" are associated with poorer outcome (100), however, analogous correlations have not been established for USC.

Management of Patients With No Residual Disease at Time of Staging

Patients with no residual cancer at time of staging can be observed. Across a median follow-up of 48 months (range: 26–68), Kelly and colleagues (2004; 101) found no recurrences in 10 patients regardless of disposition to observation vs treatment, though some critics caution that the lack of residual disease may simply reflect more the aggressiveness of preoperative endometrial curettage as opposed to intrinsic biologic behavior (57,102). Similarly the presence of microscopic foci of serous disease against a background of endometrioid grade 1 or 2 disease in patients with Stage I disease without lymphovascular space invasion managed expectantly does not appear to affect outcomes (103).

■ EMERGING THERAPIES

Immunotherapy

Targeted immunotherapy represents a promising strategy for USC. Monoclonal antibodies (mAb) result in tumor lysis through antibody-dependent cellular cytotoxicity (ADCC) or complement-dependent cytotoxicity (CDC). Both pathways begin with recognition and binding of the mAb to tumor antigen. The Fc region may then be recognized by Fc receptors located on natural killer cells, monocytes, macrophages, or granulocytes to initiate ADCC or by C1 (the first component of the complement cascade) to activate the classic pathway of CDC ending in osmotic lysis through the membrane–attack complex (MAC). Currently, the two most promising targets are HER2/Neu and vascular endothelial growth factor (VEGF).

The human epidermal growth factor receptor (EGFR) family consists of four members: EGFR (*ErbB1*), HER2/Neu (*ErbB2*), HER-3 (*ErbB3*), and HER-4 (*ErbB4*). Ligand binding induces hetero- or homo-dimerization and subsequent activation of pathways integral to proliferation pathways (104). Amplification of HER2/Neu has been documented in 26%–62% of USC cases (17,18,105–107). Overexpression has been linked to poor prognosis in endometrial cancer (18,108) and molecular profiling studies have shown *ErbB2* to be one of the most overexpressed genes to distinguish uterine serous from ovarian serous tumors (109).

Trastuzumab (Herceptin®; Genentech, San Francisco, CA) is a humanized monoclonal IgG1 antibody that works both through recruitment of natural killer cells, initiation of ADCC, as well as abrogation of downstream effectors (110). Despite encouraging case reports (111–113) when evaluated as a single-agent, trastuzumab 4 mg/kg in week 1 then 2 mg/kg weekly until disease progression in Stage III/IV or recurrent endometrial cancers at the phase II level in GOG-181B failed to demonstrate significant activity (114). These findings have been criticized as inconclusive given that 45.5% of treated patients did not have definitive HER2/Neu amplification and on the basis of slow accrual leading to premature closure (115). A phase II study of carboplatin/paclitaxel with or without trastuzumab in patients with advanced or recurrent uterine papillary serous carcinoma designated HER2/Neu-positive by 3+ IHC or FISH is currently underway (NCT01367002; 116).

VEGF is a homodimeric glycoprotein that induces pathologic neoangiogenesis in a variety of human cancers. In endometrial cancers, VEGF-A expression has been associated with advanced grade, lymphovascular space invasion, lymphatogenous spread, poor prognosis (117,118), and p53 upregulation (119). Bevacizumab (Avastin®; Genentech) is a recombinant human monoclonal IgG1 antibody that neutralizes all isoforms of VEGF (120). In a phase II study of recurrent endometrial cancer (GOG 229E; 121), bevacizumab 15 mg/kg every 3 weeks produced clinical response rate of 13.5%, including 1 complete and 6 partial responses. Median progression-free and overall survival rates were 4.2 and 10.5 months, respectively. Notably, despite representing only 27% of the

study population, serous histology was observed in 100% of complete responses and 50% of partial responses. Presently, bevacizumab in combination with paclitaxel and carboplatin is under study for advanced endometrial cancer (NCT00513786; 122). Another three-arm phase II trial is investigating carboplatin/paclitaxel/bevacizumab, carboplatin/paclitaxel/temsirolimus, and carboplatin/ixabepilone/bevacizumab (NCT00977574; 123). VEGF Trap (Afibercept®; Sanofi-Aventis, Paris, France), a fusion protein containing receptor components and fully human immunoglobulin constant region, is also under evaluation (NCT00462826; 124).

Other candidate target antigens for immunotherapeutic strategies include epithelial cell adhesion molecule (EpCAM; 125), trophoblast cell surface marker (Trop-2; 126), and αV integrins (127). Modulation of membrane complement regulatory proteins may augment cytotoxicity (128).

Novel Cytotoxic Chemotherapies

Over the past quarter century, the GOG has evaluated over 25 novel cytotoxic agents at the phase II level for use in endometrial cancers and exceedingly few of these have proceeded to phase III testing (129). Resistance to paclitaxel has been linked to overexpression of the class III beta isoform of tubulin (130) given preferential binding of paclitaxel to class III beta-tubulin isoforms (131). Class III tubulin differs from class I tubulin at paclitaxel-binding sites involving amino acid positions 175 (Ser→Ala) and 364–5 (Ala-Val→Ser-Ser; 132). Class III beta-tubulin overexpression correlates with poor clinical outcome in a variety of human cancers, including ovarian (133, 134), lung (135), and breast (136).

Epothilones (EPOxide THIazoLe ketONEs) are novel microtubule-stabilizing macrolides isolated from *Sorangium cellulosum* (137) with activity in paclitaxel-resistant malignancies, and the unique ability to bind class III and I isoforms with at least equal affinity (131). Patupilone (Novartis, Basel, Switzerland) and ixabepilone (Ixempra®/BMS-247550; Bristol-Meyers-Squibb, Princeton, NJ) are notable members of this group who vary from each other in structure by only a single moiety.

In vitro, patupilone is highly effective relative to paclitaxel against USC cell lines that express high levels of both tubulin beta III (138) and HER2/Neu (139), a known poor prognostic factor (18,106). This drug has been studied at the phase I, II, and III level in ovarian but not endometrial carcinomas (140–142; NCT00262990; 143).

In parallel, ixabepilone has been FDA-approved for treatment of locally advanced/metastatic breast cancer with capecitabine after failure of anthracycline/taxane therapy or as monotherapy after failure of anthracyclines, taxanes, and capecitabine. Applications for gynecologic malignancies are underway. In GOG-126M, an overall response rate of 14.3% and disease stabilization rate of 40.8% was achieved in 49 patients with platinum/taxane-resistant recurrent ovarian cancer using 20 mg/m² on days 1, 8, 15 of a 28-day cycle (144). GOG-129P evaluated 50 patients with recurrent or persistent endometrial cancer who received one prior line of taxane-based chemotherapy including 40% with serous and 2% with clear cell histology. An overall response rate of 12% was achieved using 40 mg/m² every 21 days; disease stabilization for at least 8 weeks occurred in 60%. Median progression-free and overall survival was 2.9 months and 8.7 months, respectively (145). Ixabepilone is currently under evaluation investigation as first-line therapy with carboplatin and bevacizumab in Stage III/IV primary or recurrent endometrial cancers (GOG-86P; NCT977574; 146).

Small Molecule Inhibitors

Small molecule inhibitors occupy binding pockets to block intracellular signaling pathways important to differentiation and proliferation among tumor cells. Tyrosine kinase inhibitors (TKIs) against EGFR (reviewed by Gehrig and Bae Jump, 2010 [147]) and fibroblast growth factor receptor (FGFR; 148) that result in selective death of endometrial cancer cells that carry activating mutations are under evaluation for efficacy in endometrial cancer (NCT01379534; 149). The PTEN/PI3KCA/AKT/mTOR (mammalian target of rapamycin) pathway is also of significance for treatment of Type II endometrial cancers. *PIK3CA*, downstream of EGFR and FGFR, encodes the catalytic p110-α subunit of phosphatidylinositol 3-kinase (PI3K), which phosphorylates phosphatidyl inositol-3,4-diphosphate (PIP2) to generate phosphatidyl inositol-3,4,5-triphosphate (PIP3). This subsequently activates the AKT–mTOR oncogenic pathway (150). *PIK3CA* mutations promote oncogenesis and have been observed in as many as 15% of USC (151). Inhibitors of mTOR are under evaluation in the treatment of endometrial cancers (152–158). Additionally, whole exome sequencing has recently identified several potential novel therapeutic targets for this disease (159).

■ SUMMARY

USC is an aggressive variant of endometrial cancer that accounts for a disproportionate number of deaths and warrants a multimodal treatment approach. Given unique patterns of spread, complete surgical staging is essential. Adjuvant platinum-based combination chemotherapy with or without radiation is indicated in patients with advanced-stage disease; many patients with early-stage disease should also receive platinum-based chemotherapy with consideration for vaginal cuff brachytherapy given the high risk of recurrence. Further elucidation of the molecular pathogenesis underlying this entity remains key to the development of novel therapeutic approaches.

■ REFERENCES

1. Siegel R, Naishadham D, Jemal A. Cancer statistics, 2013. *CA Cancer J Clin.* 2013;63:11–30.
2. Kosary, CL. Cancer of the Corpus Uteri. In: Ries LAG, Young JL, Keel GE, Eisner MP, Lin YD, Horner M-J (eds), *SEER Survival Monograph—Cancer Survival Among Adults: U.S. SEER Program, 1988–2001, Patient and Tumor Characteristics.* National Cancer Institute, SEER Program, NIH. Bethesda, MD: NIH Pub. No. 07–6215; 2007.
3. Bohkman JV. Two pathogenetic types of endometrial carcinoma. *Gynecol Oncol.* 1983;15(1):10–17.
4. Amant F, Moerman P, Neven P, Timmerman D, Van Limbergen E, Vergote I. Endometrial cancer. *Lancet.* 2005;366 (9484):491–505.
5. Felix AS, Weissfeld JL, Stone RA, et al. Factors associated with Type I and Type II endometrial cancer. *Cancer Causes Control.* 2010;21(11):1851–1856.
6. Lax SF, Pizer ES, Ronnett BM, Kurman RJ. Comparison of estrogen and progesterone receptor, Ki-67, and p53 immunoreactivity in uterine endometrioid carcinoma and endometrioid carcinoma with squamous, mucinous, secretory, and ciliated cell differentiation. *Hum Pathol.* 1998;29(9):924–931.
7. Creasman WT, Odicino F, Maisonneuve P, et al. Carcinoma of the corpus uteri. FIGO 26th Annual Report on the Results of Treatment in Gynecological Cancer. *Int J Gynaecol Obstet.* 2006;(95 Suppl 1):S105–S143.
8. Sherman ME. Theories of endometrial carcinogenesis: a multidisciplinary approach. *Mod Pathol.* 2000;13(3):295–308.
9. Hecht JL, Mutter GL. Molecular and pathologic aspects of endometrial carcinogenesis. *J Clin Oncol.* 2006;24(29):4783–4791.
10. Voss MA, Ganesan R, Ludeman L, et al. Should grade 3 endometrioid endometrial carcinoma be considered a type 2 cancer-a clinical and pathological evaluation. *Gynecol Oncol.* 2012;124(1):15–20.
11. Goff BA, Kato D, Schmidt RA, et al. Uterine papillary serous carcinoma: patterns of metastatic spread. *Gynecol Oncol.* 1994; 54(3):264–268.
12. Hameed K, Morgan DA. Papillary adenocarcinoma of endometrium with psammoma bodies. Histology and fine structure. *Cancer.* 1972;29(5):1326–1335.
13. Wilson TO, Podratz KC, Gaffey TA, Malkasian GD Jr, O'Brien PC, Naessens JM. Evaluation of unfavorable histologic subtypes in endometrial adenocarcinoma. *Am J Obstet Gynecol.* 1990;162(2):418–423; discussion 423.
14. Tashiro H, Isacson C, Levine R, Kurman RJ, Cho KR, Hedrick L. p53 gene mutations are common in uterine serous carcinoma and occur early in their pathogenesis. *Am J Pathol.* 1997; 150(1):177–185.
15. Emons G, Fleckenstein G, Hinney B, Huschmand A, Heyl W. Hormonal interactions in endometrial cancer. *Endocr Relat Cancer.* 2000;7(4):227–242.
16. Holcomb K, Delatorre R, Pedemonte B, McLeod C, Anderson L, Chambers J. E-cadherin expression in endometrioid, papillary serous, and clear cell carcinoma of the endometrium. *Obstet Gynecol.* 2002;100(6):1290–1295.
17. Santin AD, Bellone S, Van Stedum S, et al. Determination of HER2/neu status in uterine serous papillary carcinoma: comparative analysis of immunohistochemistry and fluorescence in situ hybridization. *Gynecol Oncol.* 2005;98(1):24–30.

18. Santin AD, Bellone S, Van Stedum S, et al. Amplification of c-erbB2 oncogene: a major prognostic indicator in uterine serous papillary carcinoma. *Cancer.* 2005;104(7):1391–1397.

19. Llauradó M, Ruiz A, Majem B, et al. Molecular bases of endometrial cancer: new roles for new actors in the diagnosis and the therapy of the disease. *Mol Cell Endocrinol.* 2012;358(2):244–255.

20. Wiegand KC, Lee AF, Al-Agha OM, et al. Loss of BAF250a (ARID1A) is frequent in high-grade endometrial carcinomas. *J Pathol.* 2011;224(3):328–333.

21. Nagendra DC, Burke J 3rd, Maxwell GL, Risinger JI. PPP2R1A mutations are common in the serous type of endometrial cancer. *Mol Carcinog.* 2012;51(10):826–831.

22. Chan JK, Manuel MR, Cheung MK, et al. Breast cancer followed by corpus cancer: is there a higher risk for aggressive histologic subtypes? *Gynecol Oncol.* 2006;102(3):508–512.

23. Lavie O, Ben-Arie A, Segev Y, et al. BRCA germline mutations in women with uterine serous carcinoma–still a debate. *Int J Gynecol Cancer.* 2010;20(9):1531–1534.

24. Goshen R, Chu W, Elit L, et al. Is uterine papillary serous adenocarcinoma a manifestation of the hereditary breast-ovarian cancer syndrome? *Gynecol Oncol.* 2000;79(3):477–481.

25. McCluggage WG, Sumathi VP, McManus DT. Uterine serous carcinoma and endometrial intraepithelial carcinoma arising in endometrial polyps: report of 5 cases, including 2 associated with tamoxifen therapy. *Hum Pathol.* 2003;34(9):939–943.

26. Silva EG, Tornos CS, Follen-Mitchell M. Malignant neoplasms of the uterine corpus in patients treated for breast carcinoma: the effects of tamoxifen. *Int J Gynecol Pathol.* 1994;13(3):248–258.

27. Magriples U, Naftolin F, Schwartz PE, Carcangiu ML. High-grade endometrial carcinoma in tamoxifen-treated breast cancer patients. *J Clin Oncol.* 1993;11(3):485–490.

28. Bland AE, Calingaert B, Secord AA, et al. Relationship between tamoxifen use and high risk endometrial cancer histologic types. *Gynecol Oncol.* 2009;112(1):150–154.

29. Fisher B, Costantino JP, Wickerham DL, et al. Tamoxifen for the prevention of breast cancer: current status of the National Surgical Adjuvant Breast and Bowel Project P-1 study. *J Natl Cancer Inst.* 2005;97(22):1652–1662.

30. Wagoner JK. Leukemia and other malignancies following radiation therapy for gynecological disorders. In: Boice JF, Fraumeni JD. eds *Radiation Carcinogenesis: Epidemiology and Biological Significance.* New York, NY: Raven Press; 2007:153–159.

31. Gallion HH, van Nagell JR Jr, Donaldson ES, Powell DE. Endometrial cancer following radiation therapy for cervical cancer. *Gynecol Oncol.* 1987;27(1):76–83.

32. Pothuri B, Ramondetta L, Martino M, et al. Development of endometrial cancer after radiation treatment for cervical carcinoma. *Obstet Gynecol.* 2003;101(5 Pt 1):941–945.

33. Behtash N, Tehranian A, Ardalan FA, Hanjani P. Uterine papillary serous carcinoma after pelvic radiation therapy for cancer of the cervix. *J Obstet Gynaecol.* 2002;22(1):96–97.

34. Parkash V, Carcangiu ML. Uterine papillary serous carcinoma after radiation therapy for carcinoma of the cervix. *Cancer.* 1992;69(2):496–501.

35. Fader AN, Boruta D, Olawaiye AB, Gehrig PA. Uterine papillary serous carcinoma: epidemiology, pathogenesis and management. *Curr Opin Obstet Gynecol.* 2010;22(1):21–29.

36. CA, Cheung MK, Osann K, et al. Uterine papillary serous and clear cell carcinomas predict for poorer survival compared to grade 3 endometrioid corpus cancers. *Br J Cancer* 2006; 94(5): 642–646.

37. Boruta DM 2nd, Gehrig PA, Fader AN, Olawaiye AB. Management of women with uterine papillary serous cancer: a Society of Gynecologic Oncology (SGO) review. *Gynecol Oncol.* 2009;115(1):142–153.

38. Mittal KR, Tavassoli FA, Prat J, et al. Tumours of the ovary and peritoneum. In: *World Health Organization—Tumours of the Breast and Female Genital System.* Lyon, France: IARC Press; 2003:113–145.

39. Carcangiu ML, Chambers JT. Uterine papillary serous carcinoma: a study on 108 cases with emphasis on the prognostic significance of associated endometrioid carcinoma, absence of invasion, and concomitant ovarian carcinoma. *Gynecol Oncol.* 1992;47(3):298–305.

40. Boruta DM 2nd, Gehrig PA, Groben PA, et al. Uterine serous and grade 3 endometrioid carcinomas: is there a survival difference? *Cancer.* 2004;101(10):2214–2221.

41. Lim YK, Padma R, Foo L, et al. Survival outcome of women with synchronous cancers of endometrium and ovary: a 10 year retrospective cohort study. *J Gynecol Oncol.* 2011;22(4):239–243.

42. Baergen RN, Warren CD, Isacson C, Ellenson LH. Early uterine serous carcinoma: clonal origin of extrauterine disease. *Int J Gynecol Pathol.* 2001;20(3):214–219.

43. Koss LG, Schreiber K, Oberlander SG, Moukhtar M, Levine HS, Moussouris HF. Screening of asymptomatic women for endometrial cancer. *CA Cancer J Clin.* 1981;31(5):300–317.

44. Goldstein RB, Bree RL, Benson CB, et al. Evaluation of the woman with postmenopausal bleeding: Society of Radiologists in Ultrasound-Sponsored Consensus Conference statement. *J Ultrasound Med.* 2001;20(10):1025–1036.

45. Grigoriou O, Kalovidouros A, Papadias C, Antoniou G, Antonaki V, Giannikos L. Transvaginal sonography of the endometrium in women with postmenopausal bleeding. *Maturitas.* 1996;23(1):9–14.

46. Wang J, Wieslander C, Hansen G, Cass I, Vasilev S, Holschneider CH. Thin endometrial echo complex on ultrasound does not reliably exclude type 2 endometrial cancers. *Gynecol Oncol.* 2006;101(1):120–125.

47. Faratian D, Stillie A, Busby-Earle RM, Cowie VJ, Monaghan H. A review of the pathology and management of uterine papillary serous carcinoma and correlation with outcome. *Int J Gynecol Cancer.* 2006;16(3):972–978.

48. Lampe B, Kürlz R, Hantschmann P. Reliability of tumor typing of endometrial carcinoma in pre-hysterectomy curettage. *Int J Gynecol Pathol.* 1995;14:2–6.

49. Schwartz PE. The management of serous papillary uterine cancer. *Curr Opin Oncol.* 2006;18(5):494–499.

50. Gupta D, Gunter MJ, Yang K, et al. Performance of serum CA125 as a prognostic biomarker in patients with uterine papillary serous carcinoma. *Int J Gynecol Cancer.* 2011;21(3):529–534.

51. Price FV, Chambers SK, Carcangiu ML, Kohorn EI, Schwartz PE, Chambers JT. CA 125 may not reflect disease status in patients with uterine serous carcinoma. *Cancer.* 1998;82(9):1720–1725.

52. Cocco E, Bellone S, El-Sahwi K, et al. Serum amyloid A (SAA): a novel biomarker for uterine serous papillary cancer. *Br J Cancer.* 2009;101(2):335–341.

53. Santin AD, Diamandis EP, Bellone S, et al. Human kallikrein 6: a new potential serum biomarker for uterine serous papillary cancer. *Clin Cancer Res.* 2005;11(9):3320–3325.

54. Santin AD, Diamandis EP, Bellone S, et al. Overexpression of kallikrein 10 (hK10) in uterine serous papillary carcinomas. *Am J Obstet Gynecol.* 2006;194(5):1296–1302.

55. Dizon DS. Treatment options for advanced endometrial carcinoma. *Gynecol Oncol.* 2010;117(2):373–381.

56. Goff BA, Kato D, Schmidt RA, et al. Uterine papillary serous carcinoma: patterns of metastatic spread. *Gynecol Oncol.* 1994;54(3):264–268.

57. Goff BA. Uterine papillary serous carcinoma: what have we learned over the past quarter century? *Gynecol Oncol.* 2005;98(3):341–343.

58. Gehrig PA, Groben PA, Fowler WC Jr, Walton LA, Van Le L. Noninvasive papillary serous carcinoma of the endometrium. *Obstet Gynecol.* 2001;97(1):153–157.

59. Gehrig PA, Van Le L, Fowler WC Jr. The role of omentectomy during the surgical staging of uterine serous carcinoma. *Int J Gynecol Cancer.* 2003;13(2):212–215.

60. Chan JK, Loizzi V, Youssef M, et al. Significance of comprehensive surgical staging in noninvasive papillary serous carcinoma of the endometrium. *Gynecol Oncol.* 2003;90(1):181–185.

61. Geisler JP, Geisler HE, Melton ME, Wiemann MC. What staging surgery should be performed on patients with uterine papillary serous carcinoma? *Gynecol Oncol.* 1999;74(3):465–467.

62. Walker JL, Piedmonte MR, Spirtos NM, et al. Recurrence and survival after random assignment to laparoscopy versus laparotomy for comprehensive surgical staging of uterine cancer: Gynecologic Oncology Group LAP2 Study. *J Clin Oncol.* 2012;30(7):695–700.

63. Gallion HH, Brunetto VL, Cibull M, et al.; Gynecologic Oncology Group Study. Randomized phase III trial of standard timed doxorubicin plus cisplatin versus circadian timed doxorubicin plus cisplatin in stage III and IV or recurrent endometrial carcinoma: a Gynecologic Oncology Group study. *J Clin Oncol.* 2003;21(20):3808–3813.

64. Fleming GF, Brunetto VL, Cella D, et al. Phase III trial of doxorubicin plus cisplatin with or without paclitaxel plus filgrastim in advanced endometrial carcinoma: a Gynecologic Oncology Group study. *J Clin Oncol.* 2004;22(11):2159–2166.

65. Fleming GF, Filiaci VL, Bentley RC, et al. Phase III randomized trial of doxorubicin + cisplatin versus doxorubicin + 24-h paclitaxel + filgrastim in endometrial carcinoma: a Gynecologic Oncology Group study. *Ann Oncol.* 2004;15(8):1173–1178.

66. Thigpen JT, Brady MF, Homesley HD, et al. Phase III trial of doxorubicin with or without cisplatin in advanced endometrial carcinoma: a Gynecologic Oncology Group study. *J Clin Oncol.* 2004;22(19):3902–3908.

67. Homesley HD, Filiaci V, Gibbons SK, et al. A randomized phase III trial in advanced endometrial carcinoma of surgery and volume directed radiation followed by cisplatin and doxorubicin with or without paclitaxel: a Gynecologic Oncology Group study. *Gynecol Oncol.* 2009;112(3):543–552.

68. Miller D, Filiaci V, Fleming G, et al. Randomized phase III non-inferiority trial of first-line chemotherapy for metastatic or recurrent endometrial carcinoma: a Gynecologic Oncology Group study (late-breaking abstract). *Annual Meeting of the Society of Gynecologic Oncologists.* 2012, Mar 24–7, Austin, TX.

69. Sovak MA, Hensley ML, Dupont J, et al. Paclitaxel and carboplatin in the adjuvant treatment of patients with high-risk stage III and IV endometrial cancer: a retrospective study. *Gynecol Oncol.* 2006;103(2):451–457.

70. National Comprehensive Cancer Network. Practice Guidelines: Uterine Neoplasms, v 3.2012. Available at http://www.nccn.org/professionals/physician_gls/pdf/uterine.pdf.

71. Moller KA, Gehrig PA, Van Le L, Secord AA, Schorge J. The role of optimal debulking in advanced stage serous carcinoma of the uterus. *Gynecol Oncol.* 2004;94(1):170–174.

72. Resnik E, Taxy JB. Neoadjuvant chemotherapy in uterine papillary serous carcinoma. *Gynecol Oncol.* 1996;62(1):123–127.

73. Le TD, Yamada SD, Rutgers JL, DiSaia PJ. Complete response of a stage IV uterine papillary serous carcinoma to neoadjuvant chemotherapy with Taxol and carboplatin. *Gynecol Oncol.* 1999;73(3):461–463.

74. Price FV, Amin RM, Sumkin J. Complete clinical responses to neoadjuvant chemotherapy for uterine serous carcinoma. *Gynecol Oncol.* 1999;73(1):140–144.

75. Lupe K, D'Souza DP, Kwon JS, et al. Adjuvant carboplatin and paclitaxel chemotherapy interposed with involved field radiation for advanced endometrial cancer. *Gynecol Oncol.* 2009;114(1):94–98.

76. Einstein MH, Frimer M, Kuo DY, et al. Phase II trial of adjuvant pelvic radiation "sandwiched" between combination paclitaxel and carboplatin in women with uterine papillary serous carcinoma. *Gynecol Oncol.* 2012;124(1):21–25.

77. Sutton G, Axelrod JH, Bundy BN, et al. Adjuvant whole abdominal irradiation in clinical stages I and II papillary serous or clear cell carcinoma of the endometrium: a phase II study of the Gynecologic Oncology Group. *Gynecol Oncol.* 2006;100(2):349–354.

78. Frank AH, Tseng PC, Haffty BG, et al. Adjuvant whole-abdominal radiation therapy in uterine papillary serous carcinoma. *Cancer.* 1991;68(7):1516–1519.

79. Fader AN, Drake RD, O'Malley DM, et al.; Uterine Papillary Serous Carcinoma (UPSC) Consortium. Platinum/taxane-based chemotherapy with or without radiation therapy favorably impacts survival outcomes in stage I uterine papillary serous carcinoma. *Cancer.* 2009;115(10):2119–2127.

80. Dietrich CS, Modesitt SC, DePriest PD, et al. The efficacy of adjuvant platinum-based chemotherapy in stage I uterine papillary serous carcinoma (UPSC). *Gynecol Oncol.* 2005;99:557–563.

81. Boren TP, Miller DS. Should all patients with serous and clear cell endometrial carcinoma receive adjuvant chemotherapy? *Womens Health (Lond Engl).* 2010;6(6):789–795.

82. Hamilton CA, Liou WS, Osann K, et al. Impact of adjuvant therapy on survival of patients with early-stage uterine papillary serous carcinoma. *Int J Radiat Oncol Biol Phys.* 2005;63(3):839–844.

83. Kelly MG, O'Malley DM, Hui P, et al. Improved survival in surgical stage I patients with uterine papillary serous carcinoma (UPSC) treated with adjuvant platinum-based chemotherapy. *Gynecol Oncol.* 2005;98(3):353–359.

84. Alektiar KM, Makker V, Abu-Rustum NR, et al. Concurrent carboplatin/paclitaxel and intravaginal radiation in surgical stage I-II serous endometrial cancer. *Gynecol Oncol.* 2009;112(1):142–145.

85. Silva EG, Jenkins R. Serous carcinoma in endometrial polyps. *Mod Pathol.* 1990;3(2):120–128.

86. Trahan S, Têtu B, Raymond PE. Serous papillary carcinoma of the endometrium arising from endometrial polyps: a clinical, histological, and immunohistochemical study of 13 cases. *Hum Pathol.* 2005;36(12):1316–1321.

87. Wheeler DT, Bell KA, Kurman RJ, Sherman ME. Minimal uterine serous carcinoma: diagnosis and clinicopathologic correlation. *Am J Surg Pathol.* 2000;24(6):797–806.

88. Hui P, Kelly M, O'Malley DM, Tavassoli F, Schwartz PE. Minimal uterine serous carcinoma: a clinicopathological study of 40 cases. *Mod Pathol.* 2005;18(1):75–82.

89. Slomovitz BM, Burke TW, Eifel PJ, et al. Uterine papillary serous carcinoma (UPSC): a single institution review of 129 cases. *Gynecol Oncol.* 2003;91(3):463–469.

90. Ambros RA, Sherman ME, Zahn CM, Bitterman P, Kurman RJ. Endometrial intraepithelial carcinoma: a distinctive lesion specifically associated with tumors displaying serous differentiation. *Hum Pathol.* 1995;26(11):1260–1267.

91. Soslow RA, Pirog E, Isacson C. Endometrial intraepithelial carcinoma with associated peritoneal carcinomatosis. *Am J Surg Pathol.* 2000;24(5):726–732.

92. Giuntoli RL 2nd, Gerardi MA, Yemelyanova AV, et al. Stage I noninvasive and minimally invasive uterine serous carcinoma: comprehensive staging associated with improved survival. *Int J Gynecol Cancer.* 2012;22(2):273–279.

93. Kadar N, Homesley HD, Malfetano JH. Positive peritoneal cytology is an adverse factor in endometrial carcinoma only if there is other evidence of extrauterine disease. *Gynecol Oncol.* 1992;46(2):145–149.

94. Fadare O, Mariappan MR, Hileeto D, Wang S, McAlpine JN, Rimm DL. Upstaging based solely on positive peritoneal washing does not affect outcome in endometrial cancer. *Mod Pathol.* 2005;18(5):673–680.

95. Preyer O, Obermair A, Formann E, et al. The impact of positive peritoneal washings and serosal and adnexal involvement on survival in patients with stage IIIA uterine cancer. *Gynecol Oncol.* 2002;86(3):269–273.

96. Havrilesky LJ, Cragun JM, Calingaert B, et al. The prognostic significance of positive peritoneal cytology and adnexal/serosal metastasis in stage IIIA endometrial cancer. *Gynecol Oncol.* 2007;104(2):401–405.

97. Chang YN, Zhang Y, Wang YJ, Wang LP, Duan H. Effect of hysteroscopy on the peritoneal dissemination of endometrial cancer cells: a meta-analysis. *Fertil Steril.* 2011;96(4):957–961.

98. Benevolo M, Vocaturo A, Novelli F, et al. Prognostic value of HER2 and progesterone receptor expression in endometrial carcinoma with positive peritoneal washing. *Anticancer Res.* 2007;27(4C):2839–2844.

99. Szpak CA, Creasman WT, Vollmer RT, Johnston WW. Prognostic value of cytologic examination of peritoneal washings in patients with endometrial carcinoma. *Acta Cytol.* 1981;25(6):640–646.

100. Yanoh K, Takeshima N, Hirai Y, et al. Morphologic analyses of positive peritoneal cytology in endometrial carcinoma. *Acta Cytol.* 1999;43(5):814–819.

101. Kelly MG, O'Malley D, Hui P, et al. Patients with uterine papillary serous cancers may benefit from adjuvant platinum-based chemoradiation. *Gynecol Oncol.* 2004;95(3):469–473.

102. Alobaid A, Bruchim I, Verkooijen H, Gauthier P, Petignat P. Adjuvant therapy for patients with stage I papillary serous endometrial cancer. *Eur J Surg Oncol.* 2006;32(3):358–362.

103. Aquino-Parsons C, Lim P, Wong F, Mildenberger M. Papillary serous and clear cell carcinoma limited to endometrial curettings in FIGO stage 1a and 1b endometrial adenocarcinoma: treatment implications. *Gynecol Oncol.* 1998;71(1):83–86.

104. Yarden Y, Sliwkowski MX. Untangling the ErbB signalling network. *Nat Rev Mol Cell Biol.* 2001;2(2):127–137.

105. Slomovitz BM, Broaddus RR, Burke TW, et al. Her-2/neu overexpression and amplification in uterine papillary serous carcinoma. *J Clin Oncol.* 2004;22(15):3126–3132.

106. Grushko TA, Filiaci VL, Mundt AJ, Ridderstråle K, Olopade OI, Fleming GF; Gynecologic Oncology Group. An exploratory analysis of HER-2 amplification and overexpression in advanced endometrial carcinoma: a Gynecologic Oncology Group study. *Gynecol Oncol.* 2008;108(1):3–9.

107. Díaz-Montes TP, Ji H, Smith Sehdev AE, et al. Clinical significance of Her-2/neu overexpression in uterine serous carcinoma. *Gynecol Oncol.* 2006;100(1):139–144.

108. Berchuck A, Rodriguez G, Kinney RB, et al. Overexpression of HER-2/neu in endometrial cancer is associated with advanced stage disease. *Am J Obstet Gynecol.* 1991;164(1 Pt 1):15–21.

109. Santin AD, Zhan F, Bellone S, et al. Discrimination between uterine serous papillary carcinomas and ovarian serous papillary tumours by gene expression profiling. *Br J Cancer.* 2004;90(9):1814–1824.

110. Arnould L, Gelly M, Penault-Llorca F, et al. Trastuzumab-based treatment of HER2-positive breast cancer: an antibody-dependent cellular cytotoxicity mechanism? *Br J Cancer.* 2006;94(2):259–267.

111. Santin AD, Bellone S, Roman JJ, McKenney JK, Pecorelli S. Trastuzumab treatment in patients with advanced or recurrent endometrial carcinoma overexpressing HER2/neu. *Int J Gynaecol Obstet.* 2008;102(2):128–131.

112. Jewell E, Secord AA, Brotherton T, Berchuck A. Use of trastuzumab in the treatment of metastatic endometrial cancer. *Int J Gynecol Cancer.* 2006;16(3):1370–1373.

113. Villella JA, Cohen S, Smith DH, Hibshoosh H, Hershman D. HER-2/neu overexpression in uterine papillary serous cancers and its possible therapeutic implications. *Int J Gynecol Cancer.* 2006;16(5):1897–1902.

114. Fleming GF, Sill MW, Darcy KM, et al. Phase II trial of trastuzumab in women with advanced or recurrent, HER2-positive endometrial carcinoma: a Gynecologic Oncology Group study. *Gynecol Oncol.* 2010;116(1):15–20.

115. Santin AD. Letter to the Editor referring to the manuscript entitled: "Phase II trial of trastuzumab in women with advanced or recurrent HER-positive endometrial carcinoma: a Gynecologic Oncology Group study" recently reported by Fleming et al., (Gynecol Oncol., 116;15–20;2010). *Gynecol Oncol.* 2010;118(1):95–96; author reply 96.

116. NIH Clinical Trials. Evaluation of carboplatin/paclitaxel with or without trastuzumab (Herceptin) in uterine serous cancer. http://clinicaltrials.gov/ct2/show/NCT01367002. Accessed August, 2012.

117. Kamat AA, Merritt WM, Coffey D, et al. Clinical and biological significance of vascular endothelial growth factor in endometrial cancer. *Clin Cancer Res.* 2007;13(24):7487–7495.

118. Hirai M, Nakagawara A, Oosaki T, et al. Expression of vascular endothelial growth factors (VEGF-A/VEGF-1and VEGF-C/VEGF-2) in postmenopausal uterine endometrial carcinoma. *Gyneol Oncol.* 2011;80:180–188.

119. Mazurek A, Pierzynski P, Kuc P, et al. Evaluation of angiogenesis, p-53 tissue protein expression and serum VEGF in patients with endometrial cancer. *Neoplasma.* 2004;51(3):193–197.

120. Gerber HP, Ferrara N. Pharmacology and pharmacodynamics of bevacizumab as monotherapy or in combination with cytotoxic therapy in preclinical studies. *Cancer Res.* 2005;65(3):671–680.

121. Aghajanian C, Sill MW, Darcy KM, et al. Phase II trial of bevacizumab in recurrent or persistent endometrial cancer: a Gynecologic Oncology Group study. *J Clin Oncol.* 2011;29(16):2259–2265.

122. NIH Clinical Trials. Evaluation of carboplatin/paclitaxel/bevacizumab in the treatment of advanced stage endometrial carcinoma. http://clinicaltrials.gov/ct2/show/NCT00513786. Accessed August, 2012.

123. Paclitaxel, carboplatin, and bevacizumab or paclitaxel, carboplatin, and temsirolimus or ixabepilone, carboplatin, bevacizumab in treating patients with stage III, stage IV, or recurrent endometrial cancer. http://clinicaltrials.gov/ct2/show/NCT00977574. Accessed August, 2012.

124. NIH Clinical Trials. VEGF Trap in treating patients with recurrent or persistent endometrial cancer. http://clinicaltrials.gov/ct2/show/NCT00462826. Accessed August, 2012.

125. El-Sahwi K, Bellone S, Cocco E, et al. Overexpression of EpCAM in uterine serous papillary carcinoma: implications for EpCAM-specific immunotherapy with human monoclonal antibody adecatumumab (MT201). *Mol Cancer Ther.* 2010;9(1):57–66.

126. Varughese J, Cocco E, Bellone S, et al. Uterine serous papillary carcinomas overexpress human trophoblast-cell-surface marker (Trop-2) and are highly sensitive to immunotherapy with hRS7, a humanized anti-Trop-2 monoclonal antibody. *Cancer.* 2011;117(14):3163–3172.

127. Bellone M, Cocco E, Varughese J, et al. Expression of aV-integrins in uterine serous papillary carcinomas; implications for targeted therapy with intetumumab (CNTO 95), a fully human antagonist anti-aV-integrin antibody. *Int J Gynecol Cancer.* 2011;21(6):1084–1090.

128. Bellone S, Roque D, Cocco E, et al. Down-regulation of membrane complement inhibitors CD55 and CD59 by siRNA sensitizes uterine serous carcinoma overexpressing HER2/neu to complement and antibody-dependent-cell-cytotoxicity in vitro: implications for trastuzumab-based immunotherapy. *Br J Cancer.* 2012;106(9):1543–1550.

129. McMeekin DS, Filiaci VL, Thigpen JT, Gallion HH, Fleming GF, Rodgers WH; Gynecologic Oncology Group study. The relationship between histology and outcome in advanced and recurrent endometrial cancer patients participating in first-line chemotherapy trials: a Gynecologic Oncology Group study. *Gynecol Oncol.* 2007;106(1):16–22.

130. Kavallaris M, Kuo DY, Burkhart CA, et al. Taxol-resistant epithelial ovarian tumors are associated with altered expression of specific beta-tubulin isotypes. *J Clin Invest.* 1997;100(5):1282–1293.

131. Magnani M, Ortuso F, Soro S, Alcaro S, Tramontano A, Botta M. The betaI/betaIII-tubulin isoforms and their complexes with antimitotic agents. Docking and molecular dynamics studies. *FEBS J.* 2006;273(14):3301–3310.

132. Ferlini C, Raspaglio G, Cicchillitti L, et al. Looking at drug resistance mechanisms for microtubule interacting drugs: does TUBB3 work? *Curr Cancer Drug Targets.* 2007;7(8):704–712.

133. Ferrandina G, Zannoni GF, Martinelli E, et al. Class III beta-tubulin overexpression is a marker of poor clinical outcome in advanced ovarian cancer patients. *Clin Cancer Res.* 2006;12(9):2774–2779.

134. Roque DM, Bellone S, Buza N, et al. Class III β-tubulin overexpression in ovarian clear cell and serous carcinoma as a maker for poor overall survival after platinum/taxane chemotherapy and sensitivity to patupilone. *Am J Obstet Gynecol.* 2013;209(1): 62–64.)

135. Sève P, Isaac S, Trédan O, et al. Expression of class III {beta}-tubulin is predictive of patient outcome in patients with non-small cell lung cancer receiving vinorelbine-based chemotherapy. *Clin Cancer Res.* 2005;11(15):5481–5486.

136. Paradiso A, Mangia A, Chiriatti A, et al. Biomarkers predictive for clinical efficacy of taxol-based chemotherapy in advanced breast cancer. *Ann Oncol.* 2005;16 (Suppl 4):14–19.

137. Bollag DM, McQueney PA, Zhu J, et al. Epothilones, a new class of microtubule-stabilizing agents with a taxol-like mechanism of action. *Cancer Res.* 1995;55(11):2325–2333.

138. Roque DM, Bellone S, English DP, et al. Tubulin-β-III overexpression by uterine serous carcinomas is a marker for poor overall survival after platinum/taxane chemotherapy and sensitivity to epothilones. *Cancer.* 2013 Jul 15;119(14):2582–2589.

139. Paik D, Cocco E, Bellone S, et al. Higher sensitivity to patupilone versus paclitaxel chemotherapy in primary uterine serous papillary carcinoma cell lines with high versus low HER-2/neu expression *in vitro. Gynecol Oncol.* 2010;119(1):140–145.

140. Rubin EH, Rothermel J, Tesfaye F, et al. Phase I dose-finding study of weekly single-agent patupilone in patients with advanced solid tumors. *J Clin Oncol.* 2005;23(36):9120–9129.

141. Ten Bokkel Huinink WW, Sufliarsky J, Smit WM, et al. Safety and efficacy of patupilone in patients with advanced ovarian, primary fallopian, or primary peritoneal cancer: a phase I, open-label, dose-escalation study. *J Clin Oncol.* 2009;27(19):3097–3103.

142. Bystricky B, Chau I. Patupilone in cancer treatment. *Expert Opin Investig Drugs.* 2011;20(1):107–117.

143. NIH Clinical Trials. Patupilone versus doxorubicin in patients with ovarian, primary fallopian, or peritoneal cancer. http://clinicaltrials.gov/ct2/show/NCT00262990. Accessed August, 2012.

144. De Geest K, Blessing JA, Morris RT, et al. Phase II clinical trial of ixabepilone in patients with recurrent or persistent platinum- and taxane-resistant ovarian or primary peritoneal cancer: a gynecologic oncology group study. *J Clin Oncol.* 2010;28(1): 149–153.

145. Dizon DS, Blessing JA, McMeekin DS, Sharma SK, Disilvestro P, Alvarez RD. Phase II trial of ixabepilone as second-line treatment in advanced endometrial cancer: gynecologic oncology group trial 129-P. *J Clin Oncol.* 2009;27(19):3104–3108.

146. Paclitaxel, carboplatin, and bevacizumab or paclitaxel, carboplatin, and temsirolimus or ixabepilone, carboplatin, bevacizumab in treating patients with stage III, stage IV, or recurrent endometrial cancer. http://clinicaltrials.gov/ct2/show/NCT00977574. Accessed August, 2012.

147. Gehrig PA, Bae-Jump VL. Promising novel therapies for the treatment of endometrial cancer. *Gynecol Oncol.* 2010;116(2): 187–194.

148. Byron SA, Gartside MG, Wellens CL, et al. Inhibition of activated fibroblast growth factor receptor 2 in endometrial cancer cells induces cell death despite PTEN abrogation. *Cancer Res.* 2008;68(17):6902–6907.

149. NIH Clinical Trials. A Phase II study to evaluate the efficacy of TKI258 for the treatment of patients with FGFR2 mutated or wild-type advanced and/or metastatic endometrial cancer. http://clinicaltrials.gov/ct2/show/NCT01379534. Accessed August, 2012.

150. Hayes MP, Douglas W, Ellenson LH. Molecular alterations of EGFR and PIK3CA in uterine serous carcinoma. *Gynecol Oncol.* 2009;113(3):370–373.

151. Bader AG, Kang S, Vogt PK. Cancer-specific mutations in PIK3CA are oncogenic in vivo. *Proc Natl Acad Sci USA.* 2006; 103(5):1475–1479.

152. Oza AM, Elit L, Biagi J, et al. Molecular correlates associated with a phase II study of temsirolimus (CCI-779) in patients with metastatic or recurrent endometrial cancer-NCICIND 160. *J Clin Oncol.* 2006;24 (Suppl):abstract 3003.

153. Oza AM, Elit L, Provencher D, et al. A phase II study of temsirolimus (CCI-779) in patients with metastatic and/or locally advanced recurrent endometrial cancer previously treated with chemotherapy: NCIC GTC INC 160b. *J Clin Oncol.* 2008;26(Suppl):abstract 5516.

154. Fleming GF, Filiaci VL, Hanjani P, et al. Hormone therapy plus temsirolimus for endometrial carcinoma (EC): a Gyencologic Oncology Group trial (#248). *J Clin Oncol.* 2011;29(Suppl): abstract 5014.

155. Gold MA, Brady WE, Lankes HA, et al. A phase II study of a urokinase-derived peptide (A6) in the treatment of persistent or recurrent epithelial ovarian, fallopian tube, or primary peritoneal carcinoma: a Gynecologic Oncology Group study. *Gynecol Oncol.* 2012;125(3):635–639.

156. Slomovitz BM, Brown J, Johnston TA, et al. A phase II study of everolimus and letrozole in patients with recurrent endometrial carcinoma. *J Clin Oncol.* 2011;29(Supple):abstract 5012.

157. Mackay H, Welch S, Tsao MS, et al. Phase II study of oral ridoforolimus in patients with metastatic and/or locally advanced recurrent endometrial cancer: NCIC CTG IND 192. *J Clin Oncol.* 2011;29(Suppl):abstract 5013.

158. Oza AM, Poveda A, Clamp AR, et al. A randomized phase II trial of ridaforolimus compared with progestin or chemotherapy in female adult patients with advanced endometrial carcinoma. *J Clin Oncol.* 2011;29(Suppl); abstract 5009.

159. Zhao S, Choi M, Overton JD, et al. Landscape of somatic single-nucleotide and copy-number mutations in uterine serous carcinoma. *Proc Natl Acad Sci USA.* 2013;110(8):2916–2921.

12 Multidisciplinary Approach to Diagnosis and Treatment of Uterine Sarcomas

MATTHEW L. ANDERSON

NONNA KOLOMEYEVSKAYA

Uterine sarcomas are rare but potentially aggressive cancers. This review focuses on the uterine sarcomas most commonly encountered by oncologists: uterine leiomyosarcoma (ULMS) and endometrial stromal sarcomas (ESS). Emphasis will be placed on the diagnosis and current management of these diseases. Recent translational insights will also be discussed with an eye toward understanding emerging treatment options. A summary of the World Health Organization (WHO) classification for these tumors is presented in Table 12.1.

■ UTERINE LEIOMYOSARCOMA

The human myometrium retains a singular capacity to undergo dramatic cycles of remodeling throughout the reproductive life span of a woman. Perhaps reflecting this retained plasticity, benign proliferations of uterine smooth muscle, known as leiomyomas, can be found in as many as 80% of women (1). Clinically, leiomyomas frequently cause problems with pelvic pain and vaginal bleeding, and are the leading indication for hysterectomy in the United States. In contrast, ULMS is a relatively rare disease. According to the Surveillance Epidemiology and End Results (SEER) database, the incidence of ULMS is approximately 0.8 per 100,000 women (2). This means that ULMS accounts for approximately 1% of all uterine cancers. Similar to leiomyomas, ULMS occur more commonly in African American women. Symptoms associated with ULMS include abdominal pain (35%), abnormal vaginal bleeding (53%), and a palpable abdominal mass (14%; 3).

Diagnosis

Most ULMS are diagnosed only after a woman has undergone surgery for management of intractable symptoms such as vaginal bleeding that are thought to be due to benign causes, such as leiomyomas or even adenomyosis.

Unfortunately, the clinical tools currently used to evaluate vaginal bleeding are not typically able to diagnose leiomyosarcoma prior to surgery. As discussed below, imaging modalities may identify a uterine mass but often cannot reliably distinguish leiomyomas from a leiomyosarcoma (4). Ultimately, diagnosis of ULMS relies exclusively on the presence of a limited number of histologic features. These include an elevated mitotic tumor index (typically greater than 10 mitoses per 10 high power fields [hpf]), atypia, and coagulative tumor necrosis (5). These criteria can be subjective and their histologic presentation often makes differentiating leiomyomas from leiomyosarcomas surprisingly difficult. The ability to establish a firm diagnosis can be further complicated by the fact that bland smooth muscle proliferations can behave similarly to a cancer, invading vascular spaces (intravascular leiomyomatosis), or presenting at distant sites (benign metastasizing leiomyomas; 6,7). This situation has led to a plethora of diagnostic categories over the years that can be best summarized by dividing uterine smooth muscle tumors into three broad categories: atypical leiomyomas, smooth muscle tumors of uncertain malignant potential (STUMP), and leiomyosarcomas (Table 12.1). Not infrequently, atypia or even a mildly elevated mitotic rate (less than 5/10 hpf) can be found in leiomyomas. Under these circumstances, surgical excision of the mass is usually sufficient to prevent its recurrence (8). This appears to be true even in situations where conservative surgery such as myomectomy has been used. In contrast, mitotic rates as high as 80 to 100 mitoses per 10 hpf can be observed in ULMS. In the context of greater than or equal to 10 mitoses per 10 hpf, the presence of both coagulative tumor necrosis and atypical cells with irregular nuclei establish the diagnosis. Coagulative tumor necrosis is characterized by an abrupt transition from viable to necrotic tissue and lacks the hyalinized transition found when leiomyomas undergo degeneration. The histologic features characteristic of ULMS can often be subtle. Clinical evidence suggests that many uterine smooth muscle tumors with questionable features may be associated with more benign outcomes than those observed with ULMS. These tumors are now categorized as smooth muscle tumors of uncertain malignant potential (STUMP). At our institution, we utilize

■ **Table 12.1** Classification of uterine sarcomas and mesenchymal tumors

Smooth Muscle Tumors
    Leiomyoma
        Histologic Variants
            Mitotically Active
            Cellular
            Epithelioid
            Myxoid
            Atypical
            Lipoleiomyoma
        Growth Variants
            Intravenous
            Metastasizing
            Dissecting
    Smooth Muscle Tumor of Uncertain Malignant Potential
      (STUMP)
    Leiomyosarcoma
        Epithelioid
        Myxoid
Endometrial Tumors
    Endometrial Stromal Nodule
    Endometrial Stromal Sarcoma
    Undifferentiated Endometrial Sarcoma
Miscellaneous
    Perivascular Epithelioid Cell
    Adenomatoid
    Other

a system for diagnosing STUMP tumors as outlined by Malpica and colleagues (9). These criteria include smooth muscle proliferation with tumor cell necrosis, no atypia, and fewer than 10 mitoses per 10 hpf; masses with diffuse atypia, no tumor cell necrosis, and fewer than 10 mitoses per 10 hpf; masses with fewer than 20 mitoses per 10 hpf without tumor cell necrosis, or atypia; masses with cellularity/hypercellularity and more than 4 mitoses per 10 hpf and irregular margins, or vascular invasion at the periphery of the tumor. This system is based on the criteria established by Peters in his initial description of STUMP (10). STUMP also correspond to the category of "low grade" ULMS frequently described by Hensley and collaborators in the literature (11). Regardless of terminology, however, clinical outcomes for STUMP or low grade ULMS appear good. Recurrence rates are typically low, ranging from 5% to 8%, but can occur many years after the initial diagnosis (12). In one recent case series, only three of 42 patients diagnosed with STUMP experienced a recurrence of their disease. On an average, these recurrences occurred 43months (range 19–67 months) from the time of diagnosis (9). Two of these recurrences were histologically similar to the initial tumor, while one appeared most consistent with leiomyosarcoma. However, long-term survival was good for all patients (greater than 120 months), including women diagnosed with ULMS at recurrence. These experiences as well as the experiences

of other investigators, suggest that the natural history of STUMP is much less aggressive than true leiomyosarcoma. Importantly, outcomes appeared equally good for women who initially underwent myomectomy or hysterectomy as their initial treatment. Thus, reoperation following myomectomy may not be necessary when a woman has been diagnosed with STUMP, providing options for fertility preservation for women diagnosed with this disease. However, even in the case series reported by Guntupalli et al (9), all women who initially underwent myomectomy were subsequently treated with hysterectomy within 6 months of their initial surgery. As a result, these data must be interpreted with caution. There are also no data to suggest that additional procedures such as oophorectomy improve outcomes for STUMP. Overall, data evaluating more conservative treatment options for STUMP are quite limited and a consensus on these issues has not been achieved.

Imaging

Both ultrasound and endometrial biopsy are commonly used to evaluate women experiencing problems with pelvic pain or vaginal bleeding. As mentioned above, these tests function poorly in their ability to prospectively diagnose ULMS. Sonographically, ULMS are described as heterogeneous tumors with irregular echotexture. Doppler has also been used to evaluate uterine masses as an adjunct to standard sonography. In particular, ULMS have been associated with low-impedance vessels with high-peak systolic velocities distributed irregularly throughout a myometrial mass (13). However, many of these features can also be observed in benign leiomyomas. Thus, there are no sonographic features that reliably distinguish ULMS from leiomyomas.

More recently, a number of investigators have examined the utility of MRI for differentiating leiomyosarcomas from leiomyomas. This strategy is attractive, mainly because MRI provides much more detailed information regarding soft tissue morphology than either ultrasound or CT. A number of features have been proposed to differentiate ULMS from benign uterine leiomyomas. These include the presence of a lobulated uterine mass with ill-defined or invasive margins and heterogeneous signal intensity on T1-weight images (14). Intermediate to high-signal intensity can also be observed on T2-weighted images, reflecting central necrosis. The presence of this radiographic feature has been proposed to differentiate ULMS from benign leiomyomas. This is because leiomyomas are much less likely to present with necrosis and are much more likely to be characterized by low signal intensity of T2-weighted images. However, none of these features can be considered specific to ULMS as degenerating leiomyomas may also present with necrosis and many ULMS demonstrate low signal intensity (15). ^{18}F-fluorodeoxyglucose-positron emission tomography (FDG-PET) imaging has also been tested as a tool for diagnosing ULMS. Limited data indicate that ULMS accumulate FDG avidly. Although FDG-PET has shown both high sensitivity and specificity for diagnosing recurrent ULMS, there is currently little evidence to indicate that this technique can be reliably used to prospectively identify ULMS (16). More recently, FLT-PET has been explored as a tool for differentiating leiomyosarcomas from leiomyomas. Although results are encouraging, further work is needed to validate this strategy prior to its widespread clinical application (17).

Treatment

Surgery plays a central role in the management of ULMS. The criteria for International Federation of Gynecology and Obstetrics FIGO clinical staging of ULMS are summarized in Table 12.2. Currently, standard of care for nearly all patients includes hysterectomy along with a thorough surgical exploration of the abdominal cavity. Typically, bilateral salpingo-oophorectomy is also performed. Most (approximately 70%) of ULMS are diagnosed at an early stage, typically as a solitary uterine mass. For these tumors, retroperitoneal lymph node metastases or even microscopic metastases to the tubo–ovarian complex are relatively infrequent (18). In one recent case series, microscopic ovarian metastases were detected in 4 of 108 patients (3.9%; 19). Similarly, microscopic metastases were found in 3 of 37 patients (8.1%) who underwent comprehensive retroperitoneal lymphadenectomy. Other investigators have reported similar observations (20,21). Thus, routine surgical staging appears to offer only limited benefit for women with early stage disease. Many gynecologic oncologists no longer utilize these procedures unless suspicious lymphadenopathy is identified at the time of laparotomy. For premenopausal women, oophorectomy may be omitted (22).

Use of adjuvant therapy for women with early stage ULMS is hotly debated. Much of the earlier evidence supporting the use of adjuvant radiation and chemotherapy cannot be confirmed in larger retrospective analyses (20). However, recent studies suggest that a combination of gemcitabine and docetaxel may improve outcomes for women with early stage ULMS. One recent prospective study has reported that 59% of women with Stage I or II ULMS receiving this combination were progression free 2 years after completing therapy (23). Long-term survival has also recently been reported for patients undergoing intraoperative radiation therapy for locally advanced disease (24). However, randomized trials comparing gemcitabine/docetaxel combination to other adjuvant therapies have not been reported.

In the setting of widely metastatic disease, surgical debulking appears to provide a survival benefit (25). Secondary cytoreduction of recurrent disease should also

■ Table 12.2 FIGO staging for uterine leiomyosarcomas

Stage	Definition
I	Tumor limited to uterus
IA	<5 cm
IB	>5 cm
II	Tumor extends to the pelvis
IIA	Adnexal involvement
IIB	Tumor extends to extrauterine pelvic tissue
III	Tumor invades abdominal tissues
IIIA	One site
IIIB	More than one site
IIIC	Metastasis to pelvic and/or para-aortic lymph nodes
IV	Distant disease
IVA	Tumor invades bladder and/or rectum
IVB	Other distant metastasis

be considered, as available evidence, although limited, suggests that debulking select patients improves survival (26). The benefit of resecting recurrent ULMS appears to be most robust for women with pulmonary recurrences (27,28). For advanced stage, inoperable or recurrent disease, treatment typically relies on the use of systemic chemotherapy (29). Agents used to treat this disease include Adriamycin, docetaxel, and gemcitabine. In the United States, combination therapy with gemcitabine and docetaxel has emerged as a frequent choice for frontline therapy following optimal resection of widespread disease (23). This combination has also been shown to be effective in treating metastatic disease that has not been debulked (30). Regimens that rely on Adriamycin, ifosfamide, or temozolamide are also frequently used (31–33). Radiation therapy is typically reserved for the treatment of isolated metastases or to achieve local control in select circumstances.

Outcomes

Despite aggressive treatment, outcomes for women diagnosed with ULMS remain poor (20,34). Recurrence rates for women initially diagnosed with early stage disease (FIGO Stage I) have been reported as high as 70%. Survival for women with advanced stage or recurrent disease is typically poor, averaging approximately 2 years. However, it is interesting that a subset of patient with ULMS do well as evidenced by long-term survival (34). Unfortunately, this group of patients represents fewer than 20% of all patients diagnosed with ULMS. A number of clinicians have hypothesized that response to treatment and prognosis for ULMS are different from leiomyosarcomas at other anatomic sites. However, there is currently little concrete data to support this belief. Furthermore, the reasons why some women do well, while others do not are unknown. Although it has not yet been possible to delineate clinical features of those women destined to do well, prognostic algorithms based on clinical features are being developed and refined (35). In the future, incorporation of these algorithms into routine clinical care may help to identify women for whom ambitious treatment strategies, such as the resection of recurrent disease, are most likely to prove beneficial.

Recent Advances

ULMS is considered a genetically heterogeneous disease with few features that can be consistently exploited to clinical advantage. This conclusion remains correct in that it has not yet been possible to identify one or two key molecular events, such as a translocation or mutation, uniquely associated with this disease. Nonetheless, significant progress has been recently made toward better understanding ULMS and developing more effective strategies for its diagnosis and treatment.

A number of investigators have begun to explore the utility of targeted molecular therapies, such as sorafenib in treating soft tissue sarcomas (36). For the most part, results of these studies have been disappointing. Other novel strategies are also being explored. For example, recent transcriptional profiling has shown that a subset of leiomyosarcomas are characterized by high levels of CD163 and CD68 as well as macrophage infiltration (37). These features are associated with worse clinical outcomes in nongynecologic leiomyosarcomas, suggesting that tumor-specific interactions with the immune system are important for determining survival. The concept of using immune-based therapies to target sarcomas is now being explored. Recently, monoclonal antibodies targeting interactions between CD47 and signal regulatory protein alpha (SIRPα) have been shown to prevent or treat metastasis with the possibility of eliminating smaller tumors. These observations suggest that solid human tumors, including leiomyosarcomas, require expression of CD47 to prevent phagocytosis (38). Given these observations, blockade of CD47 function may be a viable option for potentiating endogenous immune responses and improving treatment responses for sarcomas in the future.

Alternatively, it may be possible to exploit key features of leiomyosarcomas that are shared with other human cancers, including carcinomas. When compared to benign leiomyomas and myometrium, the dominant molecular phenotype of leiomyomas appears to be the widespread overexpression of gene products regulating the G2-M and spindle assembly cell cycle checkpoints (39). Of the 50 gene products most overexpressed in ULMS, 26 have been previously implicated in regulating the G2-M cell cycle checkpoint. The mechanisms responsible for this phenotype are not currently known (34). However, a large array of small molecular inhibitors have been synthesized during the past 10 years with the goal of targeting breast, lung, and other human cancers. Recent data indicate that these small molecule inhibitors can be used to arrest ULMS growth and induce apoptosis both in vitro and in vivo (39). This strategy may be particularly useful when combined with mTORC1 inhibitors such as rapamycin (40). These studies indicate that the efficacy of small molecule inhibitors targeting Aurora A kinase are potentiated by combining them at low dose with mTORC1 inhibitors. Use of this or a similar combination may be an effective strategy not only in terms of efficacy but also for reducing the incidence of side effects.

■ ENDOMETRIAL STROMAL SARCOMAS

ESS are histologically bland proliferations of mesenchymal cells that resemble endometrial stroma. ESS are relatively rare cancers, accounting for only 0.2%–1% of all uterine cancers and 6%–20% of uterine sarcomas (41–43). The annual incidence of ESS is less than 2:100,000 women (22). Although usually diagnosed as a mass originating within the uterine cavity, ESS can also occur primary to other reproductive tract tissues, such as rectovaginal septum. Reports of ESS originating in extrauterine implants of endometriosis have also been described (44). Mean age at diagnosis for women with this disease is 52 years. Predisposing risk factors include unopposed estrogen or tamoxifen use and polycystic ovarian syndrome.

Most patients diagnosed with ESS present with uterine bleeding. However, patients can also present with symptoms of pelvic pain, dysmenorrhea, and an enlarged uterine mass. Similar to ULMS, a diagnosis of ESS is made unexpectedly only after a woman has undergone hysterectomy for presumed uterine fibroids (leiomyomata) or adenomyosis. Unfortunately, as many as 25% of women with ESS remain asymptomatic and are only diagnosed after the disease has spread widely.

Diagnosis

WHO recognizes three categories of endometrial stromal neoplasms: endometrial stromal nodules (ESN), ESS, and undifferentiated endometrial sarcoma (UES). Histologically, ESS are composed of uniform small cells with scant cytoplasm and oval-to-round nuclei reminiscent of normal stroma of proliferative endometrium. Cytologic atypia and more than 5 mitoses per 10 hpf are not typically seen. Differentiation of ESN from ESS is made primarily by examining surgical specimens for features such as myometrial invasion. Although ESS can present as single or multiple uterine masses, only ESS are characterized by infiltrating margins and lymphovascular invasion not found in the benign stromal nodules. Not infrequently, ESS extend worm-like projections into the myometrium that can extend to the serosal surface of the uterus. These projections may also invade extrauterine vasculature. In contrast, ESN are fleshy, well-circumscribed masses with clearly defined margins. Grossly, ESN can grow quite large and tumors with diameters up to 22 cm have been reported (45). Occasionally, ESN can have slightly more irregular margins with focal areas of invasion into adjacent tissue (45). However, these areas typically extend no more than 3 mm from the tumor margin. Mitotic rates in ESN are typically less than 5 per 10 hpf. Roughly 50% of ESN display evidence of metaplasia, demonstrating histologic patterns similar to smooth muscle, cystic degeneration, sex cord–like differentiation, and necrosis (45). Unfortunately, it is not uncommon to miss a diagnosis of ESS in endometrial curettings.

Multiple immunohistochemical markers have been examined for their ability to distinguish ESS from other soft-tissue neoplasia including highly cellular leiomyomas, adenomyosis, other types of uterine cancers such low-grade Mullerian adenocarcinomas, or even an endometrial polyp. ESS are frequently characterized by high levels of estrogen receptors (ER) and progesterone receptors (PR), with 71% and 95% of tumors expressing these receptors, respectively (46). Cell surface neutral endopeptidase, CD10, and inhibin are also frequently expressed, further helping to distinguish ESS from its benign counterparts that express h-caldesmon, desmin, and the oxytocin receptor (47).

Imaging

Although no current imaging technique is currently capable of prospectively identifying ESS, preoperative evaluation of women for whom this diagnosis is being considered may be aided by MRI (48). T2-weighted MRI images are capable of uncovering tongue-like projections of low-signal intensity that represent tumor invading the myometrium. Unfortunately, pelvic ultrasound is unable to precisely distinguish ESS from adenomyosis or conventional fibroids. However, suspicion should be increased when an endometrial lesion is identified with a heterogenous appearance with both high-intensity and hypoechoic areas scattered throughout the myometrium (49). Further interrogation with transvaginal Doppler ultrasound often demonstrates low impedance flow.

Treatment

Treatment of ESS depends on the clinical stage at which it has been diagnosed (Table 12.3). However, the specific strategies used to manage this disease often vary widely between institutions. This variation is largely due to the rarity of this disease and the fact that most information guiding treatment is scattered across numerous small retrospective studies. In general, ESS are less aggressive neoplasms associated with high survival rates when caught early. Similar to leiomyosarcoma, surgery is the primary

■ **Table 12.3** FIGO staging for endometrial stromal sarcomas

Stage	Definition
I	Tumor limited to uterus
IA	Tumor limited to endometrium/endocervix
IB	Invasion ≤ one-half myometrial thickness
IC	Invasion > one-half myometrial thickness
II	Tumor extends to the pelvis
IIA	Adnexal involvement
IIB	Tumor extends to extrauterine pelvic tissue
III	Tumor invades abdominal tissues
IIIA	One site
IIIB	More than one site
IIIC	Metastasis to pelvic and/or para-aortic lymph nodes
IV	Distant disease
IVA	Tumor invades bladder and/or rectum
IVB	Other distant metastasis

treatment used to manage ESS. The typical approach for perimenopausal women includes total hysterectomy and bilateral salpingo-oophorectomy. Many clinicians also favor surgical staging for these tumors and perform pelvic and para-aortic lymphadenectomies. Proponents of surgical staging emphasize that the rate of lymph node metastases ranges from 10% to 45% (22,50). It is worth noting that even patients with lymph node metastases demonstrate 5-year survival of 86% vs 95% for those with no evidence of nodal spread. However, Feng et al recently evaluated the efficacy of radical hysterectomy combined with staging lymphadenectomy and omentectomy in patients with ESS. They concluded that none of these surgical approaches influenced survival. Similarly, Chan et al studied 831 patients with ESS and found a 10% rate of lymph node metastases in those women who underwent lymph node dissection (43). However, they found no difference in 5-year disease-specific survival among patients who underwent lymph node dissection and those who did not (73.8% vs 77.6%, P = .351). Other investigators have also reported decreased survival for patients with nodal metastases compared to those without nodal spread. Regardless of whether staging lymphadenectomies confers a survival benefit, information gained from these procedures potentially facilitate adjuvant treatment planning (43).

The decision to perform bilateral salpingo-oophorectomy has also recently become an area of controversy. On one hand, bilateral salpingo-oophorectomy is frequently recommended in light of the fact that ESS are frequently hormone-sensitive tumors. However, the potentially devastating impact of premature menopause has prompted further studies into the feasibility of ovarian conservation in young women with early stage disease. Li et al reported that bilateral salpingo-oophorectomy did not significantly increase prolonged disease-free interval (PFS) or overall survival (OS) in patients with Stage I ESS and could be omitted in younger patients (51). In this study, patterns and rate of recurrence were similar in both treatment groups (cases and controls) reaching 33% vs 42%, $P = .82$, respectively. The study authored by Chan et al also confirmed that ovarian-sparing surgery in women younger than 50 years and early stage disease had no adverse impact on survival (43). Conflicting reports on this topic are seen in the other studies. For example, Malouf et al analyzed 84 patients with Stage I-II ESS and concluded that surgery without bilateral salpingo-oopherectomy (BSO) was an adverse prognostic factors in multivariate analysis, with the others being deep (greater than 1/2) myometrial invasion, and lack of adjuvant therapy (52). Amant and colleagues have also reported recurrence rates of 25% and 17% in women with Stage I-II disease who underwent hysterectomy with and without BSO, respectively (53). The decision regarding oophorectomy becomes particularly important considering that hormone replacement therapy is contraindicated in patients with ESS. Chu et al demonstrated 80% recurrence rate in patients who received estrogen replacement therapy (54). At present, thorough counseling taking into account the existing data on the risks and benefits of BSO in younger patients is recommended.

High recurrence rates make adjuvant therapy an important consideration for women diagnosed with ESS. Age, race, and clinical stage have also been shown to be important prognostic features of this disease at the time of its initial diagnosis and may help to shape these decisions (43). Despite the scattered information found in the literature, a key theme that emerges is that repeat resections of isolated recurrences prolong survival and improve quality of life. However, surgical management of recurrent disease is often insufficient. Although most recurrences are local (92%), distant spread is seen in 46% of cases. This observation implies that micro-metastases occur early and that systemic chemotherapy should be considered in high-risk patients following hysterectomy. In the report authored by Malouf et al, the authors emphasized that patients with early stage disease, but deep myometrial invasion would benefit from adjuvant therapy most, given their significant risk for lung recurrences.

As ESS are slow-growing tumors with only a small fraction of cells undergoing mitotic cell division, these cancers are relatively insensitive to traditional cytotoxic chemotherapy. This would seem to potentially limit choices for adjuvant therapy. However, the robust expression of ER and PR allow the use of hormone therapy for the treatment of advanced or recurrent disease, or adjuvant therapy of early stage disease. Three regimens have been used in this regard, each with good efficacy: high-dose progestins, gonadotropin-releasing hormone (GnRH) analogues, and aromatase inhibitors. Each of these agents ultimately create a sustained hypoestrogenic state decreasing endometrial gland and stromal proliferation. Perhaps most importantly, durable responses to hormone therapy have been documented in patients with early and advanced disease after adjuvant therapy as well as recurrent disease. For example, Piver et al documented a response rate of 46% in patients with relapsed ESS treated with progestins, as opposed to 17% in those treated with other types of cytotoxic chemotherapy (55). Chu et al reported decreased recurrence rates in patients treated with progestins in the adjuvant setting (31% vs 67%; 54). These investigators recommended megestrol for patients with Stage I disease, as 75% of treated patients had no recurrence, as opposed to 29% in the untreated group that had surgery alone. The same authors successfully used progestins in patients with relapse ultimately achieving stable disease in 88% of cases and complete response in 50% of cases. Amant et al also observed decreased recurrence rates in patients with Stage III-IV ESS treated with hormonal therapy (20% vs 75%). Strikingly, they found that patients with Stage I disease who did not receive adjuvant therapy had the same recurrence rate (20%) as compared to patients with Stage III and Stage IV disease who had completed adjuvant therapy (53).

Radiotherapy has been extensively used in patients with both advanced and recurrent disease. Consideration of this modality is particularly worthwhile in the context of recurrent disease since many recurrences of ESS are confined to the pelvis. Both external beam radiation with or without brachytherapy have been employed. Similar to hormonal therapy and surgical staging, current recommendations on the use of radiotherapy are derived from retrospective studies of small numbers of patients accrued over a long period of time. Data may be conflicting and should be judged accordingly. However, available evidence indicates that radiotherapy tends to improve local control without improving overall survival. Valduvieco et al reported local control rate of 88.9% in patients treated with adjuvant radiotherapy, whereas lack of adjuvant therapy resulted in the local control rate of only 50% (56). Weitmann et al recommend adjuvant radiotherapy based on 5-year survival of 62% in patients treated with adjuvant radiotherapy, compared to 46% in those treated with surgery alone. Even more impressive is the overall local control rate of 93% at 5 years (57,58). However, Barney et al did not see any increase in survival in patients who received postoperative radiotherapy: 5-year OS: 72.2% vs 83.2%, cause-specific survival: 80.1% vs 90.7% (59).

Outcomes

Outcomes for women diagnosed with ESN and ESS are good. Cure rates for ESN should be high with surgery alone. Despite its more invasive nature, outcomes for endometrial stromal sarcoma should also be good when caught at an early stage. Five-year survival for patients with Stage

I disease ranges from 54% to 100%, whereas survival for Stage II patients is typically reported as approximately 30%. Patients with more advanced disease do even more poorly, with 5-year survival for Stage III and IV disease less than 11% (60). However, it is not unusual to have PFS in ESS with 5- and 10-year PFS approaching 73% and 62%, respectively. This is because patients with disease relapse can often be effectively managed with one of the modalities discussed above, with selection of a strategy dependent on disease location, size, resectability, and prior treatment.

Undifferentiated Endometrial Sarcoma

UES are a genetically heterogeneous category of uterine sarcomas that lack histologically defining features. In general, the degree of cytologic atypia observed in these tumors obscures their origin in the endometrium. Although UES have been reported to occur as synchronous or metachronous lesions with ESS, they lack the gene-specific fusions that have recently been identified in ESS or activating mutations in c-KIT or PDGFRA found in gastrointestinal stromal tumors (GIST). These latter observations suggest that the pathophysiologic mechanisms leading to ESS and UES are distinct. Clinically, UES are aggressive tumors with high rates of recurrence (greater than 85%) following hysterectomy. Five-year survival rates are significantly lower than those observed for ESS and have been reported to be approximately 65% (61).

Recent Advances

Over the past several years, it has become increasingly clear that a binary system for categorizing ESS into low-grade (ESS) and high-grade lesions (UES) does not adequately reflect the complexity of this disease. Understanding the molecular basis of this complexity has potentially important implications for both prognostication and treatment of the disease. Perhaps the most significant discovery regarding ESS in the past decade has been the identification of genomic rearrangements that occur at high frequency in ESS specimens (62,63). Very robust evidence indicates that more than 50% of classic "low grade" ESS lesions harbor rearrangements of genes (JAZF1, SUZ12, PHF1, EPC1) involved in the epigenetic remodeling of chromatin (64). Most frequently, these rearrangements are a translocation t(7;17; p14;q21) that results in a fusion between the JAZF1-SUZ12 gene products. Approximately one-third of ESS are associated with rearrangements that impact the JAZF1 gene, suggesting that these events may be a key driver for ESS. However, similar rearrangements are also found in more than 50% of ESN (64). Thus, the JAZF1-SUZ12 fusion product may be insufficient to malignantly transform cells by itself. Additional work will be necessary to better understand the role of translations impacting the JAZF1 gene product in endometrium.

More recently, investigators have identified a novel genomic translocation t(10;17; q22;p13) that also occurs in the endometrial stromal sarcoma. An identical translocation has been identified in clear cell carcinomas of the kidney and produces an in-frame fusion between YWHAE (exons 1 to 5) and either FAM22A or FAM22B (exons 2 to 7). In humans, FAM22A and B encode highly homologous gene products of unknown function. However, YWHAE (also known as 14–3-3ε) belongs to the 14–3-3 family of gene products, which mediate signal transduction by binding to phosphoserine- and phosphotyrosine-containing proteins. Individual members of the 14–3-3 family are highly conserved across both plant and animal species and have been shown to be a key integration point for pathways regulating proliferation, apoptosis, and metabolic stress (65). In particular, YWHAE has been shown to interact with CDC25 phosphatases, RAF1, and IRS1, reflecting its diverse roles in regulating cell division and insulin sensitivity (66,67). YWHAE has also been shown to integrate E2F activity with the DNA damage repair response by regulating gene transcription (68).

Subsequent clinical follow-up has confirmed that tumors harboring t(10;17; q22;p13) and consequently expressing the unique fusion protein generated by this translocation product are more likely to harbor focal areas of morphologically high-grade cells arranged in nests with a delicate stromal capillary network. These tumors are also much more likely to have a high mitotic index (greater than 10 mitoses/10 hpf) and present at an advanced stage (Stage II to III) when compared to ESS characterized by JAZF1 fusions (69). This observation suggests that t(10;17; q22;p13)can be used to clinically classify ESS and denotes disease behavior intermediate between ESS and UES. In the future, this knowledge may help to triage patients into specific treatment regimens personalized to the molecular context of their tumors. Furthermore, they create a unique opportunity to selectively target subsets of ESS using the unique fusion product expressed only in their cancer. It may also be possible to use similar strategies to treat women whose cancers harbor other types of translocation-dependent fusion products involving JAZF1.

■ OTHER SARCOMAS

Gastrointestinal Stromal Sarcomas (GIST)

GIST are relatively rare mesenchymal tumors that typically originate in the appendix or other parts of the gastrointestinal tract. Rare cases of GIST have been identified outside of the gastrointestinal tract, including the uterus (70). Histologically, the appearance of GIST is very similar to leiomyosarcoma. However, at a molecular level, most GIST (approximately 85%) are characterized mutations in the KIT (CD-117) or PDGFRA genes that result in their oncogenic activation. Evaluation of c-KIT as been used as a tool to differentiate GIST from ULMS (71). Accurate diagnosis of GIST is important, because conventional chemotherapy and radiation have little impact on this disease. Imatinib, an inhibitor of the KIT and PDGFR-α tyrosine kinases, can be used to treat GIST patients with disease carries an activating mutation in these genes (72). Mutational analyses is highly recommended prior to treatment, as the detection of specific KIT mutations are highly predictive of a response to therapy (73). In the absence of these mutations, alternative treatments or enrollment in a clinical trial should be considered.

■ CONCLUSIONS

Uterine sarcomas are uncommon cancers whose prognosis varies widely. Accurate diagnosis and timely treatment are critical for optimizing patient outcomes. Scientific understanding of these tumors is advancing rapidly, hopefully opening new doors for more effective diagnosis and treatment in the near future.

■ REFERENCES

1. Stewart EA. Uterine fibroids. *Lancet*. 2001;357(9252):293–298.
2. Brooks SE, Zhan M, Cote T, Baquet CR. Surveillance, epidemiology, and end results analysis of 2677 cases of uterine sarcoma 1989–1999. *Gynecol Oncol*. 2004;93(1):204–208.
3. Wu TI, Chang TC, Hsueh S, et al. Prognostic factors and impact of adjuvant chemotherapy for uterine leiomyosarcoma. *Gynecol Oncol*. 2006;100(1):166–172.
4. Shah SH, Jagannathan JP, Krajewski K, O'Regan KN, George S, Ramaiya NH. Uterine sarcomas: then and now. *AJR Am J Roentgenol*. 2012;199(1):213–223.
5. Ip PP, Cheung AN. Pathology of uterine leiomyosarcomas and smooth muscle tumours of uncertain malignant potential. *Best Pract Res Clin Obstet Gynaecol*. 2011;25(6):691–704.
6. Lewis EI, Chason RJ, Decherney AH, Armstrong A, Elkas J, Venkatesan AM. Novel hormone treatment of benign metastasizing leiomyoma: an analysis of five cases and literature review. *Fertil Steril*. 2013 Jun;99(7):2017–2024.
7. Tresukosol D, Kudelka AP, Malpica A, Varma DG, Edwards CL, Kavanagh JJ. Leuprolide acetate and intravascular leiomyomatosis. *Obstet Gynecol*. 1995;86(4 Pt 2):688–692.
8. Sung CO, Ahn G, Song SY, Choi YL, Bae DS. Atypical leiomyomas of the uterus with long-term follow-up after myomectomy with immunohistochemical analysis for p16INK4A, p53, Ki-67, estrogen receptors, and progesterone receptors. *Int J Gynecol Pathol*. 2009;28(6):529–534.
9. Guntupalli SR, Ramirez PT, Anderson ML, Milam MR, Bodurka DC, Malpica A. Uterine smooth muscle tumor of uncertain malignant potential: a retrospective analysis. *Gynecol Oncol*. 2009;113(3):324–326.
10. Peters WA 3rd, Howard DR, Andersen WA, Figge DC. Uterine smooth-muscle tumors of uncertain malignant potential. *Obstet Gynecol*. 1994;83(6):1015–1020.
11. Veras E, Zivanovic O, Jacks L, Chiappetta D, Hensley M, Soslow R. "Low-grade leiomyosarcoma" and late-recurring smooth muscle tumors of the uterus: a heterogenous collection of frequently misdiagnosed tumors associated with an overall favorable prognosis relative to conventional uterine leiomyosarcomas. *Am J Surg Pathol*. 2011;35(11):1626–1637.
12. Ip PP, Cheung AN, Clement PB. Uterine smooth muscle tumors of uncertain malignant potential (STUMP): a clinicopathologic analysis of 16 cases. *Am J Surg Pathol*. 2009;33(7):992–1005.
13. Szabó I, Szánthó A, Csabay L, Csapó Z, Szirmai K, Papp Z. Color Doppler ultrasonography in the differentiation of uterine sarcomas from uterine leiomyomas. *Eur J Gynaecol Oncol*. 2002;23(1):29–34.
14. Wu TI, Yen TC, Lai CH. Clinical presentation and diagnosis of uterine sarcoma, including imaging. *Best Pract Res Clin Obstet Gynaecol*. 2011;25(6):681–689.
15. Cornfeld D, Israel G, Martel M, Weinreb J, Schwartz P, McCarthy S. MRI appearance of mesenchymal tumors of the uterus. *Eur J Radiol*. 2010;74(1):241–249.
16. Kao YH, Saad U, Tan AE, Magsombol BM, Padhy AK. Fluorine-18-fluorodeoxyglucose PET/CT for the evaluation of suspected recurrent uterine leiomyosarcomas. *Acta Radiol*. 2011;52(4):463–466.
17. Yamane T, Takaoka A, Kita M, Imai Y, Senda M. 18F-FLT PET performs better than 18F-FDG PET in differentiating malignant uterine corpus tumors from benign leiomyoma. *Ann Nucl Med*. 2012;26(6):478–484.
18. Kapp DS, Shin JY, Chan JK. Prognostic factors and survival in 1396 patients with uterine leiomyosarcomas: emphasis on impact of lymphadenectomy and oophorectomy. *Cancer*. 2008;112(4):820–830.
19. Leitao MM, Sonoda Y, Brennan MF, Barakat RR, Chi DS. Incidence of lymph node and ovarian metastases in leiomyosarcoma of the uterus. *Gynecol Oncol*. 2003;91(1):209–212.
20. Giuntoli RL 2nd, Metzinger DS, DiMarco CS, et al. Retrospective review of 208 patients with leiomyosarcoma of the uterus: prognostic indicators, surgical management, and adjuvant therapy. *Gynecol Oncol*. 2003;89(3):460–469.
21. Goff BA, Rice LW, Fleischhacker D, et al. Uterine leiomyosarcoma and endometrial stromal sarcoma: lymph node metastases and sites of recurrence. *Gynecol Oncol*. 1993;50(1):105–109.
22. Gadducci A, Cosio S, Romanini A, Genazzani AR. The management of patients with uterine sarcoma: a debated clinical challenge. *Crit Rev Oncol Hematol*. 2008;65(2):129–142.
23. Hensley ML, Ishill N, Soslow R, et al. Adjuvant gemcitabine plus docetaxel for completely resected stages I-IV high grade uterine leiomyosarcoma: Results of a prospective study. *Gynecol Oncol*. 2009;112(3):563–567.
24. Barney BM, Petersen IA, Dowdy SC, Bakkum-Gamez JN, Haddock MG. Long-term outcomes with intraoperative radiotherapy as a component of treatment for locally advanced or recurrent uterine sarcoma. *Int J Radiat Oncol Biol Phys*. 2012;83(1):191–197.
25. Leitao MM Jr, Zivanovic O, Chi DS, et al. Surgical cytoreduction in patients with metastatic uterine leiomyosarcoma at the time of initial diagnosis. *Gynecol Oncol*. 2012;125(2):409–413.
26. Giuntoli RL 2nd, Garrett-Mayer E, Bristow RE, Gostout BS. Secondary cytoreduction in the management of recurrent uterine leiomyosarcoma. *Gynecol Oncol*. 2007;106(1):82–88.
27. Paramanathan A, Wright G. Pulmonary metastasectomy for sarcoma of gynaecologic origin. *Heart Lung Circ*. 2013;22(4):270–275.
28. Levenback C, Rubin SC, McCormack PM, Hoskins WJ, Atkinson EN, Lewis JL Jr. Resection of pulmonary metastases from uterine sarcomas. *Gynecol Oncol*. 1992;45(2):202–205.
29. Gupta AA, Yao X, Verma S, Mackay H, Hopkins L; Sarcoma Disease Site Group and the Gynecology Cancer Disease Site Group. Systematic chemotherapy for inoperable, locally advanced, recurrent, or metastatic uterine leiomyosarcoma: a systematic review. *Clin Oncol (R Coll Radiol)*. 2013;25(6):346–355.
30. Hensley ML, Blessing JA, Mannel R, Rose PG. Fixed-dose rate gemcitabine plus docetaxel as first-line therapy for metastatic

uterine leiomyosarcoma: a Gynecologic Oncology Group phase II trial. *Gynecol Oncol.* 2008;109(3):329–334.

31. Omura GA, Blessing JA, Major F, et al. A randomized clinical trial of adjuvant adriamycin in uterine sarcomas: a Gynecologic Oncology Group Study. *J Clin Oncol.* 1985;3(9):1240–1245.

32. Boyar MS, Hesdorffer M, Keohan ML, Jin Z, Taub RN. Phase II Study of Temozolomide and Thalidomide in Patients with Unresectable or Metastatic Leiomyosarcoma. *Sarcoma.* 2008;2008:412–503.

33. Sleijfer S, Ouali M, van Glabbeke M, et al. Prognostic and predictive factors for outcome to first-line ifosfamide-containing chemotherapy for adult patients with advanced soft tissue sarcomas: an exploratory, retrospective analysis on large series from the European Organization for Research and Treatment of Cancer-Soft Tissue and Bone Sarcoma Group (EORTC-STBSG). *Eur J Cancer.* 2010;46(1):72–83.

34. Lusby K, Savannah KB, Demicco EG, et al. Uterine Leiomyosarcoma Management, Outcome, and Associated Molecular Biomarkers: A Single Institution's Experience. *Ann Surg Oncol.* 2013 Jul;20(7):2364–2372.

35. Zivanovic O, Jacks LM, Iasonos A, et al. A nomogram to predict postresection 5-year overall survival for patients with uterine leiomyosarcoma. *Cancer.* 2012;118(3):660–669.

36. von Mehren M, Rankin C, Goldblum JR, et al. Phase 2 Southwest Oncology Group-directed intergroup trial (S0505) of sorafenib in advanced soft tissue sarcomas. *Cancer.* 2012;118(3):770–776.

37. Lee CH, Espinosa I, Vrijaldenhoven S, et al. Prognostic significance of macrophage infiltration in leiomyosarcomas. *Clin Cancer Res.* 2008;14(5):1423–1430.

38. Willingham SB, Volkmer JP, Gentles AJ, et al. The CD47-signal regulatory protein alpha (SIRPa) interaction is a therapeutic target for human solid tumors. *Proc Natl Acad Sci USA.* 2012;109(17):6662–6667.

39. Shan W, Akinfenwa PY, Savannah KB, et al. A small-molecule inhibitor targeting the mitotic spindle checkpoint impairs the growth of uterine leiomyosarcoma. *Clin Cancer Res.* 2012;18(12):3352–3365.

40. Brewer Savannah KJ, Demicco EG, Lusby K, et al. Dual targeting of mTOR and aurora-A kinase for the treatment of uterine Leiomyosarcoma. *Clin Cancer Res.* 2012;18(17):4633–4645.

41. Larson B, Silfversward C, Nilsson B, Pettersson F. Endometrial stromal sarcoma of the uterus. A clinical and histopathological study. The Radiumhemmet series 1936–1981. *Eur J Obstet Gynecol Reprod Biol.* 1990;35(2–3):239–249.

42. Harlow BL, Weiss NS, Lofton S. The epidemiology of sarcomas of the uterus. *J Natl Cancer Inst.* 1986;76(3):399–402.

43. Chan JK, Kawar NM, Shin JY, et al. Endometrial stromal sarcoma: a population-based analysis. *Br J Cancer.* 2008;99(8):1210–1215.

44. Rosca E, Venter A, Mutiu G, Dragan A, Coroi M, Rosca DM. Endometrial stromal sarcoma developed on outer endometriosis foci. *Rom J Morphol Embryol.* 2011;52(1 Suppl):489–492.

45. Dionigi A, Oliva E, Clement PB, Young RH. Endometrial stromal nodules and endometrial stromal tumors with limited infiltration: a clinicopathologic study of 50 cases. *Am J Surg Pathol.* 2002;26(5):567–581.

46. Reich O, Regauer S, Urdl W, Lahousen M, Winter R. Expression of oestrogen and progesterone receptors in low-grade endometrial stromal sarcomas. *Br J Cancer.* 2000;82(5):1030–1034.

47. Zhu XQ, Shi YF, Cheng XD, Zhao CL, Wu YZ. Immunohistochemical markers in differential diagnosis of endometrial stromal sarcoma and cellular leiomyoma. *Gynecol Oncol.* 2004;92(1):71–79.

48. Koyama T, Togashi K, Konishi I, et al. MR imaging of endometrial stromal sarcoma: correlation with pathologic findings. *AJR Am J Roentgenol.* 1999;173(3):767–772.

49. Cacciatore B, Lehtovirta P, Wahlström T, Ylöstalo P. Ultrasound findings in uterine mixed müllerian sarcomas and endometrial stromal sarcomas. *Gynecol Oncol.* 1989;35(3):290–293.

50. Riopel J, Plante M, Renaud MC, Roy M, Têtu B. Lymph node metastases in low-grade endometrial stromal sarcoma. *Gynecol Oncol.* 2005;96(2):402–406.

51. Li AJ, Giuntoli RL 2nd, Drake R, et al. Ovarian preservation in stage I low-grade endometrial stromal sarcomas. *Obstet Gynecol.* 2005;106(6):1304–1308.

52. Malouf GG, Duclos J, Rey A, et al. Impact of adjuvant treatment modalities on the management of patients with stages I-II endometrial stromal sarcoma. *Ann Oncol.* 2010;21(10):2102–2106.

53. Amant F, De Knijf A, Van Calster B, et al. Clinical study investigating the role of lymphadenectomy, surgical castration and adjuvant hormonal treatment in endometrial stromal sarcoma. *Br J Cancer.* 2007;97(9):1194–1199.

54. Chu MC, Mor G, Lim C, Zheng W, Parkash V, Schwartz PE. Low-grade endometrial stromal sarcoma: hormonal aspects. *Gynecol Oncol.* 2003;90(1):170–176.

55. Piver MS, Rutledge FN, Copeland L, Webster K, Blumenson L, Suh O. Uterine endolymphatic stromal myosis: a collaborative study. *Obstet Gynecol.* 1984;64(2):173–178.

56. Valduvieco I, Rovirosa A, Colomo L, De San Juan A, Pahisa J, Biete A. Endometrial stromal sarcoma. Is there a place for radiotherapy? *Clin Transl Oncol.* 2010;12(3):226–230.

57. Weitmann HD, Knocke TH, Kucera H, Pötter R. Radiation therapy in the treatment of endometrial stromal sarcoma. *Int J Radiat Oncol Biol Phys.* 2001;49(3):739–748.

58. Weitmann HD, Kucera H, Knocke TH, Pötter R. Surgery and adjuvant radiation therapy of endometrial stromal sarcoma. *Wien Klin Wochenschr.* 2002;114(1–2):44–49.

59. Barney B, Tward JD, Skidmore T, Gaffney DK. Does radiotherapy or lymphadenectomy improve survival in endometrial stromal sarcoma? *Int J Gynecol Cancer.* 2009;19(7):1232–1238.

60. Puliyath G, Nair MK. Endometrial stromal sarcoma: A review of the literature. *Indian J Med Paediatr Oncol.* 2012;33(1):1–6.

61. Schick U, Bolukbasi Y, Thariat J, et al. Outcome and prognostic factors in endometrial stromal tumors: a Rare Cancer Network study. *Int J Radiat Oncol Biol Phys.* 2012;82(5):e757–e763.

62. Micci F, Panagopoulos I, Bjerkehagen B, Heim S. Consistent rearrangement of chromosomal band 6p21 with generation of fusion genes JAZF1/PHF1 and EPC1/PHF1 in endometrial stromal sarcoma. *Cancer Res.* 2006;66(1):107–112.

63. Micci F, Walter CU, Teixeira MR, et al. Cytogenetic and molecular genetic analyses of endometrial stromal sarcoma: nonrandom involvement of chromosome arms 6p and 7p and confirmation of JAZF1/JJAZ1 gene fusion in t(7;17). *Cancer Genet Cytogenet.* 2003;144(2):119–124.

64. Chiang S, Ali R, Melnyk N, et al. Frequency of known gene rearrangements in endometrial stromal tumors. *Am J Surg Pathol.* 2011;35(9):1364–1372.

65. Gardino AK, Yaffe MB. 14-3-3 proteins as signaling integration points for cell cycle control and apoptosis. *Semin Cell Dev Biol.* 2011;22(7):688–695.

66. Kim J, Parrish AB, Kurokawa M, et al. Rsk-mediated phosphorylation and 14-3-3? binding of Apaf-1 suppresses cytochrome c-induced apoptosis. *EMBO J.* 2012;31(5):1279–1292.

67. Craparo A, Freund R, Gustafson TA. 14-3-3 (epsilon) interacts with the insulin-like growth factor I receptor and insulin receptor substrate I in a phosphoserine-dependent manner. *J Biol Chem.* 1997;272(17):11663–11669.

68. Milton AH, Khaire N, Ingram L, O'Donnell AJ, La Thangue NB. 14-3-3 proteins integrate E2F activity with the DNA damage response. *EMBO J.* 2006;25(5):1046–1057.

69. Lee CH, Mariño-Enriquez A, Ou W, et al. The clinicopathologic features of YWHAE-FAM22 endometrial stromal sarcomas: a histologically high-grade and clinically aggressive tumor. *Am J Surg Pathol.* 2012;36(5):641–653.

70. Wingen CB, Pauwels PA, Debiec-Rychter M, van Gemert WG, Vos MC. Uterine gastrointestinal stromal tumour (GIST). *Gynecol Oncol.* 2005;97(3):970–972.

71. Foster R, Solano S, Mahoney J, Fuller A, Oliva E, Seiden MV. Reclassification of a tubal leiomyosarcoma as an eGIST by molecular evaluation of c-KIT. *Gynecol Oncol.* 2006;101(2):363–366.

72. Blanke CD, Rankin C, Demetri GD, et al. Phase III randomized, intergroup trial assessing imatinib mesylate at two dose levels in patients with unresectable or metastatic gastrointestinal stromal tumors expressing the kit receptor tyrosine kinase: S0033. *J Clin Oncol.* 2008;26(4):626–632.

73. Demetri GD, Benjamin RS, Blanke CD, et al. NCCN Task Force report: management of patients with gastrointestinal stromal tumor (GIST)—update of the NCCN clinical practice guidelines. *J Natl Compr Canc Netw.* 2007;(5 Suppl 2):S1–29; quiz S30.

Epithelial Ovarian Cancer

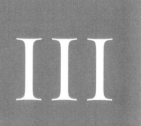

13 Molecular Pathogenesis of Ovarian Cancer

PREMAL H. THAKER

ANIL K. SOOD

■ INTRODUCTION

Ovarian cancer remains the most lethal of all gynecologic malignancies due to the lack of effective screening strategies, nonspecific symptoms at presentation, advanced stage at time of diagnosis, and its ability to rapidly develop resistance to chemotherapy (1). Epithelial ovarian neoplasms are the most common malignant ovarian neoplasm (2) and are molecularly heterogeneous. Based on histopathology and molecular/genetic alterations, epithelial ovarian carcinomas (EOC) are divided into five main types: high-grade serous (70%), endometrioid (10%), clear cell (10%), mucinous (3%), and low-grade serous carcinomas (less than 5%; 3). These pathologic subtypes are essentially distinct diseases, as evidenced by differences in epidemiological and genetic risk factors, precursor lesions, patterns of spread, and molecular events during oncogenesis, response to chemotherapy, and prognosis. This chapter will review the existing science in characterizing the molecular pathogenesis of EOC.

■ ETIOLOGY OF SPORADIC EPITHELIAL OVARIAN CARCINOMA

During embryogenesis, the coelomic layer develops into the peritoneal mesothelium that surrounds the ovary and later differentiates through metaplasia to an epithelial layer (4). Contrary to other malignancies, as the ovarian epithelium acquires a malignant phenotype, it becomes more, rather than less, differentiated. This plasticity may explain its ability to transform into any cell type found in the Mullerian tract (5). Germline mutations in *BRCA1*, *BRCA2*, and mismatch repair genes account for approximately 10% of ovarian malignancies.

For carcinogenesis to occur, the progenitor cell must overcome the physiologic checks and balances in order to become a clinically evident tumor. Examples of such mechanisms include impairment of apoptosis, insensitivity to antigrowth signaling, limitless cell proliferation, sustained angiogenesis, and metastasis (6). Multiple hypotheses have been proposed with regard to the possible origins of ovarian cancer. Since there is positive correlation between the number of ovulatory cycles with the risk of ovarian cancer, Fathalla proposed the incessant ovulation hypothesis (7). According to this hypothesis, with every ovulatory cycle there is damage to the ovarian surface epithelial cells and subsequently through repair mechanism the cells are predisposed to the development of mutations and later malignancies. The deficiencies in the incessant ovulation theory and the evidence of increased risk among women using fertility drugs for conception led to the gonadotropin hypothesis, which states that ovarian epithelial cells are more likely to undergo malignant transformation after exposure to follicle-stimulating hormone (FSH) and luteinizing hormone (LH). Since there are conflicting study results (8), it is the state of infertility rather than the gonadotropin medical therapy that increases the risk of EOC (9). Hormones, especially testosterone, have also been implicated in ovarian carcinogenesis; however, there is no strong evidence that exposure to androgens induces malignant transformation. Additionally, there is growing interest in the role of inflammation as a causative etiology for EOC. Inflammation accompanies each ovulation, with an associated influx of inflammatory cells, cytokine release, and tissue reconstruction (9). All these events stress the ovarian surface epithelial (OSE) cells such that they are predisposed to genetic damage and carcinogenesis. The more recent etiology of EOC arising from the fimbriated end of the fallopian tube will be discussed later in the chapter.

Although any of the above mechanisms may play a role in ovarian carcinogenesis in some patients, the modest association with each suggests that multiple other processes are involved, which cannot be predicted by clinically recognizable conditions. Therefore to detect early EOC or high-risk patients, more research is required for identifying genetic or epigenetic conditions.

■ EARLIEST RECOGNIZABLE PROCESSES IN TUMOR PROGRESSION

Similar to most cancers, EOCs are thought to arise from a single multidysfunctional cell. Supporting evidence for the clonality of ovarian cancer comes from studies showing common loss of heterozygosity (LOH), X-chromosome inactivation, and DNA mutation between the primary and metastatic lesions (10). The difficulty in describing the earliest biological events in EOC is due to the lack of early-stage tumors, heterogeneity among individuals, and the genetic instability of the tumors, which makes it difficult to know if the mutations are early or late occurrences.

Genomic Comparison of Early- Versus Late-Stage High-Grade Ovarian Cancers

Genomic analysis of high-grade tumors has revealed the amplification and/or overexpression of numerous genes thought to be responsible for the cancer development and predicting clinical outcome. With the emergence of new genomic technologies such as comparative genomic hybridization (CGH) and microarray expression profiling, many early genetic events such as the identification of individual genes and dominant pathways have been discovered (11,12).

Shridhar and colleagues compared normal ovarian epithelial cells to early- and late-stage cancers and found multiple differentially expressed genes between normal and cancerous tissues (13). Interestingly the early- and late-stage cancers were remarkably similar, which seems in contradiction to the concept that early-stage tumors evolve into late-stage ones. However, the authors found that CGH analysis demonstrated acquired gene abnormalities in late-stage cancers, which were more congruent with tumor evolution theory (13). Recently this has been substantiated by a European consortium as well (14). Another study analyzing malignant specimens from the ovary and omentum identified a 27-gene signature that can be used to distinguish the primary from metastatic cells (15). The main genes found to be altered were in the p53 pathway, suggesting the importance of this pathway in peritoneal metastasis. The Cancer Genome Atlas Research Network performed an integrated genomic analysis of 489 high-grade serous carcinomas, which revealed 96% prevalence of TP53 mutations in high-grade serous tumors. The high-grade serous cancers have a large degree of genomic disarray with a high frequency of somatic copy number alterations (16). Further validation studies are needed with larger power and micro-dissected samples to differentiate the tumoral and stromal alterations in early vs advanced ovarian cancers.

Inherited Disorders

Studying women with genetic disorders can give great insight as to the etiology and early events in carcinogenesis, but hereditary genetic disorders account for approximately 10% of ovarian cancers. The majority of inherited ovarian cancers may be due to BRCA1 and BRCA2 mutations, which predispose women to a lifetime risk of ovarian cancer of 56% and 27%, respectively (17). Gene profiling of BRCA1 and BRCA2 mutant and sporadic tumors revealed that the greatest contrast in expression patterns was between that of the BRCA1 and BRCA2 mutant tumors, and that the sporadic tumors had characteristics of both (18). Based on this study, BRCA1 and BRCA2 tumors may have different pathways in carcinogenesis and sporadic tumors may develop as result of changes in either pathway. Although patients with BRCA mutations have highly proliferative tumors, clinically they have more favorable outcomes when adjusted for stage (19). RAD51 genes (RAD51C and RAD51D) involved in DNA repair have been also established as germline mutation leading to ovarian cancer (20).

BRCA genes are mutated in 11%–15.3% of sporadic ovarian cancer, but through epigenetic changes, alternate splicing, and other genetic factors, BRCA function may be affected in as many as 82% of sporadic cancers (21–24). BRCA1 and BRCA2 proteins are essential components of the homologous recombination (HR) DNA system required to repair DNA double-strand breaks and play key roles in the induction of apoptosis and the monitoring of cell cycle checkpoints (25–27,44). Lack of functional BRCA in cells cause them to have increased aneuploidy, centrosome amplification, and chromosomal aberrations, which lead to susceptibility to further mutations. Additionally, BRCA is an important cofactor for a variety of transcription factors, including p53, STAT, c-Myc, JunB, ATF-1, and others (28). With the discovery of tubal intraepithelial carcinoma (TIC) in risk reducing salpingo-oophorectomy specimens in women with BRCA mutations and/or a strong family history of ovarian cancer has resulted in extensive research in the role of fallopian tube in pelvic serous carcinogenesis (29–31). BRCA1 mutation occurs early in the development of TIC but after tumor protein p53 mutation (32). It is possible that germline mutations in BRCA1 act as a promoter for the development of TIC (31). Interestingly, patients with BRCA2 mutation but not BRCA1 deficiency have improved survival, improved chemotherapy response, and genome instability compared to BRCA wild-type (33).

Defects in mismatch repair in patients with Lynch syndrome or hereditary nonpolyposis colon cancer (HNPCC) account for approximately 10% of the hereditary ovarian cancers. Patients with this syndrome have an approximately 12% risk of developing ovarian cancer (34). The defects in mismatch repair lead to genetic instability that places the cell at risk for mutation. However, the exact mechanism for ovarian carcinogenesis has not been further elucidated beyond a description of mismatch repair defects. Other rare familial syndromes associated with increased risk of ovarian cancer include Peutz–Jeghers syndrome (mutation in the *STK11* gene, 21% lifetime risk) and Gorlin syndrome (mutation in *PTCH*, 20% lifetime risk), but these tumors are usually stromal cancers and fibromas, respectively (35).

Two-Pathway Model of Ovarian Cancer

Since ovarian tumors are heterogeneous and present with a wide spectrum of disease states, there is growing clinical, translational, and genetic evidence that support at least two broad categories of carcinogenesis (36). High-grade malignancies tend to grow rapidly, be chemosensitive, and do not have a precursor lesion. Conversely, low-grade tumors grow more slowly, are less chemoresponsive, and share molecular characteristics with low-malignant potential (LMP) neoplasms. In a large series of 112 patients, Gershenson et al found the average age of diagnosis was 43 years compared to 61 for all cancers and the median survival to be 81 months, which is much longer than the 57- to 65-month survival observed in standard of care defining Phase III clinical trials (37–40). Pathologic review has demonstrated that approximately 60% of low-grade serous carcinomas are associated with serous LMP tumors compared to 2% of high-grade carcinomas. Additionally, LMP tumors recur as low-grade carcinoma in 75% of cases (41,42).

Molecular profiling of these two types of tumors substantiates the different pathogenesis. *KRAS* and *BRAF* mutations are detected in 20% of high-grade invasive carcinomas but are present in 30% to 50% of LMP tumors, low-grade adenocarcinomas, and in adjacent benign epithelium (37,42–44). Conversely, p53 are mutated in greater than 80% of high-grade tumors and rarely in LMP (45–48). HER2 and AKT are overexpressed in 20%– 67% and 12%–30% of high-grade carcinomas, respectively (49,50). Human leukocyte antigen-G has been reported in 61% of high-grade tumors and may provide an immune escape for the tumor, but is absent in low-grade or LMP tumors (51).

Whole genome approaches have differentiated developmental relatedness of various ovarian tumors. Using this approach and hierarchal clustering, LMP tumors show closer grouping to normal ovarian epithelium than to invasive ovarian cancers (52,53). Low-grade invasive cancers were more similar to borderline tumor than to high-grade invasive cancers. In LMP and low-grade cancers there is a functional wild-type p53 pathway, which is absent in the high-grade invasive cancers (52). Hence, the inactivation of the p53 pathway is a critical transition point in which a dysfunctional p53 leads to invasive high-grade cancers while an intact p53 pathway leads to LMP/low-grade cancers. In genomic studies such as LOH and CGH analyses, benign cystadenomas, LMP tumors, and

mucinous adenocarcinomas have similar gene expression indicating a sequential transformation from adenoma to LMP, and then to adenocarcinoma (54,55).

Pothuri and colleagues performed molecular, genetic, and morphologic analyses of early ovarian tumors and normal ovarian tissues and concluded that EOC may originate from the epithelial inclusion cyst, and there are dysplastic precursor lesions within these cysts (56). This quasi-neoplastic signature found in the ovarian cystic epithelium and not the ovarian surface epithelium involved signal transduction, cell-cycle control, and mitotic spindle formation. These cells had increased cell proliferation, decreased apoptosis, and aneuploidy. This study supports that at least some EOCs arise from ovarian inclusion cysts.

Another model is that the distal fallopian tube is the early precursor for the pelvic serous tumors. Evidence for this theory is supported by pathologic review of specimens from prophylactic bilateral salpingo-oophorectomy in *BRCA*-positive patients showing the presence of premalignant lesions/early serous carcinomas in the distal fallopian tubes. Moreover, these same findings were seen in more than 50% of patients with an unknown *BRCA* status and a pelvic serous carcinoma thereby further substantiating the critical link between the fallopian tube and pelvic serous cancer. Adjacent pelvic serous carcinoma and TIC show shared missense and frameshift/splicing/junction p53 mutations (57,58) thus supporting the origin to be in the distal fallopian tube (59,60). Przybycin and colleagues found that 60% of nonuterine high-grade serous carcinomas are associated with TIC (61). Recently, a Dicer-PTEN double knockout model was developed that shows the fallopian tube as the origin of high-grade serous cancer (62); however, it is unclear whether this model is truly reflective of human disease. Further molecular studies are needed to confirm the TIC as the earliest form of cancer and then more effective treatment and screening strategies can be developed (60).

■ GENETIC AND PROTEIN ALTERATIONS IN OVARIAN CANCER

Since most ovarian cancers are found at advanced stages, the study of genetic and protein alterations have been done in late-stage cancers. However, it is important to examine early-stage cancers to understand the earliest genetic alterations. For a cancer cell to become a clinically evident tumor it must undergo proliferation, inhibition of apoptosis, angiogenesis, stromal invasion, separation and survival away from the primary tumor, and implantation and growth within new tissues (63). Next, we will discuss these processes in the context of ovarian cancer (Table 13.1).

■ **Table 13.1** Select contributors to ovarian carcinogenesis

Protein	Function	Rate in EOC
Growth promotion		
EGFR(HER-1)	Membrane TK receptor, promotes growth	35%–70%
HER-2	Membrane TK receptor, promotes growth	20%–66% (HGS)
Src	TK, promotes growth, angiogenesis, survival	80%–90%
CSF-1/fms	Ligand/receptor, inhibits anoikis	50%–70%
ILGF/ILGFR	Peptide hormone/receptor, promotes growth	21%–25%
KRAS	G-protein, promotes growth through MAP kinase pathway	30%–50% (LGS)
BRAF	Promotes growth through MAP kinase pathway	30%–50% (LGS)
Insensitivity to anti-growth signals		
TGF-β	Ligand, inhibits growth through Rb activation	Lost in 40%
myc	Transcription factor, cell cycle mediator	30%
Cyclin D/Cdk4/6	Advance from G1 to S phase	30%–90%
Cyclin E/Cdk2	Advance from G1 to S phase	30%–70%
Cyclin B/Cdk1	Advance cell cycle into M phase	80%
p16	Inhibits cyclin D/Cdk4/6	Lost in 30%
p27 (kip-1)	Inhibits cyclin E/Cdk2	Lost in 55%
p21 (WAF-1)	Inhibits cyclin B/Cdk1	Lost in 25–40%
NFκB	Transcription factor, effector of many survival pathways	Unknown
NOEY(ARHI)	GTPase tumor suppressor, induces apoptosis through p21	40% LOH
Inhibition of apoptosis and immune surveillance		
PIP3/Akt	Akt (activated by PIP3) inhibits apoptosis	12%–18% (HGS)
PTEN	Decrease Akt	20% (Endo)
p53	Promotes cell cycle arrest/apoptosis with DNA damage	50%–90% (HGS)
BRCA1	Cofactor for transcription factors, "caretaker" of genome	6%–82%[a]
BRCA2	Cofactor for transcription factors, "caretaker" of genome	1%–3%
RAD51	Repairs DNA double strand breaks, tumor suppressor	0.9%–5.1%
MLH1/MSH2	Mediates mismatch repair, promotes genetic stability	30% (Endo)
Fas ligand	Produced by tumor cells to induce apoptosis of T-cells	50%–80%
HLA-G	Secreted by tumor cells to inhibit cytotoxic immune cells	61% (HGS)
Limitless replicative potential		
hTERT	Subunit of telomerase, maintains telomere length	80%–85%
Enhanced angiogenesis		
VEGF/VEGFR	Ligand/receptor complex induces angiogenesis	40%–100%
IL-8	Cytokine promoting angiogenesis	Unknown
EphA2	TK promotes angiogenesis and vasculogenic mimicry	76%
Promotion of invasion and metastasis		
MMPs	Matrix metalloproteinases degrade extracellular matrix	40%–100%
αvβ3	Integrin, promotes survival, and angiogenesis	95%
FAK	Cofactor TK promotes adhesion, proliferation, survival	70%
E-cadherin	Promotes adhesion	90%–100%

[a]Inherited mutation in 6% to 7% of all cancers; may play a role in up to 82% of sporadic cancers.
Endo, endometrioid; EOC, epithelial ovarian carcinoma; HGS, high-grade serous; LGS, low-grade serous; LOH, loss of heterozygosity; TK, tyrosine kinase.
Adapted from *Horm Cancer.* 2010 December; with permission Microenvironment and Pathogenesis of Epithelial Ovarian Cancer Antonio F. Saad, Wei Hu, and Anil K. Sood, 1(6): 277–290.

Self-Sufficiency of Growth Signals

Several oncogenes have been identified in ovarian cancer that enables the cells to proliferate independent from the host's signals. A nonreceptor tyrosine kinase src was one of the first oncoproteins described in ovarian carcinogenesis, and it is critical in promoting proliferation, adhesion, cell survival, and angiogenesis (64–66). Src overexpression has been demonstrated in 93% of advanced-stage ovarian cancers and numerous cell lines (67). Additionally, this oncoprotein promotes both chemoresistance to platinum and taxane agents in cell lines (68). Although inhibition of src with antisense or small molecule inhibitors have reduced ovarian cancer growth in preclinical mice models (64), Phase I study of dasatinib in combination with paclitaxel and carboplatin found a clinical response rate of 40% in ovarian cancer patients (69).

The Type I tyrosine kinase receptor family HER (i.e., Erb) consists of four monomers: EGFR (i.e., ERb1/HER1), HER2 (encoded by the proto-oncogene *neu*), HER3, and HER4. By immunohistochemistry EGFR is expressed on normal human ovarian surface epithelium and is overexpressed in 35%–70% of EOCs (70). Although HER2 has no extracellular ligand-binding domain, it is activated when dimerized with other Type I receptors. HER2 overexpression in ovarian cancer is 20%–30% (71). To date the monoclonal antibodies and tyrosine kinase inhibitors to HER/Erb family in ovarian cancer patients have shown only marginal activity as single agents, but have shown some improved benefit when added to platinum chemotherapy in recurrent EOC patients (72).

RAS, an oncoprotein, is a G-protein that is activated by many tyrosine kinase receptors. Activated RAS turns on a series of serine/threonine and tyrosine non-receptor kinases leading to phosphorylation of Erk1 and Erk2 transcription factors that initiate signals of cell growth and proliferation. *KRAS* mutations have variable frequency in different histologic subtypes: 61% of LMP tumors, 68% of low-grade tumors, 50% of mucinous adenocarcinomas, and in 5% of high-grade serous carcinomas (44,73). Wong and colleagues found that only 19% of low-grade serous carcinoma patients had a *KRAS* mutation, and these patients do much better clinically (74).

Resistance to Antigrowth Signals

For early malignant transformation to occur, antigrowth signals must be overcome. Although there is limited data regarding the specific sequence of genetic events required in carcinogenesis, there is evidence for abnormalities in cell cycle proteins. Examples of such critical cell cycle mediators include cyclins, cyclin-dependent kinases (CDK), CDK-inhibitors that inhibit cyclin/CDK complexes, and transcription factors such as pRB, TP53, and E2F. The G1 phase checkpoint (the restriction point) is the step at which the cell is committed to divide and is controlled by cyclin D and E's regulation of E2F release by Rb. Cyclin E is expressed by 9% of benign tumors, 48% of borderline tumors, and 70% of malignant tumors and is associated with poor outcome (75). CDK2 is another protein involved in the G1-S transition with cyclin E and is more frequently expressed in malignant compared to benign or LMP tumors (75). Cyclin D1 is found abundantly in the cytoplasm (89%) and nucleus (30%) of ovarian cancer cells, but not in the normal epithelial ovarian cells (76). CDK1/cyclin B complex regulates entry to M phase and CDK1 is highly expressed in 80% of malignant cells (77).

Another protein that controls the cell cycle is myc, which is an oncogenic transcription factor that is activated by the RAS-RAF pathway. Myc is overexpressed in approximately 30% of ovarian cancers. *AHRI* or *NOEY2* is a GTPase tumor suppressor gene present in normal epithelial ovarian cells but completely lost in almost all ovarian cancers (78,79). Due to the multiplicity of genetic anomalies in cell-cycle regulation, ovarian cancer cells gain a survival advantage facilitating unchecked growth.

Surviving Apoptosis

Avoiding cell death is thought to be the most critical step in carcinogenesis. Many genes and proteins play a role in cell death evasion. Among these is P53, which usually detects damaged DNA, promotes cell cycle arrest, initiates repair mechanisms, or directs the cell cycle into the pathway of apoptosis (80,81). Due to the importance of the *TP53* gene, it has been hypothesized that cancers that do not have *TP53* gene mutations must have alterations in the function of p53 in other ways, such as enhanced degradation through ubiquitination or the production of p53-binding proteins. In ovarian cancer most *TP53* gene mutations are missense (82). Null mutations may play a role in producing a more metastatic phenotype as evidenced by the fact that they are not found in Stage I ovarian cancers. *TP53* mutations are detected in ovarian inclusion cysts adjacent to microscopic cystadenocarcinomas and in tubular intraepithelial carcinomas removed in risk-reducing salpingo-oophorectomy specimens of *BRCA* patients (58,83,84). There is mounting evidence that p53 inactivation may be a relatively early event in ovarian carcinogenesis.

The PI3-kinase/AKT pathway is upregulated in approximately 30% of ovarian cancers (50). Activation of this pathway leads to inhibition of apoptosis, increase in neoangiogenesis, enhanced invasion, and increase in chemoresistance (85). *PTEN* controls this pathway by causing dephosphorylation of PIP3 back to PIP2 thereby promoting apoptosis. The *PTEN* mutation is frequently found in endometrioid ovarian cancer and may be an early event in this histotype (86).

The SWI–SNF complex is present in all eukaryotes and is involved in the cellular development, differentiation, proliferation, DNA repair, and tumor suppression (87). The complex utilizes adenosine triphosphate (ATP) to mobilize the nucleosome and thereby control accessibility of promoters to transcriptional activation or repression. BAF250A is a protein encoded by AT-rich interactive domain-containing protein 1A (*ARID1A*) and is one of the accessory subunits of the SWI–SNF complex that provides specificity of in gene expression regulation. Wiegand and colleagues performed RNA sequencing to detect *ARID1A* mutations in 46% of clear cell ovarian and 30% of endometrioid ovarian cancers; however, it was not present in high-grade serous ovarian cancers (88). Therefore,

ARID1A is a new potential tumor suppressor gene that may play an early role in the transformation of endometriosis to clear cell or endometrioid ovarian carcinomas.

Nuclear factor-kappa B (NFκB) is the main member of a family of transcription factors that deliver signals to the nucleus that result in proliferation and inhibition of apoptosis. Activated NFκB results in upregulation of *Bcl-2* family members, inhibition of apoptosis proteins, and expression of additional genes such as *ephrin-A1* that may play a role in ovarian cancer pathogenesis and aggressiveness (89,90). NFκB blockade also decreases interleukin-8 (IL-8) and vascular endothelial growth factor (VEGF) expression resulting in diminished malignant potential in ovarian cancer cell lines (91).

Cell Immortality

Normal cells can only divide a finite number of times before they achieve senescence and ultimately apoptosis. The timing of this phenomenon relies on telomere caps, which are on the end of chromosomes and are made up of DNA and various proteins. If the telomere protection is lost, the chromosomes are exposed to defects, which allow p53 and other proteins to initiate apoptosis. Beesley and colleagues demonstrated a direct association between functional single nucleotide polymorphisms in the TERT promoter, which decreased the risk of ovarian cancer and ultimately reduced telomerase reverse transcriptase (TERT) promoter activity. The decreased levels of TERT result in gradual telomere shortening and the onset of senescence, which ultimately suppress tumorigenesis (92).

Using telomerase-specific fluorescence in situ hybridization, 82% of Serous tubal intraepithelial carcinoma (STIC) lesions were found to have short telomeres compared to normal tubal epithelium; however, high-grade serous carcinomas had longer telomeres than the precursor lesion STIC. Based on this evidence, Kuhn and colleagues concluded that not only is telomerase activity an important event but also an early event in ovarian tumorigenesis (93). Additionally, telomere length varies by histologic type of ovarian cancer such that clear cell ovarian carcinomas have longer telomere lengths and the changes in telomere length may have an important role in the development and progression of ovarian cancer (94). The majority of ovarian cancers overcome the apoptosis pathway by producing telomerase, which is a reverse transcriptase composed of an RNA component (hTR) and a catalytic subunit (hTERT; 95). hTERT expression increases with tumorigenicity suggesting that this is the rate-limiting step in telomerase activity (96). The findings that P53 knockdown and hTERT expression alone can transform ovarian surface epithelial cells and that functional *BRCA* inhibits telomerase activity implicates telomerase activation as an early and necessary event for carcinogenesis (97,98).

DNA is continually being damaged, requiring repair of the double-strand breaks through nonhomologous end-joining and HR. HR defects in ovarian cancer due to *BRCA* deficiency confer sensitivity to poly ADP-ribose polymerase inhibitors in ovarian cancer (99).

Early Events in the Tumor Microenvironment: Angiogenesis, Invasion, and Metastasis

Although genetic events in tumor cells themselves are crucial, the interplay between host and stromal factors in the tumor microenvironment are equally important. This communication between tumor cells and normal tissue dictates angiogenesis, invasion into the surrounding stroma, penetration of lymphatic and vascular spaces, and adhesion and metastasis. In ovarian cancer, peritoneal and stromal alterations may be permissive for cancer spread (100) and by understanding these factors, unique targets for therapy may be developed.

Oxygen and nutrients are critical for benign, malignant, or normal cells, which must be within 100 μm of a capillary in order to survive (101). Angiogenesis enables the tumor to grow beyond approximately 1 mm^3 and requires a balance between pro- and anti-angiogenic influences within the tumor microenvironment. VEGF-A is not only a key mediator of angiogenesis, but also has multiple functions: increases vascular permeability, stimulates endothelial cell proliferation and migration, alters endothelial gene expression, and protects endothelial cells from apoptosis (102–105). In preclinical studies, VEGF expression induces ovarian cancer cell lines to induce carcinomatosis and ascites, and increased circulating and tumor VEGF levels are associated with the clinical outcome of ovarian cancer patients (106–108).

Mediators of angiogenesis include tumor-derived and host stromal factors. IL-8 plays a significant role in new vessel formation and ovarian cancer growth as well as being elevated in patients with all stages of ovarian cancer, and preclinically IL-8 gene silencing causes decreased tumor growth through anti-angiogenic mechanisms (109–111). Recently, it has been identified as a key adipokine that facilitates migration and invasion of ovarian cancer cells to the omentum (112). The integrin αvβ3 integrin mainly expressed on newly developing vascular endothelial cells as well as on ovarian tumor cells (113). The tyrosine kinase receptor EphA2 is overexpressed by 75% of ovarian cancers (114) and its inhibition reduces tumor growth in part by blocking angiogenesis (115,116). From a personalized medicine perspective, the patient-specific tumor microenvironment characteristics may influence the response to a particular anti-angiogenic therapy (117,118).

The critical step for metastasis is invasion of the basement membrane. Invasion of malignant cells through the basement membrane and endothelial cell migration for angiogenesis requires degradation of the extracellular matrix (ECM). Matrix metalloproteinases (MMPs) digest collagen and other ECM components and promote angiogenesis through VEGF (119). MMP-2 and MMP-9 are overexpressed in ovarian tumors and this increased expression correlates with clinical stage and patient survival (120–122). Huang et al showed that host-derived MMP-9 expression appears to play a major role in angiogenesis and progression in human ovarian tumors compared to MMPs from tumor cells (123). Another potentiator of metastasis is host production of catecholamines through chronic stress. Chronic sympathetic activation can directly promote tumor growth and metastasis (e.g., angiogenesis, anoikis via a stimulation of beta-adrenergic receptors; 124–126). Additionally, epidemiologic studies show that patients with poor social support and increased stress are at greater risk for cancer progression (127).

Inflammatory cells and associated cytokines play significant roles in the tumor microenvironment. Tumor cells produce proteins that are recognized as abnormal which then induce an immune response resulting in tumor cell death. In an effort to evade recognition by the immune system, tumor cells have acquired the ability to produce Fas ligand that induces lymphocytic apoptosis as well as the secretion of HLA-G that can inhibit NK cell activity (51,128,129). Cytokine production by mesenchymal cells stimulates ovarian epithelium and processes that activates malignant transformation (130). Cytokine production by tumor cells promotes growth and inhibits apoptosis (131). Demonstrating the importance of the host antitumor immune response, increased T-cell infiltration into the tumor is associated with increased survival (132). The exact role of the specific immune cell populations in controlling vs promoting tumor growth is still to be delineated in ovarian cancer, but there are promising data in melanoma (133,134).

Traditionally the definition of an advanced stage cancer required the metastatic spread of cancer cells; however, recent evidence suggests that metastasis could be a relatively early event (135). Very few (less than 0.01%) of shed malignant cells are capable of metastasizing. Even circulating cancer cells in the vasculature does not guarantee invading and proliferating in distant sites (136). Unlike other cancers, EOC has a different pattern of metastasis, and only 30% of Stage I cancers have positive cytology (137). Due to the shedding capability of ovarian cancer cells, an early role may be played by cell survival promoters such as focal adhesion kinase (FAK) and E-cadherin (138–140). Recently, adrenergic modulation of FAK has protected human ovarian cancer cells from anoikis, thereby promoting metastasis (126). Moreover, E-cadherin is expressed in ovarian cancer, low-malignant potential tumors, benign inclusion cysts, but not in normal surface epithelium (141).

Proposed Model of Ovarian Carcinogenesis and Conclusion

With the improving understanding and identification of key molecules and pathways in the early development of ovarian carcinogenesis, better-targeted therapies can be developed. We believe that not only are early genetic events important but also that the stroma with its inflammatory cells, MMPs, immunomodulators, and integrin ligands plays an important role in tumorigenesis. Although the sequence of events is variable, certain genetic alterations lead to specific tumor types. For example, *KRAS* mutations lead to LMP, while a *TP53* or *BRCA* mutation can lead to high-grade carcinomas. Both low- and high-grade pathways share the ability to evade the immune surveillance, invasion into the stroma, survival in the peritoneal cavity, attachment to the intraperitoneal sites, and continued growth and angiogenesis. Although many similarities exist in both pathways, every cancer is unique and many genetic alterations are yet unidentified. The real challenge is to identify the initial alterations in ovarian carcinogenesis in order to develop better early detection methods and to target key target pathways to ultimately improve cure rates.

■ REFERENCES

1. Siegel R, Naishadham D, Jemal A. Cancer statistics, 2012. *CA Cancer J Clin.* 2012;62(1):10–29.
2. Koonings PP, Campbell K, Mishell DR Jr, Grimes DA. Relative frequency of primary ovarian neoplasms: a 10-year review. *Obstet Gynecol.* 1989;74(6):921–926.
3. Prat J. Ovarian carcinomas: five distinct diseases with different origins, genetic alterations, and clinicopathological features. *Virchows Arch.* 2012;460(3):237–249.
4. Auersperg N, Wong AS, Choi KC, Kang SK, Leung PC. Ovarian surface epithelium: biology, endocrinology, and pathology. *Endocr Rev.* 2001;22(2):255–288.
5. Naora H. Developmental patterning in the wrong context: the paradox of epithelial ovarian cancers. *Cell Cycle.* 2005;4(8):1033–1035.
6. Hanahan D, Weinberg RA. The hallmarks of cancer. *Cell.* 2000;100(1):57–70.
7. Fathalla MF. Incessant ovulation–a factor in ovarian neoplasia? *Lancet.* 1971;2(7716):163.
8. Brinton LA, Lamb EJ, Moghissi KS, et al. Ovarian cancer risk after the use of ovulation-stimulating drugs. *Obstet Gynecol.* 2004;103(6):1194–1203.
9. Ness RB, Cottreau C. Possible role of ovarian epithelial inflammation in ovarian cancer. *J Natl Cancer Inst.* 1999;91(17): 1459–1467.
10. Duggan BD, Dubeau L. Genetics and biology of gynecologic cancer. *Curr Opin Oncol.* 1998;10(5):439–446.
11. Donninger H, Bonome T, Radonovich M, et al. Whole genome expression profiling of advance stage papillary serous ovarian cancer reveals activated pathways. *Oncogene.* 2004;23(49): 8065–8077.
12. Bild AH, Yao G, Chang JT, et al. Oncogenic pathway signatures in human cancers as a guide to targeted therapies. *Nature.* 2006;439(7074):353–357.
13. Shridhar V, Lee J, Pandita A, et al. Genetic analysis of early- versus late-stage ovarian tumors. *Cancer Res.* 2001;61(15):5895–5904.
14. Zaal A, Peyrot WJ, Berns PM, et al.; EORTC GCG Translational Research Group. Genomic aberrations relate early and advanced stage ovarian cancer. *Cell Oncol (Dordr).* 2012;35(3):181–188.
15. Lancaster JM, Dressman HK, Clarke JP, et al. Identification of genes associated with ovarian cancer metastasis using microarray expression analysis. *Int J Gynecol Cancer.* 2006;16(5):1733–1745.
16. The Cancer Genome Atlas Research Network. Integrated genomic analyses of ovarian carcinoma. *Nature.* 2011;474:609–615.

17. Søgaard M, Kjaer SK, Gayther S. Ovarian cancer and genetic susceptibility in relation to the BRCA1 and BRCA2 genes. Occurrence, clinical importance and intervention. *Acta Obstet Gynecol Scand.* 2006;85(1):93–105.

18. Jazaeri AA, Yee CJ, Sotiriou C, Brantley KR, Boyd J, Liu ET. Gene expression profiles of BRCA1-linked, BRCA2-linked, and sporadic ovarian cancers. *J Natl Cancer Inst.* 2002;94(13):990–1000.

19. Cass I, Baldwin RL, Varkey T, Moslehi R, Narod SA, Karlan BY. Improved survival in women with BRCA-associated ovarian carcinoma. *Cancer.* 2003;97(9):2187–2195.

20. Meindl A, Hellebrand H, Wiek C, et al. Germline mutations in breast and ovarian cancer pedigrees establish RAD51C as a human cancer susceptibility gene. *Nat Genet.* 2010;42(5):410–414.

21. Merajver SD, Pham TM, Caduff RF, et al. Somatic mutations in the BRCA1 gene in sporadic ovarian tumours. *Nat Genet.* 1995;9(4):439–443.

22. Pal T, Permuth-Wey J, Betts JA, et al. BRCA1 and BRCA2 mutations account for a large proportion of ovarian carcinoma cases. *Cancer.* 2005;104(12):2807–2816.

23. Baldwin RL, Nemeth E, Tran H, et al. BRCA1 promoter region hypermethylation in ovarian carcinoma: a population-based study. *Cancer Res.* 2000;60(19):5329–5333.

24. Esteller M, Silva JM, Dominguez G, et al. Promoter hypermethylation and BRCA1 inactivation in sporadic breast and ovarian tumors. *J Natl Cancer Inst.* 2000;92(7):564–569.

25. Hilton JL, Geisler JP, Rathe JA, Hattermann-Zogg MA, DeYoung B, Buller RE. Inactivation of BRCA1 and BRCA2 in ovarian cancer. *J Natl Cancer Inst.* 2002;94(18):1396–1406.

26. Venkitaraman AR. Linking the cellular functions of BRCA genes to cancer pathogenesis and treatment. *Annu Rev Pathol.* 2009;4:461–487.

27. Yoshida K, Miki Y. Role of BRCA1 and BRCA2 as regulators of DNA repair, transcription, and cell cycle in response to DNA damage. *Cancer Sci.* 2004;95(11):866–871.

28. Boulton SJ. Cellular functions of the BRCA tumour-suppressor proteins. *Biochem Soc Trans.* 2006;34(Pt 5):633–645.

29. Rosen EM, Fan S, Pestell RG, Goldberg ID. BRCA1 gene in breast cancer. *J Cell Physiol.* 2003;196(1):19–41.

30. Piek JM, van Diest PJ, Zweemer RP, et al. Dysplastic changes in prophylactically removed Fallopian tubes of women predisposed to developing ovarian cancer. *J Pathol.* 2001;195(4):451–456.

31. Medeiros F, Muto MG, Lee Y, et al. The tubal fimbria is a preferred site for early adenocarcinoma in women with familial ovarian cancer syndrome. *Am J Surg Pathol.* 2006;30(2):230–236.

32. Folkins AK, Jarboe EA, Saleemuddin A, et al. A candidate precursor to pelvic serous cancer (p53 signature) and its prevalence in ovaries and fallopian tubes from women with BRCA mutations. *Gynecol Oncol.* 2008;109(2):168–173.

33. Yang D, Khan S, Sun Y, et al. Association of BRCA1 and BRCA2 mutations with survival, chemotherapy sensitivity, and gene mutator phenotype in patients with ovarian cancer. *JAMA.* 2011;306(14):1557–1565.

34. Bowtell DD. The genesis and evolution of high-grade serous ovarian cancer. *Nat Rev Cancer.* 2010;10(11):803–808.

35. Aarnio M, Sankila R, Pukkala E, et al. Cancer risk in mutation carriers of DNA-mismatch-repair genes. *Int J Cancer.* 1999;81(2):214–218.

36. Papageorgiou T, Stratakis CA. Ovarian tumors associated with multiple endocrine neoplasias and related syndromes (Carney complex, Peutz-Jeghers syndrome, von Hippel-Lindau disease, Cowden's disease). *Int J Gynecol Cancer.* 2002;12(4):337–347.

37. Shih IeM, Kurman RJ. Ovarian tumorigenesis: a proposed model based on morphological and molecular genetic analysis. *Am J Pathol.* 2004;164(5):1511–1518.

38. Gershenson DM, Sun CC, Lu KH, et al. Clinical behavior of stage II-IV low-grade serous carcinoma of the ovary. *Obstet Gynecol.* 2006;108(2):361–368.

39. Ozols RF, Bundy BN, Greer BE, et al.; Gynecologic Oncology Group. Phase III trial of carboplatin and paclitaxel compared with cisplatin and paclitaxel in patients with optimally resected stage III ovarian cancer: a Gynecologic Oncology Group study. *J Clin Oncol.* 2003;21(17):3194–3200.

40. Armstrong DK, Bundy B, Wenzel L, Huang HQ, Baergen R, Lele S, Copeland LJ, Walker JL, Berger RA. Intraperitoneal cisplatin and paclitaxel in ovarian cancer. *N Engl J Med* 2006;354(1):34–43.

41. Malpica A, Deavers MT, Lu K, et al. Grading ovarian serous carcinoma using a two-tier system. *Am J Surg Pathol.* 2004;28(4):496–504.

42. Crispens MA, Bodurka D, Deavers M, Lu K, Silva EG, Gershenson DM. Response and survival in patients with progressive or recurrent serous ovarian tumors of low malignant potential. *Obstet Gynecol.* 2002;99(1):3–10.

43. Mok SC, Bell DA, Knapp RC, et al. Mutation of K-ras protooncogene in human ovarian epithelial tumors of borderline malignancy. *Cancer Res.* 1993;53(7):1489–1492.

44. Teneriello MG, Ebina M, Linnoila RI, et al. p53 and Ki-ras gene mutations in epithelial ovarian neoplasms. *Cancer Res.* 1993;53(13):3103–3108.

45. Singer G, Oldt R 3rd, Cohen Y, et al. Mutations in BRAF and KRAS characterize the development of low-grade ovarian serous carcinoma. *J Natl Cancer Inst.* 2003;95(6):484–486.

46. Kohler MF, Marks JR, Wiseman RW, et al. Spectrum of mutation and frequency of allelic deletion of the p53 gene in ovarian cancer. *J Natl Cancer Inst.* 1993;85(18):1513–1519.

47. Kupryjanczyk J, Thor AD, Beauchamp R, et al. p53 gene mutations and protein accumulation in human ovarian cancer. *Proc Natl Acad Sci USA.* 1993;90(11):4961–4965.

48. Skilling JS, Sood A, Niemann T, Lager DJ, Buller RE. An abundance of p53 null mutations in ovarian carcinoma. *Oncogene.* 1996;13(1):117–123.

49. Ross JS, Yang F, Kallakury BV, Sheehan CE, Ambros RA, Muraca PJ. HER-2/neu oncogene amplification by fluorescence in situ hybridization in epithelial tumors of the ovary. *Am J Clin Pathol.* 1999;111(3):311–316.

50. Cheng JQ, Godwin AK, Bellacosa A, et al. AKT2, a putative oncogene encoding a member of a subfamily of protein-serine/threonine kinases, is amplified in human ovarian carcinomas. *Proc Natl Acad Sci USA.* 1992;89(19):9267–9271.

51. Singer G, Rebmann V, Chen YC, et al. HLA-G is a potential tumor marker in malignant ascites. *Clin Cancer Res.* 2003;9(12):4460–4464.

52. Bonome T, Lee JY, Park DC, et al. Expression profiling of serous low malignant potential, low-grade, and high-grade tumors of the ovary. *Cancer Res.* 2005;65(22):10602–10612.

53. Ouellet V, Guyot MC, Le Page C, et al. Tissue array analysis of expression microarray candidates identifies markers associated with tumor grade and outcome in serous epithelial ovarian cancer. *Int J Cancer.* 2006;119(3):599–607.

54. Heinzelmann-Schwarz VA, Gardiner-Garden M, Henshall SM, et al. A distinct molecular profile associated with mucinous epithelial ovarian cancer. *Br J Cancer.* 2006;94(6):904–913.

55. Wamunyokoli FW, Bonome T, Lee JY, et al. Expression profiling of mucinous tumors of the ovary identifies genes of clinicopathologic importance. *Clin Cancer Res.* 2006;12(3 Pt 1):690–700.

56. Pothuri B, Leitao MM, Levine DA, et al. Genetic analysis of the early natural history of epithelial ovarian carcinoma. *PLoS ONE.* 2010;5(4):e10358.

57. Crum CP. Intercepting pelvic cancer in the distal fallopian tube: theories and realities. *Mol Oncol.* 2009;3(2):165–170.

58. Kuhn E, Kurman RJ, Vang R, et al. TP53 mutations in serous tubal intraepithelial carcinoma and concurrent pelvic high-grade serous carcinoma—evidence supporting the clonal relationship of the two lesions. *J Pathol.* 2012;226(3):421–426.

59. Kindelberger DW, Lee Y, Miron A, et al. Intraepithelial carcinoma of the fimbria and pelvic serous carcinoma: Evidence for a causal relationship. *Am J Surg Pathol.* 2007;31(2):161–169.

60. Levanon K, Crum C, Drapkin R. New insights into the pathogenesis of serous ovarian cancer and its clinical impact. *J Clin Oncol.* 2008;26(32):5284–5293.

61. Przybycin CG, Kurman RJ, Ronnett BM, Shih IeM, Vang R. Are all pelvic (nonuterine) serous carcinomas of tubal origin? *Am J Surg Pathol.* 2010;34(10):1407–1416.

62. Kim J, Coffey DM, Creighton CJ, Yu Z, Hawkins SM, Matzuk MM. High-grade serous ovarian cancer arises from fallopian tube in a mouse model. *Proc Natl Acad Sci USA.* 2012; 109(10):3921–3926.

63. Hanahan D, Weinberg RA. The hallmarks of cancer. *Cell.* 2000;100(1):57–70.

64. Han LY, Landen CN, Trevino JG, et al. Antiangiogenic and antitumor effects of SRC inhibition in ovarian carcinoma. *Cancer Res.* 2006;66(17):8633–8639.

65. Ishizawar R, Parsons SJ. c-Src and cooperating partners in human cancer. *Cancer Cell.* 2004;6(3):209–214.

66. Silva CM. Role of STATs as downstream signal transducers in Src family kinase-mediated tumorigenesis. *Oncogene.* 2004;23(48):8017–8023.

67. Wiener JR, Windham TC, Estrella VC, et al. Activated SRC protein tyrosine kinase is overexpressed in late-stage human ovarian cancers. *Gynecol Oncol.* 2003;88(1):73–79.

68. Pengetnze Y, Steed M, Roby KF, Terranova PF, Taylor CC. Src tyrosine kinase promotes survival and resistance to chemotherapeutics in a mouse ovarian cancer cell line. *Biochem Biophys Res Commun.* 2003;309(2):377–383.

69. Alvarez Secord A, Teoh DK, Barry WT, Yu M, Broadwater G, Havrilesky LJ, Lee PS, Berschuck A, Lancaster J, Wenham RM. A phase I trial of dasatinib, an SRC-family kinase inhibitor, in combination with paclitaxel and carboplatin in patients with advanced or recurrent ovarian cancer. *Clin Cancer Res.* 2012;18(19):5489–5498.

70. Bartlett JM, Langdon SP, Simpson BJ, et al. The prognostic value of epidermal growth factor receptor mRNA expression in primary ovarian cancer. *Br J Cancer.* 1996;73(3):301–306.

71. Leary JA, Edwards BG, Houghton CR, Kefford RF, Friedlander ML. Amplification of HER-2/neu oncogene in human ovarian cancer. *Int J Gynecol Cancer.* 1992;2(6):291–294.

72. Gui T, Shen K. The epidermal growth factor receptor as a therapeutic target in epithelial ovarian cancer. *Cancer Epidemiol.* 2012;36(5):490–496.

73. Suzuki M, Saito S, Saga Y, Ohwada M, Sato I. Mutation of K-RAS protooncogene and loss of heterozygosity on 6q27 in serous and mucinous ovarian carcinomas. *Cancer Genet Cytogenet.* 2000;118(2):132–135.

74. Wong KK, Tsang YT, Deavers MT, et al. BRAF mutation is rare in advanced-stage low-grade ovarian serous carcinomas. *Am J Pathol.* 2010;177(4):1611–1617.

75. Sui L, Dong Y, Ohno M, et al. Implication of malignancy and prognosis of p27(kip1), Cyclin E, and Cdk2 expression in epithelial ovarian tumors. *Gynecol Oncol.* 2001;83(1):56–63.

76. Dhar KK, Branigan K, Parkes J, et al. Expression and subcellular localization of cyclin D1 protein in epithelial ovarian tumour cells. *Br J Cancer.* 1999;81(7):1174–1181.

77. Barrette BA, Srivatsa PJ, Cliby WA, et al. Overexpression of p34cdc2 protein kinase in epithelial ovarian carcinoma. *Mayo Clin Proc.* 1997;72(10):925–929.

78. Bao R, Connolly DC, Murphy M, et al. Activation of cancer-specific gene expression by the surviving promoter. *J Natl Cancer Inst.* 2002;94(7):522–528.

79. Yu Y, Xu F, Peng H, et al. NOEY2 (ARHI), an imprinted putative tumor suppressor gene in ovarian and breast carcinomas. *Proc Natl Acad Sci USA.* 1999;96(1):214–219.

80. Michalovitz D, Halevy O, Oren M. p53 mutations: gains or losses? *J Cell Biochem.* 1991;45(1):22–29.

81. Cheng JC, Auersperg N, Leung PC. Inhibition of p53 induces invasion of serous borderline ovarian tumor cells by accentuating PI3K/Akt-mediated suppression of E-cadherin. *Oncogene.* 2011;30(9):1020–1031.

82. Skilling JS, Squatrito RC, Connor JP, Niemann T, Buller RE. p53 gene mutation analysis and antisense-mediated growth inhibition of human ovarian carcinoma cell lines. *Gynecol Oncol.* 1996;60(1):72–80.

83. Marks JR, Davidoff AM, Kerns BJ, et al. Overexpression and mutation of p53 in epithelial ovarian cancer. *Cancer Res.* 1991;51(11):2979–2984.

84. Kerner R, Sabo E, Gershoni-Baruch R, Beck D, Ben-Izhak O. Expression of cell cycle regulatory proteins in ovaries prophylactically removed from Jewish Ashkenazi BRCA1 and BRCA2 mutation carriers: correlation with histopathology. *Gynecol Oncol.* 2005;99(2):367–375.

85. Hu L, Hofmann J, Lu Y, Mills GB, Jaffe RB. Inhibition of phosphatidylinositol 3'-kinase increases efficacy of paclitaxel in *in vitro* and *in vivo* ovarian cancer models. *Cancer Res.* 2002;62(4):1087–1092.

86. Dinulescu DM, Ince TA, Quade BJ, Shafer SA, Crowley D, Jacks T. Role of K-ras and Pten in the development of mouse models of endometriosis and endometrioid ovarian cancer. *Nat Med.* 2005;11(1):63–70.

87. Reisman D, Glaros S, Thompson EA. The SWI/SNF complex and cancer. *Oncogene.* 2009;28(14):1653–1668.

88. Wiegand KC, Shah SP, Al-Agha OM, et al. ARID1A mutations in endometriosis-associated ovarian carcinomas. *N Engl J Med.* 2010;363(16):1532–1543.

89. Deregowski V, Delhalle S, Benoit V, Bours V, Merville MP. Identification of cytokine-induced nuclear factor-kappaB target genes in ovarian and breast cancer cells. *Biochem Pharmacol.* 2002;64(5–6):873–881.

90. Herath NI, Spanevello MD, Sabesan S, et al. Over-expression of Eph and ephrin genes in advanced ovarian cancer: ephrin gene expression correlates with shortened survival. *BMC Cancer.* 2006;6:144.

91. Huang S, Robinson JB, Deguzman A, Bucana CD, Fidler IJ. Blockade of nuclear factor-kappaB signaling inhibits angiogenesis and tumorigenicity of human ovarian cancer cells by suppressing expression of vascular endothelial growth factor and interleukin 8. *Cancer Res.* 2000;60(19):5334–5339.

92. Beesley J, Pickett HA, Johnatty SE, et al.; kConFab Investigators; Australian Ovarian Cancer Study Group; ABCTB Investigators; Ovarian Cancer Association Consortium. Functional polymorphisms in the TERT promoter are associated with risk of serous epithelial ovarian and breast cancers. *PLoS ONE.* 2011;6(9): e24987.

93. Kuhn E, Meeker A, Wang TL, Sehdev AS, Kurman RJ, Shih IeM. Shortened telomeres in serous tubal intraepithelial carcinoma: an early event in ovarian high-grade serous carcinogenesis. *Am J Surg Pathol.* 2010;34(6):829–836.

94. Kuhn E, Meeker AK, Visvanathan K, et al. Telomere length in different histologic types of ovarian carcinoma with emphasis on clear cell carcinoma. *Mod Pathol.* 2011;24(8):1139–1145.

95. Landen CN, Klingelhutz A, Coffin JE, Sorosky JI, Sood AK. Genomic instability is associated with lack of telomerase activation in ovarian cancer. *Cancer Biol Ther.* 2004;3(12): 1250–1253.

96. Poremba C, Heine B, Diallo R, et al. Telomerase as a prognostic marker in breast cancer: high-throughput tissue microarray analysis of hTERT and hTR. *J Pathol.* 2002;198(2):181–189.

97. Yang G, Rosen DG, Mercado-Uribe I, et al. Knockdown of p53 combined with expression of the catalytic subunit of telomerase is sufficient to immortalize primary human ovarian surface epithelial cells. *Carcinogenesis.* 2007;28(1):174–182.

98. Zhou C, Liu J. Inhibition of human telomerase reverse transcriptase gene expression by BRCA1 in human ovarian cancer cells. *Biochem Biophys Res Commun.* 2003;303(1):130–136.

99. Banerjee S, Kaye SB, Ashworth A. Making the best of PARP inhibitors in ovarian cancer. *Nat Rev Clin Oncol.* 2010;7(9):508–519.

100. Wang E, Ngalame Y, Panelli MC, et al. Peritoneal and subperitoneal stroma may facilitate regional spread of ovarian cancer. *Clin Cancer Res.* 2005;11(1):113–122.

101. Folkman J. Angiogenesis in cancer, vascular, rheumatoid and other disease. *Nat Med.* 1995;1(1):27–31.

102. Folkman J. The role of angiogenesis in tumor growth. *Semin Cancer Biol.* 1992;3(2):65–71.

103. Frumovitz M, Sood AK. Vascular endothelial growth factor (VEGF) pathway as a therapeutic target in gynecologic malignancies. *Gynecol Oncol.* 2007;104(3):768–778.

104. Connolly DT, Heuvelman DM, Nelson R, et al. Tumor vascular permeability factor stimulates endothelial cell growth and angiogenesis. *J Clin Invest.* 1989;84(5):1470–1478.

105. Senger DR, Galli SJ, Dvorak AM, Perruzzi CA, Harvey VS, Dvorak HF. Tumor cells secrete a vascular permeability factor that promotes accumulation of ascites fluid. *Science.* 1983;219(4587):983–985.

106. Yoneda J, Kuniyasu H, Crispens MA, Price JE, Bucana CD, Fidler IJ. Expression of angiogenesis-related genes and progression of human ovarian carcinomas in nude mice. *J Natl Cancer Inst.* 1998;90(6):447–454.

107. Paley PJ, Staskus KA, Gebhard K, et al. Vascular endothelial growth factor expression in early stage ovarian carcinoma. *Cancer.* 1997;80(1):98–106.

108. Cooper BC, Ritchie JM, Broghammer CL, et al. Preoperative serum vascular endothelial growth factor levels: significance in ovarian cancer. *Clin Cancer Res.* 2002;8(10):3193–3197.

109. Lokshin AE, Winans M, Landsittel D, et al. Circulating IL-8 and anti-IL-8 autoantibody in patients with ovarian cancer. *Gynecol Oncol.* 2006;102(2):244–251.

110. Xu L, Fidler IJ. Interleukin 8: an autocrine growth factor for human ovarian cancer. *Oncol Res.* 2000;12(2):97–106.

111. Merritt WM, Lin YG, Spannuth WA, et al. Effect of interleukin-8 gene silencing with liposome-encapsulated small interfering RNA on ovarian cancer cell growth. *J Natl Cancer Inst.* 2008;100(5):359–372.

112. Nieman KM, Kenny HA, Penicka CV, et al. Adipocytes promote ovarian cancer metastasis and provide energy for rapid tumor growth. *Nat Med.* 2011;17(11):1498–1503.

113. Davidson B, Goldberg I, Reich R, et al. AlphaV- and beta1-integrin subunits are commonly expressed in malignant effusions from ovarian carcinoma patients. *Gynecol Oncol.* 2003;90(2):248–257.

114. Thaker PH, Deavers M, Celestino J, et al. EphA2 expression is associated with aggressive features in ovarian carcinoma. *Clin Cancer Res.* 2004;10(15):5145–5150.

115. Landen CN Jr, Chavez-Reyes A, Bucana C, et al. Therapeutic EphA2 gene targeting *in vivo* using neutral liposomal small interfering RNA delivery. *Cancer Res.* 2005;65(15):6910–6918.

116. Landen CN Jr, Lu C, Han LY, et al. Efficacy and antivascular effects of EphA2 reduction with an agonistic antibody in ovarian cancer. *J Natl Cancer Inst.* 2006;98(21):1558–1570.

117. Jung YD, Ahmad SA, Akagi Y, et al. Role of the tumor microenvironment in mediating response to anti-angiogenic therapy. *Cancer Metastasis Rev.* 2000;19(1–2):147–157.

118. Gaur P, Bose D, Samuel S, Ellis LM. Targeting tumor angiogenesis. *Semin Oncol.* 2009;36(2 Suppl 1):S12–S19.

119. Belotti D, Paganoni P, Manenti L, et al. Matrix metalloproteinases (MMP9 and MMP2) induce the release of vascular endothelial growth factor (VEGF) by ovarian carcinoma cells: implications for ascites formation. *Cancer Res.* 2003;63(17):5224–5229.

120. Naylor MS, Stamp GW, Davies BD, Balkwill FR. Expression and activity of MMPS and their regulators in ovarian cancer. *Int J Cancer.* 1994;58(1):50–56.

121. Herrera CA, Xu L, Bucana CD, et al. Expression of metastasis-related genes in human epithelial ovarian tumors. *Int J Oncol.* 2002;20(1):5–13.

122. Kamat AA, Fletcher M, Gruman LM, et al. The clinical relevance of stromal matrix metalloproteinase expression in ovarian cancer. *Clin Cancer Res.* 2006;12(6):1707–1714.

123. Huang S, Van Arsdall M, Tedjarati S, et al. Contributions of stromal metalloproteinase-9 to angiogenesis and growth of human ovarian carcinoma in mice. *J Natl Cancer Inst.* 2002;94(15):1134–1142.

124. Thaker PH, Han LY, Kamat AA, et al. Chronic stress promotes tumor growth and angiogenesis in a mouse model of ovarian carcinoma. *Nat Med.* 2006;12(8):939–944.

125. Sood AK, Bhatty R, Kamat AA, et al. Stress hormone-mediated invasion of ovarian cancer cells. *Clin Cancer Res.* 2006;12(2):369–375.

126. Sood AK, Armaiz-Pena GN, Halder J, et al. Adrenergic modulation of focal adhesion kinase protects human ovarian cancer cells from anoikis. *J Clin Invest.* 2010;120(5):1515–1523.

127. Antoni MH, Lutgendorf SK, Cole SW, et al. The influence of bio-behavioural factors on tumour biology: pathways and mechanisms. *Nat Rev Cancer.* 2006;6(3):240–248.

128. Ben-Hur H, Gurevich P, Huszar M, et al. Apoptosis and apoptosis-related proteins (Fas, Fas ligand, Blc-2, p53) in lymphoid elements of human ovarian tumors. *Eur J Gynaecol Oncol.* 2000;21(1):53–57.

129. Paul P, Rouas-Freiss N, Khalil-Daher I, et al. HLA-G expression in melanoma: a way for tumor cells to escape from immunosurveillance. *Proc Natl Acad Sci USA.* 1998;95(8):4510–4515.

130. Bukovsky A. Immune system involvement in the regulation of ovarian function and augmentation of cancer. *Microsc Res Tech.* 2006;69(6):482–500.

131. Nash MA, Ferrandina G, Gordinier M, Loercher A, Freedman RS. The role of cytokines in both the normal and malignant ovary. *Endocr Relat Cancer.* 1999;6(1):93–107.

132. Zhang L, Conejo-Garcia JR, Katsaros D, et al. Intratumoral T cells, recurrence, and survival in epithelial ovarian cancer. *N Engl J Med.* 2003;348(3):203–213.

133. Coukos G, Conejo-Garcia JR, Roden RB, Wu TC. Immunotherapy for gynaecological malignancies. *Expert Opin Biol Ther.* 2005;5(9):1193–1210.

134. Mellman I, Coukos G, Dranoff G. Cancer immunotherapy comes of age. *Nature.* 2011;480(7378):480–489.

135. Sørlie T, Perou CM, Tibshirani R, et al. Gene expression patterns of breast carcinomas distinguish tumor subclasses with clinical implications. *Proc Natl Acad Sci USA.* 2001;98(19):10869–10874.

136. Fidler IJ. The pathogenesis of cancer metastasis: the "seed and soil" hypothesis revisited. *Nat Rev Cancer.* 2003;3(6):453–458.

137. Emerich J, Konefka T, Dudziak M, Sobol A. The value of peritoneal cytology in the staging of ovarian cancer. *Ginekol Pol.* 1997;68(2):74–77.

138. Hood JD, Cheresh DA. Role of integrins in cell invasion and migration. *Nat Rev Cancer.* 2002;2(2):91–100.

139. Sunfeldt K. Cell-cell adhesion in the normal ovary and ovarian tumors of epithelial origin; an exception to the rule. *Mol Cell Endocrinol.* 2003;202:89–96.

140. Halder J, Kamat AA, Landen CN Jr, et al. Focal adhesion kinase targeting using *in vivo* short interfering RNA delivery in neutral liposomes for ovarian carcinoma therapy. *Clin Cancer Res.* 2006;12(16):4916–4924.

141. Sundfeldt K, Piontkewitz Y, Ivarsson K, et al. E-cadherin expression in human epithelial ovarian cancer and normal ovary. *Int J Cancer.* 1997;74(3):275–280.

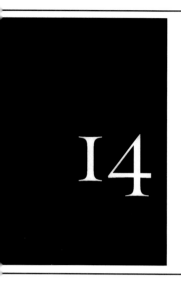

14 Current Status of Inherited Predisposition to Ovarian Cancer: Lessons From Familial Ovarian Cancer Registries in the United Kingdom and the United States

SUSAN J. RAMUS

Familial ovarian cancer registries have played an integral role in advancing our understanding of inherited predisposition to ovarian cancer. They have been key to investigating inherited ovarian cancer due to mutations in the *BRCA1* and *BRCA2* genes and are contributing, as part of large consortium projects, in the identification of moderate and low-risk susceptibility loci and modifiers of ovarian cancer risk in *BRCA1/2* mutation carriers. Additional studies utilizing these registries have included molecular pathology, epidemiology, and survival analysis based on *BRCA1/2* mutation status. To date more than 77 papers have been published that have included samples from the United Kingdom or Gilda Radner familial ovarian cancer registries.

■ INHERITED OVARIAN CANCER

A family history of the disease is the most significant known risk factor for epithelial ovarian cancer (EOC). There is a 3-fold increased risk of developing the disease for an individual with a first-degree relative affected with ovarian cancer (1). A relative with a diagnosis of EOC, before the age of 55, conveys a higher risk than those after 55 (2). Inherited EOC most often occurs as part of families with both ovarian and breast cancer cases, or in families with only multiple ovarian cancer cases. However inherited ovarian cancer is also part of Lynch syndrome or hereditary non-polyposis colorectal cancer (HNPCC), found in families with multiple cases of colon cancer. It is estimated that 5%–10% of EOC cases are due to these familial syndromes (3).

Familial Ovarian Cancer Registries

The Gilda Radner Familial Ovarian Cancer Registry (GRFOCR)

This self-referred registry was established in 1981 (4). Participants were recruited through index cases having a family history of at least one of the following criteria: (a) greater than or equal to two EOC cases; (b) one EOC case and greater than or equal to two related cancers at any other site; (c) greater than or equal to one case with greater than or equal to two primary tumors with one being EOC; (d) greater than or equal to two cancer cases with greater than or equal to one being EOC, and the other early onset (less than or equal to 45 years). The GRFOCR has enrolled over 2616 families. There are 2011 families with greater than or equal to two EOC cases, with 4987 women diagnosed with EOC.

The United Kingdom Familial Ovarian Cancer Registry (UKFOCR)

Established in 1991, this registry was formally known as the United Kingdom Coordinating Committee for Cancer Research (UKCCCR) Familial Ovarian Cancer Registry (5). The UKFOCR has recruited 391 families with greater than or equal to two EOC cases in first- or second-degree relatives. There are 1433 confirmed cancers in these families.

In both registries, termed UKFOCR and GRFOCR, data are collected on family history of cancer, reproductive history, oral contraceptive and hormone replacement therapy (HRT) use, past medical history, and tumor characteristics. In addition, women have provided blood for DNA and pathology material from ovarian and breast tumors.

Other Ovarian Cancer Families

There are a number of other familial ovarian cancer studies around the world including those from Toronto, Japan, and Poland (6–8). In addition, multiple ovarian cancer cases occur in families participating in breast or breast/ovarian cancer studies. In a review of familial ovarian cancer, 11 additional studies contained at least 60 families with one or more cases of ovarian cancer (3). There are 2678 ovarian cancer cases from 40 breast/ovarian cancer studies participating in the Consortium of Investigators of Modifiers of BRCA1/2 (CIMBA; 9). Families with two or more ovarian cancer cases are also present in population-based ovarian cancer studies. Within the 34 studies participating in the Ovarian Cancer Association Consortium (OCAC), 4149 ovarian cancer cases had data on family history and 258 (6.2%) had a first-degree family history of ovarian cancer (10). In 23 non-Ashkenazi Jewish ovarian cancer studies, 10%–47% of cases had a first- or second-degree relative with breast or ovarian cancer (3).

■ HIGH-RISK GENES

Ovarian Cancer Due to Mutations in the BRCA1/2 Genes

In 1990, a locus for hereditary breast and ovarian cancer was mapped by linkage analysis to chromosome 17q12–21 and named BRCA1 (11). An international collaboration that included the UKFOCR and GRFOCR localized BRCA1 to an interval of 1 centimorgan (cM; 12). The UKFOCR and GRFOCR also participated in the Breast Cancer Linkage Consortium study of 145 breast/ovarian cancer families, and showed a subset of families were not linked to BRCA1 (13).

The BRCA1 gene was cloned and found to have 24 exons (22 coding), spanning 80 kb of genomic DNA, and had a 7.8 kb transcript coding for an 1863 amino acid protein (14). The BRCA2 gene mapped to chromosome 13q12–13, had 27 exons (26 coding), spanning 70 kb of genomic DNA, and had an 11.4 kb transcript, and coded a 3418 amino acid protein (15).

Both genes show autosomal dominant transmission of highly penetrant germline mutations and behave as tumor suppressor genes (TSG), consistent with Knudson's two-hit hypothesis of gene inactivation, with loss of the normal allele in tumor tissue. Tumors from the UKFOCR and other studies showed allele loss at chromosome 17q12–21 in BRCA1-linked families, with loss of the wild-type chromosome (16,17). Both proteins function in the double-strand DNA break repair pathway but may have additional functions; BRCA1 functions in both checkpoint activation and DNA repair, and BRCA2 is a mediator of homologous recombination (18,19).

Mutations in BRCA1 and BRCA2 are found across the entire coding region and at splice sites. Premature protein termination mutations, such as small insertions or deletions resulting in a frameshift, nonsense mutations, or splice site alterations, are common for both genes. Some missense changes have been found to be pathogenic, but the majority are polymorphisms or are unclassified variants (UVs), also known as variants of uncertain significance (VUS). As well as the nonsynonymous coding changes, the UV include in-frame deletions that do not appear to be deleterious. The potential clinical significance of UV in BRCA1/2 are being investigated by the Evidence-based Network for the Interpretation of Germline Mutant Alleles (ENIGMA) consortium (20). A high frequency of large genomic rearrangements (LGR) have been identified in BRCA1, including founder mutations in some populations (21–23). LGR have also been detected in the BRCA2 gene (23).

In the largest study of inherited ovarian cancer, 283 families with two or more cases of EOC from the UKFOCR and GRFOCR were screened for coding sequence changes and LGR in the BRCA1 and BRCA2 genes. Deleterious BRCA1 mutations were identified in 104 families (37%) and BRCA2 mutations in 25 families (9%; 24). The extent of family history had a strong effect on mutation frequency: in families with three or more ovarian cancer cases plus breast cancer 81% had a mutation, while mutations were detected in 63% of families with three ovarian cancer cases only, and 27% in families with two ovarian cancer cases only. In other familial ovarian cancer studies, the frequency of BRCA1 mutations was 24%–66% and BRCA2 mutations 1%–17% (3). The role of BRCA1/2 founder mutations, in different populations, has been reviewed previously (3).

In a review of population-based ovarian cancer studies the frequency of BRCA1 mutations was 3%–10% and for BRCA2 0.6%–6% (3). The frequency of BRCA1 and BRCA2 mutations in the general population is estimated to be one in 800 and one in 500, respectively (25). In 17 population-based studies, 24%–100% of mutation carriers had a family history of breast or ovarian cancer (3). BRCA1 mutation carriers are diagnosed with ovarian cancer on average 7 years earlier than noncarriers (3). Screening population-based cases using family history and age of diagnosis can potentially detect more carriers than family history alone (26).

Clinical Implications of Detection of a BRCA1/2 Mutation

Based on family studies, the ovarian cancer risk by age 70 for a BRCA1 mutation carrier is 44%–63%, and for a BRCA2 mutation carriers is 27%–31% (27). The ovarian cancer risk by the age of 70 from population studies is 39% (95% confidence interval [CI]: 15–54) for BRCA1 and 11% (95% CI: 2.4–19) for BRCA2 (28). Identification of a BRCA1/2 mutation in a family allows improved clinical management and the potential for prophylactic surgery to reduce ovarian cancer risk (29). Inhibitors of poly (ADP-ribose) polymerase (PARP) exploit synthetic lethality to target DNA repair defects and are novel targeting agents for EOC. Ovarian cancer patients with BRCA1/2 mutations respond well to the PARP inhibitor olaparib, in clinical trials (30).

Further Studies of *BRCA1/2* Carriers and *BRCA1/2* Negative Cases

Screening for mutations in the *BRCA1/2* genes in the familial ovarian cancer registries provides a valuable resource of material for further studies of *BRCA1/2* mutation carriers and individuals with no identified mutations. *BRCA1/2* testing has been performed on an EOC proband from approximately 350 families from UKFOCR and GRFOCR. DNA samples from 145 families positive for *BRCA1/2* mutations and 193 *BRCA1/2* negative families have been included in additional studies and large international collaborative projects (Figure 14.1).

Mutation Position Modifies Ovarian Cancer Risk in Carriers

The position of a mutation in both *BRCA1* and *BRCA2* influences the risk of ovarian cancer (31–34). The central portion of the *BRCA2* gene was termed the ovarian cancer cluster region (OCCR) and was associated with a higher risk of ovarian cancer, than the 5′ and 3′ portion of the gene. This was confirmed in a larger study of 164 families, where the OCCR was defined from position 3059 to 6629 (35). A study of 356 families confirmed that the central portion of the *BRCA1* gene, nucleotides 2401 to 4190, was associated with significantly lower breast cancer risks and/or higher ovarian cancer risks compared to mutations elsewhere in the gene (36).

Environmental Risk Factors

Data from UKFOCR and GRFOCR showed that oral contraceptive use reduces ovarian cancer risk in *BRCA1* and *BRCA2* carriers by 5% with each year of use and with 6 or more years of use the odds ratio (OR) was 0.62 (95% CI: 0.35–1.09; 37). Another study confirmed this result and found that parity was associated with a decreased risk in *BRCA1* carriers but an increased risk in *BRCA2* carriers, while breastfeeding was associated with a decreased risk in both *BRCA1* and *BRCA2* carriers (38). Parity and/ or increased number of live births, and tubal ligation also reduces ovarian cancer risk in carriers (39,40).

Tumor Studies

There are five main histological subtypes of EOC; high-grade serous, low-grade serous, endometrioid, clear cell, and mucinous. It has been suggested by many studies, including several with data from the FOCRs, that ovarian tumors from *BRCA1* carriers are more likely to be serous compared to non-*BRCA1* tumors (41–43). Tumor profiling of UKFOCR and GRFOCR samples showed increased *TP53* mutations in *BRCA1/2* mutation carriers compared to noncarriers, and also showed differences by comparative genomic hybridization (44,45). Other groups have found different profiles for carriers and noncarriers by RNA expression analysis (46). The Cancer Genome Atlas (TCGA) performed large-scale somatic genomic analysis

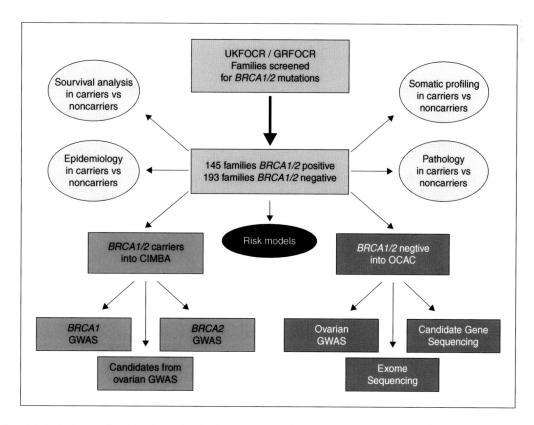

FIGURE 14.1 Inclusion of UKFOCR and GRFOCR samples in studies investigating inherited predisposition to ovarian cancer.

of 489 high-grade serous ovarian tumors and showed that 96% had mutations in *TP53* (47).

Survival in Carriers

An analysis of ovarian cancer survival in UKFOCR cases found a nonsignificant trend toward improved survival in *BRCA1* and *BRCA2* carriers compared to noncarriers (48). A large international collaboration investigated survival in *BRCA1* and *BRCA2* carriers by pooling data from 26 studies with a total of 1213 EOC cases with mutations in *BRCA1* (909) or *BRCA2* (304), and 2666 noncarriers (49). This included 176 cases from the UKFOCR and GRFOCR; 83 *BRCA1*, 9 *BRCA2*, and 84 noncarriers. *BRCA1* and *BRCA2* carriers had significantly better survival than noncarriers with hazard ratios (HRs) of 0.73 and 0.49, respectively.

Ovarian Cancer Due to Mismatch Repair Genes

Lynch syndrome or HNPCC results from mutations in the genes involved in the mismatch repair (MMR) pathway. Approximately 90% of mutations occur in the *MLH1* and *MSH2* genes. Mutations in *MSH6* and *PMS2* are less frequent and mutations in *MSH3*, *PMS1*, and *MLH3* are rare. Pedigree analysis of 226 women in the GRFOCR showed that 20 women (9%) had family histories that met the clinical criteria for HNPCC (50). The cumulative risk of ovarian cancer in Lynch syndrome is 8%–10% (51).

Seventy-seven *BRCA1/2* negative GRFOCR cases, that did not meet the Amsterdam criteria for HNPCC, were tested for germline mutations in *MLH1*, *MSH2*, and *MSH6* genes and two patients (2.6%) had deleterious mutations in the *MSH2* gene (52). Two studies have found MMR mutations in 2% of ovarian cancer unselected for age, with mutations in *MLH1*, *MSH2*, and *MSH6* genes (53,54). From two studies the lifetime risk of EOC was 7%–12% in *MLH1* or *MSH2* mutation carriers, with a higher risk for *MSH2* mutations compared to *MLH1* (55,56). Two *MSH6* Swedish founder mutations had an estimated lifetime EOC risk of 33% (57).

Other Cancers in Ovarian Cancer Families

In 143 GRFOCR families with three or more ovarian cancers, the risk of cancer at any nonovarian site in family members was 1.5 times that of the general population (58). The risk of breast and endometrial cancer in females, and prostate cancer in males was 2.5, 5, and 4.5 times the general population, respectively. The risks of other cancers, in families with *BRCA1* and *BRCA2* mutations, was reviewed previously (3). In *BRCA1* carriers there was a small increased risk of cancer overall and increased risk of pancreas, uterus, cervix, and prostate cancer. The risk of fallopian tube and peritoneal cancer was similar to ovarian cancer. *BRCA2* carriers had an increased risk of prostate and pancreatic cancer and potentially stomach, gallbladder and bile duct cancer, and malignant melanoma.

■ NON–HIGH-RISK ALLELES

The known high-penetrance susceptibility genes account for less than 40% of the excess familial risk of ovarian cancer (59). The remaining risk could be due to a combination of other high-risk genes that are probably very rare, several moderate-risk genes with a combined frequency of 5%, or multiple low-risk genes (with risks of 3 or less). In breast cancer, combining multiple, low-penetrance susceptibility alleles has a potential application in screening and early detection (60).

Common Low-Risk Alleles

Association studies, to investigate risk associated with single-nucleotide polymorphisms (SNPs), requires very large numbers of cases and controls. OCAC was established in 2005 and currently consists of 43 studies with 18,174 ovarian cancer cases and 26,134 controls. The FOCRs were not involved in the early studies of SNPs in candidate genes, which did not produce any highly significant candidate regions, reviewed previously (61). However, both studies participated in a genome-wide association study (GWAS). Stage I of the GWAS included 49 samples from UKFOCR and Stage II included 143 samples from GRFOCR. A total of six loci associated with risk of ovarian cancer have been published: 2q31, 3q25, 8q24, 9p22.2, 17q21, and 19p13.1 (Table 14.1; 10,62,63). At each region, the association was more significant in the serous only cases, reflecting the higher proportion of serous cases in the GWAS. The inclusion of individuals with a family history of ovarian cancer increased the power of the study. However, there was no significant difference in genotype frequency for cases reporting a family history of ovarian cancer compared with a negative family history (10,62). Validation of additional GWAS loci and fine mapping of the current loci is ongoing.

Genetic Modifiers of Ovarian Cancer Risk

CIMBA has shown that common genetic variants modify both breast and ovarian cancer risk (64,65). Currently within CIMBA, there are 12,599 *BRCA1* and 7132 *BRCA2* carriers. There are 2678 carriers with invasive ovarian cancer and 17,053 carriers censored as unaffected for ovarian cancer. This includes 242 (202 *BRCA1* and 40 *BRCA2*) samples from UKFOCR and GRFOCR.

CIMBA has recently performed GWAS for *BRCA1* and *BRCA2* mutation carriers (64,66). No loci were identified for ovarian cancer risk in the *BRCA1* or *BRCA2* GWAS due to small numbers of ovarian cancer cases. However, the ovarian cancer region 19p13.1 was found to modify breast cancer risk in the *BRCA1* GWAS. This region along with the additional five known ovarian cancer loci 2q31, 3q25, 8q24, 9p22.2, and 17q21 were analyzed in CIMBA in a larger sample size than the GWAS (Table 14.1; 9,65,67).

■ Table 14.1 Six common loci associated with ovarian cancer risk in the general population and modifying the risk of ovarian cancer in *BRCA1/2* mutation carriers

Chr Location—SNP	Closest Genes	OR All Invasive General Population	OR Serous General Population	HR *BRCA1* Mutation Carriers	HR *BRCA2* Mutation Carriers
9p22.2—rs3814113	*BNC2*	0.82 (0.79–0.86) $p = 5.10 \times 10^{-19}$	0.77 (0.73–0.81) $p = 4.10 \times 10^{-21}$	0.78 (0.72–0.85) $p = 4.8 \times 10^{-9}$	0.78 (0.67–0.90) $p = 5.5 \times 10^{-4}$
8q24—rs10088218	*MYC/PVT1*	0.84 (0.80–0.89) $p = 3.2 \times 10^{-9}$	0.76 (0.70–0.81) $p = 8.0 \times 10^{-15}$	0.89 (0.81–0.99) $p = 0.029$	0.81 (0.67–0.98) $p = 0.033$
3q25—rs2665390	*TIPARP*	1.19 (1.11–1.27) $p = 3.2 \times 10^{-7}$	1.24 (1.15–1.34) $p = 7.1 \times 10^{-8}$	1.25 (1.10–1.42) $p = 6.1 \times 10^{-4}$	1.48 (1.21–1.83) $p = 1.8 \times 10^{-4}$
2q31—rs717852	*HOXD1/HOXD3*	1.16 (1.12–1.21) $p = 4.5 \times 10^{-14}$	1.20 (1.14–1.25) $p = 3.8 \times 10^{-14}$	1.06 (0.98–1.14) $p = 0.16$	1.25 (1.10–1.42) $p = 6.6 \times 10^{-4}$
17q21—rs9303542	*SKAP1*	1.11 (1.06–1.16) $p = 1.4 \times 10^{-6}$	1.14 (1.09–1.20) $p = 1.4 \times 10^{-7}$	1.08 (1.00–1.17) $p = 0.06$	1.16 (1.02–1.33) $p = 0.026$
19p13.1-rs8170 *	*BABAM1*	1.12 (1.07–1.17) $p = 3.6 \times 10^{-6}$	1.18 (1.12–1.25) $p = 2.7 \times 10^{-9}$	1.15 (1.03–1.29) $p = 0.015$	1.34 (1.12–1.62) $p = 1.9 \times 10^{-3}$
19p13.1-rs2363956 *	*ANKLE1*	1.10 (1.06–1.15) $p = 1.2 \times 10^{-7}$	1.16 (1.11–1.21) $p = 3.8 \times 10^{-11}$	NA	NA
19p13.1-rs67397200 *	*ABHD8*	NA	NA	1.16 (1.05–1.29) $p = 3.8 \times 10^{-4}$	1.30 (1.10–1.52) $p = 1.8 \times 10^{-3}$

Note: CI, confidence interval; NA, not available; OR, odds ratio; SNP = single-nucleotide polymorphism. OR and 95% CI or HR and 95% CI of the rare alleles at each loci. Data from refs. (9,10,62,63,65,67). NA indicates not available as s2363956 could not be genotyped in *BRCA1/2* carriers using iPlex technology and rs67397200 was only genotyped in CIMBA samples. rs67397200 is an imputed SNP found to have a stronger association with breast cancer risk for *BRCA1* mutation carriers, $r^2 = 0.58$ with rs8170 and $r^2 = 0.37$ with rs2363956.

* Hazard Ratio for chr 19 SNPs in *BRCA1/2* carriers are competing risk values from analysis of both breast and ovarian cancer as these SNP are also associated with risk of breast cancer in *BRCA1/2* carriers. Bold indicates $< 5 \times 10^{-8}$ (genome-wide significant) for general population from GWAS study, for *BRCA1/2* < 0.05 as selected candidates for follow-up.

For each locus, the HR in mutation carriers was very similar to the OR in the general population.

A multiplicative model can be used to combine the results of several SNPs (9). With the identification of a larger panel of modifying loci, these results may have a clinical application, as the difference in absolute risk is greater in mutation carriers than in the general population. Risk prediction could combine genotyping data with mutation position and environmental risk factors known to modify ovarian cancer risk in carriers; such as oral contraceptive use, parity, and/or number of live births, and tubal ligation (37–40).

Rare Moderate-Risk Alleles

In 1997, UKFOCR and GRFOCR samples were screened for mutations in *BARD1*, as a candidate high-risk ovarian cancer gene in the *BRCA1* pathway, however no protein terminating changes were found (68). More recently, however, candidate gene sequencing has identified mutations/rare variants in 10 additional genes for EOC (50).

Mutations have been identified in four genes (*RAD51C*, *RAD51D*, *BRIP1*, and *PALB2*) that have a key role in the Fanconi Anemia (*FA*)–*BRCA* pathway. For both the *RAD51C* and *RAD51D* genes, mutations were found in approximately 1% of breast/ovarian cancer families, and

---

■ **Table 14.2** Timeline of key developments in high-risk genetic susceptibility to ovarian cancer

Year	Development	Study	Ref.
1981	*Gilda Radner Familial Ovarian Cancer Registry (GRFOCR) established	UKGRFOCR study	4
1990	***Linkage of early onset familial breast cancer to chromosome 17q21	Other study	11
1991	*UK Familial Ovarian Cancer Registry (UKFOCR) established	UKGRFOCR study	5
1992	**Allele losses at 17q12–21 of wild-type chromosome in familial OC	UKGRFOCR samples	16
1992	**Localization of *BRCA1* gene on 17q12–21 to an interval of 1 cM	UKGRFOCR samples	12
1994	***BRCA1* gene identified/cloned	Other study	14
1995	**Genetic heterogeneity in 145 breast-ovarian cancer families	UKGRFOCR samples	13
1995	*BRCA1* mutations in UKFOCR/genotype–phenotype correlation	UKGRFOCR study	31
1995	**High LOH at *BRCA1*—The Breast Cancer Linkage Consortium	UKGRFOCR samples	17
1995	*Risks of cancer among members of families in GRFOCR	UKGRFOCR study	58
1995	***BRCA2* gene identified/cloned	Other study	15
1997	*BRCA2* mutations in UKFOCR/genotype–phenotype correlation	UKGRFOCR study	33
1997	***Large Genomic Rearrangement (LGR) in *BRCA1*/Dutch founder	Other studies	21,22
1999	*Risk modeling of *BRCA1/2* in UKFOCR	UKGRFOCR study	34
1999	*High frequency of *TP53* mutations in *BRCA1/2* ovarian tumors	UKGRFOCR study	44
2000	*Histopathology *BRCA1* positive and negative ovarian tumors	UKGRFOCR study	41
2002	**Ovarian cancer risk in *BRCA1/2* carriers	UKGRFOCR samples	27
2003	*BRCA1/2* mutation status influences somatic genetic progression	UKGRFOCR study	45
2004	**Pathology of ovarian cancers in *BRCA1/2* carriers	UKGRFOCR samples	42
2004	*Oral contraceptive use and ovarian cancer risk in *BRCA1/2* carriers	UKGRFOCR study	37
2005	***Large Genomic Rearrangements (LGR) many studies	Other study	23
2006	*Role of hereditary non-polyposis colorectal cancer in familial OC	UKGRFOCR study	50
2007	*Screening of *BRCA1/2* in GRFOCR and UKFOCR including LGR	UKGRFOCR study	24
2008	***BRCA1/2* screening in population-based ovarian cancer study	Other study	26
2009	*Screening *MMR* genes in GRFOCR in *BRCA1/2* negative families	UKGRFOCR study	52
2012	**Pathology of ovarian cancers among *BRCA1/2* mutation carriers	UKGRFOCR samples	43
2012	**BRCA1* and *BRCA2* mutations and survival in ovarian cancer	UKGRFOCR samples	49

Note: * indicates UKFOCR and GRFOCR study, ** indicates inclusion of UKFOCR and GRFOCR samples, and *** indicates other studies.

no breast cancer only families and none or extremely low frequency in controls (69,70). The frequency of *RAD51D* mutations increased with number of ovarian cancer cases in the family, with 1.7% in families with two or more ovarian cases and 5.1% in families with three or more ovarian cancer cases. The relative risk (RR) of ovarian cancer in *RAD51D* carriers was 6.3 (95% CI: 2.9–13.9). Mutations in *PALB2* (FANCN) were found in 3.4% of breast cancer families and 55% of these families had family members with ovarian cancer (71). A *PALB2* founder mutation in Poland had a frequency of 0.6% in ovarian cancer cases and breast cancer cases, and 0.08% of controls (72). An Icelandic mutation in *BRIP1* (FANCJ) with a frequency of 0.41% increased the risk ovarian cancer, OR 8.1 (95% CI: 4.7–14.0), and behaved as a TSG with loss of the normal allele in tumors (73). A Spanish *BRIP1* mutation had a frequency of 1.3% in ovarian cancer cases and 0.6% in breast cancer cases, and the risk of ovarian cancer was OR 25 (95% CI: 1.8–340; 73).

Mutations in six additional genes (*BARD1*, *CHEK2*, *MRE11A*, *NBN*, *RAD50*, and *TP53*), were found by screening 21 TSG genes in 360 unselected ovarian, fallopian tube, or peritoneal cancer cases (74). Further mutations in *BRIP1*, *PALB2*, *RAD51C*, and *MSH6* were also detected.

Large case-control studies are required to determine lifetime risk estimates and average age of onset. Candidate genes sequencing is being performed on 3000 cases and 3000 controls, including 193 UKFOCR and GRFOCR

BRCA1/2 negative cases. Exome sequencing of 140 UKFOCR and GRFOCR *BRCA1/2* negative families will be used to identify novel candidate genes.

■ CONCLUSIONS

The FOCR have played a significant role in the investigation of high-risk predisposition to ovarian cancer and the identification of low- and moderate-risk genes (Tables 14.2 and 14.3). The major lesson from the familial ovarian cancer registries is the benefit of many groups collaborating in a large international consortium to identify loci involved in genetic susceptibility to ovarian cancer. The identification of common genetic susceptibility alleles and moderate-risk genes will lead to a greater understanding of disease etiology and potentially individualized therapies for ovarian cancer based on genetic pathways. PARP inhibitors are a targeted treatment for cases with *BRCA* mutations; however, they may also potentially benefit individuals with mutations in other genes in the homologous recombination or *FA-BRCA* pathways. Cells deficient for a series of proteins involved in homologous recombination and more recently *RAD51D* have shown selective sensitivity to PARP inhibitors (70,75). In the future, information on high-, moderate-, and low-risk genes as well as modifiers of risk, may be used in combined models of ovarian cancer risk, incorporating epidemiological risk factors and pathology data, to give personalized risk prediction.

■ **Table 14.3** Timeline of key developments in low/moderate-risk genetic susceptibility to ovarian cancer

Year	Development	Study	Ref.
1997	*Screening for *BARD1* mutations in UKFOCR and GRFOCR	UKGRFOCR study	68
2009	**UK ovarian GWAS chr 9p22.2	UKGRFOCR-OCAC	62
2010	**UK ovarian GWAS from serous subtypes 2q31 and 8q24	UKGRFOCR-OCAC	10
2010	**UK ovarian GWAS chr 19p13	UKGRFOCR-OCAC	63
2010	***BRCA1* GWAS breast cancer risk SNP at chr 19p13	UKGRFOCR-CIMBA	64
2010	***BRCA2* GWAS	UKGRFOCR-CIMBA	66
2010	***Moderate risk variants in *RAD51C* in ovarian cancer	Other study	69
2010	***Moderate risk variants in *PALB2* in ovarian cancer	Other study	72
2011	**CIMBA follow-up of ovarian GWAS candidate chr 9p22.2	UKGRFOCR-CIMBA	65
2011	***Moderate risk variants in *RAD51D* in ovarian cancer	Other study	70
2011	***Moderate risk variants in *BRIP1* in ovarian cancer	Other study	73
2011	***Moderate risk variants in *PALB2* in ovarian cancer	Other study	71
2011	***Screening of 21 TSG genes in unselected ovarian cancer—BROCA	Other study	74
2012	**CIMBA follow-up of ovarian GWAS chr 2q31, 3q25, 8q24, 17q21	UKGRFOCR-CIMBA	9
2012	**CIMBA follow-up of *BRCA1* GWAS and ovarian GWAS chr 19p13	UKGRFOCR-CIMBA	67

Note: * indicates UKFOCR and GRFOCR study, ** indicates inclusion of UKFOCR and GRFOCR samples, and *** indicates other studies.

■ REFERENCES

1. Stratton JF, Pharoah P, Smith SK, Easton D, Ponder BA. A systematic review and meta-analysis of family history and risk of ovarian cancer. *Br J Obstet Gynaecol.* 1998;105(5):493–499.

2. Auranen A, Pukkala E, Mäkinen J, Sankila R, Grénman S, Salmi T. Cancer incidence in the first-degree relatives of ovarian cancer patients. *Br J Cancer.* 1996;74(2):280–284.

3. Ramus SJ, Gayther SA. The contribution of BRCA1 and BRCA2 to ovarian cancer. *Mol Oncol.* 2009;3(2):138–150.

4. Piver MS, Mettlin CJ, Tsukada Y, Nasca P, Greenwald P, McPhee ME. Familial Ovarian Cancer Registry. *Obstet Gynecol.* 1984;64(2):195–199.

5. Greggi S, Ponder BA, Mancuso S. Establishment of a European registry for familial ovarian cancer. *Eur J Cancer.* 1991;27(2):113–115.

6. Narod SA, Madlensky L, Bradley L, et al. Hereditary and familial ovarian cancer in southern Ontario. *Cancer.* 1994; 74(8):2341–2346.

7. Sekine M, Nagata H, Tsuji S, et al.; Japanese Familial Ovarian Cancer Study Group. Mutational analysis of BRCA1 and BRCA2 and clinicopathologic analysis of ovarian cancer in 82 ovarian cancer families: two common founder mutations of BRCA1 in Japanese population. *Clin Cancer Res.* 2001;7(10):3144–3150.

8. Menkiszak J, Gronwald J, Górski B, et al. Hereditary ovarian cancer in Poland. *Int J Cancer.* 2003;106(6):942–945.

9. Ramus SJ, Antoniou AC, Kuchenbaecker KB, et al.; SWE-BRCA; HEBON; EMBRACE; GEMO; kConFab; OCGN; Consortium of Investigators of Modifiers of BRCA1/2 (CIMBA). Ovarian cancer susceptibility alleles and risk of ovarian cancer in BRCA1 and BRCA2 mutation carriers. *Hum Mutat.* 2012;33(4):690–702.

10. Goode EL, Chenevix-Trench G, Song H, et al.; Wellcome Trust Case-Control Consortium; Australian Cancer Study (Ovarian Cancer); Australian Ovarian Cancer Study Group; Ovarian Cancer Association Consortium (OCAC); Ovarian Cancer Association Consortium (OCAC). A genome-wide association study identifies susceptibility loci for ovarian cancer at 2q31 and 8q24. *Nat Genet.* 2010;42(10):874–879.

11. Hall JM, Lee MK, Newman B, et al. Linkage of early-onset familial breast cancer to chromosome 17q21. *Science.* 1990;250(4988):1684–1689.

12. Smith SA, DiCioccio RA, Struewing JP, et al. Localisation of the breast-ovarian cancer susceptibility gene (BRCA1) on 17q12–21 to an interval of < or = 1 cM. *Genes Chromosomes Cancer.* 1994;10(1):71–76.

13. Narod SA, Ford D, Devilee P, et al. An evaluation of genetic heterogeneity in 145 breast-ovarian cancer families. Breast Cancer Linkage Consortium. *Am J Hum Genet.* 1995;56(1):254–264.

14. Miki Y, Swensen J, Shattuck-Eidens D, et al. A strong candidate for the breast and ovarian cancer susceptibility gene BRCA1. *Science.* 1994;266(5182):66–71.

15. Wooster R, Bignell G, Lancaster J, et al. Identification of the breast cancer susceptibility gene BRCA2. *Nature.* 1995;378(6559):789–792.

16. Smith SA, Easton DF, Evans DG, Ponder BA. Allele losses in the region 17q12–21 in familial breast and ovarian cancer involve the wild-type chromosome. *Nat Genet.* 1992;2(2):128–131.

17. Cornelis RS, Neuhausen SL, Johansson O, et al. High allele loss rates at 17q12-q21 in breast and ovarian tumors from BRCAl-linked families. The Breast Cancer Linkage Consortium. *Genes Chromosomes Cancer.* 1995;13(3):203–210.

18. Roy R, Chun J, Powell SN. BRCA1 and BRCA2: different roles in a common pathway of genome protection. *Nat Rev Cancer.* 2012;12(1):68–78.

19. O'Donovan PJ, Livingston DM. BRCA1 and BRCA2: breast/ovarian cancer susceptibility gene products and participants in DNA double-strand break repair. *Carcinogenesis.* 2010;31(6):961–967.

20. Spurdle AB, Healey S, Devereau A, et al.; ENIGMA. ENIGMA–evidence-based network for the interpretation of germline mutant alleles: an international initiative to evaluate risk and clinical significance associated with sequence variation in BRCA1 and BRCA2 genes. *Hum Mutat.* 2012;33(1):2–7.

21. Puget N, Torchard D, Serova-Sinilnikova OM, et al. A 1-kb Alu-mediated germ-line deletion removing BRCA1 exon 17. *Cancer Res.* 1997;57(5):828–831.

22. Petrij-Bosch A, Peelen T, van Vliet M, et al. BRCA1 genomic deletions are major founder mutations in Dutch breast cancer patients. *Nat Genet.* 1997;17(3):341–345.

23. Mazoyer S. Genomic rearrangements in the BRCA1 and BRCA2 genes. *Hum Mutat.* 2005;25(5):415–422.

24. Ramus SJ, Harrington PA, Pye C, et al. Contribution of BRCA1 and BRCA2 mutations to inherited ovarian cancer. *Hum Mutat.* 2007;28(12):1207–1215.

25. Antoniou AC, Cunningham AP, Peto J, et al. The BOADICEA model of genetic susceptibility to breast and ovarian cancers: updates and extensions. *Br J Cancer.* 2008;98(8):1457–1466.

26. Søgaard M, KrugerKjaer S, Cox M, et al. BRCA1 and BRCA2 mutation prevalence and clinical characteristics in an ovarian cancer case population from Denmark. *Clin Cancer Res.* 2008;14(12):3761–3767.

27. Antoniou AC, Pharoah PD, McMullan G, et al. A comprehensive model for familial breast cancer incorporating BRCA1, BRCA2 and other genes. *Br J Cancer.* 2002;86(1):76–83.

28. Antoniou A, Pharoah PD, Narod S, et al. Average risks of breast and ovarian cancer associated with BRCA1 or BRCA2 mutations detected in case Series unselected for family history: a combined analysis of 22 studies. *Am J Hum Genet.* 2003;72(5):1117–1130.

29. Tinelli A, Malvasi A, Leo G, et al. Hereditary ovarian cancers: from BRCA mutations to clinical management. A modern appraisal. *Cancer Metastasis Rev.* 2010;29(2):339–350.

30. Ratner ES, Sartorelli AC, Lin ZP. Poly (ADP-ribose) polymerase inhibitors: on the horizon of tailored and personalized therapies for epithelial ovarian cancer. *Curr Opin Oncol.* 2012;24(5):564–571.

31. Gayther SA, Warren W, Mazoyer S, et al. Germline mutations of the BRCA1 gene in breast and ovarian cancer families provide evidence for a genotype-phenotype correlation. *Nat Genet.* 1995;11(4):428–433.

32. Gayther SA, Harrington P, Russell P, Kharkevich G, Garkavtseva RF, Ponder BA. Rapid detection of regionally clustered germ-line BRCA1 mutations by multiplex heteroduplex analysis. UKCCCR Familial Ovarian Cancer Study Group. *Am J Hum Genet.* 1996;58(3):451–456.

33. Gayther SA, Mangion J, Russell P, et al. Variation of risks of breast and ovarian cancer associated with different germline mutations of the BRCA2 gene. *Nat Genet.* 1997;15(1):103–105.

34. Gayther SA, Russell P, Harrington P, Antoniou AC, Easton DF, Ponder BA. The contribution of germline BRCA1 and BRCA2 mutations to familial ovarian cancer: no evidence for other ovarian cancer-susceptibility genes. *Am J Hum Genet.* 1999;65(4):1021–1029.

35. Thompson D, Easton D; Breast Cancer Linkage Consortium. Variation in cancer risks, by mutation position, in BRCA2 mutation carriers. *Am J Hum Genet.* 2001;68(2):410–419.

36. Thompson D, Easton D; Breast Cancer Linkage Consortium. Variation in BRCA1 cancer risks by mutation position. *Cancer Epidemiol Biomarkers Prev.* 2002;11(4):329–336.

37. Whittemore AS, Balise RR, Pharoah PD, et al. Oral contraceptive use and ovarian cancer risk among carriers of BRCA1 or BRCA2 mutations. *Br J Cancer.* 2004;91(11):1911–1915.

38. McLaughlin JR, Risch HA, Lubinski J, et al.; Hereditary Ovarian Cancer Clinical Study Group. Reproductive risk factors for ovarian cancer in carriers of BRCA1 or BRCA2 mutations: a case-control study. *Lancet Oncol.* 2007;8(1):26–34.

39. Milne RL, Osorio A, Ramón y Cajal T, et al. Parity and the risk of breast and ovarian cancer in BRCA1 and BRCA2 mutation carriers. *Breast Cancer Res Treat.* 2010;119(1):221–232.

40. Antoniou AC, Rookus M, Andrieu N, et al.; EMBRACE; GENEPSO; GEO-HEBON. Reproductive and hormonal factors, and ovarian cancer risk for BRCA1 and BRCA2 mutation

carriers: results from the International BRCA1/2 Carrier Cohort Study. *Cancer Epidemiol Biomarkers Prev.* 2009;18(2):601–610.

41. Werness BA, Ramus SJ, Whittemore AS, et al. Histopathology of familial ovarian tumors in women from families with and without germline BRCA1 mutations. *Hum Pathol.* 2000;31(11):1420–1424.

42. Lakhani SR, Manek S, Penault-Llorca F, et al. Pathology of ovarian cancers in BRCA1 and BRCA2 carriers. *Clin Cancer Res.* 2004;10(7):2473–2481.

43. Mavaddat N, Barrowdale D, Andrulis IL, et al.; HEBON; EMBRACE; GEMO Study Collaborators; kConFab Investigators; SWE-BRCA Collaborators; Consortium of Investigators of Modifiers of BRCA1/2. Pathology of breast and ovarian cancers among BRCA1 and BRCA2 mutation carriers: results from the Consortium of Investigators of Modifiers of BRCA1/2 (CIMBA). *Cancer Epidemiol Biomarkers Prev.* 2012;21(1):134–147.

44. Ramus SJ, Bobrow LG, Pharoah PD, et al. Increased frequency of TP53 mutations in BRCA1 and BRCA2 ovarian tumours. *Genes Chromosomes Cancer.* 1999;25(2):91–96.

45. Ramus SJ, Pharoah PD, Harrington P, et al. BRCA1/2 mutation status influences somatic genetic progression in inherited and sporadic epithelial ovarian cancer cases. *Cancer Res.* 2003;63(2):417–423.

46. Jazaeri AA, Yee CJ, Sotiriou C, Brantley KR, Boyd J, Liu ET. Gene expression profiles of BRCA1-linked, BRCA2-linked, and sporadic ovarian cancers. *J Natl Cancer Inst.* 2002;94(13):990–1000.

47 Cancer Genome Atlas Research Network. Integrated genomic analyses of ovarian carcinoma. *Nature.* 2011;474(7353):609–615.

48. Pharoah PD, Easton DF, Stockton DL, Gayther S, Ponder BA. Survival in familial, BRCA1-associated, and BRCA2-associated epithelial ovarian cancer. United Kingdom Coordinating Committee for Cancer Research (UKCCCR) Familial Ovarian Cancer Study Group. *Cancer Res.* 1999;59(4):868–871.

49. Bolton KL, Chenevix-Trench G, Goh C, et al.; EMBRACE; kConFab Investigators; Cancer Genome Atlas Research Network. Association between BRCA1 and BRCA2 mutations and survival in women with invasive epithelial ovarian cancer. *JAMA.* 2012;307(4):382–390.

50. Farrell C, Lyman M, Freitag K, Fahey C, Piver MS, Rodabaugh KJ. The role of hereditary nonpolyposis colorectal cancer in the management of familial ovarian cancer. *Genet Med.* 2006;8(10):653–657.

51. Pennington KP, Swisher EM. Hereditary ovarian cancer: beyond the usual suspects. *Gynecol Oncol.* 2012;124(2):347–353.

52. South SA, Vance H, Farrell C, et al. Consideration of hereditary nonpolyposis colorectal cancer in BRCA mutation-negative familial ovarian cancers. *Cancer.* 2009;115(2):324–333.

53. Rubin SC, Blackwood MA, Bandera C, et al. BRCA1, BRCA2, and hereditary nonpolyposis colorectal cancer gene mutations in an unselected ovarian cancer population: relationship to family history and implications for genetic testing. *Am J Obstet Gynecol.* 1998;178(4):670–677.

54. Malander S, Rambech E, Kristoffersson U, et al. The contribution of the hereditary nonpolyposis colorectal cancer syndrome to the development of ovarian cancer. *Gynecol Oncol.* 2006;101(2):238–243.

55. Aarnio M, Sankila R, Pukkala E, et al. Cancer risk in mutation carriers of DNA-mismatch-repair genes. *Int J Cancer.* 1999;81(2):214–218.

56. Watson P, Vasen HF, Mecklin JP, et al. The risk of extra-colonic, extra-endometrial cancer in the Lynch syndrome. *Int J Cancer.* 2008;123(2):444–449.

57. Cederquist K, Emanuelsson M, Wiklund F, Golovleva I, Palmqvist R, Grönberg H. Two Swedish founder MSH6 mutations, one nonsense and one missense, conferring high cumulative risk of Lynch syndrome. *Clin Genet.* 2005;68(6):533–541.

58. Jishi MF, Itnyre JH, Oakley-Girvan IA, Piver MS, Whittemore AS. Risks of cancer among members of families in the Gilda Radner Familial Ovarian Cancer Registry. *Cancer.* 1995;76(8):1416–1421.

59. Antoniou AC, Easton DF. Risk prediction models for familial breast cancer. *Future Oncol.* 2006;2(2):257–274.

60. Pharoah PD, Antoniou AC, Easton DF, Ponder BA. Polygenes, risk prediction, and targeted prevention of breast cancer. *N Engl J Med.* 2008;358(26):2796–2803.

61. Bolton KL, Ganda C, Berchuck A, Pharoah PD, Gayther SA. Role of common genetic variants in ovarian cancer susceptibility and outcome: progress to date from the Ovarian Cancer Association Consortium (OCAC). *J Intern Med.* 2012;271(4):366–378.

62. Song H, Ramus SJ, Tyrer J, et al.; Australian Cancer (Ovarian) Study; Australian Ovarian Cancer Study Group; Ovarian Cancer Association Consortium. A genome-wide association study identifies a new ovarian cancer susceptibility locus on 9p22.2. *Nat Genet.* 2009;41(9):996–1000.

63. Bolton KL, Tyrer J, Song H, et al.; Australian Ovarian Cancer Study Group; Australian Cancer Study (Ovarian Cancer); Ovarian Cancer Association Consortium. Common variants at 19p13 are associated with susceptibility to ovarian cancer. *Nat Genet.* 2010;42(10):880–884.

64. Antoniou AC, Wang X, Fredericksen ZS, et al.; EMBRACE; GEMO Study Collaborators; HEBON; kConFab; SWE-BRCA; MOD SQUAD; GENICA. A locus on 19p13 modifies risk of breast cancer in BRCA1 mutation carriers and is associated with hormone receptor-negative breast cancer in the general population. *Nat Genet.* 2010;42(10):885–892.

65. Ramus SJ, Kartsonaki C, Gayther SA, et al.; OCGN; HEBON; EMBRACE; GEMO Study Collaborators; BCFR; kConFab Investigators; Consortium of Investigators of Modifiers of BRCA1/2. Genetic variation at 9p22.2 and ovarian cancer risk for BRCA1 and BRCA2 mutation carriers. *J Natl Cancer Inst.* 2011;103(2):105–116.

66. Gaudet MM, Kirchhoff T, Green T, et al.; HEBON Study Collaborators; OCGN; kConFab; EMBRACE. Common genetic variants and modification of penetrance of BRCA2-associated breast cancer. *PLoS Genet.* 2010;6(10):e1001183.

67. Couch FJ, Gaudet MM, Antoniou AC, et al.; OCGN; SWE-BRCA; HEBON; EMBRACE; GEMO Study Collaborators; kConFab investigators; Consortium of Investigators of Modifiers of BRCA1/2. Common variants at the 19p13.1 and ZNF365 loci are associated with ER subtypes of breast cancer and ovarian cancer risk in BRCA1 and BRCA2 mutation carriers. *Cancer Epidemiol Biomarkers Prev.* 2012;21(4):645–657.

68 Ramus SJ, Baer R, Foster NA, et al. Screening for mutations in the *BARD1* gene in families with ovarian cancer. *Am J Hum Genet.* 1997;61(4):A79.

69. Meindl A, Hellebrand H, Wiek C, et al. Germline mutations in breast and ovarian cancer pedigrees establish RAD51C as a human cancer susceptibility gene. *Nat Genet.* 2010;42(5):410–414.

70. Loveday C, Turnbull C, Ramsay E, et al.; Breast Cancer Susceptibility Collaboration (UK). Germline mutations in RAD51D confer susceptibility to ovarian cancer. *Nat Genet.* 2011;43(9):879–882.

71. Casadei S, Norquist BM, Walsh T, et al. Contribution of inherited mutations in the BRCA2-interacting protein PALB2 to familial breast cancer. *Cancer Res.* 2011;71(6):2222–2229.

72. Dansonka-Mieszkowska A, Kluska A, Moes J, et al. A novel germline PALB2 deletion in Polish breast and ovarian cancer patients. *BMC Med Genet.* 2010;11:20.

73. Rafnar T, Gudbjartsson DF, Sulem P, et al. Mutations in BRIP1 confer high risk of ovarian cancer. *Nat Genet.* 2011; 43(11):1104–1107.

74. Walsh T, Casadei S, Lee MK, et al. Mutations in 12 genes for inherited ovarian, fallopian tube, and peritoneal carcinoma identified by massively parallel sequencing. *Proc Natl Acad Sci USA.* 2011;108(44):18032–18037.

75. McCabe N, Turner NC, Lord CJ, et al. Deficiency in the repair of DNA damage by homologous recombination and sensitivity to poly(ADP-ribose) polymerase inhibition. *Cancer Res.* 2006;66(16):8109–8115.

15 Surgical Management of Ovarian Cancer

JOHN O. SCHORGE

DENNIS S. CHI

■ INTRODUCTION

Epithelial ovarian cancer is unique amongst gynecologic malignancies in requiring a compassionately directed surgical approach throughout all phases of diagnosis, treatment, and palliation. Comprehensive, individualized management of each patient involves several interrelated steps. Expert knowledge of the disease process is essential to provide realistic preoperative counseling and to help guide expectations. Often, knowing when not to operate is equally important as a demonstrated willingness to intervene surgically. Absolute mastery of a broad spectrum of techniques is crucial in order to craft the type of operation best suited to addressing the clinical problem. Frequently, the findings during surgery are dramatically different than anticipated, or the frozen section histological findings are unexpected. Strict oversight of the postoperative care, including prompt identification of any complications, is also mandatory. The surgeon is routinely charged with the daunting task of achieving a perfect balance of appropriately aggressive intervention while avoiding unnecessary morbidity.

Due to the immense complexities of providing longitudinal care for patients with ovarian cancer, it is perhaps predictable that better outcomes are reported when a subspecialist is overseeing the treatment (1–3). However, the unfortunate reality is that fewer than half of such patients in the United States will be cared for by a gynecologic oncologist (3). Instead, most are managed by physicians not necessarily intimately familiar with the nuances of clinical care. For example, when confronted with an obstructing ovarian mass in the setting of unsuspected carcinomatosis, a general surgeon may simply perform a diverting colostomy. Postoperatively, the patient may be counseled about the limited benefits of palliative chemotherapy or directed to hospice. When a gynecologic oncologist is involved, patients are more likely to undergo both primary staging and surgical debulking (1,2).

Due to the high incidence of disease recurrence, additional surgery frequently needs to be at least considered, either as part of the therapeutic strategy, or for palliative purposes. Intra-abdominal tumor progression often leads inevitably to bowel obstruction. Rather than routinely proceeding with a potentially disastrous attempt at laparotomy, surgeons familiar with the course of end-stage disease might instead advise placement of a venting gastrostomy tube and initiate a hospice discussion. The aim of this chapter is to provide a comprehensive review of the surgical management of epithelial ovarian cancer from the perspective of the gynecologic oncologist.

■ PREOPERATIVE CONSIDERATIONS

Whether detected by symptoms, pelvic examination, or discovered by serendipity, any abnormal adnexal mass warrants consideration of possible malignancy. Most commonly, transvaginal sonography has demonstrated features suspicious enough for the patient to be considered for surgery. A thorough examination in the office is helpful to assess the size and texture of the mass, its mobility within the pelvis, and its association with adjacent structures. When epithelial ovarian cancer is high in the differential diagnosis, CT of at least the abdomen and pelvis is tremendously helpful for surgical planning. Especially if a minimally invasive approach is being considered, the presence of an omental cake or other obvious extra-ovarian disease would likely indicate that vertical laparotomy is a preferred option. Particularly when ovarian cancer is unexpected and not performed by a gynecologic oncologist, the initial surgical incision might otherwise be inadequate to allow complete examination of the pelvis and abdominal cavity (4).

The surgeon must incorporate all relevant concerns into the preoperative counseling session, including questions about fertility-sparing options, possible unanticipated intraoperative findings, likelihood of postsurgical complications, and the expected duration of recovery. Since ovarian cancer is surgically staged, every patient with a suspicious adnexal mass should be consented for that possibility in the event that malignancy is found. If a gynecologic oncologist is not performing the operation, then ideally he or she is available once surgery is under way. Furthermore, the operation should take place in a hospital facility that has appropriate consultative services (i.e., frozen section pathology). When a malignant ovarian tumor is discovered, a gynecologic oncologist should be consulted intraoperatively if possible. Since hospitals frequently managing ovarian cancer are more likely to provide this type of multidisciplinary support, patients may expect better long-term outcomes at higher volume centers (5,6).

If immediate consultation is not available, or if the diagnosis is only noted on final pathology, a postsurgical referral is the next best option. In these instances, the gynecologic oncologist will need to make a clinical judgment about whether there is enough information to recommend expectant management or chemotherapy. Alternatively, restaging might be advisable to better define the disease process.

■ SURGICAL STAGING

The consistent inability to reliably detect epithelial ovarian carcinoma before metastasis has occurred has proven to be an ongoing disappointment. Unfortunately, routine screening has not been shown to improve early detection or reduce mortality in either the high-risk or general populations (7,8). As a result, only one quarter of newly diagnosed women will have disease confined to the ovary. In general, surgical staging has several purposes (Table 15.1).

Patients who undergo comprehensive staging to confirm early disease have a much better prognosis than those who are thought to have disease confined to the ovary, but are inadequately staged—presumably because occult metastatic disease is not detected (9). By shifting patients with subclinical metastases from early to advanced-stage disease, the median survival for both groups is improved. In addition, treatment-related side effects or complications may be avoided. Patients with accurately defined surgical Stage I disease may not require any additional treatment, or may safely receive less chemotherapy than otherwise would be the case in unstaged patients. When occult Stage III disease is detected, patients may be treated more aggressively with intraperitoneal chemotherapy, or be eligible for clinical trial participation.

■ **Table 15.1** Purpose of surgical staging

1. Establish the diagnosis
2. Determine the extent of disease
3. Provide prognostic information
4. Remove all gross tumor

A conceptual understanding of the spread pattern of epithelial ovarian cancer is valuable to help guide the surgical staging procedure. Epithelial ovarian cancer is thought to arise within the ovarian surface epithelium, grow focally, and ultimately breach the ovarian capsule to metastasize primarily by exfoliation. Carcinomatous fluid circulating within the peritoneal cavity typically results in cancer cells implanting throughout the pelvis and upper abdomen (10). Direct extension of the ovarian mass often leads to surface involvement of the pelvic peritoneum, rectosigmoid, and adjacent structures. Lymphatic spread to the pelvic and para-aortic nodes is also commonplace.

Traditionally, surgical staging of epithelial ovarian cancer is performed via a large vertical incision that provides exposure and access to the entire abdomen (Figure 15.1). Upon entry into the peritoneal cavity, ascites is aspirated for cytology. In the absence of free fluid, cytologic washings of the pelvis and paracolic gutters are obtained. Abdominal hysterectomy and bilateral salpingo-oophorectomy is performed in the majority of patients for whom future fertility is not a concern. The contents of the peritoneal cavity, including all organs and peritoneal surfaces, are systematically inspected, a partial omentectomy is performed, and any suspicious-appearing areas are biopsied. If there is no gross evidence for extraovarian disease, then random peritoneal biopsies are valuable to detect occult microscopic implants (11).

Suspicious lymph nodes should be excised and sent for frozen section. Otherwise, bilateral pelvic and para-aortic lymphadenectomy is indicated because even if only one ovary is grossly involved, the frequency of having contralateral nodal metastases is considerable (12). In addition, the more comprehensive the dissection, the more accurate it will be in detecting subclinical Stage III disease. In a retrospective analysis of 6686 women with cancer clinically

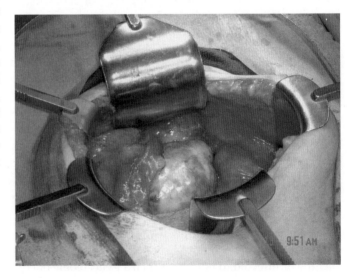

FIGURE 15.1 Vertical laparotomy with Bookwalter retractor placement provides excellent exposure to a malignant ovarian mass.

confined to the ovary, the extent of lymphadenectomy (0 nodes, less than 10 nodes, and 10 or more nodes) significantly increased the survival rates from 87% to 92% to 94%, respectively (13). Ovarian lymphatic channels follow the course of the ovarian arteries, which originate above the inferior mesenteric artery. Thus, to identify all possible nodal metastases, the para-aortic lymphadenectomy should be performed up to the level of the left renal vein. After thorough surgical evaluation, the International Federation of Gynecology and Obstetrics (FIGO) staging system is applied to guide adjuvant therapy decisions (Table 15.2).

Comprehensively staged women with Stage I disease have a cure rate exceeding 90%. Stage IA or IB patients with Grade 1 or 2 disease typically do not require any adjuvant therapy. However, those with Stage IA/B Grade 3, Stage IC or II ovarian cancer are generally treated with platinum-based adjuvant therapy. Due to the increased likelihood of occult metastases, incompletely staged patients appear to benefit the most (14). Surgical staging of apparent early-stage epithelial ovarian cancer is critically important to accurately define the true extent of disease and most appropriately guide postoperative therapy.

Minimally Invasive Surgery

The emergence of minimally invasive techniques has led to a surgical renaissance within the field of gynecologic oncology. However, since most patients with ovarian cancer are diagnosed with bulky, metastatic disease, the utility of this approach has not been as profound as in other disease types. As a result, the current literature consists mainly of case reports, small series, and cohort studies (15–17).

One disadvantage of minimally invasive surgery is the inability to fully explore the abdomen in search of tumor implants. Inherently, there are limitations in accessing the entire peritoneal cavity without a large vertical incision—no matter what other approach is used. Yet in at least one preliminary report, patients with apparent Stage I ovarian or fallopian tube cancer safely underwent laparoscopic surgical staging, with no differences in omental specimen size or number of lymph nodes removed. Estimated blood loss and hospital stay were also lower for laparoscopy, but operating time was longer (15). Overall, the limited data suggest equal efficacy of laparoscopy compared with laparotomy in both early and advanced-stage ovarian cancer. Robotic assistance has also been reported to facilitate comprehensive staging (18).

Minimally invasive surgery is postulated to increase the risk of intraoperative rupture of an ovarian cystic mass. The clinical relevance of intraperitoneal spillage is somewhat controversial, but often that is the event that triggers the indication for adjuvant chemotherapy when otherwise it might not have been required. Fortunately, the vast majority of adnexal masses can be safely detached, placed intact within a specimen retrieval bag, drained or morcellated at the abdominal wall, and removed from a trocar site without spillage. Importantly, removal of any suspicious mass without enclosure in a specimen bag is inadvisable due to the possibility of seeding the subcutaneous tissues.

Although clinically relevant, the actual rate of port-site tumor implantation after laparoscopic procedures in women with malignant disease is quite low. Almost invariably, it occurs in the setting of synchronous, advanced intra-abdominal, or distant metastatic disease. In fact, the presence of port-site implantation is a surrogate for advanced disease and should not be used as an argument against laparoscopic surgery in gynecologic malignancies (19).

Stage	Surgical-Pathologic Findings
	Table 15.2 International Federation of Gynecology and Obstetrics (FIGO) surgical staging system for ovarian cancer
IA	Growth limited to one ovary
IB	Growth limited to both ovaries
IC	Tumor limited to one or both ovaries, but with disease on the surface of one or both ovaries; or with capsule(s) ruptured; or with malignant ascites or positive peritoneal washings
IIA	Extension and/or metastases to the uterus and/or tubes
IIB	Extension to other pelvic tissues
IIC	Tumor limited to the genital tract or other pelvic tissues, but with disease on the surface of one or both ovaries; or with capsule(s) ruptured; or with malignant ascites or positive peritoneal washings
IIIA	Tumor grossly limited to the true pelvis with negative nodes, but with histologically confirmed microscopic seeding of abdominal-peritoneal surfaces
IIIB	Abdominal implants less than 2 cm in diameter with negative nodes
IIIC	Abdominal implants at least 2 cm in diameter and/or positive pelvic, paraaortic, or inguinal nodes
IV	Distant metastases, including malignant pleural effusion or parenchymal liver metastases

Fertility-Sparing Surgery

Approximately 10%–15% of epithelial ovarian cancers develop in women younger than 40 years of age, suggesting that fertility-sparing surgery may need to be considered in selected patients. When the cancer appears confined to one ovary, especially if it is low grade, it is appropriate to modify the staging procedure by leaving the uterus and the uninvolved ovary in place for younger women who wish to preserve fertility. Surgical staging otherwise proceeds as described. Although many patients will be upstaged, those with surgical Stage I disease have an excellent long-term survival with unilateral adnexectomy. Preserving the uterus and contralateral ovary does not appear to compromise the chances of cure. In some cases, postoperative chemotherapy may be required, but patients usually will retain their ability to conceive and ultimately carry a pregnancy to term (20).

■ TUMOR DEBULKING

Two-thirds of women who are newly diagnosed with epithelial ovarian cancer have Stage III or IV disease usually characterized by ascites, carcinomatosis, and omental caking (Figure 15.2). Once identified, most patients are anxious to have surgery as quickly as possible. While removal of bulky tumors as part of cancer treatment at first glance would seem to be a straightforward concept to understand, the actual clinical benefits of debulking have been harder to prove. Within the broader field of oncology, the aggressive surgical approach to widespread disease is rather unique (21).

Metastatic epithelial ovarian cancers, like other solid tumors, appear to have a small subpopulation of phenotypically distinct stem cells with self-renewal capacity to reconstitute the entire cellular heterogeneity of a tumor. As a result, ovarian cancer stem cells are thought to be responsible for tumor initiation, maintenance, and growth (22). Ineffective targeting of this cell population is thought to be responsible for the therapeutic failures and tumor recurrences currently observed (23). The elimination of potentially chemoresistant cells is one presumed benefit of surgical cytoreduction. In addition, since the probability of acquiring spontaneous mutations to drug-resistant phenotypes increases as tumor size and corresponding cell

numbers increase, removal of bulky disease would appear to make obvious clinical sense (24).

Theoretically, cytoreductive surgery should allow removal of existing resistant tumor cells and decrease the spontaneous development of additional resistant cells (21). Patients definitely do appear to benefit from *one* maximal debulking attempt, but the timing of the procedure and what defines a success have become increasingly controversial. Furthermore, the radical procedures commonly required to achieve optimal cytoreduction may at times lead to excessive morbidity, or even postoperative death. Once again, astute clinical judgment is critically important in weighing the risks and benefits of surgery.

Primary Debulking

Joe V. Meigs, a gynecologic surgeon at Massachusetts General Hospital, initially described ovarian tumor debulking in 1934 (25). However, in the absence of effective postoperative therapy, the procedure had limited utility. With the arrival of platinum drugs, the value of debulking was revisited in the mid 1970s (26). Case series and other retrospective data rapidly accrued thereafter to entrench primary cytoreductive surgery as the de facto standard of care (27–29).

The success of the operation depends on numerous factors, including patient selection, tumor location, and surgeon expertise. To achieve a survival benefit, an optimal result was initially defined as no residual tumors individually measuring more than 2 cm in size. For purposes of uniformity, the Gynecologic Oncology Group (GOG) redefined optimal debulking as residual implants less than or equal to 1 cm. For the past few decades, this criterion has served as the benchmark of success. Patients undergoing primary optimal cytoreductive surgery (less than or equal to 1 cm residual disease), followed by intraperitoneal platinum-based chemotherapy have a median overall survival of 66 months—the longest duration ever reported in a Phase III study (30). The level of success achieved in this trial is currently the gold standard for comparisons of any other sequence of treatment.

Despite the accumulated evidence supporting the importance of primary debulking, it remains controversial whether the better outcome is due to the surgeon's technical proficiency or some ill-defined, intrinsic feature of the cancer that makes the tumor implants easier to remove. Within the pelvis, rectosigmoid resection is frequently required to achieve an optimal result (31,32). In general, extensive upper abdominal disease is strongly indicative of aggressive tumor biology. Although this is a common location of unresectable disease, optimal debulking may still be achieved in many patients by performing "ultra-radical" procedures, such as splenectomy (Figure 15.3) or diaphragmatic resection (Figure 15.4; 33–35). Survival rates have been shown to improve accordingly when the

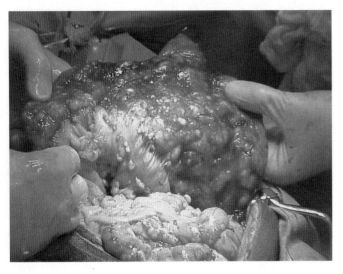

FIGURE 15.2 Omental caking in a patient with Stage IIIC ovarian cancer.

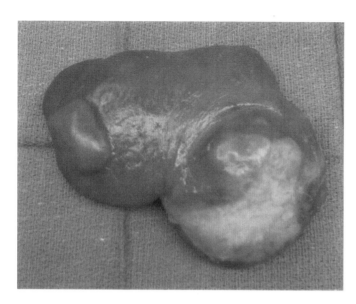

FIGURE 15.3 Spleen with 5-cm tumor implant at bottom right.

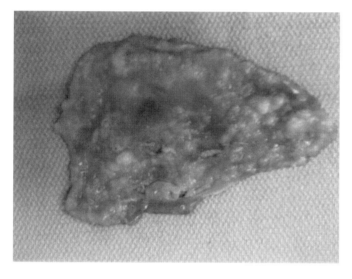

FIGURE 15.4 Peritoneal stripping of right hemidiaphragm with confluent tumor.

surgical paradigm is revised to a more aggressive philosophy incorporating these and other radical techniques. Patients referred to specialized centers where such radical procedures are commonly performed may anticipate higher rates of optimal debulking and improved survival, without additional surgery necessarily leading to increased major morbidity (36–39).

One valid criticism of cytoreductive surgery is the biased, subjective assessment of gross residual disease by the surgeon at the completion of the operation he or she performed. Due to tissue induration, inadequate exploration, radiologist overestimation, or other factors, inaccuracies of residual tumor size are common. More than half of patients deemed to have optimally debulked disease will have tumors larger than 1 cm on

early postoperative CT (40). Perhaps due to the inability to reliably quantify residual disease, a recent subanalysis of accumulated data from several prospective GOG trials demonstrated that patients with 0.1–1.0 cm residual disease had marginally improved overall survival compared to patients with greater than 1 cm residual disease for Stage III ovarian cancer and no improvement in those with Stage IV disease. In fact, dramatic survival benefit was only achieved with complete resection to microscopic residual disease (41,42).

Based on these findings and other similar reports, there is a growing consensus that optimal cytoreduction should be redefined using a more stringent criterion. Thus, the current goal of primary debulking is to achieve complete resection with no residual disease. Accordingly, the proportion of patients with Stage III-IV ovarian cancer in which this redefined optimal result can be accomplished will be diminished. For advanced disease, reports range from 15% to 30% (36,41–44). However, the clinical benefits are potentially substantial. Based on a Cochrane Database analysis of 11 retrospective studies, the suggested new terminology was optimal (no residual disease), near optimal (less than or equal to 1 cm residual), and suboptimal (greater than 1 cm; 45). Of 465 women with Stage IIIC ovarian cancer who underwent primary cytoreductive surgery at Memorial Sloan-Kettering Cancer Center, the median overall survival was 106 months for patients with no gross residual disease compared to 66 months for those with less than or equal to 0.5 cm, 48 months with 0.6–1.0 cm residual, and 33–34 months for greater than 1 cm residual disease (43). Therefore, although complete resection is often not feasible, cytoreduction to as minimal residual tumor as possible should always be the focus of aggressive surgical efforts.

Even when successful, the obvious disadvantage of radical cytoreductive surgery is that it may result in a prolonged postoperative recovery that is fraught with complications. The initiation of chemotherapy may be delayed, or worse, postponed indefinitely. When an optimal result is not possible, the surgical approach should be limited in scope to avoid unnecessary postoperative morbidity. A standardized pathway may be beneficial in decreasing some types of morbidity, reducing hospital stays, and readmissions (46,47). Special caution is indicated for women aged 75 or older, especially in the presence of other significant comorbidities (48–51). These patients, in particular, experience increased 30-day mortality. Neoadjuvant chemotherapy (NACT) should be considered in this population to reduce perioperative morbidity (52).

Diagnostic laparoscopy has been championed by some as a reliable and flexible tool to better triage patients toward debulking with improved odds at achieving an optimal result (53,54). Direct visualization of the intra-abdominal disease distribution and presence or absence of carcinomatosis would appear to improve upon physical examination and imaging tests, but is also not without potential morbidity. Occasionally, patients may be candidates for outright cytoreduction by minimally invasive techniques. Recently, laparoscopic and robotic-assisted debulking of advanced ovarian cancer each has been reported with minimal morbidity (18,55). While not typically feasible due to the extent of disease, such approaches may be warranted in selected circumstances.

Interval Debulking

Incomplete primary debulking occurs frequently in non-specialized centers. Upfront reoperation by a gynecologic oncologist before the start of chemotherapy is feasible and may be appropriate. More than half of such patients can be optimally debulked despite an initial attempt elsewhere (56). Unfortunately, no preoperative evaluation or intraoperative effort can guarantee success. As a result, many advanced ovarian cancer patients taken for surgery are not completely resected.

Two Phase III trials were conducted to determine whether a second interval debulking procedure was worthwhile after an unsuccessful initial attempt followed by a few courses of chemotherapy. A multicenter trial conducted in Europe demonstrated a 6-month median survival advantage in patients who were re-explored after three cycles of chemotherapy (57). In contrast, no survival advantage was demonstrated when a similar study was conducted in the United States (58). In the U.S. trial, virtually all patients had their initial attempt by a gynecologic oncologist, unlike the European study where relatively few had their first surgery performed by a subspecialist. Thus, interval debulking appears to yield benefit only among the patients whose primary surgery was not performed by a gynecologic oncologist, if the first try was not intended as a maximal resection of all gross disease, or if no upfront surgery was performed at all.

Some patients are too medically ill to initially undergo any type of upfront abdominal operation, whereas others have disease that is obviously too extensive to be resected by an experienced ovarian cancer surgical team. In these circumstances, NACT is routinely used, ideally after the diagnosis has been confirmed by paracentesis, CT-guided biopsy, or laparoscopy. Following three to four courses of treatment, the feasibility of surgery can be reassessed. In some series, NACT followed by interval debulking has demonstrated comparable survival outcomes to those reported for primary surgery. Fewer radical procedures may be required, the rate of achieving minimal residual disease may be higher, and patients may experience less morbidity (59). However, other reports have suggested NACT in lieu of primary debulking is associated with an inferior overall survival (60). Direct comparisons have historically been difficult to perform. Until recently, the presumed benefits of primary surgical cytoreduction in advanced ovarian cancer had not been rigorously tested.

The results of a randomized Phase III trial conducted in Europe caused the debate of how best to initially treat women with advanced ovarian cancer to resurface. In the study, 670 patients were randomized to primary debulking surgery vs NACT. After 3 courses of platinum-based treatment, NACT patients who demonstrated a response underwent interval debulking. The authors reported a median overall survival of 29 to 30 months, regardless of assigned treatment group. In the multivariate analysis, complete resection of all macroscopic disease at debulking surgery was identified as the strongest independent prognostic factor, but the timing of surgery did not seem to matter. Based on the authors' interpretation of their data, NACT and interval debulking was the preferred treatment (61). Despite these findings, most gynecologic oncologists in the United States report that they use NACT for less than 10% of advanced ovarian cancers (62).

Some European gynecologic oncologists have openly questioned what kind of evidence would be needed to convince their colleagues in the United States of the superiority of NACT (63). However, advocates of primary debulking point out that the duration of patient survival in the study was much shorter than expected. The median survival (29–30 months) was less than half that reported for optimally debulked Stage III patients receiving postoperative intraperitoneal chemotherapy (66 months; 30). Additionally, only 42% of the primary debulking operations resulted in an optimal result defined as less than or equal to 1 cm of residual disease. Since expert centers in the United States often report an optimal result in at least 75% of patients, it is feasible to think that a more aggressive initial attempt might have led to a better outcome for the group randomized to surgery.

In a provocative analysis, 316 patients undergoing primary treatment for advanced epithelial ovarian cancer at Memorial Sloan-Kettering Cancer Center over the identical period, and using the same inclusion criteria, were reviewed. Optimal cytoreduction was achieved in 71% and the median overall survival was 50 months. The authors concluded that primary debulking should continue to be the preferred initial management for patients with bulky Stage IIIC and IV disease, whereas NACT should be reserved for those who cannot tolerate primary debulking and/or for whom optimal cytoreduction is not feasible (64).

In a Cochrane Database analysis, there is yet no good evidence that NACT prior to debulking surgery is superior (65). Ultimately, a prospective Phase III trial conducted within the United States will need to be performed to sway opinion and markedly change the practice of gynecologic oncologists in this country. Meanwhile, the controversy will persist and individual patterns of care will continue.

Secondary Debulking

Although the rationale for a second debulking operation at the time of relapse is largely an extrapolation of the rationale for primary surgery, there are several reasons why the certainty of clinical benefit is even more contentious. Recurrent ovarian cancer has a much more heterogeneous disease presentation. As a result, treatment is typically more individualized. Secondary debulking is generally considered to be most effective when there is an isolated relapse, a long disease-free interval after completion of primary therapy (i.e., more than 12 months), no ascites, and a good performance status (66). In contrast, women with symptomatic ascites, carcinomatosis, early relapse (i.e., less than 6 months), and poor conditioning are least likely to benefit (67).

The clinical reality is that many patients will fall somewhere between these clinical extremes. While guidelines have been proposed (Table 15.3), each practicing gynecologic oncologist ultimately uses his or her own criteria and judgment for determining which, if any, patients are good candidates for secondary surgery. Due to the wide spectrum of relapsed disease patterns, proportionally few women undergo a second debulking operation. The previously reported retrospective series largely reflect this selection bias. Consequently, the success rates of optimal secondary debulking surgery and the corresponding survival data vary broadly. With judicious patient selection, complete resection rates of 40%–55% have been reported (66–68).

The potential for significant morbidity and the notable lack of benefit for patients who are left with residual disease emphasizes the importance of careful counseling and preoperative assessment of patients. Predictably, complete resection appears to be associated with the most prolonged postoperative survival (69). On occasion, patients with isolated relapse may also be candidates for minimally invasive secondary cytoreduction (70).

In addition to retrospective reports and prospective observational studies, a recent comparative effectiveness analysis provided additional supportive evidence of benefit in selected cases. Secondary cytoreductive surgery prolonged overall survival with a hazard ratio of 0.76 (71).

■ Table 15.3 Recommendations for secondary cytoreduction

Disease-Free Interval	Single Site of Relapse	Multiple Sites But No Carcinomatosis	Carcinomatosis
6–12 months	Offer SC	Consider SC	No SC
12–30 months	Offer SC	Offer SC	Consider SC
>30 months	Offer SC	Offer SC	Offer SC

SC, secondary cytoreduction.

Prospective randomized Phase III trials, such as the DESKTOP III and GOG protocol 213, are currently under way to evaluate the value of secondary debulking in the treatment of relapsed ovarian cancer. Unfortunately, it will be years before the results from these trials are finalized. In the meantime, practice patterns will largely continue to be guided by the results of retrospective studies and clinician experience.

Tertiary Debulking

Managing a second relapse by offering tertiary cytoreduction may offer a survival benefit in a highly select group of patients with recurrent disease. Again, the benefits appear to be greatest in patients in whom a complete gross resection can be achieved (72,73). Quaternary, or even quinternary debulking procedures may be reasonable to consider in unique circumstances (74).

■ PALLIATIVE SURGERY

Relapsed epithelial ovarian cancer patients are at risk for bowel obstruction at any point, but especially as their disease proves unresponsive to therapy and inevitably progresses within the abdomen. The diagnosis is made clinically by careful examination and confirmed by a CT scan of the abdomen that may or may not show a discrete transition point. Almost invariably, the obstruction is located in the small intestine, but occasionally the distal colon is excessively compressed by pelvic tumor. Initially, patients should be managed by nasogastric suction, intravenous hydration, supportive care, and bowel rest. Most events will resolve sufficiently to allow for hospital discharge. However, patients often develop worsening or more frequent episodes of obstruction at some point. When conservative measures fail, standard surgical teaching would ordinarily necessitate an operation to lyse adhesions and/or resect and anastomose the affected site in order to restore bowel continuity. Unfortunately, this approach does not often succeed as planned in the setting of recurrent ovarian cancer.

Whenever surgery is being considered, the decision should be incorporated into a larger discussion about future goals of care and expectations of continued therapy. There are very limited data comparing palliative surgery and medical management (75). Patients are generally in poor physical condition with a limited life expectancy, measureable in weeks (76). In fact, bowel obstruction is the most common reason for hospital admission during the last year of life and is a frequent cause of death. Therefore, maintaining quality of life and maximizing symptom control is paramount.

Endoscopic interventions may have a high likelihood of short-term success, but recurrence of symptoms is common. Gastrostomy tube placement provides the ability to drain accumulated stomach contents intermittently over days or weeks, alleviating nausea or episodes of vomiting. Unfortunately, plugging or dislodgement is a frequent cause of visits to the emergency room, or for hospital readmission. Colonic stents may allow patients with large bowel obstruction to avoid major surgery. However, the stents may erode, lead to new rectal pain, or cause other unexpected sequelae. In some situations, aggressive surgical management is a better option that may provide symptom relief while prolonging survival.

Theoretically, a colostomy, ileostomy, or bowel resection with anastomosis should allow return of reasonably normal bowel function in carefully selected patients with malignant bowel obstruction. Durable palliation and extended survival is possible with judicious use of operative intervention (77). Even in seemingly good candidates for surgery, a satisfactory result is often impossible because of extensive disease, multiple sites of partial or complete obstruction, dense adhesions resulting in visceral injury, tethering of the intestine, or other limiting factors. In addition, successful palliation is rarely achieved when the transit time is prolonged by diffuse peritoneal carcinomatosis or when the anatomy requires a bypass that results in short-bowel syndrome. However, absence of ascites is a predictor of successful palliation. About one quarter of patients will have a major complication such as an enterocutaneous fistula, peritonitis, or a venous thrombotic event. The perioperative mortality rate is significant, ranging from 5% to 20% (78).

Several clinical features have been proposed as absolute contraindications for attempted surgical correction of malignant bowel obstruction (Table 15.4; 79). While a subgroup of lower risk patients may benefit from surgery, in many end-stage patients with carcinomatosis refractory to further chemotherapy, the best approach may be placement of a palliative gastrostomy tube, pain control, hydration, and referral to hospice care. During the last 6 months of life, the majority of patients are referred for palliative care, but spend less than 30 days on hospice. Earlier referral could decrease the number of hospital admissions and procedures while providing invaluable support during this end of life transition (80).

■ **Table 15.4** Contraindications for attempted surgical correction of malignant bowel obstruction

Ileus secondary to diffuse carcinomatosis
Ascites requiring frequent paracentesis
Diffuse palpable intra-abdominal masses with liver involvement
Recent laparotomy with unsuccessful correction
Previous surgery revealing diffuse metastatic cancer
Involvement of the proximal stomach

■ CONCLUSIONS

Surgical management of the patient with epithelial ovarian cancer is a vital part of the continuum of care from diagnosis to cure, relapse, or death. Excellent clinical judgment is needed, as well as technical mastery of a wide array of procedures. Involvement of a gynecologic oncologist to oversee patient care has proven to improve outcomes for a variety of reasons. Comprehensive staging of apparent Stage I disease is critically important to provide the most accurate information in guiding postoperative decision making. Increasingly, minimally invasive techniques are being utilized that provide distinct advantages such as quicker recovery, decreased postoperative pain, and reduced morbidity.

Primary debulking surgery that achieves complete resection to no macroscopic residual disease has consistently demonstrated the best long-term survival of any treatment strategy in advanced ovarian cancer. Since ultraradical procedures are routinely required, surgically experienced centers embracing an aggressive surgical paradigm have the highest reported rates of success. Secondary debulking surgery is an option for selected patients with recurrent platinum-sensitive ovarian cancer. Tertiary, quaternary, or further cytoreductive surgery may be appropriate in very unique situations of persistent isolated relapsed disease.

The vast majority of relapsed patients will require management of bowel obstruction at some point in their course. When symptoms are not relieved with conservative management, the judicious use of palliative intervention has the potential to enhance quality of life. Surgical correction by diversion or bypass may be required, and can extend survival. End-stage patients with progressive disease represent a particular challenge. In these circumstances, the treating gynecologic oncologist must manage expectations to provide the most compassionate care.

■ REFERENCES

1. Chan JK, Kapp DS, Shin JY, et al. Influence of the gynecologic oncologist on the survival of ovarian cancer patients. *Obstet Gynecol.* 2007;109(6):1342–1350.
2. Earle CC, Schrag D, Neville BA, et al. Effect of surgeon specialty on processes of care and outcomes for ovarian cancer patients. *J Natl Cancer Inst.* 2006;98(3):172–180.
3. Carney ME, Lancaster JM, Ford C, Tsodikov A, Wiggins CL. A population-based study of patterns of care for ovarian cancer: who is seen by a gynecologic oncologist and who is not? *Gynecol Oncol.* 2002;84(1):36–42.
4. Young RC, Decker DG, Wharton JT, et al. Staging laparotomy in early ovarian cancer. *JAMA.* 1983;250(22):3072–3076.
5. Bristow RE, Zahurak ML, del Carmen MG, et al. Ovarian cancer surgery in Maryland: volume-based access to care. *Gynecol Oncol.* 2004;93(2):353–360.
6. Bristow RE, Palis BE, Chi DS, Cliby WA. The National Cancer Database report on advanced-stage epithelial ovarian cancer: impact

of hospital surgical case volume on overall survival and surgical treatment paradigm. *Gynecol Oncol.* 2010;118(3):262–267.

7. Buys SS, Partridge E, Black A, et al.; PLCO Project Team. Effect of screening on ovarian cancer mortality: the Prostate, Lung, Colorectal and Ovarian (PLCO) Cancer Screening Randomized Controlled Trial. *JAMA.* 2011;305(22):2295–2303.

8. Schorge JO, Modesitt SC, Coleman RL, et al. SGO White Paper on ovarian cancer: etiology, screening and surveillance. *Gynecol Oncol.* 2010;119(1):7–17.

9. Committee Opinion No. 477: the role of the obstetrician-gynecologist in the early detection of epithelial ovarian cancer. *Obstet Gynecol.* 2011;117:742–746.

10. Fader AN, Rose PG. Role of surgery in ovarian carcinoma. *J Clin Oncol.* 2007;25(20):2873–2883.

11. Shroff R, Brooks RA, Zighelboim I, et al. The utility of peritoneal biopsy and omentectomy in the upstaging of apparent early ovarian cancer. *Int J Gynecol Cancer.* 2011;21(7):1208–1212.

12. Cass I, Li AJ, Runowicz CD, et al. Pattern of lymph node metastases in clinically unilateral stage I invasive epithelial ovarian carcinomas. *Gynecol Oncol.* 2001;80(1):56–61.

13. Chan JK, Munro EG, Cheung MK, et al. Association of lymphadenectomy and survival in stage I ovarian cancer patients. *Obstet Gynecol.* 2007;109(1):12–19.

14. Trimbos JB, Vergote I, Bolis G, et al.; EORTC-ACTION collaborators. European Organisation for Research and Treatment of Cancer-Adjuvant ChemoTherapy in Ovarian Neoplasm. Impact of adjuvant chemotherapy and surgical staging in early-stage ovarian carcinoma: European Organisation for Research and Treatment of Cancer-Adjuvant ChemoTherapy in Ovarian Neoplasm trial. *J Natl Cancer Inst.* 2003;95(2):113–125.

15. Chi DS, Abu-Rustum NR, Sonoda Y, et al. The safety and efficacy of laparoscopic surgical staging of apparent stage I ovarian and fallopian tube cancers. *Am J Obstet Gynecol.* 2005;192(5):1614–1619.

16. Lee M, Kim SW, Paek J, et al. Comparisons of surgical outcomes, complications, and costs between laparotomy and laparoscopy in early-stage ovarian cancer. *Int J Gynecol Cancer.* 2011;21(2):251–256.

17. Nezhat FR, DeNoble SM, Liu CS, et al. The safety and efficacy of laparoscopic surgical staging and debulking of apparent advanced stage ovarian, fallopian tube, and primary peritoneal cancers. *JSLS.* 2010;14(2):155–168.

18. Magrina JF, Zanagnolo V, Noble BN, Kho RM, Magtibay P. Robotic approach for ovarian cancer: perioperative and survival results and comparison with laparoscopy and laparotomy. *Gynecol Oncol.* 2011;121(1):100–105.

19. Zivanovic O, Sonoda Y, Diaz JP, et al. The rate of port-site metastases after 2251 laparoscopic procedures in women with underlying malignant disease. *Gynecol Oncol.* 2008;111(3):431–437.

20. Schilder JM, Thompson AM, DePriest PD, et al. Outcome of reproductive age women with stage IA or IC invasive epithelial ovarian cancer treated with fertility-sparing therapy. *Gynecol Oncol.* 2002;87(1):1–7.

21. Covens AL. A critique of surgical cytoreduction in advanced ovarian cancer. *Gynecol Oncol.* 2000;78(3 Pt 1):269–274.

22. Curley MD, Garrett LA, Schorge JO, Foster R, Rueda BR. Evidence for cancer stem cells contributing to the pathogenesis of ovarian cancer. *Front Biosci.* 2011;16:368–392.

23. Dean M, Fojo T, Bates S. Tumour stem cells and drug resistance. *Nat Rev Cancer.* 2005;5(4):275–284.

24. Goldie JH, Coldman AJ. A mathematic model for relating the drug sensitivity of tumors to their spontaneous mutation rate. *Cancer Treat Rep.* 1979;63(11–12):1727–1733.

25. Meigs JV. *Tumors of the Female Pelvic Organs.* New York, NY: Macmillan; 1934.

26. Griffiths CT. Surgical resection of tumor bulk in the primary treatment of ovarian carcinoma. *Natl Cancer Inst Monogr.* 1975;42:101–104.

27. Griffiths CT, Parker LM, Fuller AF Jr. Role of cytoreductive surgical treatment in the management of advanced ovarian cancer. *Cancer Treat Rep.* 1979;63(2):235–240.

28. Hacker NF, Berek JS, Lagasse LD, Nieberg RK, Elashoff RM. Primary cytoreductive surgery for epithelial ovarian cancer. *Obstet Gynecol.* 1983;61(4):413–420.

29. Piver MS, Lele SB, Marchetti DL, Baker TR, Tsukada Y, Emrich LJ. The impact of aggressive debulking surgery and cisplatin-based chemotherapy on progression-free survival in stage III and IV ovarian carcinoma. *J Clin Oncol.* 1988;6(6):983–989.

30. Armstrong DK, Bundy B, Wenzel L, et al.; Gynecologic Oncology Group. Intraperitoneal cisplatin and paclitaxel in ovarian cancer. *N Engl J Med.* 2006;354(1):34–43.

31. Peiretti M, Bristow RE, Zapardiel I, et al. Rectosigmoid resection at the time of primary cytoreduction for advanced ovarian cancer. A multi-center analysis of surgical and oncological outcomes. *Gynecol Oncol.* 2012;126(2):220–223.

32. Aletti GD, Podratz KC, Jones MB, Cliby WA. Role of rectosigmoidectomy and stripping of pelvic peritoneum in outcomes of patients with advanced ovarian cancer. *J Am Coll Surg.* 2006;203(4):521–526.

33. Aletti GD, Dowdy SC, Podratz KC, Cliby WA. Surgical treatment of diaphragm disease correlates with improved survival in optimally debulked advanced stage ovarian cancer. *Gynecol Oncol.* 2006;100(2):283–287.

34. Eisenhauer EL, Abu-Rustum NR, Sonoda Y, et al. The addition of extensive upper abdominal surgery to achieve optimal cytoreduction improves survival in patients with stages IIIC-IV epithelial ovarian cancer. *Gynecol Oncol.* 2006;103(3):1083–1090.

35. McCann CK, Growdon WB, Munro EG, et al. Prognostic significance of splenectomy as part of initial cytoreductive surgery in ovarian cancer. *Ann Surg Oncol.* 2011;18(10):2912–2918.

36. Wimberger P, Lehmann N, Kimmig R, Burges A, Meier W, Du Bois A; Arbeitsgemeinschaft Gynaekologische Onkologie Ovarian Cancer Study Group. Prognostic factors for complete debulking in advanced ovarian cancer and its impact on survival. An exploratory analysis of a prospectively randomized phase III study of the Arbeitsgemeinschaft Gynaekologische Onkologie Ovarian Cancer Study Group (AGO-OVAR). *Gynecol Oncol.* 2007;106(1):69–74.

37. Aletti GD, Dowdy SC, Gostout BS, et al. Quality improvement in the surgical approach to advanced ovarian cancer: the Mayo Clinic experience. *J Am Coll Surg.* 2009;208(4):614–620.

38. Chi DS, Eisenhauer EL, Zivanovic O, et al. Improved progression-free and overall survival in advanced ovarian cancer as a result of a change in surgical paradigm. *Gynecol Oncol.* 2009;114(1):26–31.

39. Bristow RE, Tomacruz RS, Armstrong DK, Trimble EL, Montz FJ. Survival effect of maximal cytoreductive surgery for advanced ovarian carcinoma during the platinum era: a meta-analysis. *J Clin Oncol.* 2002;20(5):1248–1259.

40. Lakhman Y, Akin O, Sohn MJ, et al. Early postoperative CT as a prognostic biomarker in patients with advanced ovarian, tubal, and primary peritoneal cancer deemed optimally debulked at primary cytoreductive surgery. *AJR Am J Roentgenol.* 2012;198(6):1453–1459.

41. Winter WE 3rd, Maxwell GL, Tian C, et al.; Gynecologic Oncology Group Study. Prognostic factors for stage III epithelial ovarian cancer: a Gynecologic Oncology Group Study. *J Clin Oncol.* 2007;25(24):3621–3627.

42. Winter WE 3rd, Maxwell GL, Tian C, et al.; Gynecologic Oncology Group. Tumor residual after surgical cytoreduction in prediction of clinical outcome in stage IV epithelial ovarian cancer: a Gynecologic Oncology Group Study. *J Clin Oncol.* 2008;26(1):83–89.

43. Chi DS, Eisenhauer EL, Lang J, et al. What is the optimal goal of primary cytoreductive surgery for bulky stage IIIC epithelial ovarian carcinoma (EOC)? *Gynecol Oncol.* 2006;103(2): 559–564.

44. Rauh-Hain JA, Growdon WB, Rodriguez N, et al. Primary debulking surgery versus neoadjuvant chemotherapy in stage IV ovarian cancer. *Gynecol Oncol.* 2011;120:S12–S13.

45. Elattar A, Bryant A, Winter-Roach BA, Hatem M, Naik R. Optimal primary surgical treatment for advanced epithelial ovarian cancer. *Cochrane Database Syst Rev.* 2011;(8): CD007565.

46. Gerardi MA, Santillan A, Meisner B, et al. A clinical pathway for patients undergoing primary cytoreductive surgery with rectosigmoid colectomy for advanced ovarian and primary peritoneal cancers. *Gynecol Oncol.* 2008;108(2):282–286.

47. Marx C, Rasmussen T, Jakobsen DH, et al. The effect of accelerated rehabilitation on recovery after surgery for ovarian malignancy. *Acta Obstet Gynecol Scand.* 2006;85(4): 488–492.

48. Langstraat C, Aletti GD, Cliby WA. Morbidity, mortality and overall survival in elderly women undergoing primary surgical debulking for ovarian cancer: a delicate balance requiring individualization. *Gynecol Oncol.* 2011;123(2):187–191.

49. Wright JD, Lewin SN, Deutsch I, et al. Defining the limits of radical cytoreductive surgery for ovarian cancer. *Gynecol Oncol.* 2011;123(3):467–473.

50. Thrall MM, Goff BA, Symons RG, Flum DR, Gray HJ. Thirty-day mortality after primary cytoreductive surgery for advanced ovarian cancer in the elderly. *Obstet Gynecol.* 2011;118(3): 537–547.

51. Aletti GD, Eisenhauer EL, Santillan A, et al. Identification of patient groups at highest risk from traditional approach to ovarian cancer treatment. *Gynecol Oncol.* 2011;120(1): 23–28.

52. Glasgow MA, Yu H, Rutherford TJ, et al. Neoadjuvant chemotherapy (NACT) is an effective way of managing elderly women with advanced stage ovarian cancer (FIGO Stage IIIC and IV). *J Surg Oncol.* 2012 May 30 (E-pub ahead of print).

53. Fagotti A, Ferrandina G, Fanfani F, et al. A laparoscopy-based score to predict surgical outcome in patients with advanced ovarian carcinoma: a pilot study. *Ann Surg Oncol.* 2006;13(8): 1156–1161.

54. Fagotti A, Ferrandina G, Fanfani F, et al. Prospective validation of a laparoscopic predictive model for optimal cytoreduction in advanced ovarian carcinoma. *Am J Obstet Gynecol.* 2008;199(6):642.e1–642.e6.

55. Fanning J, Yacoub E, Hojat R. Laparoscopic-assisted cytoreduction for primary advanced ovarian cancer: success, morbidity and survival. *Gynecol Oncol.* 2011;123(1):47–49.

56. Grabowski JP, Harter P, Hils R, et al. Outcome of immediate re-operation or interval debulking after chemotherapy at a gynecologic oncology center after initially incomplete cytoreduction of advanced ovarian cancer. *Gynecol Oncol.* 2012;126(1): 54–57.

57. van der Burg ME, van Lent M, Buyse M, et al. The effect of debulking surgery after induction chemotherapy on the prognosis in advanced epithelial ovarian cancer. Gynecological Cancer Cooperative Group of the European Organization for Research and Treatment of Cancer. *N Engl J Med.* 1995;332(10): 629–634.

58. Rose PG, Nerenstone S, Brady MF, et al.; Gynecologic Oncology Group. Secondary surgical cytoreduction for advanced ovarian carcinoma. *N Engl J Med.* 2004;351(24):2489–2497.

59. Morice P, Dubernard G, Rey A, et al. Results of interval debulking surgery compared with primary debulking surgery in advanced stage ovarian cancer. *J Am Coll Surg.* 2003;197(6):955–963.

60. Sehouli J, Savvatis K, Braicu EI, Schmidt SC, Lichtenegger W, Fotopoulou C. Primary versus interval debulking surgery in advanced ovarian cancer: results from a systematic single-center analysis. *Int J Gynecol Cancer.* 2010;20(8):1331–1340.

61. Vergote I, Tropé CG, Amant F, et al.; European Organization for Research and Treatment of Cancer-Gynaecological Cancer Group; NCIC Clinical Trials Group. Neoadjuvant chemotherapy or primary surgery in stage IIIC or IV ovarian cancer. *N Engl J Med.* 2010;363(10):943–953.

62. Dewdney SB, Rimel BJ, Reinhart AJ, et al. The role of neoadjuvant chemotherapy in the management of patients with advanced stage ovarian cancer: survey results from members of the Society of Gynecologic Oncologists. *Gynecol Oncol.* 2010;119(1): 18–21.

63. Vergote I, Amant F, Leunen K. Neoadjuvant chemotherapy in advanced ovarian cancer: what kind of evidence is needed to convince US gynaecological oncologists? *Gynecol Oncol.* 2010;119(1):1–2.

64. Chi DS, Musa F, Dao F, et al. An analysis of patients with bulky advanced stage ovarian, tubal, and peritoneal carcinoma treated with primary debulking surgery (PDS) during an identical time period as the randomized EORTC-NCIC trial of PDS vs. neoadjuvant chemotherapy (NACT). *Gynecol Oncol.* 2012;124(1):10–14.

65. Morrison J, Swanton A, Collins S, Kehoe S. Chemotherapy versus surgery for initial treatment in advanced ovarian epithelial cancer. *Cochrane Database Syst Rev.* 2007;(4):CD005343.

66. Tian WJ, Chi DS, Sehouli J, et al. A risk model for secondary cytoreductive surgery in recurrent ovarian cancer: an evidence-based proposal for patient selection. *Ann Surg Oncol.* 2012;19(2):597–604.

67. Gil-Ibáñez B, Oskay-Özcelik G, Richter R, et al.; Tumor Bank Ovarian Cancer Network (TOC); European Competence Centre for Ovarian Cancer (EKZE Berlin). Predictive factors in relapsed ovarian cancer for complete tumor resection. *Anticancer Res.* 2011;31(8):2583–2587.

68. Schorge JO, Wingo SN, Bhore R, Heffernan TP, Lea JS. Secondary cytoreductive surgery for recurrent platinum-sensitive ovarian cancer. *Int J Gynaecol Obstet.* 2010;108(2): 123–127.

69. Harter P, du Bois A, Hahmann M, et al.; Arbeitsgemeinschaft Gynaekologische Onkologie Ovarian Committee; AGO Ovarian Cancer Study Group. Surgery in recurrent ovarian cancer: the Arbeitsgemeinschaft Gynaekologische Onkologie (AGO) DESKTOP OVAR trial. *Ann Surg Oncol.* 2006;13(12):1702–1710.

70. Holloway RW, Brudie LA, Rakowski JA, Ahmad S. Robotic-assisted resection of liver and diaphragm recurrent ovarian carcinoma: description of technique. *Gynecol Oncol.* 2011;120(3):419–422.

71. Chuang CM, Chou YJ, Yen MS, et al. The role of secondary cytoreductive surgery in patients with recurrent epithelial ovarian, tubal, and peritoneal cancers: a comparative effectiveness analysis. *Oncologist.* 2012;17(6):847–855.

72. Hizli D, Boran N, Yilmaz S, et al. Best predictors of survival outcome after tertiary cytoreduction in patients with recurrent platinum-sensitive epithelial ovarian cancer. *Eur J Obstet Gynecol Reprod Biol.* 2012;163(1):71–75.

73. Shih KK, Chi DS, Barakat RR, Leitao MM Jr. Tertiary cytoreduction in patients with recurrent epithelial ovarian, fallopian tube, or primary peritoneal cancer: an updated series. *Gynecol Oncol.* 2010;117(2):330–335.

74. Shih KK, Chi DS, Barakat RR, Leitao MM Jr. Beyond tertiary cytoreduction in patients with recurrent epithelial ovarian, fallopian tube, or primary peritoneal cancer. *Gynecol Oncol.* 2010;116(3):364–369.

75. Kucukmetin A, Naik R, Galaal K, Bryant A, Dickinson HO. Palliative surgery versus medical management for bowel obstruction in ovarian cancer. *Cochrane Database Syst Rev.* 2010;(7):CD007792.

76. Sartori E, Chiudinelli F, Pasinetti B, Sostegni B, Maggino T. Possible role of palliative surgery for bowel obstruction in advanced ovarian cancer patients. *Eur J Gynaecol Oncol.* 2010;31(1): 31–36.

77. Chi DS, Phaëton R, Miner TJ, et al. A prospective outcomes analysis of palliative procedures performed for malignant intestinal obstruction due to recurrent ovarian cancer. *Oncologist.* 2009;14(8):835–839.

78. Kolomainen DF, Daponte A, Barton DP, et al. Outcomes of surgical management of bowel obstruction in relapsed epithelial ovarian cancer (EOC). *Gynecol Oncol.* 2012;125(1):31–36.

79. Ripamonti C, Bruera E. Palliative management of malignant bowel obstruction. *Int J Gynecol Cancer.* 2002;12(2):135–143.

80. Fauci J, Schneider K, Walters C, et al. The utilization of palliative care in gynecologic oncology patients near the end of life. *Gynecol Oncol.* 2012 June 24 (E-pub ahead of print).

16 Multidisciplinary Approach to Treatment of Epithelial Ovarian Carcinoma

JAY P. SHAH

DEVANSU TEWARI

■ EPIDEMIOLOGY

It is estimated by the United States National Cancer Institute (NCI) Surveillance, Epidemiology, and End Results (SEER) Cancer Statistics Review that 22,280 women will be diagnosed with and 15,500 women will die of cancer of the ovary in 2012. Thus ovarian cancer is the eighth most common and fifth most common cause of cancer death in U.S. women. In 2009, there was approximately 182,758 women alive with a history of cancer of the ovary. From 2005 to 2009, the median age at diagnosis was 63 years of age and median age of death for cancer of the ovary was 71 years of age (1).

Trends over the past few decades show 5-year survival rates modestly improving but still highlight a need for newer treatment strategies. For example, in mid 1970s 5-year SEER survivals were 33%–37% and in mid 2000s 5-year SEER survivals were 43%–45% (1). Cooperative groups studies suggest a similar improvement in survival with median survivals in some of the latest Gynecologic Oncology Group (GOG) studies exceeding 60 months (2,3).

Lifetime risk based on incidence rates until 2009, was one in 72 women or 1.38% of women born today will be diagnosed with cancer of the ovary at some time during their lifetime (1).

■ PATHOLOGY

Ovarian cancer consists of several histopathologic entities with distinct embryologic origins and differing histologic appearances and therapies. Epithelial ovarian cancer comprises the majority of malignant ovarian neoplasms (about 80%; 3).

Epithelial ovarian cancers consist of cells mimicking the surface of the ovary. There are several subtypes: serous, mucinous, endometrioid, and clear cell. Clear cell and mucinous tend to be particularly aggressive. Pathologic grading 1–3 is an important prognostic factor and may guide selection of therapy primarily for early stage disease.

■ ORIGIN/ETIOLOGY

Risk factors for ovarian cancer have been identified in epidemiologic studies. A decreased risk is associated with young age at first birth (less than 25), use of oral contraceptives (even only a few months), and/or breastfeeding (4,5). The risk of borderline ovarian cancer may be increased after ovarian stimulation for in vitro fertilization (6).

It has been suggested that the fallopian tube may be the origin of some ovarian and primary peritoneal cancers (7). However, the guidelines for therapy for the much less common fallopian tube and primary peritoneal cancers are the same as epithelial ovarian cancer.

Hereditary factors play a role in the development of ovarian cancer, but comprise only in a small percentage of all ovarian cancers. The risk of developing ovarian cancer and having an earlier onset occurs in those with a family history (two first-degree relatives with ovarian cancer), *BRCA1* and *BRCA2* genotype, or families affected by Lynch syndrome (hereditary nonpolyposis colorectal cancer [HNPCC] syndrome). In high-risk women, salpingo-oophorectomy is associated with a reduced risk of ovarian and fallopian tube cancer; however there is still a residual risk for primary peritoneal cancer in these high-risk women (8,9).

Tumor Microenvironment

Vascular endothelial growth factor (VEGF) and angiogenesis are important promoters of ovarian cancer progression. An antibody that inhibits tumor angiogenesis by blocking VEGF has been shown to be beneficial in ovarian cancer.

Angiogenesis is the process of new blood vessel development and is critical for the growth and progression of solid tumors. Tumor vasculature is highly disorganized that result in poor blood flow and high-vascular permeability.

This may lead to decreased efficacy of cytotoxic chemotherapy and increased potential for metastasis. Antiangiogenic therapy such as inhibiting VEGF normalize tumor blood vessel structure and function. This improves delivery of chemotherapeutic drugs and may decrease the metastatic potential of tumors and cause a regression of the tumor. In epithelial ovarian cancer, angiogenesis inhibitors appear to be valid targets for ovarian cancer treatment (10).

Staging

Surgical staging is based on the pattern of disease spread. It should include a complete evaluation of all visceral and parietal surfaces within the peritoneal cavity with cytology, omentectomy, and biopsy of aortic and pelvic lymph nodes (11). The ovaries, uterus, and cervix are generally removed unless a fertility sparing approach is planned. Since 1997, no significant changes have been made in the TNM and Federation of International Gynecologic and Obstetrics (FIGO) staging systems (see Tables 16.1 and 16.2; 12 adopted from NCCN.org guidelines).

Workup of Suspicious Pelvic Mass

Ultrasound and chest/abdominal/pelvic CT with an abdominal/pelvic physical examination, and appropriate laboratory studies are the primary workup of a patient with suspected ovarian cancer. The patient may have a suspicious mass detected on examination or ascites, or abdominal distention. The most commonly reported symptoms are bloating, pelvic or abdominal pain, difficulty in eating or feeling full quickly, or urinary symptoms (13). Although a fine needle aspiration may be necessary in patients with bulky disease who are not surgical candidates, in general avoiding needle biopsy of pelvic mass in those with presumed early stage will prevent rupturing the cyst and spilling malignant cells into the peritoneal cavity (14). Tumor markers typically include CA-125, and in younger women an alpha-fetoprotein (AFP), inhibin, and beta-human chorionic gonadotropin.

A Risk of ovarian malignancy algorithm (ROMA) with CA-125 and HE-4 serum markers has been Food and Drug Administration (FDA) approved for estimating the risk of ovarian cancer in women with a pelvic mass (15). Currently the National Comprehensive Cancer Network (NCCN) does not recommend the use of these biomarkers for determining the status of an undiagnosed pelvic mass. Another FDA approved test, OVA-1 uses five markers to assess which patient may benefit from referral to a gynecologic oncologist. The five markers are transthyretin, apolipoprotein A1, transferrin, beta-2 microglobulin, and CA-125. Neither the Society of Gynecologic Oncologists (SGO) nor the NCCN panel recommends its use as a screening test or triage tool. A third screening test, no longer available outside of a clinical trial, is OvaSure and used six biomarkers (leptin, prolactin, osteopontin,

insulin-like growth factor II, macrophage inhibitory factor, and CA-125). Recent data show that many markers including CA-125 and HE-4 may not rise early enough to be useful in detecting early stage ovarian cancer (16,17).

The NCCN consensus suggested that an experienced gynecologic oncologist operate all patients with ovarian cancer. American College of Obstetricians and Gynecologists (ACOG) and SGO have created criteria to direct the referral of pelvic masses but at present no biomarker has been widely accepted to determine referral to a gynecologic oncologist (18).

■ PRIMARY TREATMENT—SURGERY

Surgery when applied as part of a multidisciplinary approach provides the patient the highest likelihood of a favorable outcome. For the vast majority of patients surgery alone is not curative but may provide diagnosis, staging, symptom relief, and cytoreduction (19). Primary therapy for presumed ovarian cancer is appropriate surgical staging and cytoreduction (tumor debulking) in conjunction with subsequent systemic chemotherapy. There exists a high level of evidence and consensus that a gynecologic oncologist should perform the primary surgery (20,21).

Suspicious masses are excised intact and submitted for frozen section. If malignancy is confirmed and no grossly visible disease is found then surgical staging is undertaken. For a patient wishing to preserve fertility, a unilateral salpingo-oophorectomy with preservation of uterus and contralateral ovary may be appropriate for Stage IA or 1C. In suspected early stage epithelial ovarian cancer, a full surgical staging procedure with lymph node evaluation is still recommended since the risk of occult higher stage disease may be as high as 30% (22). Minimally invasive techniques while maintaining the same surgical principles of removal without spill and complete surgical staging may allow more rapid recovery and less complications, but requires experienced minimally invasive surgeons (23). A complete surgical staging via laparoscopy has been suggested; however it is still under investigation (24,25).

In patients with clinical Stage II, III, IV disease upfront cytoreductive surgery remains the standard approach in the United States. This is based on retrospective data that shows an advantage to achieving maximal cytoreduction to less than 1 cm residual disease or resection of all visible disease in appropriate circumstances (26–32). Surgical cytoreduction is considered optimal if the residual tumor nodules are less than 1 cm in maximum diameter or thickness (33). Recent analysis suggests that most benefits are derived for cytoreduction to no visible residual disease but the GOG definition of optimal cytoreduction has not changed (34–36). There are several hypotheses concerning benefits of aggressive primary surgical management including better perfusion of chemotherapy drugs on smaller tumor size, increased growth fraction, improvement in disease-related symptoms by removal of tumor bulk, and enhanced immunologic competence of the patient. In general expert surgeons achieve optimal cytoreduction in about 75% of cases. Limitation to optimal cytoreduction to no gross visible disease may be technical or dictated by tumor biology. Despite studies attempting to create predictive markers for optimal or suboptimal cytoreduction, no validated criteria perform well enough for clinical use to predict those patients who will undergo an optimal cytoreduction (37,38).

This primary surgery approach per NCCN guidelines includes a maximal effort to remove all gross disease. Upon entry into the abdomen, aspiration of ascites or collection of peritoneal cytology occurs unless obvious disease beyond the ovaries is found. A total hysterectomy or supracervical hysterectomy may be performed. The encapsulated mass should be removed intact if possible

---

■ Table 16.1 Staging

American Joint Committee on Cancer (AJCC)
TNM and FIGO Staging System for Ovarian Primary Peritoneal Cancer (7th ed., 2010)

Primary Tumor (T)

TNM	FIGO		TNM	FIGO	
TX		Primary tumor cannot be assessed	T3	III	Tumor involves one or both ovaries with microscopically confimed peritoneal metastasis outside the pelvis
T0		No evidence of primary tumor			
T1	I	Tumor limited to ovaries (one or both)	T3a	IIIA	Microscopic peritoneal metastasis beyond pelvis (no macroscopic tumor)
T1a	IA	Tumor limited to one ovary; capsule intact, no tumor on ovarian surface. No malignant cells in ascites or peritoneal washings	T3b	IIIB	Macroscopic peritoneal metastasis beyond pelvis 2 cm or less in greatest dimension
T1b	IB	Tumor limited to both ovaries; capsules intact, no tumor on ovarian surface. No malignant cells in ascites or peritoneal washings	T3c	IIIC	Peritoneal metastasis beyond pelvis more than 2 cm in greatest dimension and/or regional lymph node metastasis

Regional Lymph Nodes (N)

TNM	FIGO	
NX		Regional lymph nodes cannot be assessed
N0		No regional lymph node metastasis
N1	IIIC	Regional lymph node metastasis

TNM	FIGO	
T1c	IC	Tumor limited to one or both ovaries with any of the following: capsule ruptured, tumor on ovarian surface, malignant cells in ascites or peritoneal washings
T2	II	Tumor involves one or both ovaries with pelvic extension
T2a	IIA	Extension and/or implants on uterus and/or tube(s). No malignant cells in ascites or peritoneal washings
T2b	IIB	Extension to and/or implants on pelvic tissues. No malignant cells in ascites or peritoneal washings
T2c	IIC	Pelvic extension and/or implants (T2a or T2b) with malignant cells in ascites or peritoneal washings

Distant Metastasis (M)

TNM	FIGO	
M0		No distant metastasis
M1	IV	Distant metastasis (excludes peritoneal metastasis)

Note: Liver capsule metastasis is T3/stage III; liver paraenchymal metastasis, M1/stage IV. Pleural effusion must have positive cytology for M1/stage IV.

Stage Grouping

Stage 1	T1	N0	M0
Stage IA	T1a	N0	M0
Stage IB	T1b	N0	M0
Stage IC	T1c	N0	M0
Stage II	T2	N0	M0
Stage IIA	T2a	N0	M0
Stage IIB	T2b	N0	M0
Stage IIC	T2c	N0	M0
Stage III	T3	N0	M0
Stage IIIA	T3a	N0	M0
Stage IIIB	T3b	N0	M0
Stage IIIC	T3c	N0	M0
Stage IIIC	Any T	N1	M0
Stage IV	Any T	Any N	M1

The staging system for ovarian and primary peritoneal cancer is also used for malignant germ cell tumors, malignant sex cord-stromal tumors, and carcinosarcoma (malignant mixed Müllerian tumors).

Note: For histologic grade and histopathologic type, see AJCC Staging Manual.

Used with the permission of the American Joint Committee on Cancer (AJCC), Chicago Illinois. The original and primary source for this information is the AJCC Cancer Staging Manual, Seventh Edition (2010) published by Springer Science+Business Media, LLC (SBM). For complete information and data supporting the staging tables, visit www.cancerstaging.net.) Any citation or quotation of this material must be credited to the AJCC as its primary source. The inclusion of this information herein does not authorize any reuse or further distribution without the expressed, written permission of Springer SBM, on behalf of the AJCC.

■ **Table 16.2** Staging

American Joint Committee on Cancer (AJCC)
TNM and FIGO Staging System for Ovarian Primary Peritoneal Cancer (7th ed., 2010)

Primary Tumor (T)

TNM	FIGO	
TX		Primary tumor cannot be assessed
T0		No evidence of primary tumor
Tis*		Carcinoma in situ (limited to tubal mucosa)
T1	I	Tumor limited to the fallopian tube(s)
T1a	IA	Tumor limited to one tube, without penetrating the serosal surface; no ascites
T1b	IB	Tumor limited to both tubes, without penetrating the serosal surface; no ascites
T1c	IC	Tumor limited to one or both tubes with extension onto or through the tubal serosa, or with malignant cells in ascites or peritoneal washings
T2	II	Tumor involves one or both fallopian tubes with pelvic extension
T2a	IIA	Extension and/or metastasis to the uterus and/or ovaries
T2b	IIB	Extension to other pelvic structures
T2c	IIC	Pelvic extension with malignant cells in ascites or peritoneal washings

TNM	FIGO	
T3	III	Tumor involves one or both fallopian tubes, with peritoneal implants outside the pelvis
T3a	IIIA	Microscopically peritoneal metastasis outside the pelvis
T3b	IIIB	Macroscopic peritoneal metastasis outside the pelvis 2 cm or less in greatest dimension
T3c	IIIC	Peritoneal metastasis outside the pelvis and more than 2 cm in diameter

Regional Lymph Nodes (N)

NX		Regional lymph nodes cannot be assessed
N0		No regional lymph node metastasis
N1	IIIC	Regional lymph node metastasis

Distant Metastasis (M)

M0		No distant metastasis
M1	IV	Distant metastasis (excludes metastasis within the peritoneal cavity)

* Note: FIGO no longer includes stage 0 (Tis)
Note: Liver capsule metastasis is T3/stage III; liver parenchymal metastasis, M1, stage IV. Pleural effusion must have positive cytology for M1/stage IV.

Stage Grouping

Stage 0*	Tis	N0	M0
Stage 1	T1	N0	M0
Stage IA	T1a	N0	M0
Stage IB	T1b	N0	M0
Stage IC	T1c	N0	M0
Stage II	T2	N0	M0
Stage IIA	T2a	N0	M0
Stage IIB	T2b	N0	M0
Stage IIC	T2c	N0	M0
Stage III	T3	N0	M0
Stage IIIA	T3a	N0	M0
Stage IIIB	T3b	N0	M0
Stage IIIC	T3c	N0	M0
	Any T	N1	M0
Stage IV	Any T	Any N	M1

*Note: FIGO no longer includes stage 0 (Tis)
Note: For histologic grade and histopathologic type, see AJCC Staging Manual.

and all involved omentum removed. Diaphragm biopsy or cytology should be collected. Suspicious or enlarged retroperitoneal lymph nodes removed and for those with tumor nodules less than 2 cm outside the pelvis a bilateral pelvic and para-aortic lymph node dissection performed (39). Procedures considered for optimal cytoreduction include radical pelvic dissection, bowel resection, diaphragm, or other peritoneal stripping, splenectomy, partial hepatectomy, cholecystectomy, partial gastrectomy, ureteroneocystostomy, or distal pancreatectomy (37).

Quality indicators for ovarian cancer surgery have been published by the European Organization for Research and Treatment of Cancer—Gynecological Cancer Group (EORTC-GCG). For grossly early-stage disease this included a systemic pelvic and para-aortic lymphadenectomy in the presence of medium- or high-risk factors. For advanced cancer this included the documentation of the size and location of residual disease and the performance of a staging surgery, and the proportion of patients with advanced disease undergoing debulking to residual disease of 1 cm or less. The SGO recently developed two measures to assess and improve the surgical care of patients with ovarian cancer—the description of residual disease following cytoreduction and the performance of adequate surgical staging as defined by the GOG (40).

■ PRIMARY TREATMENT—NEOADJUVANT CHEMOTHERAPY

The goal of neoadjuvant chemotherapy is to reduce the tumor masses to an extent that would allow for successful surgical debulking during delayed primary cytoreduction. For patients with a poor performance status, neoadjuvant chemotherapy may lead to reduction of ascites, pleural effusions, and an improved clinical status that would allow aggressive cytoreductive surgery. Alternatively it may allow for treatment of the cancer while the patient is undergoing therapy for an acute medical comorbidity. Some commonly used criteria suggesting suboptimal cytoreduction but not validated are disease in the portahepatis, liver or pulmonary metastasis, and massive ascites (37). A recent randomized trial sponsored by EORTC-GCG and National Cancer Institute Canada—Clinical Trial Group (NCIC-CTG) assessed neoadjuvant chemotherapy with interval debulking vs upfront primary debulking surgery in patients with extensive Stage IIIC/IV ovarian, primary peritoneal, and fallopian tube carcinoma. Median overall survival was equivalent in these patient (29 vs 30 months) but patients receiving neoadjuvant chemotherapy with interval debulking surgery had fewer complications (41). A subsequent retrospective study using SEER database linked with Medicare claims showed that women treated with neoadjuvant chemotherapy vs primary surgery had fewer ostomies, bowel resections, and postoperative complications. For women with Stage III disease at 2 years, the risk of death was higher following neoadjuvant chemotherapy (relative risk [RR] 1.16, confidence interval [CI]: 1.01–1.34), and for women with Stage IV disease, there was a reduction in the risk of death at 2 years associated with neoadjuvant chemotherapy (RR 0.85, CI: 0.73–0.99; 42). Although not specifically studied, most clinicians when using neoadjuvant chemotherapy evaluate and proceed with interval debulking surgery in women who have a response or at least stable disease, after three cycles as was done in the EORTC/NCIC randomized trial. Following interval debulking surgery, this trial completed three further IV cycles of chemotherapy. Intraperitoneal chemotherapy following interval debulking in the neoadjuvant setting lacks survival benefit data and is associated with increased morbidity (43). The median overall survival in the EORTC International trial is 20 months lower than that reported in randomized studies in the United States undergoing primary cytoreductive surgery followed by IV or intraperitoneal chemotherapy. And according to current NCCN Ovarian Cancer Guidelines subcommittee, more data will be necessary prior to recommending neoadjuvant chemotherapy as upfront therapy unless a woman is not a surgical candidate.

For patients with an incomplete previous surgery or staging, or residual disease that was considered unresectable, consideration for completion surgery after three cycles appears warranted in order to remove any potentially resectable residual disease.

■ PRIMARY ADJUVANT TREATMENT—CHEMOTHERAPY

Chemotherapy plays an important role in the treatment of ovarian cancer. Only patients with Stage IA or IB, Grade 1 tumors are treated with surgery alone, and that is because the survival is greater than 90% for this group with surgical therapy alone (44). The reported survival of 60%–80% in patients who have early stage high-risk features explains the potential role for adjuvant therapy. High-risk early stage disease includes Stage IC (tumor confined to ovary with + washings) or Stage II (tumor involving the pelvis) and clear-cell histology (any stage), and high-tumor grade (Grade 3). The EORTC-Adjuvant ChemoTherapy in Ovarian Neoplasm (ACTION) trial combined with ICON1 questioned the benefit of adjuvant chemotherapy in early stage disease following complete surgical staging. At median follow-up of 10 years chemotherapy resulted in an improvement in recurrence-free survival (RFS; 70 vs 62%, hazard ratio = 0.64, CI: 0.46–0.89) and a trend toward an improvement in cancer-specific survival (82% vs 76%, hazard ratio = 0.73, CI: 0.48–1.13) but this benefit was only statistically significant in incompletely staged women (45). However, two other meta-analyses including a Cochrane review with five randomized trials define the benefit of adjuvant therapy in early stage EOC and lead to the NCCN guidelines, which recommend chemotherapy for high-risk early stage EOC (46,47). The GOG157 trial evaluated three vs six cycles of paclitaxel and carboplatin in patients with early Stage IA or IB, Grade 2 or 3; Stage IC; or Stage II disease and found no benefit to the longer regimen. But this trial found that six cycles vs three cycles had a nonsignificant trend toward lower risk of recurrence (20% vs 25%), no difference in overall survival, and more toxicity (48). A subgroup analysis subsequently done found a lower risk of recurrence with six cycles for patients with papillary serous tumors (hazard ratio = 0.33, 95% CI: 0.14–0.77) but not in other histologic types and no overall survival difference (49).

Three modalities used in the postoperative treatment of newly diagnosed advanced stage ovarian cancer are IV cytotoxic chemotherapy alone, combination of intraperitoneal and IV chemotherapy, and combination of IV cytotoxic and biologic chemotherapy. The NCCN guidelines recommend intraperitoneal chemotherapy for Stage III patients with optimally debulked (<1 cm) disease based on randomized controlled trials. The most recent published intraperitoneal trial GOG172, in which women with Stage III ovarian cancer who received intrapertioneal chemotherapy cisplatin and paclitaxel in combination with IV paclitaxel compared with standard arm IV cisplatin and paclitaxel had a 16-month increase in survival (65.6 vs 49.7 months). The intraperitoneal regimen was paclitaxel 135 mg/m^2 over 24 hours day 1; cisplatin 75 to 100 mg/m^2 intraperitoneal, day 2; and paclitaxel 60 mg/m^2 intraperitoneal, day 8 every 3 weeks for six cycles (50). A fourth GOG front line intraperitoneal trial, GOG252 has been completed but not reported and included an intraperitoneal chemotherapy arm with a 3-hour instead of 24-hour paclitaxel infusion and a lower dose of cisplatin.

For patients with suboptimal cytoreduction or not interested in intraperitoneal chemotherapy the most common recommendation remains IV paclitaxel plus carboplatin. The IV regimen includes paclitaxel, 175 mg over 3 hours followed by carboplatin dosed at an area under the curve of 5–7.5 over 1 hour given every 3 weeks for six cycles (51,52). Alternative options include IV docetaxel plus carboplatin with docetaxel 60–75 mg/m^2 over 1 hour followed by carboplatin at area under the curve (AUC) of five or six or dose-dense paclitaxel 80 mg/m^2 IV over 1 hour on days 1, 8, 15 plus carboplatin AUC 6 IV over 1 hour on day 1 every 3 weeks for six cycles (53). A long-term follow-up was recently presented at an American Society of Clinical Oncology (ASCO) meeting in abstract form with 6.4 years of median follow-up comparing the dose-dense paclitaxel and carboplatin vs conventional every 3 weeks paclitaxel and carboplatin with PFS (28.1 vs 17.5 month, hazard ratio = 0.75, 95% CI: 0.62–0.91) and overall survival at 5 years favoring the dose-dense group (58.6% vs 51%, hazard ratio = 0.79, CI: 0.63–0.99) (54).

These regimens have different toxicity profiles. Docetaxel/paclitaxel increased neutropenia; the IV paclitaxel/carboplatin with sensory peripheral neuropathy, and dose-dense paclitaxel with increased anemia. The intraperitoneal paclitaxel/cisplatin regimen is associated with myelosuppression, fatigue, renal toxicity, abdominal pain, and neurotoxicity. In the initial GOG172 study only 42% of women were able to complete all six intraperitoneal-based treatment cycles. The most common reasons for discontinuing therapy included catheter complications, nausea/vomiting/dehydration, and abdominal pain (50). Future studies such as GOG252 and GOG262 will compare the effect of weekly paclitaxel and intraperitoneal chemotherapy with biologic agent, bevacizumab.

Antiangiogenesis

A recent Phase III randomized trial GOG218 assessed bevacizumab with carboplatin/paclitaxel in the upfront setting compared to carboplatin/paclitaxel alone. The median PFS was increased in patients receiving bevacizumab upfront and as maintenance (14.1 vs 10.3 months; hazard ratio = 0.717, CI: 0.62–0.82). No benefit was found in those receiving upfront bevacizumab with placebo maintenance vs chemotherapy alone. No difference in overall survival or quality of life was reported (55). Another recent Phase III randomized trial, ICON7, also found a benefit on PFS of upfront bevacizumab followed by bevacizumab as maintenance therapy (56). In this study, the benefits in PFS was a modest 1.7 months and survival data are currently immature. However, a post hoc subset analysis suggests an overall survival advantage in patients with the most aggressive disease (suboptimal and Stage IV disease). The difference between the GOG218 and ICON7 study is that bevacizumab was available after progression of disease in the United States trial. Without an overall survival benefit or improved quality of life, no consensus currently exists regarding adding bevacizumab to upfront chemotherapy. The magnitude of the clinical benefit vs the potential for serious side effects (<3% GI perforation or fistula), and cost make its role in front line therapy unclear at this time (57).

Number of Cycles

Recommendations for patients with advanced disease are six to eight cycles whereas for early stage disease, three to six cycles are recommended. Patients with advanced disease can also have three to six cycles of chemotherapy followed by interval debulking surgery and then postoperative chemotherapy. More than six to eight cycles are required for initial therapy (58).

Radiation

Although whole abdominal radiation has been an effective adjuvant therapy in the past following optimally debulked tumors, it is no longer included in NCCN guidelines as an option for initial treatment or consolidation treatment in ovarian cancer. Palliative localized radiation therapy is an option for symptom control (59,60).

Maintenance

The majority of patients with epithelial ovarian cancer achieve a complete clinical remission with first line chemotherapy, but the majority will recur. This has lead to trials of maintenance or consolidation therapy beyond the standard and short-term high-dose strategies (six cycles of IV or intraperitoneal chemotherapy). The GOG178 trial randomly assigned patients to 3 vs 12 months of further paclitaxel (175 mg/m^2 every 4 weeks for 12 cycles) after initial chemotherapy (61). The protocol closed with all patients receiving the 175 mg/m^2 dose and a suggestion that those patients receiving 12 cycles have a PFS advantage. This approach has not been widely accepted because no overall survival data will be available and a subsequent placebo-controlled trial GOG212 is still enrolling patients. A meta-analysis of six randomized trials (n = 902 patients) concluded there was no significant improvement in 5-year overall survival to justify the administration of maintenance chemotherapy (RR 1.07, 95% CI: 0.91–1.27; 62).

Surveillance

The evaluation of women after chemotherapy generally includes a history and physical (pelvic examination) and CA-125. A second-look laparotomy to confirm pathologic response has been shown not to be associated with altered prognosis (63). If there is evidence of residual cancer by examination, computed tomography (CT), or CA-125 then women are considered platinum resistant for primary refractory epithelial ovarian cancer. The SGO guidelines recommend office visits with pelvic and physical exam every 3 to 6 months with an individualized approach to monitoring by serum CA-125. CT, complete blood counts, ultrasound only done as clinically indicated. Patients with symptoms such as bloating, pain, obstruction, weight loss, and fatigue may require imaging studies such as chest/abdominal/pelvic CT, MRI, positron emission tomography (PET) scan, PET-CT.

A recent multi-institutional European trial assessed the use of CA-125 for monitoring ovarian cancer recurrence after primary therapy. The data suggest that treating recurrences early (based on detectable CA-125 levels in asymptomatic patients) is not associated with an increase in survival and is associated with a decrease in quality of life (64,65). Despite this trial, the NCCN and SGO both confirm that the pros and cons of CA-125 monitoring (opportunity for secondary cytoreduction) be discussed individually and acknowledge that patients seem reluctant to give up monitoring (66,67).

Rising CA-125

The management of patients in a clinical complete remission who during routine surveillance are found to have an increasing CA-125 but no signs or symptoms of recurrent disease and a negative pelvic exam and negative chest/abdominal/pelvic CT scan require extensive counseling. The median time for a clinical relapse after an increase in CA-125 (biochemical relapse) is 3 months. Data suggest that immediate treatment for a biochemical relapse is not beneficial and that delaying treatment, that is, continued observation until symptoms arise, may maximize quality of life (68). Tamoxifen and other hormonally active agents are often administered to patients who have only a rising CA-125 level (69).

■ CHEMOTHERAPY FOR RECURRENT DISEASE

Management of recurrent disease is stratified based on the time that has elapsed between the completion of platinum-based treatment and the detection of relapse, known as the platinum-free interval (PFI). Platinum-sensitive women are those with a PFI of 6 months or longer. Those with a PFI of less than 6 months are considered to have platinum-resistant disease. The worse prognosis is for patients who progress after two consecutive chemotherapy regimens without ever sustaining a clinical benefit (refractory) and those whose disease recurs in less than 6 months (platinum resistant; 70).

Options for platinum-resistant patients include recurrence chemotherapy, clinical trial, and observation with best supportive care. For platinum-sensitive patients after considering secondary cytoreductive surgery, the combination platinum-based chemotherapy is preferred for first recurrence. The preferred combinations include carboplatin/paclitaxel (71), carboplatin/weekly paclitaxel (72), carboplatin/docetaxel (73), carboplatin/gemcitabine (74), carboplatin/liposomal doxorubicin (75), or cisplatin/gemcitabine (76).

For platinum-resistant disease the preferred agent is a single non–platinum-based agent. The activity of the following agents appears similar: topotecan, 20% (77); gemcitabine, 19% (78); vinorelbine, 20% (79); liposomal doxorubicin, 26% (80); oral etoposide, 27% (81); docetaxel, 22% (82); and weekly paclitaxel, 21% (83; see Table 16.3).

Other potential active agents include altretamine, capecitabine, cyclophosphamide, ifosfamide, irinotecan, melphalan, oxaliplatin, paclitaxel, nab-paclitaxel, pemetrexed, and vinorelbine.

Bevacizumab has been shown to be beneficial in two trials in combination with cytotoxic chemotherapy in the recurrent setting. The OCEANS trial with platinum-sensitive recurrent ovarian cancer showed the progression-free survival (PFS) for bevacizumab with carboplatin and gemcitabine was superior to the placebo arm with carboplatin and gemcitabine alone (hazard ratio = 0.484; 95% CI: 0.388–0.605); with median PFS of 12.4 vs 8.4 months, respectively (84).

In the AURELIA study, in platinum-resistant ovarian cancer, bevacizumab with chemotherapy provided statistically significant and clinically meaningful improvement in PFS versus chemotherapy alone (85).

Drug Reactions

Common drug-related reactions occur with carboplatin, cisplatin, docetaxel, liposomal doxorubicin, oxaliplatin, and paclitaxel. For patients with allergic reactions, various desensitization protocols have been published. Almost all patients can be desensitized usually for safety in the

■ **Table 16.3** NCCN guidelines for acceptable recurrence therapies		
	Cytotoxic Therapy	**Targeted**
Preferred agents	Platinum-sensitive combination	Bevacizumab
	Carboplatin/docetaxel	
	Carboplatin/gemcitabine	
	Carboplatin/gemcitabine/bevacizumab	
	Carboplatin/liposomal doxorubicin	
	Carboplatin/paclitaxel	
	Carboplatin/weekly paclitaxel	
	Cisplatin/gemcitabine	
	Platinum-sensitive—single agent	
	Carboplatin	
	Cisplatin	
	Platinum-resistant—single agent	
	Docetaxel	
	Gemcitabine	
	Liposomal doxorubicin	
	Oral etoposide	
	Topotecan	
	Weekly paclitaxel	
	Cytotoxic Therapy	**Hormonal**
Other potentially active agents	Altretamine	Anastrozole
	Capecitabine	Letrozole
	Cyclophosphamide	Leuprolide acetate
	Ifosfamide	Megestrol acetate
	Irinotecan	Tamoxifen
	Melphalan	
	Nab-paclitaxel	
	Oxaliplatin	
	Paclitaxel	
	Pemetrexed	
	Vinorelbine	

Adapted from Version 1.2013, 10/12/12 © National Comprehensive Cancer Network, Inc. 2012.

ICU (86). Data suggest that an extended infusion schedule and use of premedications may decrease the number of hypersensitivity reactions to even carboplatin (87).

Secondary Surgery

Secondary cytoreductive surgery may be considered for patients who recur after a long disease-free interval. The GOG213 trial required a disease-free interval of 6 months for enrollment and other retrospective studies have suggested at least a 6-month interval (88,89).

■ POLY ADP-RIBOSE POLYMERASE INHIBITORS

Recent data suggest that olaparib, which is a poly ADP-ribose polymerase (PARP) inhibitor is active in patients with DNA repair defects. Patients with *BRCA1* and *BRCA2* mutations have higher response rates than *BRCA* negative

patients (90). In a randomized open-label Phase II trial, reported in abstract form found a benefit for the addition of olaparib with chemotherapy and maintenance dosing of olaparib despite only 15% of patients having *BRCA1* and *BRCA2* mutations. Patients were assigned to treatment with carboplatin (AUC = 6) plus paclitaxel (175 mg/m²) for six cycles (repeated every 3 weeks) with or without olaparib (200 mg twice daily), followed by observation or maintenance olaparib until progression. Incorporation of olaparib to chemotherapy resulted in a significant benefit in PFS compared to chemotherapy alone (median PFS, 12 vs 10 months, hazard ratio = 0.51, 95% CI: 0.34–0.77). Overall survival data were not presented (91). Currently olaparib is only available in a clinical trial.

Resistance Assay

In vitro chemosensitivity and resistance assays are laboratory tests that have been developed to help guide the clinician's selection of chemotherapy agent. A sensitivity assay selects the optimal chemotherapy regimen and a resistance assay identifies agents to avoid or least likely to be effective. The ASCO has concluded that at this time the evidence is insufficient to justify its use outside a clinical trial setting (92,93). Instead, they recommend oncologists take into account individual patient preferences and clinical trial reports to make chemotherapy treatment recommendations (92).

Localized Control

Localized radiotherapy can also provide effective palliation when directed to specific symptomatic sites (94). Image-guided percutaneous cryotherapy for the management of symptomatic metastasis and local control have also been reported in ovarian cancer patients (95).

■ QUALITY OF LIFE

Regardless of the regimen selected reevaluation should follow after two to four cycles of chemotherapy to determine if the patient is benefitting from chemotherapy. Decisions to offer supportive care, additional therapy, and palliative care services should be made on a highly individualized basis. Quality of life evaluation is a valuable measure in optimizing care of patients with ovarian cancer (96). It appears that the majority of gynecologic oncology patients spend less than 30 days on hospice and earlier referral could decrease hospital admission and procedures while providing invaluable support during this end-of-life (EOL) transition (97). EOL care focuses on comfort, control, meaning, and support that become particularly intense when death is imminent (98). Identifying modifiable characteristics that are associated with survival offers the potential for providing support that may improve outcomes (99). Quality of life measurement is the only trial end point available to measure the benefits of disease progression delay and symptom control, thus supporting early palliative care/hospice intervention with potential improvement in quality of life indices, and further evaluation in clinical trials are encouraged (100,101).

■ REFERENCES

1. Howlader N, Noone AM, Krapcho M, et al. (eds). *SEER Cancer Statistics Review, 1975–2009* (Vintage 2009 Populations). Bethesda, MD: National Cancer Institute. http://seer.cancer.gov/csr/1975_2009_pops09/, based on November 2011 SEER data submission, posted to the SEER web site, 2012.

2. Armstrong DK, Bundy B, Wenzel L, et al.; Gynecologic Oncology Group. Intraperitoneal cisplatin and paclitaxel in ovarian cancer. *N Engl J Med.* 2006;354(1):34–43.

3. Chan JK, Cheung MK, Husain A, et al. Patterns and progress in ovarian cancer over 14 years. *Obstet Gynecol.* 2006;108(3 Pt 1):521–528.

4. Fleming GF, Ronnett BM, Seidman J. Epithelial ovarian cancer. In: Barakat RR, Markman M, Randall ME, eds. *Principles and Practice of Gynecologic Oncology.* 5th ed. Philadelphia, PA: Lippincott Williams & Wilkins, 2009:763–836.

5. The reduction in risk of ovarian cancer associated with oral-contraceptive use. The Cancer and Steroid Hormone Study of the Centers for Disease Control and the National Institute of Child Health and Human Development. *N Engl J Med.* 1987;316(11):650–655.

6. van Leeuwen FE, Klip H, Mooij TM, et al. Risk of borderline and invasive ovarian tumours after ovarian stimulation for *in vitro* fertilization in a large Dutch cohort. *Hum Reprod.* 2011;26(12):3456–3465.

7. Collins IM, Domchek SM, Huntsman DG, Mitchell G. The tubal hypothesis of ovarian cancer: caution needed. *Lancet Oncol.* 2011;12(12):1089–1091.

8. ACOG Practice Bulletin No. 103. Hereditary breast and ovarian cancer syndrome. *Obstet Gynecol.* 2009;113:957–966.

9. Domchek SM, Friebel TM, Singer CF, et al. Association of risk-reducing surgery in BRCA1 or BRCA2 mutation carriers with cancer risk and mortality. *JAMA.* 2010;304(9):967–975.

10. Burger RA. Overview of anti-angiogenic agents in development for ovarian cancer. *Gynecol Oncol.* 2011;121(1):230–238.

11. Whitney CW, Spirtos N. Gynecologic Oncology Group Surgical Procedures Manual. Philadelphia: Gynecologic Oncology Group; 2009. https://gogmember.gog.org/manuals/pdf/surgman.pdf.

12. Edge SB, Byrd DR, Compton CC, et al. AJCC Cancer Staging Manual, 7th ed. New York: Springer; 2010.

13. Goff BA, Mandel LS, Drescher CW, et al. Development of an ovarian cancer symptom index: possibilities for earlier detection. *Cancer.* 2007;109(2):221–227.

14. American College of Obstetricians and Gynecologists. ACOG Practice Bulletin. Management of adnexal masses. *Obstet Gynecol.* 2007 Jul;110(1):201–214.

15. Moore RG, Miller MC, Disilvestro P, et al. Evaluation of the diagnostic accuracy of the risk of ovarian malignancy algorithm in women with a pelvic mass. *Obstet Gynecol.* 2011;118(2 Pt 1):280–288.

16. Cramer DW, Bast RC Jr, Berg CD, et al. Ovarian cancer biomarker performance in prostate, lung, colorectal, and ovarian cancer screening trial specimens. *Cancer Prev Res (Phila).* 2011;4(3):365–374.

17. Anderson GL, McIntosh M, Wu L, et al. Assessing lead time of selected ovarian cancer biomarkers: a nested case-control study. *J Natl Cancer Inst.* 2010;102(1):26–38.

18. Earle CC, Schrag D, Neville BA, et al. Effect of surgeon specialty on processes of care and outcomes for ovarian cancer patients. *J Natl Cancer Inst.* 2006;98(3):172–180.

19. Holshneider CH, Berek JS. Cytoreductive surgery: principles and rationale. In: Bristow R, Kaplan B, Surgery for ovarian cancer. Boca Raton, FL: Taylor and Francis; 2006; 127–171.

20. du Bois A, Quinn M, Thigpen T, Vermorken J, et al; Gynecologic Cancer Intergroup; AGO-OVAR; ANZGOG; EORTC; GEICO; GINECO; GOG; JGOG; MRC/NCRI; NCIC-CTG; NCI-US; NSGO; RTOG; SGCTG; IGCS; Organizational team of the two prior International OCCC. 2004 consensus statements on the management of ovarian cancer: final document of the 3rd International Gynecologic Cancer Intergroup Ovarian Cancer Consensus Conference (GCIG OCCC 2004). *Ann Oncol.* 2005;16 (Suppl 8):viii7–viii12.

21. Giede KC, Kieser K, Dodge J, Rosen B. Who should operate on patients with ovarian cancer? An evidence-based review. *Gynecol Oncol.* 2005;99(2):447–461.

22. Stier EA, Barakat RR, Curtin JP, Brown CL, Jones WB, Hoskins WJ. Laparotomy to complete staging of presumed early ovarian cancer. *Obstet Gynecol.* 1996;87(5 Pt 1):737–740.

23. Demir RH, Marchand GJ. Adnexal masses suspected to be benign treated with laparoscopy. *JSLS.* 2012;16(1):71–84.

24. Chi DS, Abu-Rustum NR, Sonoda Y, et al. The safety and efficacy of laparoscopic surgical staging of apparent stage I ovarian and fallopian tube cancers. *Am J Obstet Gynecol.* 2005;192(5):1614–1619.

25. Nezhat FR, Ezzati M, Chuang L, Shamshirsaz AA, Rahaman J, Gretz H. Laparoscopic management of early ovarian and fallopian tube cancers: surgical and survival outcome. *Am J Obstet Gynecol.* 2009;200(1):83.e1–83.e6.

26. Fader AN, Rose PG. Role of surgery in ovarian carcinoma. *J Clin Oncol.* 2007;25(20):2873–2883.

27. Stier EA, Barakat RR, Curtin JP, Brown CL, Jones WB, Hoskins WJ. Laparotomy to complete staging of presumed early ovarian cancer. *Obstet Gynecol.* 1996;87(5 Pt 1):737–740.

28. Bristow RE, Tomacruz RS, Armstrong DK, Trimble EL, Montz FJ. Survival effect of maximal cytoreductive surgery for advanced ovarian carcinoma during the platinum era: a meta-analysis. *J Clin Oncol.* 2002;20(5):1248–1259.

29. Eisenhauer EL, Abu-Rustum NR, Sonoda Y, et al. The addition of extensive upper abdominal surgery to achieve optimal cytoreduction improves survival in patients with stages IIIC-IV epithelial ovarian cancer. *Gynecol Oncol.* 2006;103(3):1083–1090.

30. du Bois A, Reuss A, Pujade-Lauraine E, Harter P, Ray-Coquard I, Pfisterer J. Role of surgical outcome as prognostic factor in advanced epithelial ovarian cancer: a combined exploratory analysis of 3 prospectively randomized phase 3 multicenter trials: by the Arbeitsgemeinschaft Gynaekologische Onkologie Studiengruppe Ovarialkarzinom (AGO-OVAR) and the Groupe d'Investigateurs Nationaux Pour les Etudes des Cancers de l'Ovaire (GINECO). *Cancer.* 2009;115(6):1234–1244.

31. Aletti GD, Dowdy SC, Gostout BS, et al. Aggressive surgical effort and improved survival in advanced-stage ovarian cancer. *Obstet Gynecol.* 2006;107(1):77–85.

32. Eisenhauer EL, Abu-Rustum NR, Sonoda Y, Aghajanian C, Barakat RR, Chi DS. The effect of maximal surgical cytoreduction on sensitivity to platinum-taxane chemotherapy and subsequent survival in patients with advanced ovarian cancer. *Gynecol Oncol.* 2008;108(2):276–281.

33. Elattar A, Bryant A, Winter-Roach BA, et al. Optimal primary surgical treatment for advanced epithelial ovarian cancer. *Cochrane Database Syst Rev.* 2011:CD007565.

34. Chi DS, Eisenhauer EL, Lang J, et al. What is the optimal goal of primary cytoreductive surgery for bulky stage IIIC epithelial ovarian carcinoma (EOC)? *Gynecol Oncol.* 2006;103(2):559–564.

35. Winter WE 3rd, Maxwell GL, Tian C, et al.; Gynecologic Oncology Group. Tumor residual after surgical cytoreduction in prediction of clinical outcome in stage IV epithelial ovarian cancer: a Gynecologic Oncology Group Study. *J Clin Oncol.* 2008;26(1):83–89.

36. Eisenhauer EL, Abu-Rustum NR, Sonoda Y, Aghajanian C, Barakat RR, Chi DS. The effect of maximal surgical cytoreduction on sensitivity to platinum-taxane chemotherapy and subsequent survival in patients with advanced ovarian cancer. *Gynecol Oncol.* 2008;108(2):276–281.

37. Bristow RE, Lagasse LD. Cytoreductive surgery: pelvis. In: Bristow R, Kaplan B, et al. *Surgery for Ovarian Cancer.* Boca Raton, FL: Taylor and Francis; 2006:127–171.

38. Wimberger P, Lehmann N, Kimmig R, Burges A, Meier W, Du Bois A; Arbeitsgemeinschaft Gynaekologische Onkologie Ovarian Cancer Study Group. Prognostic factors for complete debulking in advanced ovarian cancer and its impact on survival. An exploratory analysis of a prospectively randomized phase III study of the Arbeitsgemeinschaft Gynaekologische Onkologie Ovarian Cancer Study Group (AGO-OVAR). *Gynecol Oncol.* 2007;106(1):69–74.

39. du Bois A, Reuss A, Harter P, Pujade-Lauraine E, Ray-Coquard I, Pfisterer J; Arbeitsgemeinschaft Gynaekologische Onkologie Studiengruppe Ovarialkarzinom; Groupe d'Investigateurs Nationaux pour l'Etude des Cancers Ovariens. Potential role of lymphadenectomy in advanced ovarian cancer: a combined exploratory analysis of three prospectively randomized phase III multicenter trials. *J Clin Oncol.* 2010;28(10):1733–1739.

40. Gogoi RP, Urban R, Sun H, Goff B. Evaluation of Society of Gynecologic Oncologists (SGO) ovarian cancer quality surgical measures. *Gynecol Oncol.* 2012;126(2):217–219.

41. Vergote I, Tropé CG, Amant F, et al.; European Organization for Research and Treatment of Cancer-Gynaecological Cancer Group; NCIC Clinical Trials Group. Neoadjuvant chemotherapy or primary surgery in stage IIIC or IV ovarian cancer. *N Engl J Med.* 2010;363(10):943–953.

42. Thrall MM, Gray HJ, Symons RG, Weiss NS, Flum DR, Goff BA. Neoadjuvant chemotherapy in the Medicare cohort with advanced ovarian cancer. *Gynecol Oncol.* 2011;123(3):461–466.

43. Le T, Latifah H, Jolicoeur L, et al. Does intraperitoneal chemotherapy benefit optimally debulked epithelial ovarian cancer patients after neoadjuvant chemotherapy? *Gynecol Oncol.* 2011;121(3):451–454.

44. Young RC, Walton LA, Ellenberg SS, et al. Adjuvant therapy in stage I and stage II epithelial ovarian cancer. Results of two prospective randomized trials. *N Engl J Med.* 1990;322(15):1021–1027.

45. Trimbos B, Timmers P, Pecorelli S, et al. Surgical staging and treatment of early ovarian cancer: long-term analysis from a randomized trial. *J Natl Cancer Inst.* 2010;102(13):982–987.

46. Elit L, Chambers A, Fyles A, Covens A, Carey M, Fung MF. Systematic review of adjuvant care for women with Stage I ovarian carcinoma. *Cancer.* 2004;101(9):1926–1935.

47. Winter-Roach BA, Kitchener HC, Lawrie TA. Adjuvant (postsurgery) chemotherapy for early stage epithelial ovarian cancer. *Cochrane Database Syst Rev.* 2012;3:CD004706.

48. Bell J, Brady MF, Young RC, et al.; Gynecologic Oncology Group. Randomized phase III trial of three versus six cycles of adjuvant carboplatin and paclitaxel in early stage epithelial ovarian carcinoma: a Gynecologic Oncology Group study. *Gynecol Oncol.* 2006;102(3):432–439.

49. Chan JK, Tian C, Fleming GF, et al. The potential benefit of 6 vs. 3 cycles of chemotherapy in subsets of women with early-stage high-risk epithelial ovarian cancer: an exploratory analysis of a Gynecologic Oncology Group study. *Gynecol Oncol.* 2010;116(3):301–306.

50. Armstrong DK, Bundy B, Wenzel L, et al.; Gynecologic Oncology Group. Intraperitoneal cisplatin and paclitaxel in ovarian cancer. *N Engl J Med.* 2006;354(1):34–43.

51. Ozols RF, Bundy BN, Greer BE, et al.; Gynecologic Oncology Group. Phase III trial of carboplatin and paclitaxel compared with cisplatin and paclitaxel in patients with optimally resected stage III ovarian cancer: a Gynecologic Oncology Group study. *J Clin Oncol.* 2003;21(17):3194–3200.

52. Pignata S, Scambia G, Ferrandina G, et al. Carboplatin plus paclitaxel versus carboplatin plus pegylated liposomal doxorubicin as first-line treatment for patients with ovarian cancer: the MITO-2 randomized phase III trial. *J Clin Oncol.* 2011;29(27):3628–3635.

53. Katsumata N, Yasuda M, Takahashi F, et al.; Japanese Gynecologic Oncology Group. Dose-dense paclitaxel once a week in combination with carboplatin every 3 weeks for advanced ovarian cancer: a phase 3, open-label, randomised controlled trial. *Lancet.* 2009;374(9698):1331–1338.

54. Katsumata N, Yasuda M, Isonishi S, et al. Japanese Gynecologic Oncology Group; Long term follow up of a randomized trial comparing conventional paclitaxel and carboplatin with dose-dense weekly paclitaxel and carboplatin in women with advanced epithelial ovarian, fallopian tube, or primary peritoneal cancer; {GOG 3016 trial}. *J Clin Oncol.* 30, 2012 (Suppl; abstract 5003).

55. Burger RA, Brady MF, Bookman MA, et al.; Gynecologic Oncology Group. Incorporation of bevacizumab in the primary treatment of ovarian cancer. *N Engl J Med.* 2011;365(26):2473–2483.

56. Perren TJ, Swart AM, Pfisterer J, et al.; ICON7 Investigators. A phase 3 trial of bevacizumab in ovarian cancer. *N Engl J Med.* 2011;365(26):2484–2496.

57. Morgan RJ Jr, Alvarez RD, Armstrong DK, et al.; National Comprehensive Cancer Network. Ovarian cancer, version 3.2012. *J Natl Compr Canc Netw.* 2012;10(11):1339–1349.

58. Bookman MA, Brady MF, McGuire WP, et al. Evaluation of new platinum-based treatment regimens in advanced-stage ovarian cancer: a Phase III Trial of the Gynecologic Cancer Intergroup. *J Clin Oncol.* 2009;27(9):1419–1425.

59. Corn BW, Lanciano RM, Boente M, Hunter WM, Ladazack J, Ozols RF. Recurrent ovarian cancer. Effective radiotherapeutic palliation after chemotherapy failure. *Cancer.* 1994;74(11):2979–2983.

60. Tinger A, Waldron T, Peluso N, et al. Effective palliative radiation therapy in advanced and recurrent ovarian carcinoma. *Int J Radiat Oncol Biol Phys.* 2001;51(5):1256–1263.

61. Markman M, Liu PY, Wilczynski S, et al.; Southwest Oncology Group; Gynecologic Oncology Group. Phase III randomized trial of 12 versus 3 months of maintenance paclitaxel in patients with advanced ovarian cancer after complete response to platinum and paclitaxel-based chemotherapy: a Southwest Oncology Group and Gynecologic Oncology Group trial. *J Clin Oncol.* 2003;21(13):2460–2465.

62. Mei L, Chen H, Wei DM, et al. Maintenance chemotherapy for ovarian cancer. *Cochrane Database Syst Rev.* 2010;(9):1–41.

63. Greer BE, Bundy BN, Ozols RF, et al. Implications of second-look laparotomy in the context of optimally resected stage III ovarian cancer: a non-randomized comparison using an explanatory analysis: a Gynecologic Oncology Group study. *Gynecol Oncol.* 2005;99(1):71–79.

64. Rustin GJ, van der Burg ME, Griffin CL, et al.; MRC OV05; EORTC 55955 investigators. Early versus delayed treatment of relapsed ovarian cancer (MRC OV05/EORTC 55955): a randomised trial. *Lancet.* 2010;376(9747):1155–1163.

65. Miller RE, Rustin GJ. How to follow-up patients with epithelial ovarian cancer. *Curr Opin Oncol.* 2010;22(5):498–502.

66. Markman M, Petersen J, Belland A, Burg K. CA-125 monitoring in ovarian cancer: patient survey responses to the results of the MRC/EORTC CA-125 Surveillance Trial. *Oncology.* 2010;78(1):1–2.

67. Morris RT, Monk BJ. Ovarian cancer: relevant therapy, not timing, is paramount. *Lancet.* 2010;376(9747):1120–1122.

68. Rustin GJ, van der Burg ME, Griffin CL, et al.; MRC OV05; EORTC 55955 investigators. Early versus delayed treatment of relapsed ovarian cancer (MRC OV05/EORTC 55955): a randomised trial. *Lancet.* 2010;376(9747):1155–1163.

69. Markman M, Webster K, Zanotti K, Rohl J, Belinson J. Use of tamoxifen in asymptomatic patients with recurrent small-volume ovarian cancer. *Gynecol Oncol.* 2004;93(2):390–393.

70. Griffiths RW, Zee YK, Evans S, et al. Outcomes after multiple lines of chemotherapy for platinum-resistant epithelial cancers of the ovary, peritoneum, and fallopian tube. *Int J Gynecol Cancer.* 2011;21(1):58–65.

71. Parmar MK, Ledermann JA, Colombo N, et al.; ICON and AGO Collaborators. Paclitaxel plus platinum-based chemotherapy versus conventional platinum-based chemotherapy in women with relapsed ovarian cancer: the ICON4/AGO-OVAR-2.2 trial. *Lancet.* 2003;361(9375):2099–2106.

72. Katsumata N, Yasuda M, Takahashi F, et al.; Japanese Gynecologic Oncology Group. Dose-dense paclitaxel once a week in combination with carboplatin every 3 weeks for advanced ovarian cancer: a phase 3, open-label, randomised controlled trial. *Lancet.* 2009;374(9698):1331–1338.

73. Strauss HG, Henze A, Teichmann A, et al. Phase II trial of docetaxel and carboplatin in recurrent platinum-sensitive ovarian, peritoneal and tubal cancer. *Gynecol Oncol.* 2007;104(3):612–616.

74. Pfisterer J, Plante M, Vergote I, et al.; AGO-OVAR; NCIC CTG; EORTC GCG. Gemcitabine plus carboplatin compared with carboplatin in patients with platinum-sensitive recurrent ovarian cancer: an intergroup trial of the AGO-OVAR, the NCIC CTG, and the EORTC GCG. *J Clin Oncol.* 2006;24(29):4699–4707.

75. Pujade-Lauraine E, Wagner U, Aavall-Lundqvist E, et al. Pegylated liposomal Doxorubicin and Carboplatin compared with Paclitaxel and Carboplatin for patients with platinum-sensitive ovarian cancer in late relapse. *J Clin Oncol.* 2010;28(20):3323–3329.

76. Rose PG. Gemcitabine reverses platinum resistance in platinum-resistant ovarian and peritoneal carcinoma. *Int J Gynecol Cancer.* 2005;15 Suppl 1:18–22.

77. Gordon AN, Tonda M, Sun S, Rackoff W; Doxil Study 30–49 Investigators. Long-term survival advantage for women treated with pegylated liposomal doxorubicin compared with topotecan in a phase 3 randomized study of recurrent and refractory epithelial ovarian cancer. *Gynecol Oncol.* 2004;95(1):1–8.

78. Ferrandina G, Ludovisi M, Lorusso D, et al. Phase III trial of gemcitabine compared with pegylated liposomal doxorubicin in progressive or recurrent ovarian cancer. *J Clin Oncol.* 2008;26(6):890–896.

79. Rothenberg ML, Liu PY, Wilczynski S, et al. Phase II trial of vinorelbine for relapsed ovarian cancer: a Southwest Oncology Group study. *Gynecol Oncol.* 2004;95(3):506–512.

80. Mutch DG, Orlando M, Goss T, et al. Randomized phase III trial of gemcitabine compared with pegylated liposomal doxorubicin in patients with platinum-resistant ovarian cancer. *J Clin Oncol.* 2007;25(19):2811–2818.

81. Rose PG, Blessing JA, Mayer AR, Homesley HD. Prolonged oral etoposide as second-line therapy for platinum-resistant and platinum-sensitive ovarian carcinoma: a Gynecologic Oncology Group study. *J Clin Oncol.* 1998;16(2):405–410.

82. Rose PG, Blessing JA, Ball HG, et al. A phase II study of docetaxel in paclitaxel-resistant ovarian and peritoneal carcinoma: a Gynecologic Oncology Group study. *Gynecol Oncol.* 2003;88(2):130–135.

83. Miller DS, Blessing JA, Krasner CN, et al. Phase II evaluation of pemetrexed in the treatment of recurrent or persistent platinum-resistant ovarian or primary peritoneal carcinoma: a study of the Gynecologic Oncology Group. *J Clin Oncol.* 2009;27(16):2686–2691.

84. Aghajanian C, Blank SV, Goff BA, et al. OCEANS: a randomized, double-blind, placebo-controlled phase III trial of chemotherapy with or without bevacizumab in patients with platinum-sensitive recurrent epithelial ovarian, primary peritoneal, or fallopian tube cancer. *J Clin Oncol.* 2012;30(17):2039–2045.

85. Pujade-Lauraine E, Hilpert F, Weber B, et al. AURELIA: a randomized phase III trial evaluating bevacizumab (BEV) plus chemotherapy (CT) for platinum (PT)-resistant recurrent ovarian cancer (OC). *J Clin Oncol.* 2012;30(Suppl; abstr LBA5002).

86. Castells MC, Tennant NM, Sloane DE, et al. Hypersensitivity reactions to chemotherapy: outcomes and safety of rapid desensitization in 413 cases. *J Allergy Clin Immunol.* 2008;122(3):574–580.

87. O'Cearbhaill R, Zhou Q, Iasonos A, et al. The prophylactic conversion to an extended infusion schedule and use of premedication to prevent hypersensitivity reactions in ovarian cancer patients during carboplatin retreatment. *Gynecol Oncol.* 2010;116(3):326–331.

88. Eisenkop SM, Friedman RL, Spirtos NM. The role of secondary cytoreductive surgery in the treatment of patients with recurrent epithelial ovarian carcinoma. *Cancer.* 2000;88(1):144–153.

89. Chi DS, McCaughty K, Diaz JP, et al. Guidelines and selection criteria for secondary cytoreductive surgery in patients with recurrent, platinum-sensitive epithelial ovarian carcinoma. *Cancer.* 2006;106(9):1933–1939.

90. Audeh MW, Carmichael J, Penson RT, et al. Oral poly(ADP-ribose) polymerase inhibitor olaparib in patients with BRCA1 or BRCA2 mutations and recurrent ovarian cancer: a proof-of-concept trial. *Lancet.* 2010;376(9737):245–251.

91. Oza Am, Cibula D, Oaknin A, et al. Olaparib plus paclitaxel plus carboplatin (P/C) followed by olaparib maintenance treatment in patients (pts) with platinum-sensitive recurrent serous ovarian cancer (PSR SOC): A randomized, open-label phase II study. *J Clin Oncol.* 2012; 30 (Suppl; abstr 5001).

92. Burstein HJ, Mangu PB, Somerfield MR, et al.; American Society of Clinical Oncology. American Society of Clinical Oncology clinical practice guideline update on the use of chemotherapy sensitivity and resistance assays. *J Clin Oncol.* 2011;29(24):3328–3330.

93. Gallion H, Christopherson WA, Coleman RL, et al. Progression-free interval in ovarian cancer and predictive value of an ex vivo chemoresponse assay. *Int J Gynecol Cancer.* 2006;16(1):194–201.

94. Tinger A, Waldron T, Peluso N, et al. Effective palliative radiation therapy in advanced and recurrent ovarian carcinoma. *Int J Radiat Oncol Biol Phys.* 2001;51(5):1256–1263.

95. Solomon LA, Munkarah AR, Vorugu VR, et al. Image-guided percutaneous cryotherapy for the management of gynecologic cancer metastases. *Gynecol Oncol.* 2008;111(2):202–207.

96. Grzankowski KS, Carney M. Quality of life in ovarian cancer. *Cancer Control.* 2011;18(1):52–58.

97. Fauci J, Schneider K, Walters C, et al. The utilization of palliative care in gynecologic oncology patients near the end of life. *Gynecol Oncol.* 2012;127(1):175–179.

98. Radwany SM, von Gruenigen VE. Palliative and end-of-life care for patients with ovarian cancer. *Clin Obstet Gynecol.* 2012;55(1):173–184.

99. von Gruenigen VE, Huang HQ, Gil KM, Frasure HE, Armstrong DK, Wenzel LB. The association between quality of life domains and overall survival in ovarian cancer patients during adjuvant chemotherapy: a Gynecologic Oncology Group study. *Gynecol Oncol.* 2012;124(3):379–382.

100. Brundage M, Gropp M, Mefti F, et al. Health-related quality of life in recurrent platinum-sensitive ovarian cancer–results from the CALYPSO trial. *Ann Oncol.* 2012;23(8):2020–2027.

101. Chase DM, Wenzel LB, Monk BJ. Quality-of-life results used to endorse changes in standard of care for recurrent platinum-sensitive ovarian cancer. *Expert Rev Pharmacoecon Outcomes Res.* 2012;12(3):279–281.

17 Recurrent Ovarian Cancer: Approach to Diagnosis and Treatment

MICHELLE M. BOISEN

ROBERT P. EDWARDS

■ INTRODUCTION

Epithelial ovarian cancer (EOC) recurs in approximately 90% of patients with advanced stage disease after complete remission. Therefore defining the approach to the diagnosis and management of recurrent ovarian cancer (ROC) will consume a major component of the physician's effort when caring for patients afflicted with advanced stage disease. The evidence that exists to validate the techniques for diagnosis and treatment of recurrent ovary cancer is limited. The management choices of patients and physicians dealing with ROC are among the most controversial aspects of the disease with high degrees of variability regionally, nationally, and internationally. The timing of detection along the disease course of persistent or recurrent disease has repeatedly been found to have little impact on disease outcomes in terms of overall survival. However, the frequency and intensity of surveillance for recurrence has a major impact on down-stream resource utilization and treatment-associated toxicity. As such, ovary cancer recurrence is an ideal model to evaluate effective utilization of resources in the age of health care reform. The current mainstay of ovarian cancer surveillance is the tumor marker CA125.

■ RECURRENT OVARIAN CANCER: DEFINING RECURRENCE

CA125

The oncofetal antigen CA125 is the most frequently used tumor marker in the evaluation of treatment response and recurrence in ROC. CA125 tumor-expression and serum elevations are seen in approximately 90% of EOCs, higher in serous, and lower in the other histologies particularly mucinous types. A persistent and progressive elevation in a recurrent EOC patient's serum CA125 is highly predictive of recurrent disease with sensitivities and specificities that exceed 90% usually several months before detection by exam, symptoms, or radiology. The Gynecologic Cancer Intergroup (GCIG) has developed a standard definition for CA125 level that defines progression of disease following first-line treatment and has been validated when compared to the use of clinical and radiographic markers for disease recurrence. In patients with either normal or elevated CA125 levels prior to treatment who normalize their CA125 levels following treatment, recurrence is defined as an elevation of CA125 to levels greater than or equal to twice the upper limit of normal on two occasions at least 1 week apart. For those patients who do not normalize their CA125 levels following treatment, recurrence is defined as an elevation of CA125 to levels greater than or equal to twice the nadir value on two occasions at least 1 week apart (1).

A recently reported trial by the European Medical Research Council has evaluated the question of using CA125 surveillance to initiate early treatment for recurrence vs treatment initiated based on clinical symptoms. Patients in clinical complete remission after platinum-based chemotherapy were followed with CA125 levels and intermittent clinical visits. Upon detection of a 2-fold elevation over the normal range, patients were randomly assigned to early platinum-based treatment for recurrence based on CA125 or continued observation until development of signs and symptoms indicative of clinical relapse. The study required almost 10 years to accrue the required subjects and is not fully mature to date. However, it does appear that early initiation of second-line therapy increases the number of chemotherapy courses, treatment toxicity, and cost but had no impact on survival. Median survival for patients randomly assigned to early treatment ($n = 265$) was 25.7 months compared with 27.1 months for those patients in the delayed-treatment group ($n = 264$; hazard ratio 0.98, 95% confidence interval [CI], 0.8–1.2). The median delay in instituting second-line and third-line chemotherapy was 4.8 and 4.6 months, respectively (2). Critical review of this study will await the mature data and yet the findings are provocative but consistent with prior data on the use of second-look laparotomy to define response; that being that early detection of persistent or recurrent subclinical disease has no impact on overall survival.

Imaging

CT

Contrast-enhanced CT is the most common imaging modality used to evaluate for the presence of disease recurrence in EOC. In one study by Sebastian and colleagues, CT effectively identified recurrent disease in 83% of total recurrences with identification of 89% of chest recurrences and 79% of abdominal recurrences (3). Several studies have correlated CT scan findings with findings at the time of second-look surgery. In a study of 35 patients clinically in remission who underwent evaluation with a CT scan prior to undergoing second-look laparotomy, the sensitivity and specificity of CT scan in the detection of disease were 42% and 85%, respectively. Overall diagnostic accuracy was 60%. CT performed poorly in the detection of mesenteric, peritoneal, and omental metastases. CT was most useful in the detection of ascites, abdominal masses, and liver metastases. False positive CT results occurred in the setting of anatomic variations and postoperative adhesions and scarring (4). A similar study performed by Clarke-Pearson and colleagues of 47 patients clinically free of disease who underwent a contrast-enhanced CT scan prior to undergoing a second-look laparotomy found a sensitivity of 32% and specificity of 77% of CT scan for the prediction of recurrent disease. In this study, CT scan performed better when foci of disease recurrence were large with only 7% of tumor nodules 1 cm or less detected by preoperative CT scan (5).

PET

Positron emission tomography (PET) with or without CT imaging may aid in the detection of relapse in patients with ovarian cancer. A study of the utility of fludeoxyglucose (FDG)-PET, conventional imaging modalities (CT or MRI), and CA125 in the evaluation of possible ROC demonstrated a sensitivity of 86%, specificity of 78%, and diagnostic accuracy of 84.8% when FDG-PET was used to detect disease recurrence. FDG-PET had a higher sensitivity, specificity, and diagnostic accuracy than either conventional imaging or CA125. FDG-PET was particularly useful in the detection of lymph node and peritoneal metastases when compared with conventional imaging modalities although both modalities missed metastatic lesions less than 5 mm (6).

PET-CT

A limitation of FDG-PET alone is the inability to correlate areas of increased FDG uptake with anatomic structures. This limitation led to the development of FDG-PET-CT devices that provide the ability so simultaneously obtain both FDG-PET and CT images. The role of FDG-PET-CT has been evaluated for utility in the setting of ovarian cancer recurrence. In an initial report by Makhija and colleagues, 62% of patients with histologically confirmed recurrent EOC had a positive FDG-PET-CT with a negative contrast-enhanced CT scan prior to undergoing second-look surgery (7). Nanni and colleagues reported a series of 41 patients who underwent evaluation for ROC with CA125 and either CT or MRI, and subsequently underwent FDG-PET-CT. They found a sensitivity of 88.2%, specificity of 71.4%, and 85.4% accuracy when FDG-PET-CT is used for the detection of ovarian cancer recurrence (8). FDG-PET-CT is thus a useful tool in the detection of ROC particularly when localization of disease for secondary cytoreductive surgery is being considered.

MRI

MRI has been used increasingly in the diagnosis of ROC. The sensitivity and specificity of MRI for the detection of ovarian cancer recurrence have ranged significantly in the literature. A retrospective study by Low and colleagues reported an overall sensitivity, specificity, and accuracy of MRI in the diagnosis of ROC of 90%, 88%, and 89%, respectively (9). Other studies have described the limitations of MRI in the detection of lymph node and omental recurrences. In a recent meta-analysis and systematic review by Gu et al, the authors found a pooled sensitivity of 75% and specificity of 87% when MRI is used in the detection of ROC. In this study, the sensitivities and specificities of diagnostic imaging modalities were compared and the authors found no significant differences between MRI and CT for these parameters (10). A potential benefit of MRI over CT scan is that MRI can be performed without contrast and does not involve radiation exposure.

Second-Look Surgery

A second-look surgery is one performed on a patient with no clinical evidence of recurrent disease at the completion of a course of therapy to assess for response to treatment. Traditionally, second-look surgery has been performed via laparotomy, however more recent data have reported on the utility of laparoscopy in this setting. At the time of second-look surgery, areas of previously documented tumor are biopsied along with multiple peritoneal surfaces, residual omentum, the diaphragm, and any sites suspicious for persistent or recurrent disease (11). It is the gold standard for diagnosis of persistent disease and disease recurrence in research settings. However, the fact that this is a potentially morbid procedure and a paucity of evidence that this surgical procedure impacts outcomes has limited its utility in recent years except in research settings. Various studies have investigated the rates of recurrence following a negative second-look surgery and have shown a recurrence rate range of 24%–54% with those patients designated as high risk (age less than or equal to 67 years, high-histologic grade, residual tumor less than 2 cm) with the highest rates of recurrence (12–14). In addition, of those patients with no evidence of macroscopic disease at the time of second-look surgery, approximately 30% will be found to have microscopic metastases (15). Although the information obtained at the time of second-look surgery can be useful in providing prognostic information to patients and their families, this procedure has not been shown to consistently impact patient survival.

Several studies have investigated the role of secondary cytoreduction at the time of second-look surgery with mixed results. Resection of persistent disease after primary platinum-based therapy followed by locoregional consolidation appears to increase treatment-free interval based on small single institution trials (16–18). Several retrospective studies have demonstrated a survival benefit in those patients who were completely cytoreduced to no visible disease followed by consolidation hyperthermic intraperitoneal intraoperative chemotherapy (HIPEC). However, no prospective trials have been completed in ovarian cancer with HIPEC used at the time of second-look surgery. Due to the lack of impact on survival as well as the high rates of recurrence following negative second-look surgery, second-look surgery has fallen out of favor somewhat in current practice. However, its utility in determining clinical response to therapy is most often used currently in patients receiving treatment on research protocols where follow-up biopsies after treatment are required.

■ RECURRENT OVARIAN CANCER: TREATMENT

Despite aggressive frontline therapy for EOC, which routinely includes a combination of surgical cytoreduction and platinum-/taxane-based chemotherapy, most patients diagnosed with advanced stage disease will experience recurrence. Treatment of disease recurrence is aimed at control of symptoms, maintenance of quality of life, and delaying time to progression.

Options for treatment of recurrent disease include secondary surgical cytoreduction, hormonal therapy, cytotoxic chemotherapy, and biologic agents. The choice of therapy should be specifically tailored to each patient based upon their disease course as well as their ability to tolerate second-line therapy.

Secondary Cytoreduction

Secondary cytoreduction is defined as a secondary surgery to debulk residual or recurrent tumor burden in the setting of persistent or recurrent disease. As discussed previously, cytoreduction may be beneficial in those patients who are clinically without evidence of disease but are found to have residual disease at the time of second-look surgery following completion of frontline cytotoxic chemotherapy. Several studies have investigated the role of secondary cytoreduction in the setting of known disease recurrence. Eisenkop and colleagues reported on their series of 106 patients with platinum-sensitive (disease-free interval greater than 6 months) disease who underwent secondary cytoreductive surgery for first recurrence of epithelial ovarian carcinoma. Multiple patient variables were evaluated for their influence on patient survival. Prior salvage chemotherapy, distribution of peritoneal recurrence, post-cytoreductive residual disease, disease-free interval, and volume of largest recurrence were found to influence patient survival. For those patients with an initial disease-free interval of greater than 36 months, 13 to 36 months, and 6 to 12 months, medial overall survival was found to be 56.8 months, 44.4 months, and 25 months, respectively. For those patients visibly free of disease at the completion of secondary surgery, median overall survival was 44.4 months; for those with visible disease following cytoreduction, median overall survival was 19.3 months. Median survival was worse for those patients who had undergone prior salvage chemotherapy. The authors postulate that this is likely related to probable higher tumor burden at the time of recurrence (19). In a similar study by Tay et al, 46 patients with first recurrence of EOC underwent secondary cytoreduction. The authors found overall survival was significantly increased for those with no macroscopic residual disease remaining at the completion of surgery with a median overall survival of 38 months for those with no residual disease, 14.5 months for those with 0 to 1 cm of residual disease, and 11 months for those with greater than 1 cm of residual disease. Similarly, the authors found a significant survival advantage in those patients with a longer disease-free interval, particularly in those with a disease-free interval of greater than 24 months (20).

Salani and colleagues performed a study of 55 patients undergoing secondary cytoreduction for first recurrence of platinum-sensitive EOC. Similar to the findings of Tay et al and Eisenkop et al, the authors found both disease-free interval and volume of residual disease to have a significant impact on median survival. In addition, the authors assessed the number of sites of recurrent disease for impact on overall survival and found that median overall survival was significantly longer in patients with one to two sites of recurrent disease as compared to those with three to five sites of recurrent disease (52 vs 12 months; 21). Similarly, Chi et al published their experience with secondary cytoreduction for first recurrence of ovarian cancer and found a significant increase in survival for those patients with a single site of recurrence as compared to those patients with multiple sites of recurrence and carcinomatosis (22).

In each of the trials discussed here, surgical morbidity was significant and ranged from 10% to 32%. Common postoperative complications include febrile morbidity, postoperative ileus, respiratory complications, and wound complications. Given the significant morbidity associated with secondary cytoreduction, this procedure should be reserved for patients most likely to benefit. Based on the available data, patients most likely to benefit from secondary cytoreduction include those patients with a sufficiently long disease-free interval (at least 12–24 months) with disease that is thought to be limited to one to two sites of recurrence amenable to optimal cytoreduction. As discussed in the previous section, PET-CT and laparoscopy appear to be beneficial in defining this optimal cohort and reducing the number of ineffective laparotomies and the comorbidity that follows such procedures. A prospective Gynecologic Oncology Group (GOG) trial is evaluating secondary cytoreduction for recurrent EOC and is currently open to accrual.

Treatment of Recurrent Disease With Cytotoxic Chemotherapy

Response rates for second-line chemotherapy agents range significantly from 10% to 40%. Response rates are dependent on multiple factors. Treatment options and treatment responses are highly dependent on the patient's response to front-line therapy. Markman and colleagues reported their experience with a cohort of patients who underwent treatment for ROC with platinum-based chemotherapy after front-line therapy with a platinum-based regimen. They found an increase in response rate for those patients with a longer platinum-free interval (23). It is important to define patients based upon their response to frontline platinum-based chemotherapy as described by the GOG. Patients who recur more than 6 months following completion of front-line chemotherapy are classified as *platinum-sensitive*. This group of patients has the highest rate of response to second-line therapy. Patients who recur within 6 months of completion of front-line chemotherapy are classified as *platinum-resistant*. Patients who experience disease progression while on chemotherapy are classified as *platinum-refractory*. This group of patients will have the lowest response rate to second-line therapy (24).

Platinum-Sensitive Disease

In patients known to have platinum-sensitive disease, standard treatment for recurrence typically involves a second platinum-based regimen. Several studies have investigated the use of cisplatin or carboplatin alone in the treatment of ROC and have demonstrated response rates from 35% to 100% (23,25–26). These studies all also found an association between duration of response

to frontline therapy and response rate in the setting of recurrence. Proponents of using single-agent platinum-containing compounds for the treatment of ROC cite increased toxicity without a significant survival advantage with the use of multiagent regimens as reasons to treat recurrent disease with platinum-containing compounds alone. This may be particularly true for elderly patients, patients with limited bone marrow reserve, or patients with medical comorbidities including prolonged postoperative morbidities.

Platinum/taxane regimens are currently the standard treatment for front-line EOC following surgical cytoreduction. Several trials have evaluated the role of combination platinum-taxane regimens for the treatment of recurrence. In an observational study, Rose and colleagues reported on their experience using carboplatin and paclitaxel for treatment of disease recurrence in patients with platinum-sensitive ovarian cancer and describe a 90% response rate in these patients with a median progression-free interval of 9.0 months (27). The use of combination platinum plus paclitaxel vs single-agent platinum has been evaluated in two large Phase III clinical trials and a randomized Phase II study. Gonzalez-Martin and colleagues reported the results of their randomized Phase II study in which patients with recurrent EOC with a treatment-free interval of at least 6 months were randomized to treatment with carboplatin or carboplatin plus paclitaxel. Their results show a statistically significant increase in response rate for those patients treated with carboplatin plus paclitaxel (75.6%) as compared to those treated with carboplatin alone (50%). Secondary outcomes in this study include both median time to progression and median overall survival, both of which were longer in the carboplatin plus paclitaxel group. Mucositis, myalgia/arthralgia, and peripheral neuropathy were all more frequent in the carboplatin plus paclitaxel group, but no differences in severe hematologic toxicity were observed (28). A report of the ICON4 and AGO-OVAR-2.2 trials describes 802 patients who were randomized to either platinum-based chemotherapy alone or platinum-based chemotherapy plus paclitaxel for first recurrence of EOC after at least a 6-month treatment-free interval. At median follow-up of 42 months, treatment with paclitaxel plus platinum-based chemotherapy was shown to confer a survival advantage (hazard ratio = 0.82, P = .02) with an absolute 2-year survival advantage of 7% (57% vs 50%) and improvement in median survival of 5 months (29 vs 24 months). Progression-free survival (PFS) was also significantly longer in the platinum-based chemotherapy plus paclitaxel group (hazard ratio = 0.76, P = .0004), which corresponds to an absolute difference in 1-year PFS of 10% (50% vs 40%) and a difference in median PFS of 3 months (13 vs 10 months). The toxicities of both regimens were relatively similar with the exception of rates of alopecia, which were higher in the platinum-based chemotherapy plus paclitaxel group, and rates of moderate or severe hematologic toxicity, which were higher in the platinum-based chemotherapy alone group (29).

The use of a combination of platinum- and taxane-based chemotherapy in the treatment of ROC has proven to confer a survival advantage when compared to treatment with platinum-based regimens alone. However, the significant risk of cumulative neurotoxicity with this combination has led investigators to investigate other combinations of chemotherapeutic agents. Several trials have investigated the role of pegylated liposomal doxorubicin (PLD) plus carboplatin in the treatment of recurrent, platinum-sensitive EOC. In a Phase II trial by Ferrero et al, the combination of PLD plus carboplatin for the treatment of platinum-sensitive EOC recurrence demonstrated a response rate of 63% with median progression-free and overall survival of 9.4 and 32.0 months, respectively (30). The promising results of this and other trials demonstrating the effectiveness of PLD in the treatment of recurrent platinum-sensitive EOC led to the development of the CALYPSO trial. In this large (n = 356), Phase III, multi-institution trial, investigators compared treatment of first or second recurrence of platinum-sensitive EOC with PLD plus carboplatin with paclitaxel plus carboplatin. In this trial, treatment with PLD plus carboplatin demonstrated statistically significant improvement in PFS as compared with the paclitaxel plus carboplatin arm (11.3 vs 9.4 months, P = .005). The overall survival data were not mature at the time of publication of the manuscript and have not yet been published. In the CALYPSO trial, severe hematologic toxicity, alopecia, hypersensitivity reactions, and sensory neuropathy all occurred significantly more frequently in the paclitaxel plus carboplatin group. Palmar-plantar erythrodysesthesia, mucositis, and nausea occurred more frequently in the PLD plus carboplatin group (31). These findings support the treatment of platinum-sensitive, recurrent EOC with combination PLD and carboplatin given the superior PFS and improved side-effect profile as compared with combination paclitaxel and carboplatin, but the overall survival data will be important in determining if this regimen becomes the standard of care.

Gemcitabine has also been investigated as a potential second-line treatment for recurrent, platinum-sensitive EOC. A study of gemcitabine plus carboplatin as compared with carboplatin alone for treatment of patients with platinum-sensitive ROC demonstrated a statistically significant improvement in PFS in the gemcitabine plus carboplatin group (8.6 vs 5.8 months, P = .0031). However, this study failed to demonstrate a difference in overall survival between the two groups. In addition, the rate of Grade 3/4 hematologic toxicities was significantly higher in the gemcitabine plus carboplatin group, although the rate of febrile neutropenia did not differ between the two treatment arms (32). Recently the OCEANS trial, a large (n = 484), Phase III, randomized, multicenter trial investigated the effectiveness of the addition of bevacizumab to gemcitabine and carboplatin in the setting of platinum-sensitive recurrent EOC. Bevacizumab had previously been investigated both for use in the setting of primary EOC and heavily pretreated patients with platinum-resistant and platinum-refractory disease. This was the first trial to investigate bevacizumab in the setting of platinum-sensitive, recurrent EOC. This trial randomized patients with first recurrence of platinum-sensitive EOC to treatment with carboplatin/gemcitabine plus placebo vs carboplatin/gemcitabine plus bevacizumab. Investigators found a statistically significant increase in PFS for those patients treated with carboplatin/gemcitabine plus bevacizumab (12.4 vs 8.4 months, hazard ratio = 0.821, P < .001). Overall response rate and duration of response were also significantly improved in the group treated with carboplatin/gemcitabine plus bevacizumab. At the time of publication of the manuscript, overall survival data were not mature and have yet to be published. Prior to this study, the safety of bevacizumab had been called into question after high rates of gastrointestinal perforation were noted when bevacizumab was used to treat women with refractory, heavily pretreated EOC. In this study, patients were carefully selected prior to receiving bevacizumab and only two gastrointestinal perforations were noted outside of the study period. Patients in the carboplatin/gemcitabine plus bevacizumab group experienced higher rates of Grade 3 hypertension and proteinuria. The rates of neutropenia and febrile neutropenia were similar between groups (33).

Based on available data, best treatment for recurrent platinum-sensitive EOC is a platinum-based doublet with the drug combination specifically tailored to the patient. For patients with intermediate platinum-sensitive disease (treatment free interval of 6-12 months), responses to platinum-based therapy are less robust and single-agent liposomal doxorubicin or gemcitabine may be considered alone or in combination with platinum depending on the cumulative previous platinum-associated toxicities such as neuropathy or renal dysfunction. Patients with poor performance status may consider abstaining from salvage therapy until symptomatic.

Platinum-Resistant and Platinum-Refractory Disease

In patients with platinum-resistant and platinum-refractory disease, treatment is typically considered palliative. Treatment with single-agent chemotherapy is often preferred in this setting to limit toxicity. Multiple agents have been investigated for utility in the treatment of platinum-resistant and platinum-refractory disease. Once EOC has become resistant to platinum, response to other agents is limited. Most active agents have shown an overall response rate of approximately 10%–20% with an overall survival of around 12 months. Currently, there are three Food and Drug Administration (FDA) approved agents for the treatment of recurrent, platinum-resistant EOC: paclitaxel, PLD, and topotecan. Other cytotoxic chemotherapy drugs that have shown to be active in platinum-resistant ovarian cancer include gemcitabine, oral etoposide, trabectedin, and pemetrexed.

Paclitaxel

Patients treated with single-agent paclitaxel have demonstrated overall response rates of 20%–30% in platinum-resistant, ROC. In a Phase II study by the GOG, investigators evaluated the role of single-agent paclitaxel dosed every 3 weeks in the treatment of both recurrent platinum-sensitive and platinum-resistant EOC. Of 27 patients in this study with platinum-resistant disease, investigators demonstrated a 34% overall response rate; however median progression-free interval was only 4 months (34). An alternative paclitaxel dosing regimen has also demonstrated benefit in platinum-resistant patients. Several studies have demonstrated clinical response of platinum-resistant EOC to weekly paclitaxel. In a Phase II study by the GOG, Markman and colleagues demonstrated an overall response rate of 20.9% in 48 patients treated with weekly paclitaxel for recurrent, platinum-resistant EOC who had also previously been treated with standard 3-week paclitaxel dosing. In this study, the most common side effect was neurologic toxicity; however this was found to be mild (35). Rosenberg and colleagues compared the efficacy of weekly dosing with every 3 week dosing of paclitaxel for the treatment of both platinum-sensitive and platinum-resistant EOC. They found no statistically significant difference in overall response rate for either platinum-sensitive or platinum-resistant patients. There was significantly more hematologic toxicity, neurologic toxicity, and arthralgias/myalgias in the group of patients receiving paclitaxel every 3 weeks (36). The improved side-effect profile of weekly dosing suggests this as the preferred dosing regimen for those undergoing treatment of recurrent EOC with single-agent paclitaxel. Nanoparticle, albumin-bound (nab) paclitaxel has also been investigated as a possible active agent in recurrent EOC. Coleman and colleagues evaluated nab-paclitaxel in the treatment of platinum-resistant EOC and found an overall response rate of 23% with an acceptable toxicity profile. The most common toxicity in this study was Grade 3 hematologic toxicity (37). A study of nab-paclitaxel for first recurrence of platinum-sensitive disease revealed an overall response rate of 64% (38).

Several taxane analogues have proven to be active agents in recurrent, platinum-resistant EOC. Docetaxel appears to have similar activity to paclitaxel in the primary treatment of EOC with less neuropathy (39). The GOG conducted a Phase II trial of docetaxel every 21 days in patients with platinum- and paclitaxel-resistant EOC who had undergone only one prior course of chemotherapy. The response rate was 22.4%, but 75% of patients experienced significant hematologic toxicity (40). In a similar study, weekly dosing of docetaxel was noted to have a response rate of 18.9% with an improved side-effect profile (41).

PLD

PLD has been shown to have activity in platinum-resistant, recurrent EOC. Several Phase II studies have shown response rates of 17%–25% for patients with recurrent, platinum-resistant EOC treated with PLD (42,43). There have been several Phase III trials that have compared PLD to other agents for the treatment of recurrent, platinum-resistant EOC. Gordon and colleagues compared the safety and efficacy of PLD to topotecan in patients with recurrent EOC. The overall response rates for PLD and topotecan were 19.7% and 17.0%, respectively, which were not statistically significantly different ($P = .390$). Median overall survival for patients treated with PLD and topotecan were 60 and 56.7 weeks, respectively. When the results were stratified by platinum sensitivity, PLD demonstrated a statistically significant improvement in both progression-free and overall survival in platinum-sensitive patients. In patients with platinum-resistant disease, a nonsignificant trend toward improvement in progression-free and overall survival was seen in favor to topotecan. In this study, significant hematologic toxicity was seen more frequently in the group of patients treated with topotecan while palmar-plantar erythrodysesthesia was seen more commonly in the PLD group (44).

Gemcitabine

Gemcitabine is an active agent in platinum-sensitive, recurrent EOC. It has also been studied for use in recurrent, platinum-resistant disease. Several Phase II trials have established gemcitabine as an active agent in the setting of recurrent disease. Two trials have compared the activity of gemcitabine with that of PLD in this patient population. Mutch and colleagues investigated the efficacy of gemcitabine as compared with PLD in patients with platinum-resistant, recurrent EOC. They found no statistically significant difference in overall response rate, progression-free, or overall survival between the two groups (45). In a similar study by Ferrandina et al, which included both platinum-sensitive and platinum-resistant patients, investigators found no significant difference in time to progression or overall survival between the gemcitabine and PLD treatment arms. In this study, hematologic side effects were more frequent in the gemcitabine arm while palmar–plantar dysesthesia was more frequent in the PLD group. Although these trials were powered for superiority, the results suggest that gemcitabine has similar efficacy of PLD in patients with platinum-resistant, recurrent EOC (46).

Topotecan

Topotecan is another agent that has been shown to have activity in recurrent EOC. Several Phase II studies have established the efficacy of topotecan in the setting of both platinum-sensitive and platinum-resistant recurrent EOC. Bookman and colleagues published a Phase II study of patients treated with topotecan for ROC after undergoing prior treatment with both platinum and paclitaxel. The overall response rate was 13.7% with a 12.4% response rate in platinum-resistant patients and a 19.2% response rate in platinum-sensitive patients. The most severe toxicities in this study were hematologic with 82% of patients experiencing Grade 4 neutropenia (47). A Phase III study comparing the efficacy of topotecan to that of paclitaxel for recurrent EOC demonstrated a response rate of 20.5% in those patients treated with topotecan and 13.2% in those patients treated with paclitaxel ($P = .138$). Median overall survival was 61 and 43 weeks in the topotecan and paclitaxel groups, respectively ($P = .515$). The results were stratified by platinum sensitivity and there was no statistically significant difference in response rate noted for either platinum-sensitive or platinum-resistant patients (48). Long-term survival of patients in this study was not statistically significant between the two groups (49).

Etoposide

Both intravenous and oral etoposide have been studied as treatments for recurrent EOC. The most promising results have been demonstrated with oral etoposide. In a GOG study of patients with both platinum-sensitive and platinum-resistant EOC treated with one prior regimen, prolonged oral etoposide demonstrated response rates of 27% and 34% for platinum-resistant and platinum-sensitive disease, respectively. The most common toxicity observed was myelosuppression (50). Despite promising results, concerns about the risk of leukemia following treatment with etoposide have limited the utility of this drug in clinical practice.

Other Cytotoxic Chemotherapy Agents

Multiple other cytotoxic agents have been investigated in the treatment of recurrent EOC. Two agents that have shown promise are trabectedin and pemetrexed. Trabectedin is a marine-derived antineoplastic agent that disrupts DNA transcription. A trial by Monk et al evaluated the addition of trabectedin to PLD for the treatment of first recurrence of EOC in platinum-sensitive and platinum-resistant patients. Patients treated with trabectedin plus PLD had a statistically significant improvement in both response rate and PFS when compared with those treated with PLD alone. When the results were stratified based on platinum sensitivity, only the patients with platinum-sensitive disease had a significant improvement in response rate and PFS (51). While not yet approved by the FDA for treatment of ovarian cancer, these results are promising for the use of trabectedin in recurrent EOC.

Pemetrexed is an antifolate metabolite which interrupts DNA replication. A Phase II study evaluated the effectiveness of pemetrexed in patients with recurrent, platinum-resistant or platinum-refractory disease. The results of the study showed an overall response rate of 21% with a PFS of 2.9 months and an overall survival of 11.4 months. Toxicities were mostly hematologic (52). These results establish pemetrexed as an active agent in ROC and further studies are warranted to further elucidate the role of this drug.

Biologic Agents

Multiple biologic agents have been evaluated for utility in the setting of ROC. The agent that has shown the most promise in the treatment of ROC is bevacizumab. Bevacizumab is a humanized anti-vascular endothelial growth factor (VEGF) monoclonal antibody that works as an antiangiogenesis drug. Several studies have investigated the role of bevacizumab in combination with other cytotoxic agents and alone for treatment of recurrent EOC. The role of bevacizumab in combination with gemcitabine and carboplatin in the treatment of platinum-sensitive, recurrent EOC has recently been demonstrated in the OCEANS trial as discussed previously. The GOG conducted a Phase II trial of single-agent bevacizumab in the treatment of recurrent EOC. Sixty-two patients with recurrent EOC underwent second- or third-line treatment with bevacizumab every 21 days. Thirty six patients in this study had platinum-resistant disease. Clinical response rate was 21% with 40.3% of patients achieving greater than or equal to 6-month progression-free interval. Prior platinum sensitivity had no impact on PFS (53). Another study performed by Cannistra and colleagues specifically investigated the role of bevacizumab in platinum-resistant EOC. Forty-four patients who had undergone no more than three prior chemotherapy regimens and had progressed or recurred within 3 months on prior treatment underwent treatment with bevacizumab every 21 days. A response rate of 15.9% was seen in this study. However, a higher than anticipated rate of gastrointestinal perforation (11%) was observed with a trend toward higher rate of gastrointestinal perforation in patients with bowel thickening or bowel obstruction, and all gastrointestinal perforations were observed in patients who had undergone three prior chemotherapy regimens. Due to the higher than anticipated rate of gastrointestinal perforation, this study was terminated prior to completion (54). Other common toxicities seen with bevacizumab include hypertension and proteinuria. Less common toxicities include vascular thrombosis, bleeding, and wound healing complications. These trials have established the activity of bevacizumab in the treatment of recurrent EOC. Given the potential for serious side effects of this drug, patients should be carefully selected to avoid potential side effects.

Other trials have investigated the role of other biologic agents in the treatment of recurrent EOC. Oregovomab, a monoclonal antibody to CA125, has been studied in the setting of EOC recurrence. Ehlen and colleagues administered oregovomab to 13 women with recurrent EOC who had received at least one prior course of platinum-based chemotherapy. They demonstrated robust immune responses in 50% of patients and disease stabilization in 3 out of 13 patients. Disease stabilization was strongly correlated with degree of immune response (55). In a similar trial by Gordon and colleagues, 20 patients with a history of recurrent EOC were treated with oregovomab plus optional cytotoxic chemotherapy. Seventy-nine percent of patients demonstrated robust immune responses. Those patients who mounted T-cell responses to CA125 and/or autologous tumor were shown to have significantly improved survival (56). Abagovomab, an anti-idiotypic antibody to CA125, has also been studied in the treatment of recurrent EOC. In a Phase I/II trial, authors investigated the role of the anti-idiotype anti-CA125 vaccine. They found an overall anti-idiotype antibody response of 68.1% and a longer overall survival in those patients who mounted this antibody response (57). Unfortunately, front-line Phase III trials with oregovomab and abagovomab failed to demonstrate a survival advantage when used as single agents for consolidation after primary therapy (58,59).

Various cytokines have also been studied in the treatment of EOC. In a Phase II study, 31 patients with recurrent, platinum-resistant or refractory EOC were treated with intraperitoneal interleukin-2 (IL-2). Clinical response was seen in 25% of patients. The authors report an association between clinical response and antitumor response (60).

Hormonal Therapy

Multiple studies have evaluated the role of tamoxifen, a selective estrogen receptor modulator, in the treatment of recurrent EOC. Hatch and colleagues investigated the role of tamoxifen in patients with persistent ROC after one prior chemotherapy regimen and found an overall response rate of 17% with an additional 38% of patients having stable disease (61). A systematic review of 18 studies that evaluated the role of tamoxifen in 638 total patients with recurrent EOC found an overall response rate of 13% and a stable disease rate of 38%. The authors postulate that the low response rate seen in this population is because the majority of the patients included in their analysis had been heavily pretreated with prior chemotherapy regimens and because treatment with tamoxifen was not determined by estrogen receptor status (62). Markman and colleagues performed a retrospective study in which patients with asymptomatic, small volume disease recurrence, defined by either elevated CA125 level only, no or minimal evidence of

recurrence on physical exam, or findings of minimal small volume disease on CT scan, were treated with tamoxifen until evidence of disease progression. Forty-two percent of patients remained on tamoxifen therapy at 6 months and 19% remained on therapy at 12 months (63). These results are promising for the treatment of small volume disease with tamoxifen, however it is difficult to determine whether the patients remaining on tamoxifen therapy is related to the therapy itself or whether it is a function of the natural history of the disease.

Intraperitoneal Chemotherapy

Recently, several large, randomized studies have established a role for intraperitoneal chemotherapy as frontline treatment for those patients with advanced stage, optimally cytoreduced EOC (64–66). Intraperitoneal chemotherapy has been studied in the setting of recurrent disease mostly in those patients with minimal disease confined to the peritoneal cavity with response rates of 20%–40%. Agents studied include: cisplatin, paclitaxel, 5-fluorouracil (5-FU), etoposide, and mitoxantrone. A recent retrospective, single institution report of experience with intraperitoneal chemotherapy for treatment of recurrent EOC found a median PFS of 10.5 months and median overall survival of 51 months in patients treated for recurrent EOC with platinum- and/or taxane-based intraperitoneal chemotherapy. More importantly, this study described an overall favorable side-effect profile (67). These data establish intraperitoneal chemotherapy as a feasible treatment option for recurrent EOC. Larger studies are needed to more firmly define the optimal use of this treatment modality for recurrent disease.

■ REFERENCES

1. Rustin GJ, Vergote I, Eisenhauer E, et al.; Gynecological Cancer Intergroup. Definitions for response and progression in ovarian cancer clinical trials incorporating RECIST 1.1 and CA 125 agreed by the Gynecological Cancer Intergroup (GCIG). *Int J Gynecol Cancer.* 2011;21(2):419–423.

2. Rustin GJ, van der Burg ME, Griffin CL, et al.; MRC OV05; EORTC 55955 investigators. Early versus delayed treatment of relapsed ovarian cancer (MRC OV05/EORTC 55955): a randomised trial. *Lancet.* 2010;376(9747):1155–1163.

3. Sebastian S, Lee SI, Horowitz NS, et al. PET-CT vs. CT alone in ovarian cancer recurrence. *Abdom Imaging.* 2008;33(1):112–118.

4. Pectasides D, Kayianni H, Facou A, et al. Correlation of abdominal computed tomography scanning and second-look operation findings in ovarian cancer patients. *Am J Clin Oncol.* 1991;14(6):457–462.

5. Clarke-Pearson DL, Bandy LC, Dudzinski M, Heaston D, Creasman WT. Computed tomography in evaluation of patients with ovarian carcinoma in complete clinical remission. Correlation with surgical-pathologic findings. *JAMA.* 1986;255(5):627–630.

6. García-Velloso MJ, Jurado M, Ceamanos C, et al. Diagnostic accuracy of FDG PET in the follow-up of platinum-sensitive epithelial ovarian carcinoma. *Eur J Nucl Med Mol Imaging.* 2007;34(9):1396–1405.

7. Makhija S, Howden N, Edwards R, Kelley J, Townsend DW, Meltzer CC. Positron emission tomography/computed tomography imaging for the detection of recurrent ovarian and fallopian tube carcinoma: a retrospective review. *Gynecol Oncol.* 2002;85(1):53–58.

8. Nanni C, Rubello D, Farsad M, et al. (18)F-FDG PET/CT in the evaluation of recurrent ovarian cancer: a prospective study on forty-one patients. *Eur J Surg Oncol.* 2005;31(7):792–797.

9. Low RN, Duggan B, Barone RM, Saleh F, Song SY. Treated ovarian cancer: MR imaging, laparotomy reassessment, and serum CA-125 values compared with clinical outcome at 1 year. *Radiology.* 2005;235(3):918–926.

10. Gu P, Pan LL, Wu SQ, Sun L, Huang G. CA 125, PET alone, PET-CT, CT and MRI in diagnosing recurrent ovarian carcinoma: a systematic review and meta-analysis. *Eur J Radiol.* 2009;71(1):164–174.

11. Berek, JS, Neville FH. *Berek & Hacker's Gynecologic Oncology.* 5th ed. Philadelphia, PA: Wolters Kluwer/Lippincott Williams & Wilkins Health; 2010.

12. Gershenson DM, Copeland LJ, Wharton JT, et al. Prognosis of surgically determined complete responders in advanced ovarian cancer. *Cancer.* 1985;55(5):1129–1135.

13. Podratz KC, Malkasian GD Jr, Wieand HS, et al. Recurrent disease after negative second-look laparotomy in stages III and IV ovarian carcinoma. *Gynecol Oncol.* 1988;29(3):274–282.

14. Rubin SC, Hoskins WJ, Saigo PE, et al. Prognostic factors for recurrence following negative second-look laparotomy in ovarian cancer patients treated with platinum-based chemotherapy. *Gynecol Oncol.* 1991;42(2):137–141.

15. Berek JS, Hacker NF, Lagasse LD, Poth T, Resnick B, Nieberg RK. Second-look laparotomy in stage III epithelial ovarian cancer: clinical variables associated with disease status. *Obstet Gynecol.* 1984;64(2):207–212.

16. Hoskins WJ, Rubin SC, Dulaney E, et al. Influence of secondary cytoreduction at the time of second-look laparotomy on the survival of patients with epithelial ovarian carcinoma. *Gynecol Oncol.* 1989;34(3):365–371.

17. Podratz KC, Schray MF, Wieand HS, et al. Evaluation of treatment and survival after positive second-look laparotomy. *Gynecol Oncol.* 1988;31(1):9–24.

18. Lippman S, Alberts D, Slymen D, et al. Second-look laparotomy in ovarian cancer: Evaluation of pathologic variables. *Am J Obstet Gynecol.* 1985;152:230–238.

19. Eisenkop SM, Friedman RL, Spirtos NM. The role of secondary cytoreductive surgery in the treatment of patients with recurrent epithelial ovarian carcinoma. *Cancer.* 2000;88(1):144–153.

20. Tay EH, Grant PT, Gebski V, Hacker NF. Secondary cytoreductive surgery for recurrent epithelial ovarian cancer. *Obstet Gynecol.* 2002;99(6):1008–1013.

21. Salani R, Santillan A, Zahurak ML, et al. Secondary cytoreductive surgery for localized, recurrent epithelial ovarian cancer: analysis of prognostic factors and survival outcome. *Cancer.* 2007;109(4):685–691.

22. Chi DS, McCaughty K, Diaz JP, et al. Guidelines and selection criteria for secondary cytoreductive surgery in patients with recurrent, platinum-sensitive epithelial ovarian carcinoma. *Cancer.* 2006;106(9):1933–1939.

23. Markman M, Rothman R, Hakes T, et al. Second-line platinum therapy in patients with ovarian cancer previously treated with cisplatin. *J Clin Oncol.* 1991;9(3):389–393.

24. Markman M, Hoskins W. Responses to salvage chemotherapy in ovarian cancer: a critical need for precise definitions of the treated population. *J Clin Oncol.* 1992;10(4):513–514.

25. Gershenson DM, Kavanagh JJ, Copeland LJ, Stringer CA, Morris M, Wharton JT. Re-treatment of patients with recurrent epithelial ovarian cancer with cisplatin-based chemotherapy. *Obstet Gynecol.* 1989;73(5 Pt 1):798–802.

26. Gore ME, Fryatt I, Wiltshaw E, Dawson T. Treatment of relapsed carcinoma of the ovary with cisplatin or carboplatin following initial treatment with these compounds. *Gynecol Oncol.* 1990;36(2):207–211.

27. Rose PG, Fusco N, Fluellen L, Rodriguez M. Second-line therapy with paclitaxel and carboplatin for recurrent disease following first-line therapy with paclitaxel and platinum in ovarian or peritoneal carcinoma. *J Clin Oncol.* 1998;16(4):1494–1497.

28. González-Martín AJ, Calvo E, Bover I, et al. Randomized phase II trial of carboplatin versus paclitaxel and carboplatin in platinum-sensitive recurrent advanced ovarian carcinoma: a GEICO (Grupo Espanol de Investigacion en Cancer de Ovario) study. *Ann Oncol.* 2005;16(5):749–755.

29. Parmar MK, Ledermann JA, Colombo N, et al.; ICON and AGO Collaborators. Paclitaxel plus platinum-based chemotherapy versus conventional platinum-based chemotherapy in women with relapsed ovarian cancer: the ICON4/AGO-OVAR-2.2 trial. *Lancet.* 2003;361(9375):2099–2106.

30. Ferrero JM, Weber B, Geay JF, et al. Second-line chemotherapy with pegylated liposomal doxorubicin and carboplatin is highly effective in patients with advanced ovarian cancer in late relapse: a GINECO phase II trial. *Ann Oncol.* 2007;18(2):263–268.

31. Pujade-Lauraine E, Wagner U, Aavall-Lundqvist E, et al. Pegylated liposomal Doxorubicin and Carboplatin compared with Paclitaxel and Carboplatin for patients with platinum-sensitive ovarian cancer in late relapse. *J Clin Oncol.* 2010;28(20):3323–3329.

32. Pfisterer J, Plante M, Vergote I, et al.; AGO-OVAR; NCIC CTG; EORTC GCG. Gemcitabine plus carboplatin compared with carboplatin in patients with platinum-sensitive recurrent ovarian cancer: an intergroup trial of the AGO-OVAR, the NCIC CTG, and the EORTC GCG. *J Clin Oncol.* 2006;24(29):4699–4707.

33. Aghajanian C, Blank SV, Goff BA, et al. OCEANS: a randomized, double-blind, placebo-controlled phase III trial of chemotherapy with or without bevacizumab in patients with platinum-sensitive recurrent epithelial ovarian, primary peritoneal, or fallopian tube cancer. *J Clin Oncol.* 2012;30(17):2039–2045.

34. Thigpen JT, Blessing JA, Ball H, Hummel SJ, Barrett RJ. Phase II trial of paclitaxel in patients with progressive ovarian carcinoma after platinum-based chemotherapy: a Gynecologic Oncology Group study. *J Clin Oncol.* 1994;12(9):1748–1753.

35. Markman M, Blessing J, Rubin S, et al. Phase II trial of weekly paclitaxel (80 mg/m^2) in platinum and paclitaxel-resistant ovarian and primary peritoneal cancers: a Gynecologic Oncology Group study. *Gynecol Oncol.* 2006;101:436–440.

36. Rosenberg P, Andersson H, Boman K, et al. Randomized trial of single agent paclitaxel given weekly versus every three weeks and with peroral versus intravenous steroid premedication to patients with ovarian cancer previously treated with platinum. *Acta Oncol.* 2002;41(5):418–424.

37. Coleman RL, Brady WE, McMeekin DS, et al. A phase II evaluation of nanoparticle, albumin-bound (nab) paclitaxel in the treatment of recurrent or persistent platinum-resistant ovarian, fallopian tube, or primary peritoneal cancer: a Gynecologic Oncology Group study. *Gynecol Oncol.* 2011;122(1):111–115.

38. Teneriello MG, Tseng PC, Crozier M, et al. Phase II evaluation of nanoparticle albumin-bound paclitaxel in platinum-sensitive patients with recurrent ovarian, peritoneal, or fallopian tube cancer. *J Clin Oncol.* 2009;27(9):1426–1431.

39. Vasey PA, Jayson GC, Gordon A, et al.; Scottish Gynaecological Cancer Trials Group. Phase III randomized trial of docetaxel-carboplatin versus paclitaxel-carboplatin as first-line chemotherapy for ovarian carcinoma. *J Natl Cancer Inst.* 2004;96(22):1682–1691.

40. Rose PG, Blessing JA, Ball HG, et al. A phase II study of docetaxel in paclitaxel-resistant ovarian and peritoneal carcinoma: a Gynecologic Oncology Group study. *Gynecol Oncol.* 2003;88(2):130–135.

41. Tinker AV, Gebski V, Fitzharris B, et al. Phase II trial of weekly docetaxel for patients with relapsed ovarian cancer who have previously received paclitaxel–ANZGOG 02-01. *Gynecol Oncol.* 2007;104(3):647–653.

42. Muggia FM, Hainsworth JD, Jeffers S, et al. Phase II study of liposomal doxorubicin in refractory ovarian cancer: antitumor activity and toxicity modification by liposomal encapsulation. *J Clin Oncol.* 1997;15(3):987–993.

43. Gordon AN, Granai CO, Rose PG, et al. Phase II study of liposomal doxorubicin in platinum- and paclitaxel-refractory epithelial ovarian cancer. *J Clin Oncol.* 2000;18(17):3093–3100.

44. Gordon AN, Fleagle JT, Guthrie D, Parkin DE, Gore ME, Lacave AJ. Recurrent epithelial ovarian carcinoma: a randomized phase III study of pegylated liposomal doxorubicin versus topotecan. *J Clin Oncol.* 2001;19(14):3312–3322.

45. Mutch DG, Orlando M, Goss T, et al. Randomized phase III trial of gemcitabine compared with pegylated liposomal doxorubicin in patients with platinum-resistant ovarian cancer. *J Clin Oncol.* 2007;25(19):2811–2818.

46. Ferrandina G, Ludovisi M, Lorusso D, et al. Phase III trial of gemcitabine compared with pegylated liposomal doxorubicin in progressive or recurrent ovarian cancer. *J Clin Oncol.* 2008;26(6):890–896.

47. Bookman MA, Malmström H, Bolis G, et al. Topotecan for the treatment of advanced epithelial ovarian cancer: an open-label phase II study in patients treated after prior chemotherapy that contained cisplatin or carboplatin and paclitaxel. *J Clin Oncol.* 1998;16(10):3345–3352.

48. ten Bokkel Huinink W, Gore M, Carmichael J, et al. Topotecan versus paclitaxel for the treatment of recurrent epithelial ovarian cancer. *J Clin Oncol.* 1997;15(6):2183–2193.

49. ten Bokkel Huinink W, Lane SR, Ross GA; International Topotecan Study Group. Long-term survival in a phase III, randomised study of topotecan versus paclitaxel in advanced epithelial ovarian carcinoma. *Ann Oncol.* 2004;15(1):100–103.

50. Rose PG, Blessing JA, Mayer AR, Homesley HD. Prolonged oral etoposide as second-line therapy for platinum-resistant and platinum-sensitive ovarian carcinoma: a Gynecologic Oncology Group study. *J Clin Oncol.* 1998;16(2):405–410.

51. Monk BJ, Herzog TJ, Kaye SB, et al. Trabectedin plus pegylated liposomal Doxorubicin in recurrent ovarian cancer. *J Clin Oncol.* 2010;28(19):3107–3114.

52. Miller DS, Blessing JA, Krasner CN, et al. Phase II evaluation of pemetrexed in the treatment of recurrent or persistent platinum-resistant ovarian or primary peritoneal carcinoma: a study of the Gynecologic Oncology Group. *J Clin Oncol.* 2009;27(16):2686–2691.

53. Burger RA, Sill MW, Monk BJ, Greer BE, Sorosky JI. Phase II trial of bevacizumab in persistent or recurrent epithelial ovarian cancer or primary peritoneal cancer: a Gynecologic Oncology Group study. *J Clin Oncol.* 2007;25(33):5165–5171.

54. Cannistra SA, Matulonis UA, Penson RT, et al. Phase II study of bevacizumab in patients with platinum-resistant ovarian cancer or peritoneal serous cancer. *J Clin Oncol.* 2007;25(33):5180–5186.

55. Ehlen TG, Hoskins PJ, Miller D, et al. A pilot phase 2 study of oregovomab murine monoclonal antibody to CA125 as an immunotherapeutic agent for recurrent ovarian cancer. *Int J Gynecol Cancer.* 2005;15(6):1023–1034.

56. Gordon AN, Schultes BC, Gallion H, et al. CA125- and tumor-specific T-cell responses correlate with prolonged survival in oregovomab-treated recurrent ovarian cancer patients. *Gynecol Oncol.* 2004;94(2):340–351.

57. Reinartz S, Köhler S, Schlebusch H, et al. Vaccination of patients with advanced ovarian carcinoma with the anti-idiotype ACA125: immunological response and survival (phase Ib/II). *Clin Cancer Res.* 2004;10(5):1580–1587.

58. Berek JS, Taylor PT, Gordon A, et al. Randomized, placebo-controlled study of oregovomab for consolidation of clinical remission in patients with advanced ovarian cancer. *J Clin Oncol.* 2004;22(17):3507–3516.

59. Pfisterer J, Berek J, Casado A, et al. Randomized double-blind placebo-controlled internation trial of abagovomab maintenance therapy in patients with advanced ovarian cancer after complete response to first-line chemotherapy: The Monoclonal Antibody Immunotherapy for Malignancies of the Ovary by Subcutaneous Abago-vomab (Mimosa) trial. *J Clin Oncol.* 2011;29 (suppl; abstr LBA5002).

60. Vlad AM, Budiu RA, Lenzner DE, et al. A phase II trial of intraperitoneal interleukin-2 in patients with platinum-resistant or platinum-refractory ovarian cancer. *Cancer Immunol Immunother.* 2010;59(2):293–301.

61. Hatch KD, Beecham JB, Blessing JA, Creasman WT. Responsiveness of patients with advanced ovarian carcinoma to tamoxifen. A Gynecologic Oncology Group study of second-line therapy in 105 patients. *Cancer.* 1991;68(2):269–271.

62. Perez-Gracia JL, Carrasco EM. Tamoxifen therapy for ovarian cancer in the adjuvant and advanced settings: systematic review of the literature and implications for future research. *Gynecol Oncol.* 2002;84(2):201–209.

63. Markman M, Webster K, Zanotti K, Rohl J, Belinson J. Use of tamoxifen in asymptomatic patients with recurrent small-volume ovarian cancer. *Gynecol Oncol.* 2004;93(2):390–393.

64. Alberts DS, Liu PY, Hannigan EV, et al. Intraperitoneal cisplatin plus intravenous cyclophosphamide versus intravenous cisplatin plus intravenous cyclophosphamide for stage III ovarian cancer. *N Engl J Med.* 1996;335(26):1950–1955.

65. Markman M, Bundy BN, Alberts DS, et al. Phase III trial of standard-dose intravenous cisplatin plus paclitaxel versus moderately high-dose carboplatin followed by intravenous paclitaxel and intraperitoneal cisplatin in small-volume stage III ovarian carcinoma: an intergroup study of the Gynecologic Oncology Group, Southwestern Oncology Group, and Eastern Cooperative Oncology Group. *J Clin Oncol.* 2001;19(4):1001–1007.

66. Armstrong DK, Bundy B, Wenzel L, et al.; Gynecologic Oncology Group. Intraperitoneal cisplatin and paclitaxel in ovarian cancer. *N Engl J Med.* 2006;354(1):34–43.

67. Skaznik-Wikiel ME, Lesnock JL, McBee WC, et al. Intraperitoneal chemotherapy for recurrent epithelial ovarian cancer is feasible with high completion rates, low complications, and acceptable patient outcomes. *Int J Gynecol Cancer.* 2012;22(2):232–237.

Borderline Ovarian Tumors

IV

18

A Multidisciplinary Approach to Diagnosis and Treatment of Borderline Ovarian Tumors

ANE GERDA ZAHL ERIKSSON

CLAES GÖRAN TROPÉ

JANNE KAERN

BEN DAVIDSON

■ INTRODUCTION

Borderline ovarian tumors (BOT) were first described as a separate group in 1929 by Taylor (1), and accepted by the International Federation of Gynecology and Obstetrics (FIGO) as carcinoma of low malignancy potential in 1971 (2). BOT are distinguished from malignant ovarian tumors on the basis of distinct histopathologic features and biologic behavior; they are epithelial tumors of the ovaries characterized by cellular proliferation and nuclear atypia without stromal invasion.

BOT account for between 10% and 20% of all epithelial ovarian malignancies (3). Ten to 15% may develop a clinically aggressive behavior as invasive carcinoma, and potentially spread beyond the ovary. They also may recur as carcinomas.

One-third of BOT arise in women under the age of 40 years. As a result, fertility-sparing surgery has increased over the last decade in this group of patients. Recurrence rates may be high, depending on stage of disease and type of initial surgery. Careful selection of candidates for conservative treatment is necessary.

■ EPIDEMIOLOGY

Pregnancies, oral contraceptives, and breastfeeding decrease the risk of BOT, whereas primary infertility and nulliparity increase the risk (4). It is currently unclear whether BRCA1 and BRCA2 mutations increase the risk of BOT (5).

■ HISTOLOGY

The vast majority of BOT are mucinous (Figures 18.1 and 18.2) or serous (Figures 18.3 and 18.4) tumors, they comprise 43%–53% and 42.5%–52% of all BOT, respectively. The remaining 4%–5% are of endometrioid, clear cell, mixed, transitional cell, or Brenner type (6–9).

■ PATHOGENESIS

Over the last few years, a new theory of carcinogenesis describing a subset of serous ovarian cystadenomas that evolve through serous BOT to low-grade epithelial ovarian cancer has been proposed (10–13; Figure 18.5). This low-grade pathway involves serous BOT as a precursor mimicking the adenocarcinoma sequence in colorectal cancer, where carcinoma evolves through a continuum of histological precursor lesions (14–16). Low-grade BOT are mostly characterized by KRAS and BRAF mutations. Only 2% of all serous BOT progress to carcinoma via the low-grade pathway (Figure 18.5). Most serous ovarian carcinomas follow the high-grade pathway, with no known precursor lesion. Tumors in the high-grade pathway are characterized by mutation of TP53 and a high level of genetic instability (11).

The sequence of malignant transformation from benign mucinous tumors to carcinoma represents transitional stages of mucinous carcinogenesis. Mucinous BOT have a higher frequency of KRAS mutation than that of mucinous cystadenoma, but a lower rate than that of mucinous carcinoma. In mucinous BOT with invasion, one can frequently identify foci suggesting in-situ malignant changes.

■ SEROUS BORDERLINE TUMORS

In approximately one-third of cases serous borderline tumors (Figure 18.6) are bilateral (6,8). They frequently spread as peritoneal implants (35%), of which 20%–25% are invasive implants (17; Figure 18.7). Most peritoneal implants remain stable or regress after removal of the primary ovarian tumor, the invasive implants may progress to invasive carcinoma (18,19). Thirty percent of patients with invasive implants develop progressive disease, compared to only 2% of those women without invasive

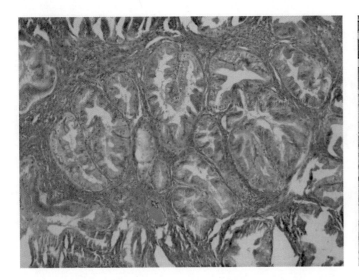

FIGURE 18.1 Hematoxylin and eosin slide, magnification 100×. Mucinous BOT with complex growth pattern, nuclear stratification, and mild atypia. BOT, borderline ovarian tumors.

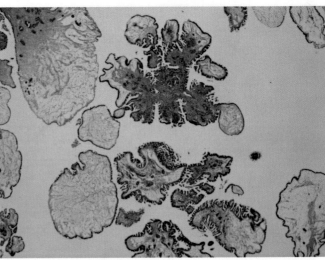

FIGURE 18.3 Hematoxylin and eosin slide. magnification 25×. Serous BOT depicting papillary growth with complex epithelial proliferation. BOT, borderline ovarian tumors.

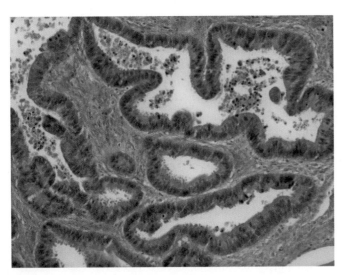

FIGURE 18.2 Hematoxylin and eosin slide, magnification 200×. Mucinous BOT with marked atypia and intracystic necrosis. BOT, borderline ovarian tumors.

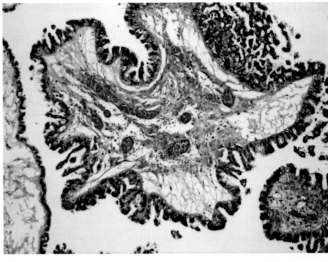

FIGURE 18.4 Hematoxylin and eosin slide, magnification 100×. Serous BOT, papillary growth with atypia. BOT, borderline ovarian tumors.

implants (20,21). Noninvasive implants (Figure 18.8) and bilaterality do not predict worse outcome compared with the presence of invasive implants (8,17,18,22). The 10-year survival in women with serous BOT without invasive implants is 95%, in women with invasive implants it is 60%–70% (5).

■ MUCINOUS BORDERLINE TUMORS

Mucinous borderline tumors are composed of two histological subtypes: intestinal (85%) and endocervical (15%; 8,23). The intestinal type of tumors is commonly unilateral and may be large (Figure 18.9). If a woman presents with a bilateral tumor of this histological subtype, she should have further workup in search of a primary intestinal tumor. Endocervical mucinous BOTs may be associated with endometriosis and mixed-BOT; they may be bilateral. Intraepithelial carcinoma can present with both subtypes (2,6).

It is not so common for mucinous BOTs to metastasize beyond the ovaries (10%–15%), if they do so it is nearly always as pseudomyxoma peritonei. This condition is commonly disseminated from a mucinous appendix tumor, appendectomy is therefore routinely performed during primary surgery for mucinous BOTs.

Any subtype of mucinous BOT can recur as invasive adenocarcinoma. The rate of recurrence is higher if only

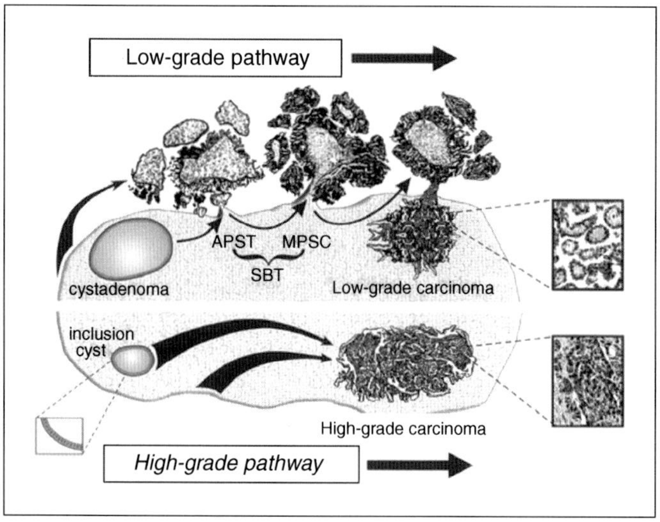

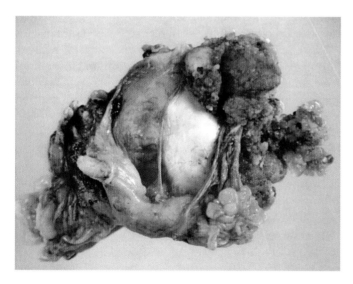

FIGURE 18.5 "Low-grade pathway": frequent *BRAF* and *KRAS* mutations (61%–68%); low cellular proliferation, gradual increase in chromosomal instability; 5-year survival about 55%. "High-grade pathway": frequent *TP53* mutations (70%); high cellular proliferation, high chromosomal instability; frequent HLA-G expression; 5-year survival about 30%. APST, atypical proliferative serous tumors; MPSC, micropapillary serous carcinoma; SBT, serous borderline ovarian tumor. Published with permission Shih and Kurman (12).

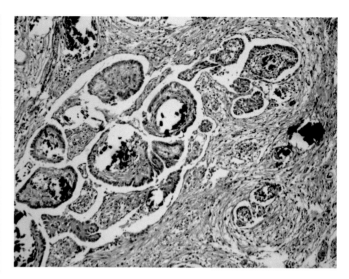

FIGURE 18.7 Hematoxylin and eosin slide, magnification 100×. Serous BOT, invasive peritoneal implant. BOT, borderline ovarian tumors.

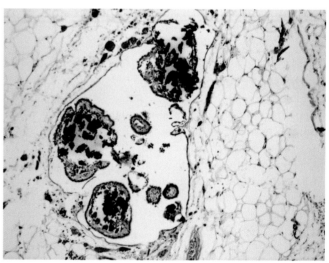

FIGURE 18.8 Hematoxylin and eosin slide, magnification 100×. BOT, noninvasive implant of the omentum. BOT, borderline ovarian tumors.

FIGURE 18.6 Mucinous BOT, macroscopic image. BOT, borderline ovarian tumors.

cystectomy, rather than salpingo-oophorectomy, has been performed. Unilateral salpingo-oophorectomy is thus recommended in mucinous BOT (4,8).

■ PROGNOSTIC FACTORS

The FIGO stage is the strongest prognostic factor for recurrence and survival for BOT. Kaern et al (24) found that the only independent prognostic factors for corrected survival were FIGO stage, ploidy, histological type, and age.

Women with aneuploid tumors had a 19-fold increased risk of dying of disease compared with patients with diploid tumors (complete follow-up of median 149 months, range 5–246 months). Based on the prognostic factors patients could be divided into risk groups: The low-risk group was characterized by Stage I disease, diploid serous BOT or mucinous BOT, and age less than 40 years; they had 100% survival. The high-risk group had a 75% or higher risk of dying of disease; they were characterized by aneuploid serous BOT or mucinous BOT, Stage II-III disease, and age more than 70 years.

For serous BOT micropapillary histology has been reported as an additional risk factor. However, this is controversial as poor prognosis is only seen when this histology is associated with invasive implants (25–28). Lymph

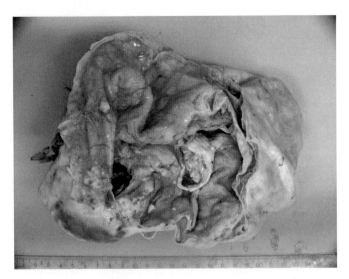

FIGURE 18.9   Serous BOT, macroscopic image

node involvement has not been confirmed as an independent risk factor (24,27,29,30).

■ SYMPTOMS

There is not much information available regarding symptoms registered by women with BOT at the time of diagnosis. In comparison to women with invasive ovarian cancer, women with BOT experience symptoms less commonly. Most patients are asymptomatic, although 75% of these women may have at least one symptom as abdominal pain or discomfort, bowel irregularity, and persisting fatigue or weight loss (31,32).

■ SURGICAL TREATMENT

The recommendation for primary surgery in BOT is removal of all macroscopic disease and proper surgical staging. This entails exploration of the entire abdominal cavity, hysterectomy, omentectomy, bilateral salpingo-oophorectomy, multiple peritoneal biopsies and peritoneal washing with cytology. Appendectomy should be performed in all patients with mucinous BOT. Lymph node involvement does not influence recurrence or survival rate (6,33), and routine lymphadenectomy is not required even in Stage II and III disease (33,34). However, enlarged lymph nodes at time of surgery should always be removed. Fewer than 50% of women with BOT will have complete surgical staging.

One cannot diagnose BOT prior to surgery, even experienced pathologists have difficulties making the diagnosis of BOT by intraoperative frozen section. Frozen section can be helpful in distinguishing BOT/epithelial ovarian cancer from benign tumors (overdiagnosed in less than 10%), but not in distinguishing BOT from epithelial ovarian cancer (underdiagnosed in 25%–30%; 35,36).

Many women with BOT are of reproductive age and desire conservative treatment to preserve their fertility. Conservative surgery is defined as complete staging in which the uterus and at least a part of one ovary are preserved (8,37). This can be performed by conventional laparotomy, or in selected cases via minimal invasive surgery. In comparison to laparotomy, laparoscopy has a shorter postoperative recovery, fewer adhesions, and improved cosmetic results (38). Laparoscopic technique is under constant development; the introduction of endo-bags provide lower risk of spillage during surgery and less port-site metastases. Despite this, cyst rupture and incomplete staging occur in 33.9% of cases during laparoscopy vs 12.4% in laparotomy (39,40). Women who wish to preserve their fertility presenting with Stage IA tumors can safely be treated with unilateral salpingo-oophorectomy after thorough surgical staging (Figure 18.10).

Early detected recurrences can be cured with repeated surgery (6,26,34). In women with recurrent disease who still have not completed childbearing one may consider conservative treatment again as long as the woman is informed about the high risk of recurrence and the need for close follow-up. Studies from the Gynecologic Oncology Group (41) and from the Norwegian Radium Hospital (6) have demonstrated that fertility-sparing surgery is feasible. Laparoscopic surgery may be used, but should be reserved for oncologic surgeons.

Relapse rates after bilateral salpingo-oophorectomy range between 0% and 20%. This rate varies between 12% and 58% for cystectomy and between 2.5% and 5.7% for radical surgery. Resection margins containing tumor cells are predictors of recurring disease (42); extensive sampling of the resection margins of ovarian cysts is important. Multifocality may be a strong predictor of failure of cystectomy (43).

■ FERTILITY AFTER CONSERVATIVE MANAGEMENT OF BORDERLINE OVARIAN TUMORS

Unilateral oophorectomy, omentectomy, and appendectomy is indicated for women wishing to preserve their fertility in Stage IA diploid mucinous BOT (24). If the primary tumor is serous, it is also safe to perform this procedure as long as the contralateral ovary is macroscopically normal. As previously mentioned, primary infertility and nulliparity increase the risk of BOT (4). As many as 10%–35% of women with BOT have been reported to have a history of infertility prior to surgery (44–46). Surgical treatment for BOT may further impair

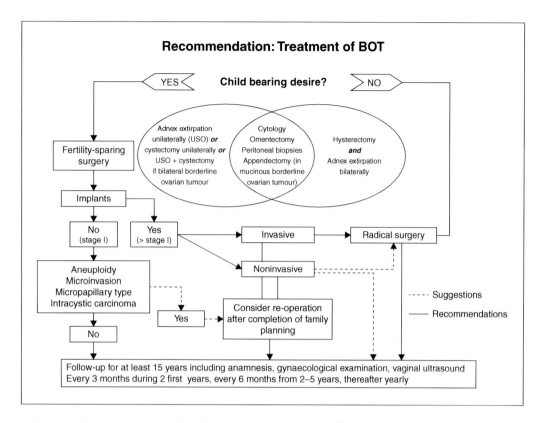

FIGURE 18.10 Recommendation: Treatment of borderline ovarian tumors. Modified from Trillsch et al (8) and Cadron et al (34) with permission.

the fertility not only by loss of ovarian tissue, but also by pelvic scarring and adhesions.

Ovulation induction is often required to conceive (47). The role of ovulation drugs and in vitro fertilization (IVF) in BOT is an ongoing debate (46–51). IVF has been shown to significantly increase the risk of BOT and epithelial ovarian cancer (52). Ovarian stimulation and exposure to high levels of estrogen do not seem to increase the risk for recurrence (46,53). Based on available literature, we recommend proceeding with caution and to only treat women with early stage BOT with IVF drugs.

Ovarian stimulation, egg retrieval, and egg freezing are options for women with reduced fertility after surgery. Approximately one-third of women having undergone conservative surgery for BOT will be able to conceive with no negative influence of pregnancy on the disease (39,46,53,54). Cryopreservation of ovarian tissue and auto transplantation provides a new option for women with premature ovarian failure (55).

■ ADJUVANT THERAPY OF BORDERLINE OVARIAN TUMORS

There is no proven benefit from adjuvant chemotherapy or radiotherapy in BOT, even in advanced stage or in the presence of invasive implants (4,21). In women with serous BOT with residual disease cisplatin-based therapy has

shown high response rates, but little effect on long-term survival (4,56). If the recurrent disease has transformed to an invasive ovarian carcinoma it is reasonable to consider platinum- and/or taxane-based chemotherapy.

■ RESTAGING

On occasion, the final histological diagnosis of BOT was not suspected at the time of surgery, and the woman has not undergone complete surgical staging. Should she undergo restaging?

Mucinous BOT confined to one ovary is unlikely to be upstaged at a restaging procedure. If there is extra-ovarian disease, complete surgical staging and appendectomy are indicated since mucinous BOT with abdominal spread arise in the appendix, or simultaneously in one or both ovaries in 50% of cases. The decision to restage any patient should be individualized, considering histology, stage, and level of concern of the patient. There is not much support in the literature that restaging will have an effect on survival (8,33,57–59).

■ FOLLOW-UP

The recommendation for follow-up is every 3 months during the first 2 years, every 6 months for the following

3 years, and annually thereafter. The follow-up visits should include pelvic examination, transvaginal ultrasound, and CA-125 measurement. If there is evidence of recurrence, a CT scan of the thorax, abdomen, and pelvis is warranted. If the patient has undergone conservative treatment, it is debatable if she should have further surgery to remove her remaining ovary once she has completed childbearing (Figure 18.10). Relapse can occur late, and has been described as late as 39 years after initial treatment (26,34). Follow-up should thus be lifelong.

■ FUTURE DIRECTION IN BORDERLINE OVARIAN TUMORS

To optimize the quality of life and survival of women with BOT, increased knowledge regarding biologic behavior, diagnostic tools, and clinical management is needed. Future research regarding epidemiology of BOT should focus on the identification of risk factors for invasive implants, recurrences, and death as well as identification of predisposing heritable factors.

Concerning pathology and molecular biology, further molecular studies assessing the relationship between serous BOT, low-grade serous carcinoma, and high-grade serous carcinoma are warranted. Molecular studies to aid in the characterization of implants, and to determine the biology of microinvasive BOT are necessary.

In regards to clinical management, improved methods for preoperative and intraoperative diagnosis should be explored. Risks associated with conservative treatment must be determined, in addition to further investigations of the role and safety of minimal invasive surgery in managing BOT (60).

■ CONCLUSION

BOT comprise 10%–20% of all epithelial ovarian tumors; they are usually associated with good prognosis, and they are frequently diagnosed in women younger than 40 years. In the past, primary treatment has been laparotomy including exploration of the entire abdominal cavity, bilateral salpingo-oophorectomy, omentectomy, complete resection of peritoneal lesions, peritoneal washing, and in the case of mucinous tumors, appendectomy. There is no proven benefit for adjuvant therapy in treating BOT. Minimal invasive surgery can be used in treating women with BOT, but this should be reserved for oncologic surgeons. The role of minimal invasive surgery in the removal of complex cysts should be explored further. Molecular studies are needed to further understand the biological behavior of BOT to potentially improve early diagnosis, management, and follow-up of these tumors.

Delayed childbearing is a trend in developed countries, and as a result, some women are nulliparous at the time of diagnosis. Fertility-sparing treatment is increasingly used in women with BOT; however improved methods to determine risks associated with conservative treatment are needed. Women undergoing conservative treatment must be informed of the risk of recurrence and need for close follow-up. All women with BOT, regardless of initial treatment, should have lifelong follow-up.

■ ACKNOWLEDGMENT

We wish to thank Mrs. Gry Seppola for technical assistance and gratefully acknowledge the financial support from the Inger and John Fredriksen Foundation for Ovarian Cancer Research.

■ REFERENCES

1. Taylor HC. Malignant and semi-malignant tumors of the ovary. *Surg Gynecol Obstet.* 1929;48:204–230.
2. Kottmeier HL, Kolstad P, McGarrity KA. Annual report on results of treatment in gynaecologic cancer, vol. 17. Statements of results obtained in 1969–1972, inclusive. FIGO. Stockholm, Sweden, Editorial office, Radiumhemmet, 1973.
3. Lenhard MS, Mitterer S, Kümper C, et al. Long-term follow-up after ovarian borderline tumor: relapse and survival in a large patient cohort. *Eur J Obstet Gynecol Reprod Biol.* 2009;145(2):189–194.
4. Tropé C, Davidson B, Paulsen T, Abeler VM, Kaern J. Diagnosis and treatment of borderline ovarian neoplasms "the state of the art." *Eur J Gynaecol Oncol.* 2009;30(5):471–482.
5. Sherman ME, Mink PJ, Curtis R, et al. Survival among women with borderline ovarian tumors and ovarian carcinoma: a population-based analysis. *Cancer.* 2004;100(5):1045–1052.
6. Kaern J, Tropé CG, Abeler VM. A retrospective study of 370 borderline tumors of the ovary treated at the Norwegian Radium Hospital from 1970 to 1982. A review of clinicopathologic features and treatment modalities. *Cancer.* 1993;71(5):1810–1820.
7. Bjørge T, Engeland A, Hansen S, Tropé CG. Trends in the incidence of ovarian cancer and borderline tumours in Norway, 1954–1993. *Int J Cancer.* 1997;71(5):780–786.
8. Trillsch F, Mahner S, Ruetzel J, et al. Clinical management of borderline ovarian tumors. *Expert Rev Anticancer Ther.* 2010;10(7):1115–1124.
9. du Bois A, Ewald-Riegler N, du Bois O, et al. Borderline tumors of the ovary: a systematic review [German]. *Geburtsh Frauenheilk.* 2009;69:807–833.
10. Kurman RJ, Shih IeM. Pathogenesis of ovarian cancer: lessons from morphology and molecular biology and their clinical implications. *Int J Gynecol Pathol.* 2008;27(2):151–160.
11. Kurman RJ, Visvanathan K, Roden R, Wu TC, Shih IeM. Early detection and treatment of ovarian cancer: shifting from early stage to minimal volume of disease based on a new model of carcinogenesis. *Am J Obstet Gynecol.* 2008;198(4):351–356.
12. Shih IeM, Kurman RJ. Ovarian tumorigenesis: a proposed model based on morphological and molecular genetic analysis. *Am J Pathol.* 2004;164:1511–1518.
13. Levanon K, Crum C, Drapkin R. New insights into the pathogenesis of serous ovarian cancer and its clinical impact. *J Clin Oncol.* 2008;26(32):5284–5293.

14. Meinhold-Heerlein I, Bauerschlag D, Hilpert F, et al. Molecular and prognostic distinction between serous ovarian carcinomas of varying grade and malignant potential. *Oncogene.* 2005;24(6):1053–1065.
15. Bonome T, Lee JY, Park DC, et al. Expression profiling of serous low malignant potential, low-grade, and high-grade tumors of the ovary. *Cancer Res.* 2005;65(22):10602–10612.
16. Mahner S, Baasch C, Schwarz J, et al. C-Fos expression is a molecular predictor of progression and survival in epithelial ovarian carcinoma. *Br J Cancer.* 2008;99(8):1269–1275.
17. Seidman JD, Horkayne-Szakaly I, Haiba M, Boice CR, Kurman RJ, Ronnett BM. The histologic type and stage distribution of ovarian carcinomas of surface epithelial origin. *Int J Gynecol Pathol.* 2004;23(1):41–44.
18. Bell DA, Weinstock MA, Scully RE. Peritoneal implants of ovarian serous borderline tumors. Histologic features and prognosis. *Cancer.* 1988;62(10):2212–2222.
19. Kurman RJ, Trimble CL. The behavior of serous tumors of low malignant potential: are they ever malignant? *Int J Gynecol Pathol.* 1993;12(2):120–127.
20. Oedegaard E. Ovarian carcinomas and borderline ovarian tumors - molecular markers and operative treatment. Dissertation, Faculty of Medicine, University of Oslo, 2008.
21. Morice P, Camatte S, Rey A, et al. Prognostic factors for patients with advanced stage serous borderline tumours of the ovary. *Ann Oncol.* 2003;14(4):592–598.
22. Tinelli R, Tinelli A, Tinelli FG, Cicinelli E, Malvasi A. Conservative surgery for borderline ovarian tumors: a review. *Gynecol Oncol.* 2006;100(1):185–191.
23. Kramer JL, Greene MH. Epidemiology of ovarian, fallopian tube, and primary peritoneal cancer. In: Gershenson DM, McGuire WP, Gore M, et al., eds, *Gynecologic Cancer. Controversies in Management.* 1st ed. Philadelphia, PA: Elsevier Churchill Livingstone; 2004:327–340.
24. Kaern J, Tropé CG, Kristensen GB, Abeler VM, Pettersen EO. DNA ploidy; the most important prognostic factor in patients with borderline tumors of the ovary. *Int J Gynecol Cancer.* 1993;3(6):349–358.
25. Prat J, De Nictolis M. Serous borderline tumors of the ovary: a long-term follow-up study of 137 cases, including 18 with a micropapillary pattern and 20 with microinvasion. *Am J Surg Pathol.* 2002;26(9):1111–1128.
26. Silva EG, Gershenson DM, Malpica A, Deavers M. The recurrence and the overall survival rates of ovarian serous borderline neoplasms with noninvasive implants is time dependent. *Am J Surg Pathol.* 2006;30(11):1367–1371.
27. Seidman JD, Kurman RJ. Ovarian serous borderline tumors: a critical review of the literature with emphasis on prognostic indicators. *Hum Pathol.* 2000;31(5):539–557.
28. Chang SJ, Ryu HS, Chang KH, Yoo SC, Yoon JH. Prognostic significance of the micropapillary pattern in patients with serous borderline ovarian tumors. *Acta Obstet Gynecol Scand.* 2008;87(4):476–481.
29. Yokoyama Y, Moriya T, Takano T, et al. Clinical outcome and risk factors for recurrence in borderline ovarian tumours. *Br J Cancer.* 2006;94(11):1586–1591.
30. Leake JF, Rader JS, Woodruff JD, Rosenshein NB. Retroperitoneal lymphatic involvement with epithelial ovarian tumors of low malignant potential. *Gynecol Oncol.* 1991;42(2):124–130.
31. Paulsen T, Kaern J, Kjaerheim K, Tropé C, Tretli S. Symptoms and referral of women with epithelial ovarian tumors. *Int J Gynaecol Obstet.* 2005;88(1):31–37.
32. Paulsen T. *Epithelial Ovarian Cancer. A Clinical Epidemiological Approach on Diagnosis and Treatment.* Dissertation, Faculty of Medicine, University of Oslo, 2007.
33. Camatte S, Morice P, Thoury A, et al. Impact of surgical staging in patients with macroscopic "stage I" ovarian borderline tumours: analysis of a continuous series of 101 cases. *Eur J Cancer.* 2004;40(12):1842–1849.
34. Cadron I, Leunen K, Van Gorp T, Amant F, Neven P, Vergote I. Management of borderline ovarian neoplasms. *J Clin Oncol.* 2007;25(20):2928–2937.
35. Tropé CG, Kristensen G, Makar A. Surgery for borderline tumor of the ovary. *Semin Surg Oncol.* 2000;19(1):69–75.
36. Tempfer CB, Polterauer S, Bentz EK, Reinthaller A, Hefler LA. Accuracy of intraoperative frozen section analysis in borderline tumors of the ovary: a retrospective analysis of 96 cases and review of the literature. *Gynecol Oncol.* 2007;107(2):248–252.
37. Cadron I, Amant F, Van Gorp T, Neven P, Leunen K, Vergote I. The management of borderline tumours of the ovary. *Curr Opin Oncol.* 2006;18(5):488–493.
38. Deffieux X, Morice P, Camatte S, Fourchotte V, Duvillard P, Castaigne D. Results after laparoscopic management of serous borderline tumor of the ovary with peritoneal implants. *Gynecol Oncol.* 2005;97(1):84–89.
39. Fauvet R, Boccara J, Dufournet C, Poncelet C, Daraï E. Laparoscopic management of borderline ovarian tumors: results of a French multicenter study. *Ann Oncol.* 2005;16(3):403–410.
40. Vandenput I, Amant F, Vergote I. Peritoneal recurrences might be less common in advanced stage serous borderline ovarian tumors that were treated by laparotomy. *Gynecol Oncol.* 2005;98(3):523; author reply 524–525.
41. Gershenson DM. Clinical management potential tumours of low malignancy. *Best Pract Res Clin Obstet Gynaecol.* 2002;16(4):513–527.
42. Leake JF, Currie JL, Rosenshein NB, Woodruff JD. Long-term follow-up of serous ovarian tumors of low malignant potential. *Gynecol Oncol.* 1992;47(2):150–158.
43. Lim-Tan SK, Cajigas HE, Scully RE. Ovarian cystectomy for serous borderline tumors: a follow-up study of 35 cases. *Obstet Gynecol.* 1988;72(5):775–781.
44. Fauvet R, Poncelet C, Boccara J, Descamps P, Fondrinier E, Daraï E. Fertility after conservative treatment for borderline ovarian tumors: a French multicenter study. *Fertil Steril.* 2005;83(2):284–290; quiz 525.
45. Morris RT, Gershenson DM, Silva EG, Follen M, Morris M, Wharton JT. Outcome and reproductive function after conservative surgery for borderline ovarian tumors. *Obstet Gynecol.* 2000;95(4):541–547.
46. Gotlieb WH, Flikker S, Davidson B, Korach Y, Kopolovic J, Ben-Baruch G. Borderline tumors of the ovary: fertility treatment, conservative management, and pregnancy outcome. *Cancer.* 1998;82(1):141–146.
47. Fasouliotis SJ, Davis O, Schattman G, Spandorfer SD, Kligman I, Rosenwaks Z. Safety and efficacy of infertility treatment after conservative management of borderline ovarian tumors: a preliminary report. *Fertil Steril.* 2004;82(3):568–572.
48. Kashyap S, Davis OK. Ovarian cancer and fertility medications: a critical appraisal. *Semin Reprod Med.* 2003;21(1):65–71.
49. Morice P, Camatte S, Wicart-Poque F, et al. Results of conservative management of epithelial malignant and borderline ovarian tumours. *Hum Reprod Update.* 2003;9(2):185–192.
50. Whittemore AS, Harris R, Itnyre J. Characteristics relating to ovarian cancer risk: collaborative analysis of 12 US case-control studies. II. Invasive epithelial ovarian cancers in white women. Collaborative Ovarian Cancer Group. *Am J Epidemiol.* 1992;136(10):1184–1203.
51. Fortin A, Morice P, Thoury A, Camatte S, Dhainaut C, Madelenat P. Impact of infertility drugs after treatment of borderline ovarian tumors: results of a retrospective multicenter study. *Fertil Steril.* 2007;87(3):591–596.
52. Burger CW, van de Swaluw A, Mooij TM, et al. Risk of borderline and invasive ovarian tumors after ovarian stimulation for in vitro fertilization in a large Dutch cohort after 15 years of follow-up. Abstracts presented for the 40th Annual Meeting of the Society of Gynecologic Oncologists February 2009 (abstract no 6). *Gynecol Oncol.* 2009;112(Suppl.):S4.

53. Morice P, Camatte S, El Hassan J, Pautier P, Duvillard P, Castaigne D. Clinical outcomes and fertility after conservative treatment of ovarian borderline tumors. *Fertil Steril.* 2001;75(1): 92–96.

54. Beiner ME, Gotlieb WH, Davidson B, Kopolovic J, Ben-Baruch G. Infertility treatment after conservative management of borderline ovarian tumors. *Cancer.* 2001;92(2):320–325.

55. Donnez J, Dolmans MM, Demylle D, et al. Livebirth after orthotopic transplantation of cryopreserved ovarian tissue. *Lancet.* 2004;364(9443):1405–1410.

56. Gershenson DM, Silva EG. Serous ovarian tumors of low malignant potential with peritoneal implants. *Cancer.* 1990;65(3): 578–585.

57. Zanetta G, Rota S, Chiari S, Bonazzi C, Bratina G, Mangioni C. Behavior of borderline tumors with particular interest to persistence, recurrence, and progression to invasive carcinoma: a prospective study. *J Clin Oncol.* 2001;19(10):2658–2664.

58. Fauvet R, Boccara J, Dufournet C, David-Montefiore E, Poncelet C, Daraï E. Restaging surgery for women with borderline ovarian tumors: results of a French multicenter study. *Cancer.* 2004;100(6):1145–1151.

59. Zapardiel I, Rosenberg P, Peiretti M, et al. The role of restaging borderline ovarian tumors: single institution experience and review of the literature. *Gynecol Oncol.* 2010;119(2):274–277.

60. Tropé CG, Kaern J, Davidson B. Borderline ovarian tumours. *Best Pract Res Clin Obstet Gynaecol.* 2012;26(3):325–336.

Germ Cell Tumors
of the Ovary

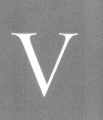

19 Germ Cell Tumors of the Ovary: Multidisciplinary Approach to Diagnosis and Treatment

MICHAEL A. BIDUS

JAY E. ALLARD

ELIZABETH A. DUBIL

■ INTRODUCTION

Germ cell tumors (GCT) represent a relatively small proportion (20%) of all ovarian tumors. There is a bimodal age distribution of GCT, with one peak occurring in infancy and a second peak occurring after the onset of puberty and extending into the second, and third decades of life. Ninety-seven percent of GCT are benign and 3% are malignant. Three percent of all malignant tumors occurring in children less than 15 years of age are GCT, with an estimated childhood incidence of 0.6 per 100,000 children less than the age of 15 (1). Unlike other ovarian malignancies, which occur predominantly in the fifth and sixth decades of life or older, GCT are far more likely to occur in reproductive age women. Not surprisingly, GCT are commonly diagnosed during pregnancy. Dysgerminomas and teratomas are the most common GCT diagnosed during pregnancy or shortly after delivery. Fortunately, malignant GCT have very favorable long-term outcomes when treated with modern surgical management and platinum-based chemotherapy. Even patients with incompletely resected or advanced stage disease are expected to have long-term survival approaching 80%. Given these clinical characteristics, the diagnosis and management of GCT involves a unique multidisciplinary approach in order to preserve reproductive potential and minimize long-term treatment-related morbidity.

■ MULTIDISCIPLINARY APPROACH TO DIAGNOSIS

Pathology

As a group, ovarian GCT consist of several histologically different tumor types that are all derived from primitive germ cells of the embryonic gonad (Figure 19.1). This classification system has evolved over the last 60 years and is based on the common histogenesis of these neoplasms, the presence of histologically different neoplastic elements within the same tumor, the presence of histologically similar neoplasms in extragonadal locations along the migratory pathway of primitive germ cells from the wall of the yolk sac to the gonadal ridge, and the relative homology between various tumors in males and females (2). In fact, this homology is illustrated no better in any other group of gonadal neoplasms (3). The similarity between the testicular seminoma and the ovarian dysgerminoma is an excellent case in point. These were the first neoplasms that were noted to originate from germ cells. Since their original description, the classification system for ovarian GCT has matured from that originally described by Teilum to one that is similar to that proposed by the World Health Organization (WHO), which divides the germ cell neoplasms into several groups and includes neoplasms composed of germ cells as well as sex-cord stromal derivatives (Table 19.1).

Two classes of GCT exist based upon their degree of differentiation. These are the undifferentiated GCT, which include dysgerminoma and gonadoblastoma and the differentiated GCT, which include all other types. Differentiated tumors are further classified based on their histologic distinction into embryonic or extraembryonic structures. Embryonic tumors include embryonal carcinoma, polyembryoma, and teratomas that may be mature, immature, or highly specialized. Extraembryonic tumors include choriocarcinoma and endodermal sinus tumor (yolk sac tumor). Additionally, it is important to note that GCT behave clinically, in part, on whether they are histologically pure, consisting of only one cell type, or mixed, consisting of multiple cell types. Clinical behavior typically follows the most aggressive histologic subtype that is present within the tumor. Treatment, therefore, needs to be tailored based upon this knowledge. Additionally, knowledge of the classification of these lesions and how the pathologist arrives at the diagnosis, as well as the clinical significance of that diagnosis, is extremely important to the practicing clinician.

Radiology

Different radiological findings are exhibited by various ovarian GCT and help to differentiate them into

161

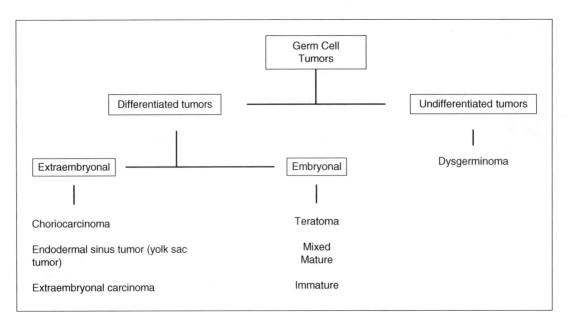

FIGURE 19.1 Classification of GCT based on differentiation

■ **Table 19.1** Classification of germ cell neoplasms of the ovary

Germ cell tumors
Dysgerminoma
Endodermal sinus tumor (yolk sac tumor)
Embryonal carcinoma
Polyembryoma
Choriocarcinoma
Teratoma
   Immature (solid, cystic, or both)
   Mature
      Solid
      Cystic
         Mature cystic teratoma (dermoid cyst)
         Mature cystic teratoma (dermoid cyst) with
           malignant transformation
   Highly specialized (monodermal)
      Struma ovarii
      Carcinoid
      Struma ovarii and carcinoid
      Other
Mixed forms (tumors composed of the above types in any
   possible combination)
Tumors composed of germ cells and sex-cord stromal
   derivatives
Gonadoblastoma
Mixed germ cell sex-cord stromal tumor

dysgerminomas and nondysgerminomas. Dysgerminomas are typically characterized as multiloculated solid masses that are divided by fibrovascular septa on CT and MRI (4). Calcifications are rare in dysgerminomas, however, when present they appear in a speckled ring-like or stippled pattern (5–7). Nondysgerminomas typically have a mixed solid and cystic pattern and are most often unilateral (8). Immature teratomas are typically large, heterogeneous, irregular masses with solid and cystic components on CT and MRI (9). Coarse calcifications can be seen in up to 40% of cases, with areas of fat and hemorrhage. Hemorrhage and necrosis are more common in choriocarcinomas and yolk sac tumors. Abdominal and pelvic lymphadenopathy, peritoneal and omental disease, and liver metastasis can be seen with all types of malignant ovarian GCT. Additionally, a radiograph of the chest is useful because of the propensity of GCT to metastasize to the lungs or mediastinum (10).

Positron emission tomography (PET scan) is a relatively new imaging modality. Although there are no studies using PET scanning in malignant ovarian GCT, there are data from the testicular GCT literature that may be applicable to their ovarian counterparts. PET is particularly useful in evaluating posttherapy residual masses in testicular GCT where the sensitivity, specificity, positive, and negative predictive values of PET scans compared to conventional CT scan are 80%, 100%, 100%, and 96%, respectively. This was seen in a study of testicular seminomas by De Santis et al (11). The low negative predictive value of the PET scan (76%) in initial staging of testicular GCT precludes its use in the initial management of GCT (12). Additionally, a negative PET scan may not have sufficient prognostic value to stratify treatment in patients with nonseminomatous testicular tumors, as shown in a study by Huddart et al (13). For this group of patients with clinical Stage I tumors, postsurgery PET identified additional disease in 21% of patients, however 40% of the patients who were PET negative and went on to surveillance subsequently relapsed. The utility of PET for evaluating ovarian GCT is still in its infancy.

■ MULTIDISCIPLINARY APPROACH TO TREATMENT

Surgery

The initial approach to patients with a suspected diagnosis of GCT is surgical. Surgery offers accurate diagnosis and in many cases is the only therapy required. The extent of surgery performed is dictated by the reproductive desires of the patient and the findings at surgery. In patients who have benign GCT, simple cystectomy with ovarian preservation is sufficient therapy. For all patients with malignant GCT, appropriate surgical management is full surgical staging according to the International Federation of Gynecologists and Obstetrician (FIGO) surgical staging guidelines. The importance of surgical staging is paramount, as additional treatment decisions are predicated in large measure by the surgical stage. For patients who have no future childbearing desires, full surgical staging with hysterectomy and bilateral salpingo-oophorectomy is usually performed.

Patients with malignant GCT who desire preservation of fertility should undergo full surgical staging followed by a unilateral salpingo-oophorectomy. The safety of this approach is well established. Recently, several investigators have evaluated the safety of ovarian cystectomy as opposed to unilateral salpingo-oophorectomy in select patients. While not considered the standard of care, early published results are promising and encouraging. Beiner et al (14) retrospectively reviewed eight cases of pure immature teratoma of all grades treated with cystectomy alone. Five of the eight cases received adjuvant therapy. After 4.7 years of follow-up, there were no recurrences and seven babies born to three of the eight patients. All patients in this series had immature teratomas, Grades 1 to 3. There is currently no evidence that cystectomy for other malignant histologic subtypes of GCT is adequate therapy or a safe surgical approach. In all cases where conservative fertility-sparing procedures are performed, the contralateral ovary must be closely inspected. Although dysgerminomas are the only malignant GCT that has the propensity to occur bilaterally (10%–20% of cases), all histologic subtypes of malignant GCT have been reported to occur bilaterally. Random contralateral ovarian biopsy and bivalving normal contralateral ovaries is no longer recommended due to concerns regarding hemorrhage and the development of adhesive disease. Only contralateral ovaries that are suspicious or grossly abnormal should undergo biopsy. (3)

Similar to epithelial ovarian cancer, the surgical tenet of maximal attempt at cytoreduction to no gross residual disease is valid for patients with advanced stage malignant GCT and should be vigorously pursued. There are no randomized trials to support this contention; however, the Gynecologic Oncology Group (GOG; 15) reported that patients with completely resected malignant GCT failed adjuvant VAC (Vincristine, Dactinomycin, Cyclophosphamide) therapy in 28% of cases compared to 68% of patients with incompletely resected disease. 82% of patients with bulky residual disease failed therapy compared with 55% of patients who had minimal residual disease. In another GOG trial (16), patients without measurable disease at the conclusion of surgery remained progression free in 65% of cases, compared to 34% with measurable disease (in spite of all patients receiving PVB—Cisplatin, Vinblastine, Bleomycin). These trials are interesting; however, neither PVB nor VAC are first-line chemotherapeutic regimens of choice in modern practice. The only published trial utilizing BEP (Bleomycin, Etoposide, Cisplatin) showed that completely resected Stage II and III patients with GCT who were treated with adjuvant BEP, had the same outcomes as patients whose disease was confined to the ovary (17). These three trials all support maximal attempts at cytoreduction.

Patients who desire fertility preservation but who are found at surgery to have bulky metastatic disease may have preservation of the uterus and contralateral ovary if these organs are uninvolved with disease. Multiple clinical trials have shown that such an approach is safe and that the ability to conceive is preserved. In Tangir's series (18), 10 patients with Stage III disease had fertility preserving surgery. Eight of the 10 patients went on to conceive. Zanetta et al reported on 81 patients with GCT of advanced stage, all received fertility-sparing surgery and were treated with postoperative chemotherapy (19). Fifty-seven similar patients received radical surgery. Overall survival was comparable between the two groups. Low et al reported on 15 patients with Stage III or IV disease treated conservatively. Ninety-four percent of patients were alive after 52 months of follow-up, similar to historical controls (20).

Similar to epithelial ovarian cancer, the value of second-look laparotomy (SLL) is unknown. Unfortunately, limited literature is available to explore the merits of SLL. The GOG reported their experience with SLL in GCT (21). Forty-three out of 45 patients who had complete tumor resection at initial surgery followed by BEP chemotherapy had either no disease on SLL, or mature elements only. Of the patients who had incompletely resected disease without teratomatous elements (48 patients), 45 were found to have no disease on SLL. The three patients with residual disease all died from disease. Second-look laparotomy is a meaningful procedure only when adequate additional therapy is available should the SLL procedure be positive for residual disease. Therefore, there is clearly no benefit of SLL in either of these two subsets of patients. Only patients who had incomplete resection at primary surgery and who had immature elements on primary pathology were found to have possibly benefitted from SLL. It is this subset of patients who, upon finding residual mature teratomas or bulky disease, may benefit from secondary cytoreduction surgery.

Secondary cytoreduction in malignant GCT patients has not been studied. As noted in the following section on chemotherapy, malignant GCT are usually responsive to combination chemotherapy even in the recurrent setting. As a result, it is unlikely that secondary cytoreduction would offer substantial benefit over additional chemotherapy alone. For patients with isolated recurrences secondary cytoreduction is likely to be beneficial. There is no known value of secondary cytoreduction for patients with platinum-resistant disease.

Chemotherapy

The current standard of care for malignant ovarian GCT is complete surgical staging and debulking followed by chemotherapy. In select GCT (Stage 1A Grade 1 immature teratomas and Stage 1A dysgerminomas) chemotherapy may be safely omitted as the recurrence risk is negligible and recurrence, when it occurs, is highly salvageable with chemotherapy. All other GCT require adjuvant chemotherapy. The most commonly used chemotherapeutic regimen is three to four cycles of BEP (Table 19.2; 17,22). Historically, the overall survival rate for malignant GCT, regardless of modality of treatment, was 30% (23). The first advancement in chemotherapeutic treatment for GCT came from the development of effective chemotherapy for testicular GCT (24,25). Subsequently, VAC or VAC-like regimens were adopted for treatment of ovarian GCT. Cure rates, however, although high in Stage I tumors, were only 50% for women with advanced-stage tumors (26) and 32% for women with incompletely resected tumors (15).

The second advancement came from the addition of platinum-based chemotherapy, showing a 70% 4-year overall survival rate, which was an improvement over VAC chemotherapy (16). PVB became the standard chemotherapeutic regimen. However, despite improvements in overall survival, recurrences still occurred in not only patients with poor prognostic features, but also those with favorable characteristics. PVB was eventually abandoned for a less neurotoxic combination of BEP.

Not surprisingly, BEP has been associated with significant toxicity. Reducing chemotherapy to two drugs, etoposide and cisplatin (EP) for four cycles has proven equivalent efficacy to three cycles of BEP in testicular cancer (27,28). The Southeastern Cancer Study Group and

Indiana University compared three cycles of BEP to four cycles in minimal to moderate extent disseminated GCT proving the two regimens to be equivalent with regards to disease-free status and relapses (29). Dimopoulos used three cycles in 48 patients with Stage I to Stage III ovarian tumors and showed an overall 95% 5-year disease-free survival (DFS; 30). Not all studies however, have shown equivalency. De Wit et al evaluated the importance of bleomycin in a randomized study of 395 patients with good prognosis nonseminomatous testicular tumors. Two hundred patients received BEP compared to 195 patients with EP only. Both regimens showed equivalent rates of progression and survival but a decreased complete response in the EP arm (87%) compared to the BEP arm (95%; 31). Clearly controversial, most oncologists treating malignant ovarian GCT recognize the importance of bleomycin and are reticent to jettison bleomycin in the absence of compelling clinical efficacy data in the ovarian GCT population. It is notable that despite cited evidence for testicular GCT, there are no studies comparing EP to BEP in ovarian tumors. EP exposes patients to a higher cumulative cisplatin dose with resultant long-term side effects. The only benefit to the EP regimen is avoiding possible pulmonary fibrosis, which in patients without baseline lung dysfunction, is rare (32). Grade 3 and Grade 4 pulmonary toxicity was reported to occur in 1%–2% of patients (over 800 patients treated) with three cycles of BEP (33).

The addition of paclitaxel to BEP (T-BEP) showed favorable results in a Phase I/II trial (34,35); however, in Phase III testing, statistical superiority of T-BEP could not be shown due to inclusion of good prognosis and poor prognosis patients. Eligibility criteria was defined as intermediate-prognosis metastatic GCT according to International Germ Cell Cancer Consensus (Table 19.3). There were also accrual difficulties with this trial for multiple reasons cited in the original paper. Of the needed 498 patients, 377 were enrolled. PFS at 3 years with

---

■ Table 19.3 Intermediate-prognosis metastatic germ cell tumors

Nonseminoma	Seminoma
• A testis or retroperitoneal primary tumor	• Any primary site
• AFP >1000 but <10,000 U/L, hcG >5000 but <50,000 U/L, or LDH >1.5 but <10× the upper limit of normal	• Any LDH, any hcG
• No liver, bone, brain, or other nonpulmonary visceral metastases	• Nonpulmonary visceral metastases present
	• AFP within normal range

AFP, alpha fetoprotein; hcG, human chorionic gonadotropin; LDH, lactate dehydrogenase.

■ Table 19.2 BEP regimen

Cisplatin	20 mg/m^2 days 1–5
Etoposide	100 mg/m^2 days 1–5
Bleomycin	30 units weekly

Note: Three to four cycles given at 21-day intervals.

(intention to treat) was 79.4% in the T-BEP arm and 71% in the BEP arm, which was not statistically significant. However, when a secondary analysis that excluded good and poor prognosis patients was done, T-BEP showed a 12% superior 3-year progression-free survival (PFS) 82% vs 70%. Hematopoietic growth factors should be used if this regimen is attempted (36). There is currently no defined role for a more aggressive regimen of chemotherapy for GCT patients.

Patients With Intermediate or Poor Prognosis Tumor

Patients with metastatic disease (advanced stage), incompletely resected disease, and high tumor markers show a worse prognosis with PFS in all GCT except dysgerminoma; however, there is no dependable risk-stratification schema for ovarian tumor patients (30,37–39).

Residual and Recurrent Disease

Disease recurrence in the germ cell setting is classified as platinum resistant/refractory and platinum sensitive. Platinum sensitive is defined as disease recurrence greater than 4 weeks from the completion of primary chemotherapy. There is no universally accepted definition in malignant GCT for platinum resistance; however, inability to achieve a complete response to BEP therapy or relapse within 4 weeks of platinum-based therapy is a useful clinical definition for resistance. Platinum-resistant disease is not thought to be curable, with only a 30% complete remission rate with high-dose salvage therapy as opposed to 60% or better in platinum sensitive tumors (22). Additionally, long-term survival in the platinum-resistant setting is rare, occurring in less than 10% of cases.

Most (90%) recurrences of malignant GCT usually occur within 2 years of primary therapy and are salvageable. Patients who recur and have never been treated with chemotherapy should be treated with standard BEP. Active second-line therapies after failure to cure with BEP include cisplatin and ifosfamide plus either vinblastine (40) or paclitaxel (41), or high-dose chemotherapy with marrow or peripheral stem cell transplantation (HDCT; 42). HDCT is more commonly used in patients who are cisplatin refractory. Refractory or resistant patients should be enrolled in clinical trials of new agents whenever possible, as outcomes with current regimens are poor. Patients who progress after second-line therapy or HDCT can be treated with paclitaxel and gemcitabine salvage therapy. In a Phase II trial published by Einhorn et al, complete response was achieved in 18.7% with 31% of patients achieving objective responses (43).

Immediate and Long-Term Toxicity

Treatable immediate toxicities of chemotherapies for GCT include bone marrow suppression, febrile neutropenia, and nausea. Nausea can be easily prevented and treated with a thorough antiemetic regimen. Patients with poor hematologic parameters are typically given treatment regardless of laboratory values as cycle timing has been associated with outcomes in testicular tumors. Hematopoietic growth factors are typically not needed as most patients will not develop fever or infection (44). If fever or infection develops, or if HDCT is used, it is reasonable to use growth factors as opposed to dose reduction.

Late complications of chemotherapy must be considered as a large number of patients achieve cure. Acute myelogenous leukemia (AML) has been associated with etoposide use and is dose and schedule dependent. AML has rarely been associated with less than three cycles or cumulative dose less than 2000 mg/m^2 with an incidence of 0.4% (45,46). Studies of AML risk with HDCT also show a cumulative incidence of 0.5%–1.3%, which for most is an acceptably low risk-to-benefit ratio for high-dose etoposide-based therapy (47,48).

Bleomycin has been associated with pulmonary toxicity. In one study of 96 patients, 14.6% developed pulmonary toxicity, equally distributed between pulmonary fibrosis, pneumonia, and nonspecific interstitial pneumonitis. A significant relationship was found between these toxicities and age, cumulative dose, and starting GFR (49). Patients older than 50, heavy tobacco use, or patients with creatinine higher than 2 mg/100 mL are at higher risk for toxicity and may benefit from EP therapy only (32). Mitigating pulmonary toxicity risk by dropping bleomycin from the combination regimen must be balanced with the potential for decreased complete response to treatment.

Women who have fertility-sparing surgery can, for the most part, expect return of menstrual function and minimal effect on gonadal function, even in adolescents undergoing treatment prior to menarche (50). However, persistent amenorrhea occurs in 2%–15% of patients (Table 19.4). The risk of persistent amenorrhea is thought to be related to ovarian reserve at the beginning of therapy; however, there are no studies evaluating causes of persistent amenorrhea. In an attempt to avoid chemotherapy induced persistent amenorrhea, all patients should be give ovarian suppression during therapy. Hormonal suppression can be achieved with daily oral contraceptive pills (51), or subcutaneous and intramuscular gonadotropin-releasing hormone (GnRH) agonists. Intranasal GnRH agonists have not proven effective for ovarian protection. (52)

There are many options available for women with diminished ovarian reserve prior to chemotherapy who desire future fertility. These include ovarian tissue freezing (if the contralateral ovary was not affected) with reimplantation, oocyte freezing, embryo freezing, donor egg, surrogacy, in vitro fertilization (IVF), and adoption. Patients should be referred to a reproductive endocrinologist for

■ Table 19.4 Oncologic and obstetric outcomes in patients with malignant germ cell tumors treated conservatively

Author	Patients	Resumption of Menses (%)	Pregnancies	Live Births	SAB (% of Pregnancies)	Recurrences	Deaths	Chemo
Gershenson (67)	40	67	22	22		3	2	VAC
Kanazawa et al (68)	21	85	11	9	18	1	1	Multiple
Low et al. (69)	74	91	19	14		7	2	
Gershenson et al (55)	71	87	37	30	5.5	10	4	BEP, PVB
Zanetta et al (19)	138	99	41	28	22	16	3	
Perrin et al (70)	45		8	7		4	2	
Tangir et al (18)	64		47	38	4.2	5	3	VAC, BEP, PVB
De La Motte et al (54)[a]	41	97	19	12	11	4	3	BEP
Nishio et al (50)	30	93	8	7		0	0	VAC, BEP, PVB
Weinberg et al (51)	40	100	11	14	0	3	0	BEP, VAC
Total	564		223 (40%)	181 (81%)		53 (9%)	20 (3.5%)	

[a]Yolk sac tumors only.

Modified from Eskander et al (66).

management. Success rates and costs vary from center to center. The feasibility of the above options must be weighed against the need for immediate surgery or treatment.

Obstetrical outcomes for patients treated with fertility-sparing surgery and chemotherapy appear to be similar to that of the normal population. The spontaneous abortion rate in pregnancies occurring after the completion of chemotherapy ranges from 4.2% to 22%, no higher than in the general population, which is 12% for women younger than 20 years and 26% for women over 40 years old (53). Only one study reported associated fetal malformations (19). Although all other reports documented normal infants, several made reference to elective termination rates ranging from 3% to 20% (18,19,54,55), but did not comment on reason for termination, so it is unknown if identified malformations contributed to the termination rates in these studies.

Pediatric Considerations

In the pediatric population, a strong case has been made for a "watch and wait" protocol for all Stage I tumors regardless of histology by the United Kingdom Children's Cancer Study Group's second GCT study (GCII). Fifty-four patients in this series had ovarian GCT. Of those, 9 were treated initially with surgery alone for Stage I tumors. Six patients were cured by surgery alone and 3 recurred and were all salvaged by chemotherapy (56).

In the pediatric population, new advances have been made with less toxic first-line adjuvant therapy, and withholding adjuvant therapy in any Stage I tumors. Unlike adult testicular and GCT, pediatric GCT tend to act similarly regardless of location of tumor, and generalization between testicular and ovarian tumors can more readily be made. Although many similarities exist between adult testicular and ovarian tumors, not all data are translational. Identical treatment algorithms and outcomes cannot be assumed.

Children with GCT have an excellent chance of being cured and more consideration needs to be given to the long-term side effects of chemotherapy. Cisplatin has been associated with hearing loss and renal toxicity. Rates of hearing loss range from 10% to 58% (57,58). Renal impairment is reported to range from 25% to 45% (57,59). In an attempt to eliminate cisplatin-related toxicity, the United Kingdom Children's Cancer Study investigated the substitution of carboplatin for cisplatin (Table 19.5). Thus far, there has been one report of severe deafness and no reports of significant renal toxicity, although the late-effects have not been published to date (56). Carboplatin was also substituted for pediatric tumors in the French GCT TGM90 study and was found to be inferior to cisplatin; however, a dose of 400 mg/m^2 was given once every 6 weeks in that study (60). Cisplatin is now used as a relapse treatment instead of first line in certain pediatric centers (56).

■ **Table 19.5** United Kingdom Children's Cancer Study Group Regimen: Carboplatin, etoposide, bleomycin (JEB)

Etoposide	120 mg/m² IV given over 1 hour on days 1 through 3
Carboplatin	600 mg/m² or 6× [uncorrected GFR + (15× surface area)] IV given over 1 hour on day 2. ªTarget: AUC 6
Bleomycin	15 mg/m² IV given over 15 minutes on day 3

ªFormulation has changed (65).
AUC, area under the curve; GFR, glomerular filtration rate.

Carboplatin has been shown to be inferior for adult GCT of the testis (61,62). Limited case series and retrospective reviews in adult GCT have shown no difference in outcome measures; however, there has been no prospective noninferiority trial (63,64).

■ **REFERENCES**

1. Kaatsch P, Kaletsch U, Michaelis J. *Annual Report of the German Childhood Cancer Registry.* I. Main, Germany: Deutsches Kinderkrebsregister; 2002.
2. Talerman A. Germ cell tumors of the ovary. In: Kurman RJ, ed. *Blaustein's Pathology of the Female Genital Tract*, 5th ed. New York, NY: Springer-Verlag; 2002:967–1033.
3. Bidus MA, Zahn CM, Rose GS. Germ cell, stromal, and other ovarian tumors. In: Disaia PJ, Creasman WT, eds. *Clinical Gynecologic Oncology*, 7th ed. Philadelphia, PA: Elsevier; 2007:369.
4. Ueno T, Tanaka YO, Nagata M, et al. Spectrum of germ cell tumors: from head to toe. *Radiographics*. 2004;24(2):387–404.
5. Brammer HM 3rd, Buck JL, Hayes WS, Sheth S, Tavassoli FA. From the archives of the AFIP. Malignant germ cell tumors of the ovary: radiologic-pathologic correlation. *Radiographics*. 1990;10(4):715–724.
6. Tanaka Y, Sasaki Y, Tachibana K, et al. Gonadal mixed germ cell tumor combined with a large hemangiomatous lesion in a patient with Turner's syndrome and 45,X/46,X, +mar karyotype. *Arch Pathol Lab Med*. 1994;118(11):1135–1138.
7. Rosado-de-Christenson ML, Templeton PA, Moran CA. From the archives of the AFIP. Mediastinal germ cell tumors: radiologic and pathologic correlation. *Radiographics*. 1992;12(5),1013–1030.
8. Parkinson CA, Hatcher HM, Earl HM, Ajithkumar TV. Multidisciplinary management of malignant ovarian germ cell tumours. *Gynecol Oncol*. 2011;121(3):625–636.
9. Levitt RG, Husband JE, Glazer HS. CT of primary germ-cell tumors of the mediastinum. *AJR Am J Roentgenol*. 1984;142(1):73–78.
10. Berek JS, Friedlander M, Hacker NF. Germ cell and other non-epithelial ovarian cancers. In: Berek JS, Hacker NF, eds. *Berek & Hacker's Gynecologic Oncology*, 5th ed. Philadelphia, PA: Lippincott Williams & Wilkins, 2010:509–535.
11. De Santis M, Becherer A, Bokemeyer C, et al. 2–18fluoro-deoxy-D-glucose positron emission tomography is a reliable predictor for viable tumor in postchemotherapy seminoma: an update of the prospective multicentric SEMPET trial. *J Clin Oncol*. 2004;22(6):1034–1039.
12. de Wit M, Hartmann M, Kotzerke J, et al. 18F-FDG-PET in clinical stage I and II non-seminomatous germ cell tumors: first results of the German Multicenter Trial. *J Clin Oncol*. 2005;23(16S):4504.
13. Huddart RA, O'Doherty MJ, Padhani A, et al.; NCRI Testis Tumour Clinical Study Group. 18fluorodeoxyglucose positron emission tomography in the prediction of relapse in patients with high-risk, clinical stage I nonseminomatous germ cell tumors: preliminary report of MRC Trial TE22–the NCRI Testis Tumour Clinical Study Group. *J Clin Oncol*. 2007;25(21):3090–3095.
14. Beiner ME, Gotlieb WH, Korach Y, et al. Cystectomy for immature teratoma of the ovary. *Gynecol Oncol*. 2004;93(2):381–384.
15. Slayton RE, Park RC, Silverberg SG, Shingleton H, Creasman WT, Blessing JA. Vincristine, dactinomycin, and cyclophosphamide in the treatment of malignant germ cell tumors of the ovary. A Gynecologic Oncology Group Study (a final report). *Cancer*. 1985;56(2):243–248.
16. Williams SD, Blessing JA, Moore DH, Homesley HD, Adcock L. Cisplatin, vinblastine, and bleomycin in advanced and recurrent ovarian germ-cell tumors. A trial of the Gynecologic Oncology Group. *Ann Intern Med*. 1989;111(1):22–27.
17. Williams S, Blessing JA, Liao SY, Ball H, Hanjani P. Adjuvant therapy of ovarian germ cell tumors with cisplatin, etoposide, and bleomycin: a trial of the Gynecologic Oncology Group. *J Clin Oncol*. 1994;12(4):701–706.
18. Tangir J, Zelterman D, Ma W, Schwartz PE. Reproductive function after conservative surgery and chemotherapy for malignant germ cell tumors of the ovary. *Obstet Gynecol*. 2003;101(2):251–257.
19. Zanetta G, Bonazzi C, Cantù M, et al. Survival and reproductive function after treatment of malignant germ cell ovarian tumors. *J Clin Oncol*. 2001;19(4):1015–1020.
20. Low JJ, Perrin LC, Crandon AJ, Hacker NF. Conservative surgery to preserve ovarian function in patients with malignant ovarian germ cell tumors. A review of 74 cases. *Cancer*. 2000;89(2):391–398.
21. Williams SD, Blessing JA, DiSaia PJ, Major FJ, Ball HG 3rd, Liao SY. Second-look laparotomy in ovarian germ cell tumors: the gynecologic oncology group experience. *Gynecol Oncol*. 1994;52(3):287–291.
22. Barakat RR, Markman M, Randall M, *Principles and Practice of Gynecologic Oncology*, 5th ed. Philadelphia, PA: Wolters Kluwer Health/Lippincott Williams & Wilkins, 2009:1072.
23. Li MC, Hsu KP. Combined drug therapy for ovarian carcinoma. *Clin Obstet Gynecol*. 1970;13(4):928–944.
24. Einhorn LH, Donohue J. Cis-diamminedichloroplatinum, vinblastine, and bleomycin combination chemotherapy in disseminated testicular cancer. *Ann Intern Med*. 1977;87(3):293–298.
25. Williams SD, Birch R, Einhorn LH, Irwin L, Greco FA, Loehrer PJ. Treatment of disseminated germ-cell tumors with cisplatin, bleomycin, and either vinblastine or etoposide. *N Engl J Med*. 1987;316(23):1435–1440.
26. Gershenson DM, Copeland LJ, Kavanagh JJ, et al. Treatment of malignant nondysgerminomatous germ cell tumors of the ovary with vincristine, dactinomycin, and cyclophosphamide. *Cancer*. 1985;56(12):2756–2761.
27. Kondagunta GV, Bacik J, Bajorin D, et al. Etoposide and cisplatin chemotherapy for metastatic good-risk germ cell tumors. *J Clin Oncol*. 2005;23(36):9290–9294.
28. Xiao H, Mazumdar M, Bajorin DF, et al. Long-term follow-up of patients with good-risk germ cell tumors treated with etoposide and cisplatin. *J Clin Oncol*. 1997;15(7):2553–2558.
29. Einhorn LH, Williams SD, Loehrer PJ, et al. Evaluation of optimal duration of chemotherapy in favorable-prognosis disseminated germ cell tumors: a Southeastern Cancer Study Group protocol. *J Clin Oncol*. 1989;7(3):387–391.
30. Dimopoulos MA, Papadimitriou C, Hamilos G, et al. Treatment of ovarian germ cell tumors with a 3-day bleomycin, etoposide, and cisplatin regimen: a prospective multicenter study. *Gynecol Oncol*. 2004;95(3):695–700.
31. de Wit R, Stoter G, Kaye SB, et al. Importance of bleomycin in combination chemotherapy for good-prognosis testicular non-seminoma: a randomized study of the European Organization for

Research and Treatment of Cancer Genitourinary Tract Cancer Cooperative Group. *J Clin Oncol.* 1997;15(5):1837–1843.

32. Einhorn LH, Foster RS. Bleomycin, etoposide, and cisplatin for three cycles compared with etoposide and cisplatin for four cycles in good-risk germ cell tumors: is there a preferred regimen? *J Clin Oncol.* 2006;24(16):2597–8; author reply 2598.

33. de Wit R, Roberts JT, Wilkinson PM, et al. Equivalence of three or four cycles of bleomycin, etoposide, and cisplatin chemotherapy and of a 3- or 5-day schedule in good-prognosis germ cell cancer: a randomized study of the European Organization for Research and Treatment of Cancer Genitourinary Tract Cancer Cooperative Group and the Medical Research Council. *J Clin Oncol.* 2001;19(6):1629–1640.

34. de Wit R, Louwerens M, de Mulder PH, Verweij J, Rodenhuis S, Schornagel J. Management of intermediate-prognosis germ-cell cancer: results of a phase I/II study of Taxol-BEP. *Int J Cancer.* 1999;83(6):831–833.

35. Mardiak J, Sálek T, Sycová-Milá Z, et al. Paclitaxel, bleomycin, etoposide, and cisplatin (T-BEP) as initial treatment in patients with poor-prognosis germ cell tumors (GCT): a phase II study. *Neoplasma.* 2007;54(3):240–245.

36. de Wit R, Skoneczna I, Daugaard G, et al. Randomized phase III study comparing paclitaxel-bleomycin, etoposide, and cisplatin (BEP) to standard BEP in intermediate-prognosis germ-cell cancer: intergroup study EORTC 30983. *J Clin Oncol.* 2012;30(8):792–799.

37. Gershenson DM, Copeland LJ, del Junco G, Edwards CL, Wharton JT, Rutledge FN. Second-look laparotomy in the management of malignant germ cell tumors of the ovary. *Obstet Gynecol.* 1986;67(6):789–793.

38. Norris HJ, Zirkin HJ, Benson WL. Immature (malignant) teratoma of the ovary: a clinical and pathologic study of 58 cases. *Cancer.* 1976;37(5):2359–2372.

39. Murugaesu N, Schmid P, Dancey G, et al. Malignant ovarian germ cell tumors: identification of novel prognostic markers and long-term outcome after multimodality treatment. *J Clin Oncol.* 2006;24(30):4862–4866.

40. Loehrer PJ Sr, Gonin R, Nichols CR, Weathers T, Einhorn LH. Vinblastine plus ifosfamide plus cisplatin as initial salvage therapy in recurrent germ cell tumor. *J Clin Oncol.* 1998;16(7):2500–2504.

41. Kondagunta GV, Bacik J, Donadio A, et al. Combination of paclitaxel, ifosfamide, and cisplatin is an effective second-line therapy for patients with relapsed testicular germ cell tumors. *J Clin Oncol.* 2005;23(27):6549–6555.

42. Bhatia S, Abonour R, Porcu P, et al. High-dose chemotherapy as initial salvage chemotherapy in patients with relapsed testicular cancer. *J Clin Oncol.* 2000;18(19):3346–3351.

43. Einhorn LH, Brames MJ, Juliar B, Williams SD. Phase II study of paclitaxel plus gemcitabine salvage chemotherapy for germ cell tumors after progression following high-dose chemotherapy with tandem transplant. *J Clin Oncol.* 2007;25(5):513–516.

44. Oncology, A.S.o.C. Update of recommendations for the use of white blood cell growth factors: an evidence-based clinical practice guideline. *J Clin Oncol.* 2006;24(19):3187–3205.

45. Pedersen-Bjergaard J, Daugaard G, Hansen SW, Philip P, Larsen SO, Rørth M. Increased risk of myelodysplasia and leukaemia after etoposide, cisplatin, and bleomycin for germ-cell tumours. *Lancet.* 1991;338(8763):359–363.

46. Nichols CR, Breeden ES, Loehrer PJ, Williams SD, Einhorn LH. Secondary leukemia associated with a conventional dose of etoposide: review of serial germ cell tumor protocols. *J Natl Cancer Inst.* 1993;85(1):36–40.

47. Wierecky J, Kollmannsberger C, Boehlke I, et al. Secondary leukemia after first-line high-dose chemotherapy for patients with advanced germ cell cancer. *J Cancer Res Clin Oncol.* 2005;131(4):255–260.

48. Kollmannsberger C, Beyer J, Droz JP, et al. Secondary leukemia following high cumulative doses of etoposide in patients treated for advanced germ cell tumors. *J Clin Oncol.* 1998;16(10):3386–3391.

49. Usman M, Faruqui ZS, ud Din N, Zahid KF. Bleomycin induced pulmonary toxicity in patients with germ cell tumours. *J Ayub Med Coll Abbottabad.* 2010;22(3):35–37.

50. Nishio S, Ushijima K, Fukui A, et al. Fertility-preserving treatment for patients with malignant germ cell tumors of the ovary. *J Obstet Gynaecol Res.* 2006;32(4):416–421.

51. Weinberg LE, Lurain JR, Singh DK, Schink JC. Survival and reproductive outcomes in women treated for malignant ovarian germ cell tumors. *Gynecol Oncol.* 2011;121(2):285–289.

52. Chen H, Li J, Cui T, Hu L. Adjuvant gonadotropin-releasing hormone analogues for the prevention of chemotherapy induced premature ovarian failure in premenopausal women. *Cochrane Database Syst Rev.* 2011;9(11):CD008018.

53. Cunningham FG, Williams JW. *Williams Obstetrics.* 23rd ed. New York, NY: McGraw-Hill Medical; 2010:1385.

54. de La Motte Rouge T, Pautier P, Duvillard P, et al. Survival and reproductive function of 52 women treated with surgery and bleomycin, etoposide, cisplatin (BEP) chemotherapy for ovarian yolk sac tumor. *Ann Oncol.* 2008;19(8):1435–1441.

55. Gershenson DM, Miller AM, Champion VL, et al.; Gynecologic Oncology Group. Reproductive and sexual function after platinum-based chemotherapy in long-term ovarian germ cell tumor survivors: a Gynecologic Oncology Group study. *J Clin Oncol.* 2007;25(19):2792–2797.

56. Mann JR, Raafat F, Robinson K, et al. The United Kingdom Children's Cancer Study Group's second germ cell tumor study: carboplatin, etoposide, and bleomycin are effective treatment for children with malignant extracranial germ cell tumors, with acceptable toxicity. *J Clin Oncol.* 2000;18(22):3809–3818.

57. Mann JR, Pearson D, Barrett A, Raafat F, Barnes JM, Wallendszus KR. Results of the United Kingdom Children's Cancer Study Group's malignant germ cell tumor studies. *Cancer.* 1989;63(9):1657–1667.

58. Hale GA, Marina NM, Jones-Wallace D, et al. Late effects of treatment for germ cell tumors during childhood and adolescence. *J Pediatr Hematol Oncol.* 1999;21(2):115–122.

59. Göbel U, Calaminus G, Teske C, et al. [BEP/VIP in children and adolescents with malignant non-testicular germ cell tumors. A comparison of the results of treatment of therapy studies MAKEI 83/86 and 89P/89]. *Klin Padiatr.* 1993;205(4):231–240.

60. Baranzelli MC, Patte C, Bouffet E, et al. An attempt to treat pediatric intracranial alphaFP and betaHCG secreting germ cell tumors with chemotherapy alone. SFOP experience with 18 cases. Société Française d'Oncologie Pédiatrique. *J Neurooncol.* 1998;37(3):229–239.

61. Horwich A, Sleijfer DT, Fosså SD, et al. Randomized trial of bleomycin, etoposide, and cisplatin compared with bleomycin, etoposide, and carboplatin in good-prognosis metastatic nonseminomatous germ cell cancer: a Multiinstitutional Medical Research Council/European Organization for Research and Treatment of Cancer Trial. *J Clin Oncol.* 1997;15(5):1844–1852.

62. Bokemeyer C, Köhrmann O, Tischler J, et al. A randomized trial of cisplatin, etoposide and bleomycin (PEB) versus carboplatin, etoposide and bleomycin (CEB) for patients with "good-risk" metastatic non-seminomatous germ cell tumors. *Ann Oncol.* 1996;7(10):1015–1021.

63. Cheung MM, Lau WH, Chan M, et al. Experience with the management of ovarian germ cell tumors in Chinese patients. *Gynecol Oncol.* 1994;52(3):306–312.

64. Dimopoulos MA, Papadopoulou M, Andreopoulou E, et al. Favorable outcome of ovarian germ cell malignancies treated with cisplatin or carboplatin-based chemotherapy: a Hellenic Cooperative Oncology Group study. *Gynecol Oncol.* 1998;70(1):70–74.

65. Newell DR, Pearson AD, Balmanno K, et al. Carboplatin pharmacokinetics in children: the development of a pediatric dosing

formula. The United Kingdom Children's Cancer Study Group. *J Clin Oncol.* 1993;11(12):2314–2323.

66. Eskander RN, Randall LM, Berman ML, Tewari KS, Disaia PJ, Bristow RE. Fertility preserving options in patients with gynecologic malignancies. *Am J Obstet Gynecol.* 2011;205(2):103–110.

67. Gershenson DM. Menstrual and reproductive function after treatment with combination chemotherapy for malignant ovarian germ cell tumors. *J Clin Oncol.* 1988;6(2):270–275.

68. Kanazawa K, Suzuki T, Sakumoto K. Treatment of malignant ovarian germ cell tumors with preservation of fertility:

reproductive performance after persistent remission. *Am J Clin Oncol.* 2000;23(3):244–248.

69. Low JJ, Perrin LC, Crandon AJ, Hacker NF. Conservative surgery to preserve ovarian function in patients with malignant ovarian germ cell tumors. A review of 74 cases. *Cancer.* 2000;89(2):391–398.

70. Perrin LC, Low J, Nicklin JL, Ward BG, Crandon AJ. Fertility and ovarian function after conservative surgery for germ cell tumours of the ovary. *Aust N Z J Obstet Gynaecol.* 1999;39(2): 243–245.

20 | *Nonepithelial Ovarian Cancer*

WILLIAM E. WINTER, III

■ INTRODUCTION

Whereas epithelial ovarian cancers (EOC) make up the vast majority of the more than 20,000 new cases of ovarian cancer annually (1), there are a wide variety of rare ovarian cancers that together account for less than 10% of these cancers (2). These include germ cell, sex-cord stromal, and exceedingly rare ovarian tumors, such as lipoid tumors, ovarian sarcomas, and small cell carcinoma. This latter group makes up 0.1% of all ovarian malignancies and will not be covered in this chapter. Nonepithelial ovarian tumors share the same International Federation of Gynecology and Obstetrics (FIGO) staging system as their more common epithelial counterparts. The purpose of this chapter is to briefly describe the clinical presentation and current management of these rare ovarian tumors (see Chapter 19 for germ cell tumors of the ovary).

■ SEX-CORD STROMAL TUMORS

These uncommon tumors make up about 5% of all ovarian malignancies (2–5). Granulosa cell tumors (GCTs) are typically indolent tumors. Most thecomas and fibromas are benign, but can demonstrate sarcomatous characteristics. These are all derived from female mesenchymal tissue, whereas Sertoli-Leydig cell tumors resemble male mesenchymal tissue.

Granulosa Cell Tumors

GCTs are diagnosed in all age groups, even before puberty in 5% of cases (5,6). Most prepubertal girls exhibit sexual pseudoprecocity due to these estrogen-secreting tumors (5). GCTs are found in association with endometrial hyperplasia in about 20% and cancer in 5% of patients (3,5,6).

Women typically present with a unilateral ovarian mass. While CA125 may be elevated, there are two other useful markers—inhibin and Müllerian inhibitory substance (MIS) (7). MIS has a high specificity for GCT (8). Most GCTs are early stage at diagnosis. Though they tend to be indolent in nature, GCTs may still recur up to 30 years after original diagnosis (9). Estradiol levels have little utility in diagnosing or following these tumors. Initial management of these patients is surgical resection. In premenopausal women, fertility-sparing surgery (i.e., unilateral salpingo-oophorectomy) is recommended if they have not completed childbearing (9). If the uterus is spared dilatation and curettage is recommended to rule out concurrent endometrial cancer (6). In postmenopausal women or those who do not desire future fertility, standard of care is hysterectomy, bilateral salpingo-oophorectomy, and possible surgical staging. There is considerable debate regarding reoperating for complete staging, specifically lymph node dissection, on patients with incidentally diagnosed GCTs. Furthermore, there is some retrospective evidence that questions the need for standard lymph dissection even at the initial surgical diagnosis of clinically early stage tumors (10,11). It is reasonable to base this decision on the risk and clinical factors present for metastatic disease. Most oncologists recommend approaching clinically advanced disease similar to those with EOC—surgical cytoreduction—as complete resection of disease portends for improved clinical outcomes (10,12).

Given the rare incidence of GCTs, it is difficult to design randomized trials to definitively evaluate the efficacy of adjuvant therapy. Most gynecologic oncologists agree that there is no evidence of benefit for adjuvant therapy in Stage I patients, with the debatable exception of those patients with large tumor size, high mitotic rate, and/or tumor rupture (12). Clinical observation is recommended in low-risk early-stage patients. In terms of advanced or recurrent disease, radiation therapy may be useful in the treatment of pelvic recurrences, but is not typically recommended as adjuvant therapy for GCTs given mixed results (12). Chemotherapy has demonstrated significant improvement in progression-free survival (PFS) in the recurrent setting (13) and a trend toward improvement in the adjuvant setting, reaching significance in optimally debulked Stage III/IV patients receiving all of their planned therapy (10). However, adjuvant chemotherapy has yet to show an overall survival benefit (14). Regimens that have demonstrated activity are all platinum-based—bleomycin, etoposide, and cisplatin (BEP), etoposide and cisplatin (EP), and carboplatin/paclitaxel (10,12,15).

Prognosis of GCTs is associated with initial stage (5,6,10,12). Poor prognosis and early recurrences are also associated with cellular atypia, high mitotic rate, and the absence of Call-Exner bodies (11). Stage I tumors have up to a 92% cure rate (16), but can present with late recurrences as previously stated (6,17). Five-year overall survival rates of patients with Stage I disease is over 90%, while that of Stage II to Stage IV tumors is just above 50% (12).

Sertoli-Leydig Tumors

Sertoli-Leydig tumors (SLTs) are extremely rare and typically found as a benign incidental finding (3). Most malignant SLTs are low grade and follow an indolent course. Those rare tumors with high-grade histology tend to follow a more aggressive clinical course. These androgen-secreting tumors cause clinically evident virilization in over 25%–70% of patients (18,19).

Management of malignant SCTs includes unilateral salpingo-oophorectomy in premenopausal patients who desire future fertility. The incidence of bilateral tumors is less than 5% (4). In postmenopausal patients or those who have completed childbearing, hysterectomy and bilateral salpingo-oophorectomy is standard of care. Metastasis or recurrence in the lymph nodes is rare (20). Therefore, the necessity of standard lymph node dissection is questionable. Five-year survival is as high as 90% in Stage I tumors and, unlike GCTs, with very few late recurrences. Grades 2 and 3 histology are associated with poorer survival (18).

■ CONCLUSIONS

In addition to these tumors there are others to note. Small cell tumors and sarcomas have a particularly poor prognosis. There is also a reasonable incidence of metastatic tumors to the ovaries. Most commonly, other gynecologic tumors may metastasize to the ovary—tubal, endometrial, and less commonly cervical cancer. Nongynecologic tumors may also metastasize. Ovarian metastases from other nongynecologic tumors are seen in 7%–8% of patients thought to have a primary ovarian malignancy (21,22). In one series of 59 nongenital tract metastases, the authors found colon (32%), appendiceal (20%), and primary of unknown origin (17%) to be the most common nongynecologic malignancies metastatic to the ovary. Breast, gastric, small bowel, pancreatic, urinary bladder, and gallbladder should also be considered (21).

In conclusion, it will be difficult for one or a small number of institutions to perform clinically meaningful research to help outline the most appropriate management of these patients given the uncommon to rare incidence of these tumors. In recent years, co-operative groups, such as the Gynecologic Oncology Group (GOG), have started to focus on developing trials and studies of rare nonepithelial tumors. Until we are able to design an effective trial or prospective longitudinal study on a larger population, management of these patients will be the subject of continued debate.

■ REFERENCES

1. Siegel R, Ward E, Brawley O, Jemal A. Cancer statistics, 2011: the impact of eliminating socioeconomic and racial disparities on premature cancer deaths. *CA Cancer J Clin.* 2011;61(4):212–236.
2. Chen LM, Berek JS. Ovarian and fallopian tubes. In: Haskell CM, ed. *Cancer treatment.* 5th ed. Philadelphia, PA: WB Saunders; 2000:900–932.
3. Scully PE, Young RH, Clement RB. Surface epithelial-stromal tumors. In: *Tumors of the ovary, maldeveloped gonads, fallopian tube, and broad ligament.* Washington, DC: Armed Force Institute of Pathology; 1998:169–498.
4. Gershenson DM. Management of early ovarian cancer: germ cell and sex cord-stromal tumors. *Gynecol Oncol.* 1994;55(3 Pt 2):S62–S72.
5. Segal R, DePetrillo AD, Thomas G. Clinical review of adult granulosa cell tumors of the ovary. *Gynecol Oncol.* 1995;56(3):338–344.
6. Cronjé HS, Niemand I, Bam RH, Woodruff JD. Review of the granulosa-theca cell tumors from the Emil Novak Ovarian Tumor Registry. *Am J Obstet Gynecol.* 1999;180:323–327.
7. Hildebrandt RH, Rouse RV, Longacre TA. Value of inhibin in the identification of granulosa cell tumors of the ovary. *Hum Pathol.* 1997;28(12):1387–1395.
8. Matias-Guiu X, Pons C, Prat J. Müllerian inhibiting substance, alpha-inhibin, and CD99 expression in sex cord-stromal tumors and endometrioid ovarian carcinomas resembling sex cord-stromal tumors. *Hum Pathol.* 1998;29(8):840–845.
9. Malmström H, Högberg T, Risberg B, Simonsen E. Granulosa cell tumors of the ovary: prognostic factors and outcome. *Gynecol Oncol.* 1994;52:50–55.
10. Park JY, Jin KL, Kim DY, et al. Surgical staging and adjuvant chemotherapy in the management of patients with adult granulosa cell tumors of the ovary. *Gynecol Oncol.* 2012;125(1):80–86.
11. Thrall MM, Paley P, Pizer E, Garcia R, Goff BA. Patterns of spread and recurrence of sex cord-stromal tumors of the ovary. *Gynecol Oncol.* 2011;122(2):242–245.
12. Schumer ST, Cannistra SA. Granulosa cell tumor of the ovary. *J Clin Oncol.* 2003;21(6):1180–1189.
13. Uygun K, Aydiner A, Saip P, et al. Clinical parameters and treatment results in recurrent granulosa cell tumor of the ovary. *Gynecol Oncol.* 2003;88(3):400–403.
14. Al-Badawi IA, Brasher PM, Ghatage P, Nation JG, Schepansky A, Stuart GC. Postoperative chemotherapy in advanced ovarian granulosa cell tumors. *Int J Gynecol Cancer.* 2002;12:119–123.
15. Brown J, Shvartsman HS, Deavers MT, et al. The activity of taxanes compared with bleomycin, etoposide, and cisplatin in the treatment of sex cord-stromal ovarian tumors. *Gynecol Oncol.* 2005;97(2):489–496.
16. Lauszus FF, Petersen AC, Greisen J, Jakobsen A. Granulosa cell tumor of the ovary: a population-based study of 37 women with stage I disease. *Gynecol Oncol.* 2001;81(3):456–460.
17. Miller BE, Barron BA, Wan JY, Delmore JE, Silva EG, Gershenson DM. Prognostic factors in adult granulosa cell tumor of the ovary. *Cancer.* 1997;79(10):1951–1955.

18. Sigismondi C, Gadducci A, Lorusso D, et al. Ovarian Sertoli-Leydig cell tumors. a retrospective MITO study. *Gynecol Oncol.* 2012;125(3):673–676.

19. Roth LM, Anderson MC, Govan AD, Langley FA, Gowing NF, Woodcock AS. Sertoli-Leydig cell tumors: a clinicopathologic study of 34 cases. *Cancer.* 1981;48(1):187–197.

20. Brown J, Sood AK, Deavers MT, Milojevic L, Gershenson DM. Patterns of metastasis in sex cord-stromal tumors of the ovary: can routine staging lymphadenectomy be omitted? *Gynecol Oncol.* 2009;113(1):86–90.

21. Moore RG, Chung M, Granai CO, Gajewski W, Steinhoff MM. Incidence of metastasis to the ovaries from nongenital tract primary tumors. *Gynecol Oncol.* 2004;93(1):87–91.

22. Ulbright TM. Germ cell tumors of the gonads: a selective review emphasizing problems in differential diagnosis, newly appreciated, and controversial issues. *Mod Pathol.* 2005;18 Suppl 2:S61–S79.

■ RESOURCES

Bajorin DF, Sarosdy MF, Pfister DG, et al. Randomized trial of etoposide and cisplatin versus etoposide and carboplatin in patients with good-risk germ cell tumors: a multiinstitutional study. *J Clin Oncol.* 1993;11(4):598–606.

Fujita M, Inoue M, Tanizawa O, Minagawa J, Yamada T, Tani T. Retrospective review of 41 patients with endodermal sinus tumor of the ovary. *Int J Gynecol Cancer.* 1993;3(5):329–335.

Gershenson DM. Update on malignant ovarian germ cell tumors. *Cancer.* 1993;71(4 Suppl):1581–1590.

Kanazawa K, Suzuki T, Sakumoto K. Treatment of malignant ovarian germ cell tumors with preservation of fertility: reproductive performance after persistent remission. *Am J Clin Oncol.* 2000;23(3):244–248.

Krege S, Beyer J, Souchon R, et al. European consensus conference on diagnosis and treatment of germ cell cancer: a report of the second meeting of the European Germ Cell Cancer Consensus group (EGCCCG): part I. *Eur Urol.* 2008;53(3):478–496.

Kurman RJ, Scardino PT, McIntire KR, Waldmann TA, Javadpour N, Norris HJ. Malignant germ cell tumors of the ovary and testis. An immunohistologic study of 69 cases. *Ann Clin Lab Sci.* 1979;9(6):462–466.

Loehrer PJ Sr, Johnson D, Elson P, Einhorn LH, Trump D. Importance of bleomycin in favorable-prognosis disseminated germ cell tumors: an Eastern Cooperative Oncology Group trial. *J Clin Oncol.* 1995;13(2):470–476.

Nawa A, Obata N, Kikkawa F, et al. Prognostic factors of patients with yolk sac tumors of the ovary. *Am J Obstet Gynecol.* 2001;184(6):1182–1188.

Norris HJ, Zirkin HJ, Benson WL. Immature (malignant) teratoma of the ovary: a clinical and pathologic study of 58 cases. *Cancer.* 1976;37(5):2359–2372.

O'Connor DM, Norris HJ. The influence of grade on the outcome of stage I ovarian immature (malignant) teratomas and the reproducibility of grading. *Int J Gynecol Pathol.* 1994;13:283–289.

O'Sullivan JM, Huddart RA, Norman AR, Nicholls J, Dearnaley DP, Horwich A. Predicting the risk of bleomycin lung toxicity in patients with germ-cell tumors. *Ann Oncol.* 2003;14:91–96.

Patterson DM, Murugaesu N, Holden L, Seckl MJ, Rustin GJ. A review of the close surveillance policy for stage I female germ cell tumors of the ovary and other sites. *Int J Gynecol Cancer.* 2008;18:43–50.

Schwartz PE, Chambers SK, Chambers JT, Kohorn E, McIntosh S. Ovarian germ cell malignancies: the Yale University experience. *Gynecol Oncol.* 1992;45:26–31.

Tangjitgamol S, Manusirivithaya S, Leelahakorn S, Thawaramara T, Suekwatana P, Sheanakul C. The growing teratoma syndrome: a case report and a review of the literature. *Int J Gynecol Cancer.* 2006;16 (Suppl 1):384–390.

Ulbright TM, Roth LM, Stehman FB. Secondary ovarian neoplasia. A clinicopathologic study of 35 cases. *Cancer.* 1984;53(5):1164–1174.

Williams S, Blessing JA, Liao SY, Ball H, Hanjani P. Adjuvant therapy of ovarian germ cell tumors with cisplatin, etoposide, and bleomycin: a trial of the Gynecologic Oncology Group. *J Clin Oncol.* 1994;12:701–706.

Williams SD, Blessing JA, DiSaia PJ, Major FJ, Ball HG 3rd, Liao SY. Second-look laparotomy in ovarian germ cell tumors. *Gynecol Oncol.* 1994;52:287–291.

Williams SD, Kauderer J, Burnett AF, Lentz SS, Aghajanian C, Armstrong DK. Adjuvant therapy of completely resected dysgerminoma with carboplatin and etoposide: a trial of the Gynecologic Oncology Group. *Gynecol Oncol.* 2004:5, 496–499.

Cancer of the Vulva

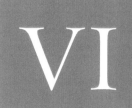

21   *Precancerous Lesions of the Vulva*

COLLEEN McCORMICK

The incidence of vulvar intraepithelial neoplasia has increased by over 400% in the last four decades (1). Nevertheless, vulvar intraepithelial neoplasia remains relatively rare, with an incidence of 2.86 cases per 100,000 women (1).

Over the years, vulvar dysplasia has gone by many names, but increasing understanding of the biology has led to simplification and consolidation of the terminology. Previously vulvar dysplasia was separated out into vulvar intraepithelial neoplasia (VIN) 1, 2, and 3. However, as there was no biological evidence that VIN1 was a precursor to cancer, and no evidence that there was a biological progression from VIN1 to VIN3; in 2004, this classification was dropped. VIN should now be reserved only for high-grade squamous lesions (those previously classified as VIN2 or VIN3). The term VIN1 should no longer be used (2). However, many publications and clinical reports continue to classify lesions in the old schema.

Additionally, further understanding of the biology of vulvar neoplasia and vulvar cancer has shown that there are two distinct pathways of vulvar dysplasia. VIN, usual type (also called warty, basaloid, or mixed type) is related to human papillomavirus (HPV) infection and leads to invasive vulvar squamous carcinoma of the warty or basaloid type. A review of worldwide cases of vulvar cancer of the warty or basaloid subtype showed that 86% of these lesions demonstrated high-risk type HPV DNA (3). These lesions tend to occur in younger women and are often multifocal due to the field effect of HPV infection. Tobacco abuse and immunosuppression have also been shown to be risk factors.

VIN differentiated type is associated with lichen sclerosis and leads to keratinizing vulvar squamous cell carcinoma. These lesions tend to occur in older women and are often isolated lesions. These lesions do not appear to be associated with HPV infection, as high-risk HPV DNA was identified in only 6.4% of keratinizing vulvar cancers (3). Lichen sclerosus presents as well-demarcated, white, wrinkled, atrophic patches, and is often associated with

significant pruritus. Often anatomical landmarks can be obliterated. Treatment is aimed at preventing progression to cancer, avoiding anatomical changes, and alleviating itching. High-dose topical steroid ointment is recommended. The risk of vulvar cancer associated with lichen sclerosis is unknown, but is likely less than 5%. Yearly examination to screen for VIN and cancer is recommended (4).

Despite our improved understanding of the biology of vulvar dysplasia, the true risk of progression to cancer remains unknown, and likely will remain so, since it would be unethical to perform an observational trial on lesions that are considered precancerous. Reported rates of cancer in untreated women vary widely from 9% to close to 90% (5,6). The risk of progression to cancer in previously treated women is approximately 2%–4% (5–7).

Women with VIN can present with vulvar pruritus or a lesion that they have noticed. Many women are asymptomatic, however, and lesions are discovered by palpation or visual inspection at the time of gynecologic examination. On examination, VIN often appears as a raised, white, or verrucous area. Colposcopy can aid in the evaluation and should be performed on women with vulvar dysplasia to evaluate for other simultaneous areas of disease. Acetowhite changes and vascular punctuations can be seen with colposcopy. All concerning areas should be biopsied. Diagnosis of vulvar dysplasia and vulvar cancer is often delayed, both by a woman's reluctance to present to the gynecologist and then by delays in biopsying lesions.

Treatment should be individualized. Traditionally, simple vulvectomy was used for treatment, but such extensive surgery has a significant functional and psychological impact on a woman. Instead, treatment should be individualized to the extent and location of the disease, and the concern for underlying malignancy. Treatment options include excision, laser ablation, and topical therapies.

Wide local excision has the advantage of providing tissue for pathological diagnosis and should be the treatment of choice if there is any concern about an underlying malignancy. The goal of an excisional procedure should be a 1 cm margin and deep enough to remove the epidermis. The rate of occult carcinoma found at the time of excisional procedure varies from 3% to 21% (6,8), but clearly is dependent on patient selection and individual practitioners experience in colposcopic evaluation. The rate of recurrence depends on the status of the margins, with a reported 11% risk of recurrence in women with negative margins and a 32% risk of recurrence in cases of positive margins, and a 26% overall risk of recurrence (7).

Laser ablation is another option for treatment, but is only appropriate where there is no concern for an underlying malignancy as there is no tissue available for pathological evaluational. However, this approach is often well suited for larger or multifocal lesions where an excisional procedure would have significant disfiguring effect. Laser ablation should be to a depth of 1 mm in hair-free areas and to a depth of 3 mm in hair-bearing areas. Recurrence rates of 40%–45% are reported (7,9). However, the higher rate of recurrence seen with this modality should take into consideration that these studies were observational and often larger, multifocal lesions are the ones that are selected for treatment with laser ablation.

Topical therapy with imiquimod (Aldara®) is another treatment option. Imiquimod is an immune response modifier. It is applied directly onto the lesion by the patient, two to three times per week over a 16-week course. This approach has the advantage of preserving normal anatomy. However, some patients are not capable of applying the cream or do not feel comfortable doing so. Additionally, treatment can lead to significant blistering and discomfort. No tissue is available for pathological evaluation either, so this modality should not be employed in cases where there is concern for a possible invasive carcinoma. Forty-six percent of women treated with imiquimod have a partial response, and 35% have a complete response (10). Recurrence risk after imiquimod therapy is 14% (7).

In the past topical 5-fluorouracil (5-FU) has been used, which causes desquamation. However, this approach is more painful than imiquimod and has mostly been abandoned.

Overall, imiquimod therapy appears to provide the lowest risk of recurrence and preserves normal anatomy. However, in cases where there is concern for a possible occult malignancy, wide local excision should be employed. An increased recurrence risk is seen with large lesions and positive margins.

In women with HIV, treatment of their underlying disease is an important component of therapy of VIN, as continued immunodeficiency is associated with increased risk of persistent and progressive disease.

Tobacco cessation is also an important component of preventing recurrence. Tobacco abuse is a known risk factor for developing VIN and continued tobacco use has been shown to be associated with increased risk of recurrence (7).

Due to the risk of recurrence and the risk of progression to cancer continued follow-up with visual inspection is recommended, although the optimal schedule for such follow-up is not know. Examination every 6 months after treatment for several years and then transitioning to yearly follow-up is reasonable.

■ REFERENCES

1. Judson PL, Habermann EB, Baxter NN, Durham SB, Virnig BA. Trends in the incidence of invasive and in situ vulvar carcinoma. *Obstet Gynecol.* 2006;107(5):1018–1022.

2. Sideri M, Jones RW, Wilkinson EJ, et al. Squamous vulvar intraepithelial neoplasia: 2004 modified terminology, ISSVD Vulvar Oncology Subcommittee. *J Reprod Med.* 2005;50(11):807–810.

3. Smith JS, Backes DM, Hoots BE, Kurman RJ, Pimenta JM. Human papillomavirus type-distribution in vulvar and vaginal cancers and their associated precursors. *Obstet Gynecol.* 2009;113(4):917–924.

4. Neill SM, Lewis FM, Tatnall FM, Cox NH; British Association of Dermatologists. British Association of Dermatologists' guidelines for the management of lichen sclerosus 2010. *Br J Dermatol.* 2010;163(4):672–682.

5. Jones RW, Rowan DM, Stewart AW. Vulvar intraepithelial neoplasia: aspects of the natural history and outcome in 405 women. *Obstet Gynecol.* 2005;106(6):1319–1326.

6. van Seters M, van Beurden M, de Craen AJ. Is the assumed natural history of vulvar intraepithelial neoplasia III based on enough evidence? A systematic review of 3322 published patients. *Gynecol Oncol.* 2005;97(2):645–651.

7. Wallbillich JJ, Rhodes HE, Milbourne AM, et al. Vulvar intraepithelial neoplasia (VIN 2/3): comparing clinical outcomes and evaluating risk factors for recurrence. *Gynecol Oncol.* 2012;127(2):312–315.

8. Husseinzadeh N, Recinto C. Frequency of invasive cancer in surgically excised vulvar lesions with intraepithelial neoplasia (VIN 3). *Gynecol Oncol.* 1999;73(1):119–120.

9. Hillemanns P, Wang X, Staehle S, Michels W, Dannecker C. Evaluation of different treatment modalities for vulvar intraepithelial neoplasia (VIN): CO(2) laser vaporization, photodynamic therapy, excision and vulvectomy. *Gynecol Oncol.* 2006;100(2):271–275.

10. van Seters M, van Beurden M, ten Kate FJ, et al. Treatment of vulvar intraepithelial neoplasia with topical imiquimod. *N Engl J Med.* 2008;358(14):1465–1473.

22

Multidisciplinary Approach to Diagnosis and Treatment of Early Cancer

KATHERINE C. FUH

JONATHAN S. BEREK

Vulvar cancer is the fourth most common gynecologic cancer and comprises 5% of the malignancies of the female genital tract (1). Squamous cell carcinoma of the vulva is predominantly a disease of postmenopausal women with a mean age at diagnosis of approximately 65 years. The diagnosis is often made after years of symptoms of pruritus associated with vulvar dystrophy. The lesion is usually raised and may be fleshy, ulcerated, leukoplakic, or warty in appearance. Most squamous cell carcinomas of the vulva occur on the labia majora, but the labia minora, clitoris, and the perineum may be primary sites.

Vulvar cancer is surgically staged based on pathologic evaluation of a vulvar lesion and of the inguinofemoral lymph nodes. A complete clinical assessment will help guide the surgical and medical approach to treatment. In particular, the diameter of the primary tumor should be measured, and the inguinal, axillary, and supraclavicular lymph nodes should be palpated. Due to the multifocal nature of squamous intraepithelial lesions, cervical cytology and colposcopy of the cervix, vagina, and vulva should be performed. Imaging such as an abdominal/pelvic computed tomography may be performed for women with tumors 2 cm or larger to detect suspected metastases to lymph node or other distant sites.

Diagnosis requires a biopsy specimen, which can be taken in the office. The biopsy specimen must include underlying dermis and connective tissue so that depth and stromal invasion can be evaluated. Staging and primary surgical treatment are typically performed as a single procedure. Staging should include the evaluation for factors related to prognosis: tumor size, depth of invasion, lymph node metastases, and distant metastases.

■ STAGING

Staging historically was based on clinical factors using the tumor node metastasis (TNM) classification adopted by the International Federation of Gynecology and Obstetrics

(FIGO) in 1969. This staging was focused on a clinical evaluation of the primary tumor, the regional lymph nodes, and a limited search for distant metastases. However, clinical evaluation of inguinofemoral lymph nodes is inaccurate in approximately 25%–30% of the cases (2–4). The percentage of error in clinical staging compared to surgical staging increased from 18% for Stage I disease to 44% for Stage IV disease (5). In 1988, surgical staging for vulvar cancer was introduced and updated FIGO staging occurred in 2008 with most recent updated report in 2012 (see Table 22.1). Surgical staging is mandated because the diagnosis of inguinofemoral lymph node metastasis is the most important predictor of overall prognosis.

Pathology

Squamous Cell Carcinoma

Over 90% of vulvar malignancies are squamous cell carcinomas. There are two subtypes, both of which usually occur on the labia or vestibule. The keratinizing, differentiated, or simplex type is more common. It occurs in older women and it is not related to human papillomavirus (HPV) infection, but is associated with vulvar dystrophies such as lichen sclerosus and in developing countries, chronic venereal granulomatous disease. The classic, warty, or Bowenoid type is predominantly associated with HPV16, HPV18, and HPV33, and is found in younger women (6,7). These patients tend to present with early-stage disease, although several cases of Stage III/IV disease in HIV-infected women have been reported. Verrucous carcinoma is a variant of squamous cell carcinoma that has distinct features. Although cauliflower-like in appearance, it is differentiated from squamous cell carcinoma with a verrucous configuration. The lesion grows slowly and rarely metastasizes to lymph nodes but it may be locally destructive.

Melanoma

Melanoma is the second most common vulvar cancer histology, accounting for approximately 5% for primary vulvar neoplasms. Melanoma of the vulva occurs predominantly in postmenopausal white non-Hispanic women at a median age of 68 years (8). Vulvar melanoma is usually a

■ **Table 22.1** FIGO (International Federation of Gynecology and Obstetrics) Staging of cancer of the vulva

FIGO Stage	Description
I	Tumor confined to the vulva
IA	Lesions ≤ 2cm in size, confined to the vulva or perineum and with stromal invasion ≤ 1.0 mm², no nodal metastasis
IB	Lesions > 2 cm in size or with stromal invasion > 1.0 mm², confined to the vulva or perineum, with negative nodes
II	Tumor of any size with extension to adjacent perineal structures (lower third of urethra, lower third of vagina, anus) with negative nodes
III	Tumor of any size with or without extension to adjacent perineal structures (lower third of urethra, lower third of vagina, anus) with positive inguinotemoral nodes
IIIA	(i) With 1 lymph node metastasis (≥ 5 mm), or
	(ii) With 1-2 lymph node metastasis(es) (< 5 mm)
IIIB	(i) With 2 or more lymph node metastases (≥ 5 mm), or
	(ii) With 3 or more lymph node metastases (< 5 mm)
IIIC	With positive nodes with extracapsular spread
IV	Tumor invades other regional (upper 2/3 urethra, upper 2/3 vagina), or distant structures
IVA	Tumor invades any of the following:
	(i) upper urethral and/or vaginal mucosa, bladder mucosa, rectal mucosa, or fixed pelvic bone, or
	(ii) fixed or ulcerated inguinofemoral lymph nodes
IVB	Any distant metastasis including pelvic lymph nodes

[a] The depth of invasion is defined as the measurement of the tumor from the epithelial-stromal junction of the adjacent most superficial dermal papilla to the deepest point of invasion.
From Hacker N., Eifel P., van der Velden J. *International Journal of Gynecology and Obstetrics* 2012: S90-S96.

pigmented lesion, but amelanotic lesions also occur. Most arise de novo on the clitoris or labia minora, but can also develop within pre-existing junctional or compound nevi.

Basal Cell Carcinoma

Two percent of vulvar cancers are basal cell cancers and 2% of basal cell cancers occur on the vulva (9). They usually affect postmenopausal Caucasian women and may be locally invasive, although usually non-metastasizing. The typical appearance is that of a "rodent" ulcer with rolled edges and central ulceration; the lesion may be pigmented or pearly and gray. They are often asymptomatic, but pruritus, bleeding, or pain may occur. Basal cell carcinomas are associated with a high incidence of antecedent or concomitant malignancy elsewhere in the body (10). A thorough search for primary malignancies should be performed.

Sarcoma

Soft tissue sarcomas, such as leiomyosarcomas, rhabdomyosarcomas, liposarcomas, angiosarcomas, neurofibrosarcomas, fibrous histiocytomas, and epithelioid sarcomas, constitute 1%–2% of vulvar malignancies. As with soft tissue sarcomas located elsewhere on the extremities and trunk, high-grade lesions that are larger than 5 cm in diameter, with infiltrating margins and a high mitotic rate, are most likely to recur.

Adenocarcinoma

Most primary adenocarcinomas of the vulva occur in the Bartholin gland. This gland is composed of columnar epithelium; ducts are lined by stratified squamous epithelium, which changes to transitional cell epithelium as the terminal ducts are reached. Cancers arising in the Bartholin gland are most often adenocarcinomas or squamous cell carcinomas, but transitional cell carcinomas, adenosquamous, and adenoid cystic cell carcinomas may also develop (11,12). Median age is 57 and enlargement of the Bartholin gland in a postmenopausal woman is worrisome for malignancy since benign inflammatory disease usually does not occur in the age group. The gland should be biopsied in older (over 40 years of age) women with a mass in this location, even if the lesions appear cystic or abscessed. Metastatic disease is common in cancers of the Bartholin gland due to the rich vascular and lymphatic network.

Invasive adenocarcinoma may be present within or beneath the surface intraepithelial lesion known as Paget's disease (13,14). This is a very uncommon malignancy. Most patients are in their 60s and 70s and Caucasian. Pruritus is the most common symptom, present in 70% of patients. The lesion has an eczematoid appearance; it is well demarcated, and has slightly raised edges and a red background, often dotted with small, pale islands. It is usually multifocal and may occur anywhere on the vulva, mons, perineum/perianal area, or inner thigh. Vulvar biopsy should be performed in patients with suspicious lesions, including those

■ Table 22.2 Treatment based on size of lesion, depth of invasion, and laterality

Size of lesion	Depth of invasion	Location	Operation	Inguinal-femoral lymphadenectomy or sentinel lymph node evaluation*1
T1 (<2cm) or T2 (>2cm)	<1mm	Lateral+ or central	Radical local excision	No
T1 or T2	≥1mm	Lateral+	Radical local excision	Ipsilateral
		Central	Radical local excision	Bilateral
T2		Central	Radical local excision or modified radical**	Bilateral
Any size with extension to adjacent perineal structures (lower/distal 1/3 urethra, lower/distal 1/3 vagina, anal involvement	—	—	Modified radical and selected chemoradiation	Bilateral
Extensive T3 to T4 disease (spread to the urethra, anus, bladder, rectum, or pelvic bone)	—	—	Neoadjuvantchemoradiation# and selected surgery	—

+Further than 1 cm from midline.
*Sentinel node biopsy can be considered as an alternative to inguinofemoral lymphadenectomy in all cases that require a lymphadenectomy.
1Bilateral lymphadenectomy is performed if unilateral nodal specimen is positive.
**Modified radical vulvectomy (terminology includes radical hemivulvectomy, anterior or posterior modified radical vulvectomy).
#Can consider chemoradiation as primary treatment or postoperative radiation for patients with high-risk of local recurrence (those with Stage IVA disease, positive or close margins, and a large number of groin nodes).

with persistent pruritic eczematous lesions that fail to resolve within 6 weeks of appropriate antieczema therapy. Women with Paget's disease should be evaluated for the possibility of synchronous neoplasms as approximately 4%–5% of these patients have a noncontiguous carcinoma involving the breast, rectum, bladder, urethra, cervix, or ovary.

■ MANAGEMENT OF STAGE I AND STAGE II VULVAR CANCER

The modern approach to the management of patients with early-stage vulvar carcinoma should be individualized. In considering the appropriate operation, it is necessary to determine independently the appropriate management of the primary lesion and the inguinofemoral lymph nodes (15, 16).

Management of the Primary Tumor

Several factors have led to modifications from the *en bloc* radical vulvectomy and bilateral inguinofemoral, and pelvic lymphadenectomy. These factors include the more frequent presentation of smaller tumors at diagnosis in younger women, the concern of postoperative morbidity and associated long-term hospitalization, the

psychosexual effects from distortion of the vulva, and the problem of lymphedema. Alternative and less radical surgical approaches that remove less of the vulva and the surrounding skin are most commonly performed.

Two factors should be taken into consideration: age and condition of the remainder of the vulva. Since the 1980s, several investigators have advocated for a radical local excision rather than a radical vulvectomy for the primary lesion in patients with T_1 (2 cm or less) or T_2 (larger than 2 cm). It is desirable to conserve as much of the vulva as possible. For Stage II disease, the most conservative excision technique should be used that results in at least a 1 cm tumor-free margin. Depending on the size, location, and depth of invasion of the lesion, this may necessitate radical local excision, or modified radical vulvectomy, and the separate incision technique of an inguinofemoral lymphadenectomy (16; Table 22.2)

Radical Local Excision

Radical local excision or modified radical vulvectomy (removal of part or the entire vulva unilaterally, also called modified radical hemivulvectomy) is most appropriate for the lesions on the lateral or posterior aspects of the vulva where preservation of the clitoris is feasible. For anterior lesions, clitoral sparing modified radical vulvectomy can be an option. However, the depth of the resection, from the skin to the urogenital diaphragm, is the same as in standard radical vulvectomy (17).

In a retrospective study including 41 patients with squamous carcinoma of the anterior vulva not involving the clitoris, 13 patients had clitoral sparing modified radical vulvectomy and 28 had radical vulvectomy. The 13 patients who had clitoral sparing surgery included 8 with Stage I, 2 with Stage II, 2 with Stage III, and 1 with Stage IV disease. After a median follow-up of 59 months, none of the 13 patients having conservative surgery had locoregional failure. In another study, 122 patients with lateral T_1 and T_2 lesions were studied: half of these patients had radical vulvectomy and the other half a radical hemivulvectomy. Disease-free survival at 5 years was 98% and 93%, respectively. Local or distant recurrence was not more common in patients treated by radical vulvectomy or radical hemivulvectomy (18). Another published experience at the Royal Hospital for Women in Sydney reported on 116 patients with FIGO Stages I and II vulvar cancer who underwent radical local excision. The patients who had radical vulvectomy were because the tumor was multifocal. With a median follow-up of 84 months, the overall 5-year survival of patients with radical local excision was 96.4% (19).

Technique for Radical Local Excision

Radical local excision implies a deep excision of the primary tumor. The surgical margins should be at least 1 cm and should be drawn using a marking pen with the vulva in its natural state. The incision should be carried down to the inferior fascia of the urogenital diaphragm, which is coplanar with the fascia lata and the fascia over the pubic symphysis. The surgical defect is closed in two layers. *For perineal lesions*, proximity to the anus may preclude adequate surgical margins, and consideration should be given to preoperative radiation. *For periurethral lesions*, the distal half of the urethra may be resected without loss of continence (Figure 22.1).

For all types of vulvar excisions, a tumor-free margin of at least 1 cm appears to decrease the risk of local recurrence (17,20,21). A retrospective case series ($n = 135$) reported a decrease in the rate of local recurrence in cases with normal tissue margin of 1 cm or greater compared with less than 8 mm (0% vs 50%; 22). Therefore, a surgical margin of at least 1 cm accounts for the 20% tissue shrinkage with formalin fixation. Care should be taken to ensure the skin incision is made without tension.

Management of Inguinofemoral Lymph Nodes

Appropriate management of the regional lymph nodes is the single most important factor in decreasing mortality from early vulvar cancer. The only patients who are not at significant risk of lymph node metastases are those with a T_1 tumor that invades the stroma to a depth of no

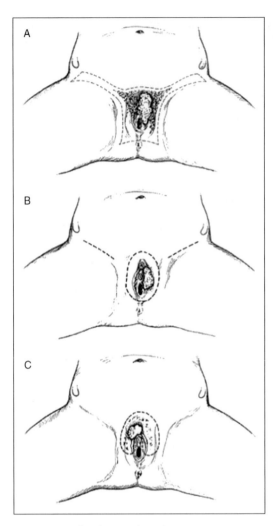

FIGURE 22.1 Surgical techniques for vulvar carcinoma. (A) Modified butterfly incision. (B) Triple incision technique—a skin bridge is left between the radical vulvectomy and the groin incisions. (C) Anterior horseshoe incision. Courtesy of Elkas and Berek.

greater than 1 mm. If tumor is less than 2 cm in diameter, the entire lesion should be locally excised and analyzed histologically to determine the depth of invasion. Depth of invasion is measured from the most superficial dermal papilla adjacent to the tumor to the deepest focus of invasion.

If recurrence occurs in the undissected inguinofemoral lymph nodes, there is a very high mortality rate. Pelvic lymphadenectomy, removal of iliac and obturator nodes, is not required for staging or therapy and has not been shown to improve survival. The choice of approach for lymphadenectomy depends on the size and location of the lesion as well as the presence of bulky positive nodes.

Tumor thickness is also measured and the average difference between tumor thickness and depth of invasion has been found to be 0.3 mm (23–25). If the invasive focus is less than 1 mm, inguinofemoral lymphadenectomy may be omitted given the incidence of nodal metastases is essentially nil (15, 26–29). All patients with a more deeply invasive T_1 or a T_2 tumor require surgical removal of inguinofemoral lymph nodes or sentinel node evaluation. The Gynecologic Oncology Group (GOG) reported 6 inguinofemoral recurrences among 121 patients with T_1N_0 or T_1N_1 tumors after a superficial (inguinal) dissection, even though the inguinal nodes were reported as negative, although it is unclear whether all these recurrences were in femoral nodes (30). Therefore, this approach has now been abandoned in favor of either a complete inguinofemoral lymphadenectomy or a sentinel lymph node assessment.

Separate Incision Technique

The separate incision technique allows for radical excision of the primary lesion and the unilateral or bilateral pathologic analysis of the inguinofemoral lymph nodes. This operation can be performed in modified dorsal lithotomy position using Allen stirrups. In this manner, the surgeon can modify the degree of exposure for the vulvectomy and the inguinofemoral lymphadenectomy to maximize the exposure during each portion of the operation. The radical local excision is performed to remove the primary tumor with at least 1 cm margin.

Ipsilateral Inguinofemoral Lymph Node Assessment

The surgical evaluation of the ipsilateral inguinofemoral lymph nodes is suitable for lateralized primary lesions, when there are no metastases in the ipsilateral inguinofemoral lymph nodes. A study of 163 patients with a unilateral vulvar cancer of whom 48 had positive inguinofemoral lymph nodes, 3 of the patients with positive contralateral nodes had negative ipsilateral nodes. In this study, the only independent risk factor for contralateral lymph node involvement is the total number of positive ipsilateral inguinofemoral lymph nodes. With each positive lymph node, the possibility of having bilateral inguinofemoral lymph node involvement increases by 84%. Central, nonlateralized lesions should have bilateral surgical assessment (31). Ipsilateral lymphadenectomy was associated with less than 1% risk of contralateral inguinofemoral node metastases for Stage IB disease that are unifocal, lateral at least 1 cm from vulvar midline, not located in the anterior portion of the labia minora (area just posterior to the clitoris), no palpable lymphadenopathy in either inguinofemoral region, and no lymph node metastases found at time of unilateral lymphadenectomy (30,31). Bilateral lymphadenectomy is performed for midline tumors or if lymph node metastases are discovered at unilateral lymphadenectomy. The rate of bilateral inguinofemoral metastases in women with lesions with unilateral lesions with stromal invasion 3 mm or deeper is 2.8% or higher (32). If an inguinal lymphadenectomy is being performed, it should include the femoral lymph nodes because so-called superficial lymphadenectomy has been associated with a high rate of inguinofemoral recurrence (30).

Given the diagnosis of a vulvar malignancy can be particularly distressing, the current treatment recommendations for less disfiguring surgery can provide tremendous relief. Moving away from the historic "butterfly" radical vulvectomy and instead toward radical local excision with adequate margins has proven to be equally effective and less psychologically harmful. With the multidisciplinary team of gynecologic oncologists and pathologists, the appropriate treatment of early-stage vulvar cancer will continue to result in optimal care for our patients.

■ REFERENCES

1. Jemal A, Bray F, Center MM, Ferlay J, Ward E, Forman D. Global cancer statistics. *CA Cancer J Clin.* 2011;61(2):69–90.
2. Way S. Carcinoma of the vulva. *Am J Obstet Gynecol.* 1960;79:692–697.
3. Monaghan JM. Vulvar carcinoma: the case for individualization of treatment. *Baillieres Clin Obstet Gynaecol.* 1987;1(2): 263–276.
4. Hoffman JS, Kumar NB, Morley GW. Prognostic significance of groin lymph node metastases in squamous carcinoma of the vulva. *Obstet Gynecol.* 1985;66(3):402–405.
5. Homesley HD, Bundy BN, Sedlis A, et al. Assessment of current International Federation of Gynecology and Obstetrics staging of vulvar carcinoma relative to prognostic factors for survival (a Gynecologic Oncology Group study). *Am J Obstet Gynecol.* 1991;164(4):997–1003; discussion 1003–1004.
6. Hildesheim A, Han CL, Brinton LA, Kurman RJ, Schiller JT. Human papillomavirus type 16 and risk of preinvasive and invasive vulvar cancer: results from a seroepidemiological case-control study. *Obstet Gynecol.* 1997;90(5):748–754.
7. Iwasawa A, Nieminen P, Lehtinen M, Paavonen J. Human papillomavirus in squamous cell carcinoma of the vulva by polymerase chain reaction. *Obstet Gynecol.* 1997;89(1):81–84.
8. Sugiyama VE, Chan JK, Shin JY, Berek JS, Osann K, Kapp DS. Vulvar melanoma: a multivariable analysis of 644 patients. *Obstet Gynecol.* 2007;110(2 Pt 1):296–301.
9. de Giorgi V, Salvini C, Massi D, Raspollini MR, Carli P. Vulvar basal cell carcinoma: retrospective study and review of literature. *Gynecol Oncol.* 2005;97(1):192–194.
10. Benedet JL, Miller DM, Ehlen TG, Bertrand MA. Basal cell carcinoma of the vulva: clinical features and treatment results in 28 patients. *Obstet Gynecol.* 1997;90(5):765–768.
11. Felix JC, Cote RJ, Kramer EE, Saigo P, Goldman GH. Carcinomas of Bartholin's gland. Histogenesis and the etiological role of human papillomavirus. *Am J Pathol.* 1993;142(3):925–933.
12. Copeland LJ, Sneige N, Gershenson DM, McGuffee VB, Abdul-Karim F, Rutledge FN. Bartholin gland carcinoma. *Obstet Gynecol.* 1986;67(6):794–801.
13. Parker LP, Parker JR, Bodurka-Bevers D, et al. Paget's disease of the vulva: pathology, pattern of involvement, and prognosis. *Gynecol Oncol.* 2000;77(1):183–189.
14. Fanning J, Lambert HC, Hale TM, Morris PC, Schuerch C. Paget's disease of the vulva: prevalence of associated vulvar adenocarcinoma, invasive Paget's disease, and recurrence after surgical excision. *Am J Obstet Gynecol.* 1999;180(1 Pt 1):24–27.
15. Hacker NF, Berek JS, Lagasse LD, Nieberg RK, Leuchter RS. Individualization of treatment for stage I squamous cell vulvar carcinoma. *Obstet Gynecol.* 1984;63(2):155–162.

16. Hacker NF, Leuchter RS, Berek JS, Castaldo TW, Lagasse LD. Radical vulvectomy and bilateral inguinal lymphadenectomy through separate groin incisions. *Obstet Gynecol.* 1981; 58(5):574–579.

17. Rouzier R, Haddad B, Atallah D, Dubois P, Paniel BJ. Surgery for vulvar cancer. *Clin Obstet Gynecol.* 2005;48(4):869–878.

18. DeSimone CP, Van Ness JS, Cooper AL, et al. The treatment of lateral T1 and T2 squamous cell carcinomas of the vulva confined to the labium majus or minus. *Gynecol Oncol.* 2007;104(2):390–395.

19. Tantipalakorn C, Robertson G, Marsden DE, Gebski V, Hacker NF. Outcome and patterns of recurrence for International Federation of Gynecology and Obstetrics (FIGO) stages I and II squamous cell vulvar cancer. *Obstet Gynecol.* 2009;113(4):895–901.

20. Farias-Eisner R, Cirisano FD, Grouse D, et al. Conservative and individualized surgery for early squamous carcinoma of the vulva: the treatment of choice for stage I and II (T1–2N0–1M0) disease. *Gynecol Oncol.* 1994;53(1):55–58.

21. Chan JK, Sugiyama V, Pham H, et al. Margin distance and other clinico-pathologic prognostic factors in vulvar carcinoma: a multivariate analysis. *Gynecol Oncol.* 2007;104(3):636–641.

22. Heaps JM, Fu YS, Montz FJ, Hacker NF, Berek JS. Surgical-pathologic variables predictive of local recurrence in squamous cell carcinoma of the vulva. *Gynecol Oncol.* 1990;38(3):309–314.

23. Wilkinson EJ, Rico MJ, Pierson KK. Microinvasive carcinoma of the vulva. *Int J Gynecol Pathol.* 1982;1(1):29–39.

24. Magrina JF, Webb MJ, Gaffey TA, Symmonds RE. Stage I squamous cell cancer of the vulva. *Am J Obstet Gynecol.* 1979;134(4):453–459.

25. Sedlis A, Homesley H, Bundy BN, et al. Positive groin lymph nodes in superficial squamous cell vulvar cancer. A Gynecologic Oncology Group study. *Am J Obstet Gynecol.* 1987;156(5): 1159–1164.

26. Hacker NF, Van der Velden J. Conservative management of early vulvar cancer. *Cancer.* 1993;71(4 Suppl):1673–1677.

27. Atamdede F, Hoogerland D. Regional lymph node recurrence following local excision for microinvasive vulvar carcinoma. *Gynecol Oncol.* 1989;34(1):125–128.

28. Van Der Velden J, Kooyman CD, Van Lindert AC, Heintz AP. A stage Ia vulvar carcinoma with an inguinal lymph node recurrence after local excision. A case report and literature review. *Int J Gynecol Cancer.* 1992;2(3):157–159.

29. Vernooij F, Sie-Go DM, Heintz AP. Lymph node recurrence following stage IA vulvar carcinoma: two cases and a short overview of literature. *Int J Gynecol Cancer.* 2007;17(2): 517–520.

30. Stehman FB, Bundy BN, Dvoretsky PM, Creasman WT. Early stage I carcinoma of the vulva treated with ipsilateral superficial inguinal lymphadenectomy and modified radical hemivulvectomy: a prospective study of the Gynecologic Oncology Group. *Obstet Gynecol.* 1992;79(4):490–497.

31. Iversen T, Aas M. Lymph drainage from the vulva. *Gynecol Oncol.* 1983;16(2):179–189.

32. Homesley HD, Bundy BN, Sedlis A, et al. Prognostic factors for groin node metastasis in squamous cell carcinoma of the vulva (a Gynecologic Oncology Group study). *Gynecol Oncol.* 1993;49(3):279–283.

23 The Role of Sentinel Lymph Node Mapping

ELENA DIAZ

OLIVER DORIGO

The concept of sentinel lymph node biopsy (SLNB) relies on the hypothesis that lymphatic drainage from the primary tumor occurs in a predictable and nonrandom fashion to a preferred nodal basin. The sentinel lymph node (SLN) is defined as the first draining lymph node from the primary tumor. The pathology on this SLN is thought to be representative of the pathology in the non-SLNs. Ideally, the absence of metastatic disease in the SLN should predict the absence of disease in other non-SLNs (1). A high negative predictive value for SLNB ideally negates the need for an extensive lymphadenectomy and therefore reduces surgical morbidity.

The identification of a SLN was first pioneered by Cabanas in 1977 using lymphangiography in the evaluation of penile carcinoma. This early study suggested that the SLN was the first site of metastasis (2). The modern SLNB using isosulfan blue dye was first described by Morton et al in 1992 in the treatment of early cutaneous melanoma (1). Since then, SLNB has become an accepted and routinely utilized technique in the management of cutaneous melanoma and breast cancer (3,4).

Standard treatment for vulvar cancer with at least 1 mm invasion currently includes wide radical excision of the tumor and inguinofemoral lymphadenectomy (5). Despite the use of modern aseptic surgical techniques, about half of women undergoing treatment for vulvar cancer will experience a wound complication in particular at the site of the lymphadenectomy (6). Although many of these complications may be short-term, lymphedema and cellulitis may become chronic lifelong conditions with significant associated morbidity.

Currently, there are two techniques utilized for mapping of SLNs: injection of isosulfan blue dye or preoperative lymphoscintigraphy. In the technique using isosulfan blue dye, the peritumoral area or the area around the scar if a prior wide local excision has been performed, is injected with dye. A groin incision is subsequently made and carried down to Camper's fascia to identify blue afferent lymphatic channels leading to blue SLNs (7). The technique using preoperative lymphoscintigraphy involves injection of technetium-99-labeled radiocolloid (^{99m}Tc) into the peritumoral or area around the scar prior to surgery. The radiocolloid traffics to the sentinel lymph nodes in the inguinal area and can be visualized on a radiograph. Intraoperatively, a sterile handheld gamma counter is passed over the groin to identify the lymph nodes that emit a radioactive signal. These lymph nodes are considered the sentinel lymph nodes (7).

Several studies have evaluated the sensitivity and specificity of each of these techniques alone or in combination. In a multi-institutional study, Ansink and colleagues used injection of patent blue V dye before radical vulvectomy and inguinal-femoral lymphadenectomy in 51 patients with vulvar cancer (8). The investigators identified SLN in 56% of the 93 groins dissected. There were 2 false-negative SLN with a negative predictive value of 0.953. The authors concluded that the blue dye technique was sufficiently sensitive to detect SLN. However, the negative predictive value was considered too low and therefore it was recommended that further studies should combine the blue dye technique with radiocolloid injection.

Following this study, Levenback et al published a single-institution study in which 52 patients were enrolled and injected with isosulfan blue dye alone to identify SLN followed by complete inguinofemoral lymphadenectomy (9). They reported a much higher rate of SLN identification at 88%, and there were no false-negative sentinel nodes. In contrast to Ansink et al, these authors concluded that lymphatic mapping with blue dye alone successfully identifies SLNs in vulvar cancer.

Other investigators have focused on lymphoscintigraphy using radiocolloid for SLN mapping. Sideri and colleagues reported on peritumoral administration of ^{99m}Tc in 44 patients with the use of an intraoperative gamma detecting probe to detect SLNs during surgery (10). Using this technique, the investigators identified sentinel nodes in all of the groins studied. Thirteen cases had positive nodes and the sentinel node was positive in all of them. There were no false-negative SLN detected. They concluded that lymphoscintigraphy and SLNB under gamma detecting probe guidance is an easy and reliable method for detection of SLN in early vulvar cancer.

Other groups have investigated the use of combining both blue dye and lymphoscintigraphy in SLNB for vulvar cancer. De Hullu et al used a combination of preoperative lymphoscintigraphy with ^{99m}Tc and intraoperative injection of blue dye in 59 patients with vulvar cancer (11). SLNs were identified in all patients with at least one of these techniques and in 95 (89%) of total 107 groins dissected. The negative predictive value for a negative SLN was 100%, which is in concordance with the results published by other investigators using this technique (12,13). These authors stated that they relied mainly on the gamma probe to identify SLNs intraoperatively and that the blue dye was visible in only 60% of sentinel nodes.

Rob et al investigated the use of blue dye and ^{99m}Tc in 59 women with vulvar cancers less than 4 cm in size (14). Blue dye alone was used in the first 16 women (Group A) and a combination of lymphoscintigraphy and blue dye were used for the remaining 43 women (Group B). The SLN detection rate and false-negative rate when both mapping techniques were used was 100% and 0% respectively, compared to 68.8% and 6.3% when blue dye only was used. The authors concluded that the combined use of ^{99m}Tc and blue dye was superior to blue dye alone for the detection of SLN.

The multi-institutional study Gronigen International Sentinel Nodes Vulva (GROINSS-V) was conducted primarily in the Netherlands. This observational study included women with primary tumor less than 4 cm who had negative findings on SLNB performed after mapping with combined radioactive tracer and blue dye (15). Patients were followed for 2 years at intervals of every 2 months for groin recurrence. Of the 403 women enrolled in the study, eight women had groin relapse. Based on the assumption that these patients represent false-negative findings on SLNB, the false-negative rate in this study was calculated to 5.9% (16). In addition, the investigators found that short-term and long-term morbidity was decreased in patients after sentinel node dissection only compared with patients with a positive sentinel node who underwent a complete inguinofemoral lymphadenectomy (wound breakdown in groin: 11.7% vs 34%, respectively, $P < .0001$; cellulitis: 4.5% vs 21.3%, respectively, $P < .0001$; recurrent erysipelas: 0.4% vs 16.2%, respectively, $P < .0001$; and lymphedema of the legs: 1.9% vs 25.2%, respectively, $P < .0001$). The authors concluded that SLN dissection is safe with minimal morbidity and should be part of the standard treatment in selected patients with early-stage vulvar cancer.

In 2008, the International Sentinel Node Society issued an expert panel statement regarding SLNB in patients with gynecologic cancers (16). The panel considered use of a combination of radiocolloid and blue dye as the best technique for SLN identification. Good candidates for SLN procedure were considered to be patients with squamous cell carcinoma of the vulva with greater than 1 mm of invasion and a tumor diameter less than 4 cm, as well as those with vulvar melanoma. Given the wide variation of pathology resources available in different practices, panelists felt that the decision to perform a frozen section analysis of the SLN should be guided by the surgical pathologist. The panel recommended that an individual gynecologic oncologist perform at least 10 consecutive cases with successful SLN identification and no false-negative results before performing SLNB without lymphadenectomy. When a SLN is not identified intraoperatively, a complete inguinal-femoral lymphadenectomy should be performed. With regard to the proper treatment for patients with a positive SLNB, the panel was unable to reach a consensus. They referenced the Gronigen International Study on Sentinel Nodes in Vulvar Cancer (GROINSS-V) II study discussed below as an opportunity to answer this question and concluded that the panel enthusiastically supports clinical trials that incorporate SLNB into new treatment strategies for vulvar cancer.

Most recently, the long-awaited results of Gynecologic Oncology Group (GOG) 173 have been published (17). This multi-institutional study enrolled patients at 47 GOG-affiliated institutions between 1999 and 2009. Women were eligible if they had invasive squamous cell carcinoma of the vulva with at least 1 mm depth of invasion, a primary tumor size of greater than 2 cm and less than 6 cm, and no evidence of inguinal lymph node metastasis on physical exam. All women underwent intraoperative lymphatic mapping with isosulfan blue dye. At the beginning of the study, preoperative lymphoscintigraphy and intraoperative radiolocalization were optional. However, within 2 years of entry into the study, the combination of both techniques was required. The results showed that at least one SLN was identified in 92.5% of patients. SLN were both blue and radioactive in 61% of women, blue only in 24% of women, and radioactive only in 15% of women. Interestingly, the rate of identification of the SLN was not statistically different in women who had a prior wide local excision with dye and radiocolloid injected around the scar compared to those that received the injections around the primary tumor. There were 132 women with positive nodes, including 11 (8.3%) false-negative nodes. Twenty-three percent of true-positive patients were only detected after immunohistochemical analysis of the SLN. The sensitivity was 91.7% and the false-negative predictive value 3.7%. In women with tumors less than 4 cm, the false-negative predictive value was 2%. The authors pointed out the fact that these results closely replicate the results of the GROINSS-V trial and concluded that these data together provide adequate evidence that SLNB is a reasonable alternative to inguinal-femoral lymphadenectomy in selected women with squamous cell carcinoma of the vulva.

Currently, the GOG has joined GROINSS-V in GOG 270/GROINSS-V II, which will address the management of SLN-positive women (18). Other aims of this study include investigating the safety of omitting complete inguinofemoral lymphadenectomy in patients with a negative sentinel node, to evaluate the morbidity associated with the SLN procedure, and to evaluate the role of frozen section, immunohistochemical staining, and multiple sectioning in the accuracy of detecting lymph node metastases. In this prospective observational study, SLN will be identified by both radiocolloid and blue dye. If the sentinel node is negative by morphology and immunohistochemical staining, no further treatment will follow. Any positive groin lymph nodes identified either by morphology or immunohistochemistry will be regarded as metastatic disease. Adjuvant radiation will be used in case of a metastasis less than or equal to 2 mm. In case of a metastasis greater than 2 mm, an inguinofemoral lymphadenectomy will be performed. In contrast to the protocol in GOG 173, this study will include preoperative imaging, assessment of surgeons' experience, and central pathology review.

In summary, SLNB in the treatment of early-stage vulvar cancer appears to be a safe option with minimal morbidity in properly selected patients. Combining the use of blue dye and radiocolloid has been the most successful strategy in identifying SLNs in prospective trials. Patients are best treated at high-volume centers where gynecologic oncologists are proficient at performing the procedure. The results of ongoing clinical trials involving SLNB in vulvar cancer will be anxiously awaited to help answer unresolved questions regarding the best use of this technique.

■ REFERENCES

1. Morton DL, Wen DR, Wong JH, et al. Technical details of intraoperative lymphatic mapping for early stage melanoma. *Arch Surg.* 1992;127(4):392–399.
2. Cabanas RM. An approach for the treatment of penile carcinoma. *Cancer.* 1977;39(2):456–466.
3. Balch CM, Cascinelli N. Sentinel-node biopsy in melanoma. *N Engl J Med.* 2006;355(13):1370–1371.
4. Singletary SE, Allred C, Ashley P, et al. Revision of the American Joint Committee on Cancer staging system for breast cancer. *J Clin Oncol.* 2002;20(17):3628–3636.
5. Moore DH, Koh WJ, McGuire WP, Wilkinson EJ. Vulva. In: Barakat R, Markman M, Randall ME, eds. *Principles and Practice of Gynecologic Oncology.* Philadelphia, PA: Lippincott Williams & Wilkins, 2009:571–572.
6. Gaarenstroom KN, Kenter GG, Trimbos JB, et al. Postoperative complications after vulvectomy and inguinofemoral lymphadenectomy using separate groin incisions. *Int J Gynecol Cancer.* 2003;13(4):522–527.
7. Fuh KC, Berek JS. Current management of vulvar cancer. *Hematol Oncol Clin North Am.* 2012;26(1):45–62.
8. Ansink AC, Sie-Go DM, van der Velden J, et al. Identification of sentinel lymph nodes in vulvar carcinoma patients with the aid of a patent blue V injection: a multicenter study. *Cancer.* 1999;86(4):652–656.
9. Levenback C, Coleman RL, Burke TW, Bodurka-Bevers D, Wolf JK, Gershenson DM. Intraoperative lymphatic mapping and sentinel node identification with blue dye in patients with vulvar cancer. *Gynecol Oncol.* 2001;83(2):276–281.
10. Sideri M, De Cicco C, Maggioni A, et al. Detection of sentinel nodes by lymphoscintigraphy and gamma probe guided surgery in vulvar neoplasia. *Tumori.* 2000;86(4):359–363.
11. de Hullu JA, Hollema H, Piers DA, et al. Sentinel lymph node procedure is highly accurate in squamous cell carcinoma of the vulva. *J Clin Oncol.* 2000;18(15):2811–2816.
12. Hauspy J, Beiner M, Harley I, Ehrlich L, Rasty G, Covens A. Sentinel lymph node in vulvar cancer. *Cancer.* 2007;110(5):1015–1023.
13. Nyberg RH, Iivonen M, Parkkinen J, Kuoppala T, Mäenpää JU. Sentinel node and vulvar cancer: a series of 47 patients. *Acta Obstet Gynecol Scand.* 2007;86(5):615–619.
14. Rob L, Robova H, Pluta M, et al. Further data on sentinel lymph node mapping in vulvar cancer by blue dye and radiocolloid Tc99. *Int J Gynecol Cancer.* 2007;17(1):147–153.
15. Van der Zee AG, Oonk MH, De Hullu JA, et al. Sentinel node dissection is safe in the treatment of early-stage vulvar cancer. *J Clin Oncol.* 2008;26(6):884–889.
16. Levenback CF, van der Zee AG, Rob L, et al. Sentinel lymph node biopsy in patients with gynecologic cancers Expert panel statement from the International Sentinel Node Society Meeting, February 21, 2008. *Gynecol Oncol.* 2009;114(2):151–156.
17. Levenback CF, Ali S, Coleman RL, et al. Lymphatic mapping and sentinel lymph node biopsy in women with squamous cell carcinoma of the vulva: a Gynecologic Oncology Group study. *J Clin Oncol.* 2012;30(31):3786–3791.
18. GOG 270 Study Protocol. *GROningen INternational Study on Sentinel Nodes in Vulvar Cancer (GROINSS-V) II, an Observational Study.* Version 7, May 2011. https://gogmember.gog.org/documents/protocols/pdf/0270.pdf.

Gestational Trophoblastic Disease

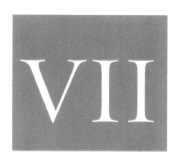

24 Choriocarcinoma

ROSHAN AGARWAL

NEIL J. SEBIRE

MICHAEL J. SECKL

■ INTRODUCTION

Gestational trophoblastic disease (GTD) consists of the premalignant complete and partial hydatidiform moles (CHM and PHM), and the malignant disorders, invasive mole, gestational choriocarcinoma (CC), placental site trophoblastic tumor (PSTT), and epithelioid trophoblastic tumors (ETT; 1). The malignant conditions are also known as gestational trophoblastic tumors (GTT) or neoplasia (GTN). Both CHM and PHM can develop into invasive moles, CC, and PSTT/ETT, but CC and PSTT/ETT can also develop after any type of pregnancy including term delivery, miscarriage, and an ectopic implantation (2–4). While survival rates for women with malignant change following a molar pregnancy is currently running at around 100% in the United Kingdom, patients with CC following nonmolar pregnancies are still not always cured (5,6). The reason for the high-success rates reside in centralized patients registration, human chorionic gonadotrophin (hCG) monitoring, pathology review, genetics, and clinical management with careful long-term follow-up. The reasons for failure to cure reside in early deaths from late presentation of advanced CC, the subsequent development of multidrug-resistant disease, or the distinct diseases of PSTT/ETT (covered in a separate chapter; 6,7). This chapter will review the epidemiology, pathology, hCG monitoring, diagnosis, and management of CC and cover some of our latest advances that have helped to improve outcomes.

Epidemiology

Although choriocarcinoma can arise following any type of pregnancy, CHM is probably the most common antecedent with an estimated 3% of CHMs developing into choriocarcinomas (7). In contrast, the incidence of choriocarcinoma following term delivery without a history of CHM is approximately 1:50,000 (Figure 24.1). Given a frequency of CHM of approximately one in 1000 pregnancies, this equates to an overall incidence of choriocarcinoma of approximately three in 50,000 pregnancies, with a 2.5:1 ratio of choriocarcinoma following molar to nonmolar pregnancy. CCs can also arise from PHMs, albeit with a very low frequency (≈0.25%; 4). In contrast to CHM, there are no clear international geographical trends in the incidence of choriocarcinoma, but the effect of age remains important.

Pathology

Choriocarcinoma is a highly malignant tumor, which appears as a soft purple largely hemorrhagic mass (8). Microscopically it mimics the appearances of an early implanting blastocyst with central cores of mononuclear cytotrophoblast surrounded by a rim of multinucleated syncytiotrophoblast and a distinct absence of chorionic villi. The surrounding areas are usually necrotic and hemorrhagic and tumor is frequently seen within venous sinuses. Genetic analysis frequently demonstrates multiple karyotype anomalies, but none as yet are specific for choriocarcinoma (8). However, where the preceding pregnancy was either a CHM or PHM, it has been possible to show that the resulting CC shares genetic identity either being androgenetic or triploid, respectively (4).

Choriocarcinomas are highly metastatic, and the majority of patients have high-risk disease at presentation (International Federation of Gynecology and Obstetrics [FIGO] score greater than 6, discussed below), and about 28% have ultra-high-risk disease (FIGO score greater than 12; Table 24.1; 6). In a recent analysis of high-risk patients from our center, six of seven deaths were in patients with choriocarcinomas, all of whom had nonmolar choriocarcinomas (three postterm deliveries and four abortions/undefined antecedent; 6).

The remainder of this chapter while touching on the general management of GTD will focus on the management of high-risk, and in particular ultra-high-risk, patients.

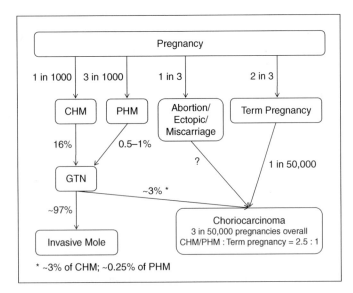

FIGURE 24.1 Incidence of choriocarcinoma.

Human Chorionic Gonadotrophin

The ability of serial measurements of hCG revolutionized the management of GTD and it remains the first and one of the most important tumor markers in oncology (9). hCG has a half-life of 24 to 36 hours and is the most sensitive and specific marker for trophoblastic tissue. The amount of hCG produced correlates with tumor volume so that a serum hCG of 5 IU/L corresponds to approximately 10^4 to 10^5 viable tumor cells. Consequently, these assays are several orders of magnitude more sensitive than the best imaging modalities available today. In addition, hCG levels can be used to determine prognosis (10). Serial measurements allow progress of the disease or response to therapy to be monitored (Figure 24.2). Development of drug resistance can be detected at an early stage that facilitates appropriate changes in management and estimates may be made of the time for which chemotherapy should be continued after hCG levels are undetectable in serum to reduce the tumor volume to zero. For these reasons, hCG is the best tumor marker known. A number of different commercial assays are available for hCG measurement for pregnancy, but their utility varies with respect to GTN management. For GTN management, tests with high sensitivity and specificity, and those able to detect all forms of hCG (intact, nicked, beta, and hyperglycosylated) equally well are ideal (11).

However, hCG production is not confined to pregnancy and GTD. Indeed, hCG is produced by any trophoblastic tissue found, for example, in germ cell tumors and in up to 15% of epithelial malignancies (9). The hCG levels in such cases can be just as high as those seen in GTD or in pregnancy. Therefore, measurements of hCG do not reliably discriminate between pregnancy, GTD, or non-GTT. It is conceivable that in the future we will discover hCG forms that are more specific for distinct disease processes. Hyperglycosylated hCG has been suggested to fit this bill but the underlying supporting data are insufficient for managing clinicians to have confidence in this approach so far and a commercial assay is not yet available (1).

Postmolar Choriocarcinoma: Presentation, Surveillance, and Diagnosis

The management of patients with potential choriocarcinoma often starts following a CHM or PHM. These usually present with threatened or missed abortions during the first trimester (12). Intraperitoneal bleeding can occur and occasionally this is catastrophic. Other presentations are those related to very high hCG levels such as toxaemia, hyperemesis, hyperthyroidism, and theca luteal cysts, or the finding of an excessively large uterus for dates. Symptoms related to pulmonary, vaginal, and cervical metastasis can also occur, although these may spontaneously disappear following evacuation of the mole. Trophoblastic embolization and disseminated intravascular coagulation (DIC) are now rarely seen (13).

The primary treatment for these patients is prompt evacuation of the uterine contents using gentle suction dilatation and curettage (D&C; 12). Prostanoids to ripen a nulliparous cervix are not recommended as this may induce uterine contractions and trigger trophoblastic embolization. The latter may be fatal and is probably also the explanation for why there is a higher risk of needing subsequent chemotherapy if medical or other surgical methods are used to evacuate the uterus.

Once diagnosed, all patients with GTD are registered with one of three centers located in Dundee, Sheffield, and the Charing Cross Hospital in London, which together form the United Kingdom GTD national follow-up service (5). These patients and their gynecologists then receive an information pack and the histology is requested for central review. All patients then send 2 weekly blood and urine samples to one of the three centers for serial hCG estimations. In the majority of cases any residual molar tissue regresses and the hCG levels return to normal (less than or equal to 4 IU/L). If the hCG has fallen to normal within 8 weeks of evacuation then marker follow-up can be safely reduced to 6 months from the date of evacuation. However, in patients whose hCG levels are still elevated beyond 8 weeks from the date of evacuation, follow-up is currently continued for 6 months of normal values. As patients who have had a previous mole or GTN are at an increased risk of developing reactivation of previous disease, hCG levels are measured at 6 and 10 weeks following the completion of each subsequent pregnancy.

Failure of the hCG to normalize, either with a plateau (over three values) or a rise (on two consecutive values), heralds the development of GTN and is an indication for chemotherapy in patients with a CHM or PHM as shown

■ **Table 24.1** Presenting characteristics of high-risk patients with biopsy-proven choriocarcinoma, compared to non-choriocarcinoma/non-biopsied patients (PTD)

| | | Total | High Risk GTN | | | | |
| | | | Choriocarcinoma | | PTD | | |
		n = 149	n = 72	%	n = 68	%	*p* value
WHO Age Score	0	98	56	78%	42	62%	.039
	1	42	16	22%	26	38%	
WHO Pregnancy Score	0	69	11	15%	58	85%	.000
	1	23	16	22%	7	10%	
	2	48	45	63%	3	4%	
WHO Interval Score	0	83	29	40%	54	79%	.000
	1	20	14	19%	6	9%	
	2	7	6	8%	1	1%	
	4	30	23	32%	7	10%	
WHO hCG Score	0	5	3	4%	2	3%	.236
	1	12	9	13%	3	4%	
	2	24	14	19%	10	15%	
	4	99	46	64%	53	78%	
WHO No. of Mets Score	0	44	17	24%	27	40%	.013
	1	44	19	26%	25	37%	
	2	15	11	15%	4	6%	
	4	37	25	35%	12	18%	
Lungmets	N	42	19	26%	23	34%	.337
	Y	98	53	74%	45	66%	
Livermets	N	136	69	96%	67	99%	.339
	Y	4	3	4%	1	1%	
Brainmets	N	123	57	79%	66	97%	.001
	Y	17	15	21%	2	3%	
WHO Mets Score	0	116	54	75%	62	91%	.019
	1	2	0	0%	2	3%	
	2	2	2	3%	0	0%	
	4	19	15	21%	4	6%	
	6	1	1	1%	0	0%	
WHO Large Mass Score	0	21	17	24%	4	6%	.004
	1	27	16	22%	11	16%	
	2	92	39	54%	53	78%	
FIGO Total Score	≤12	120	52	72%	68	100%	.000
	>12	20	20	28%	0	0%	
Dead	No	133	66	92%	67	99%	.063
	Yes	7	6	8%	1	1%	

Note: Decisions to biopsy were based on clinical assessment of risk and diagnostic uncertainty.

in Table 24.2. Where previous D&C or biopsy has demonstrated evidence of choriocarcinoma, these patients should be treated immediately with chemotherapy. However, for the majority of patients with postmolar plateau or rise in hCG levels, a biopsy to confirm the development of invasive mole or choriocarcinoma is not performed due to the risk of life-threatening hemorrhage, and the similarity in the management of patients. Chemotherapy is therefore started in most patients without any further histological confirmation and is guided by hCG levels and other prognostic features. Unlike the FIGO criteria, in the United Kingdom, there are some additional reasons why patients may start chemotherapy following a molar pregnancy (Table 24.2). Thus, for example, women with hCG values

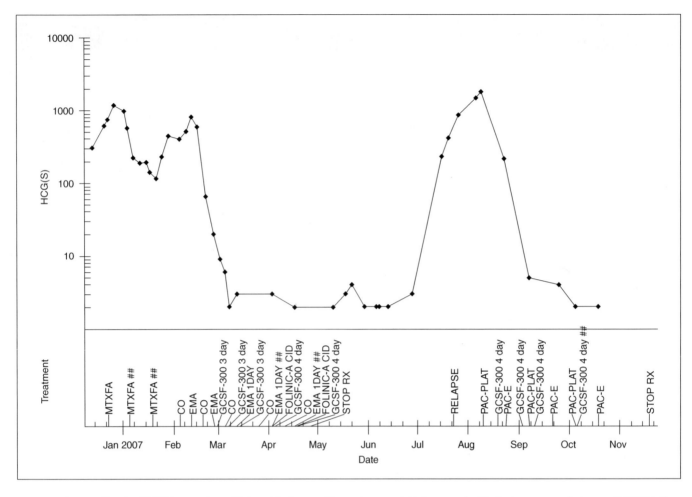

FIGURE 24.2 Graph of hCG in a patient with low risk disease. The patient was initially treated with single-agent methotrexate (MTX-FA), then changed to combination EMA/CO chemotherapy due the development of drug resistance, as indicated by the rise in hCG levels, and then on relapsed was salvaged with paclitaxel, etoposble/paclitaxel, cisplatinum (TE/TP) chemotherapy. EMA/CO, etoposide, methotrexate, actinomycin D, cyclophosphamide, vincristine; hCG, human chorionic gonadotrophin.

■ **Table 24.2** Indications for chemotherapy

Plateaued or rising hCG concentration after evacuation

Heavy vaginal bleeding or evidence of gastrointestinal or intraperitoneal hemorrhage

Histological evidence of choriocarcinoma

Evidence of metastases in brain, liver, or gastrointestinal tract, or radiological opacities larger than 2 cm on chest radiograph

Serum hCG concentration of 20,000 IU/L or more

4 Weeks or more after evacuation, because of the risk of uterine perforation

Raised hCG concentration 6 months after evacuation, even when still decreasing

Note: Any of the above are indications to treat following the diagnosis of GTD.
GTD, gestational trophoblastic disease; hCG, human chorionic gonadotrophin.

greater than 20,000 IU/L 4 weeks after evacuation of a mole, are at increased risk of uterine perforation or severe hemorrhage. These complications can be life threatening and the risk can be reduced by starting chemotherapy. Overall, in the United Kingdom, about 16% of patients with CHMs and 0.5%–1% with PHMs ultimately require chemotherapy for invasive mole, and approximately 3% will have an underlying choriocarcinoma (Figure 24.1; 1).

Choriocarcinoma Following Nonmolar Pregnancy

Choriocarcinoma can also present following an apparently normal pregnancy or nonmolar abortion (Figure 24.1; 1,2). This usually presents within a year of delivery, very rarely it can occur within the pregnancy, and in the Charing Cross series the longest interval to date has been greater than 20 years after the last known pregnancy. It is therefore perhaps unsurprising that in these diverse settings, the diagnosis of CC can be much more challenging. Table 24.1 summarizes the differences in the presenting features in a cohort of high-risk patients treated at our center between 1995 and 2010 by tumor histology. While the presenting features of choriocarcinoma can be similar to hydatidiform moles with vaginal bleeding, abdominal pain, pelvic mass, and symptoms due to a high serum hCG, one-third of all patients with choriocarcinomas present without gynecological features. Instead, a greater proportion of patients present with symptoms and signs associated with metastases. Pulmonary, cerebral, and hepatic deposits are most frequent, but any site may be involved including the cauda equina, gums, bones, and skin (Figure 24.3 and Table 24.1). In these cases, lives can be saved by remembering to include choriocarcinoma in the differential diagnosis of metastatic malignancy presenting in a woman of childbearing age.

Gestational Versus Nonchoriocarcinomas

In the absence of a clear antecedent molar or other recent pregnancy, despite the vascularity of these tumors, excision biopsy of a metastasis should be considered where it can be safely achieved. This not only enables histological confirmation of the diagnosis but more critically permits genetic analysis to differentiate between gestational and non-CCs (14). While the prognosis of CCs is excellent and the majority are cured (greater than 90%), most patients with non-CCs have at best brief responses to chemotherapy (6). Indeed, the latter cases with the exception of germ cell tumors have a very poor long-term survival that is best related to the tissue of origin. Where biopsy is not possible, the diagnosis is made on the clinical history and other investigation findings.

The International Federation of Gynecology and Obstetrics Staging

Where a histological diagnosis is not available, patients with suspected GTN following a molar pregnancy should undergo pelvic Doppler ultrasound scan (USS), to determine the uterine volume and vascularity, hCG estimation in serum and/or urine, and chest radiography (CXR) to look for pulmonary metastases. In contrast, all patients with suspected or a histologically proven diagnosis of choriocarcinoma should have a whole body CT, MRI brain and pelvis, and Doppler USS pelvis, due to the higher risks of metastases and potential for nongestational origin (1,12). Where pathology is available, genetic diagnosis to confirm a gestational origin through the presence of paternal genes is helpful in guiding subsequent management but should not delay the institution of life-saving chemotherapy (15,16). The use of 18-fluoro-deoxyglucose-positron emission tomography (FDG-PET/CT) imaging is still experimental but appears to be helpful in the subsequent

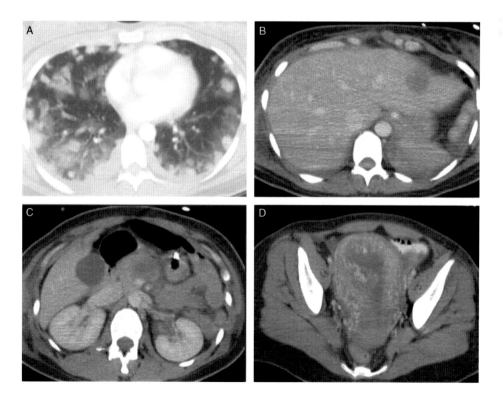

FIGURE 24.3 Staging CT scan of a high-risk choriocarcinoma patient with (A) pulmonary, (B) hepatic, and (C) para-aortic metastases, and extensive intrauterine disease (D). CT, computed tomography.

management of drug resistant disease rather than initial staging.

In addition, a full blood count, coagulation screen, group and save, urea, creatinine, electrolytes, and liver function tests are performed prior to starting chemotherapy. Following MRI imaging of the brain, provided no intracranial metastases are identified, cerebrospinal fluid (CSF) is obtained for hCG estimation (a hCG ratio of greater than 1:60 CSF: blood indicates CNS involvement; 17).

The information from these staging investigations is then used in the international FIGO scoring system (Table 24.3), to determine whether patients have disease that is at low or high risk of becoming resistant to single drug therapy with either methotrexate and folinic acid, or dactinomycin (18).

Chemotherapy

Low Risk

Patients with low-risk disease (less than 7 on the new FIGO system) are treated at Charing Cross Hospital with single-agent methotrexate with folinic acid rescue (MTX-FA; 5). The methotrexate (50 mg) is given intramuscularly, alternating daily with oral folinic acid (15 mg) 24 hours later for 1 week followed by a week of rest prior to recommencing treatment (Table 24.4). Chemotherapy shrinks the disease very rapidly, and this predisposes the patient to an increased risk of tumor hemorrhage. The other principal side effects

occurring in about 2% of patients are mucosal ulceration, conjunctivitis, and occasionally serositis. For these reasons, patients remain in hospital for the first 1 to 3 weeks of treatment. Overall, methotrexate therapy is very well tolerated, does not induce alopecia, and can be completed at a local health center. Given the higher rate of metastases, the majority of patients with CC have high-risk disease and only a minority receive single-agent chemotherapy based on a low-risk FIGO score at our center. However, due to the aggressiveness of CC it has been argued by some groups that irrespective of the FIGO score, CC patients should receive upfront combination agent chemotherapy (19).

High Risk

Patients with a FIGO score greater than or equal to 7 at presentation, have a high risk of resistance to single-agent therapy with, for example, methotrexate (greater than 60%), and at many centers in the world receive "high-risk" IV combination chemotherapy comprising etoposide, methotrexate, and actinomycin-D (EMA) alternating weekly with cyclophosphamide and vincristine (CO), instead of the MTX-FA regime (Table 24.4) (6,20). Acute side effects include myelosuppression, alopecia, peripheral neuropathy, and those associated with single-agent methotrexate therapy. This treatment requires an overnight stay in hospital every 2 weeks and 70% of the patients require granulocyte colony-stimulating factor injections to help maintain a sufficient neutrophil count and treatment intensity.

■ Table 24.3 FIGO scoring system for gestational trophoblastic tumors

FIGO Scoring	0	1	2	4
Age	<40	≥40	—	—
Antedecent pregnancy	Mole	Abortion	Term	—
Interval months from index pregnancy	<4	4–<7	7–<13	≥13
Pretreatment serum hCG (IU/L)	<10^3	10^3–<10^4	10^4–<10^5	≥10^5
Largest tumor size (including uterus) cm	<3	3–<5	≥5	—
Size of metastases	Lung	Spleen, Kidney	Gastrointestinal	Liver, brain
Number of metastases	—	1–4	5–8	>8
Previous failed chemotherapy	—	—	Single drug	Two or more drugs

hCG, human chorionic gonadotrophin.

■ Table 24.4 Common chemotherapy regimes used in GTN

Single-agent methotrexate (MTX-FA)

Methotrexate 50 mg IM D1, 3, 5 and 7, with folinic acid 15 mg PO D 2, 4, 6 and 8, every 14 days

Single-agent dactinomycin

Dactinomycin 0.5 mg IV D1–5, every 14 days

EMA/CO chemotherapy (every 14 days)

D1

    Etoposide 100 mg/m² by IV infusion for 30 minutes

    Methotrexate 300 mg/m² by IV infusion for 12 hours

    Actinomycin-D 0.5 mg IV bolus

D2

    Etoposide 100 mg/m² by IV infusion for 30 minutes

    Dactinomycin 0·5 mg IV bolus

    Folinic acid rescue 15 mg IV or orally every 12 hours for four doses commencing 24 hour post-starting methotrexate

D8

    Cyclophosphamide 600 mg/m² IV infusion for 30 minutes

    Vincristine (Oncovin) 1 mg/m² IV bolus (maximum 2 mg)

IM, intramuscular

Ultra High Risk

Patients with a FIGO score greater than 12 at presentation are considered to have ultra-high-risk disease, and usually all have choriocarcinomas (Table 24.1; 6). Historically due to the large disease burden, these patients frequently died within 4 weeks of treatment initiation due to catastrophic tumor hemorrhage and/or tumor-associated oedema, and organ failure, precipitated by chemotherapy. This was responsible for about 5% of all deaths in patients with high-risk GTN (20). However, we have recently shown, that the risk of early death can be almost completely eliminated in these patients with the use of induction of low-dose etoposide and cisplatinum (EP; E 100 mg/m^2 and P 20 mg/m^2 days 1 and 2 weekly for 1–3 weeks), prior to EMA/CO chemotherapy to achieve a more gradual reduction in tumor burden without precipitating catastrophic hemorrhage and respiratory failure (6). These ultra-high-risk patients, should also be considered for upfront full dose EP/EMA chemotherapy (discussed below), instead of EMA/CO, following induction low-dose EP.

Treatment with MTX-FA, EMA/CO, and/or EP/EMA is continued in all patients until the hCG has normalized, followed by a further 6 to 8 weeks of consolidation chemotherapy (Figure 24.2; 6). During this time the serum hCG is measured twice a week, so that the tumor response can be closely monitored and appropriate treatment changes made promptly.

Patient Follow Up and Relapse

On completion of their chemotherapy, patients are advised to use adequate sun-block to minimize the effect of therapy induced skin photosensitivity (1,12). They should also avoid pregnancy for 1 year to reduce the risk of teratogenicity due to chemotherapy, disease reactivation, and the inability to detect recurrent disease in the presence of high hCG levels due to pregnancy. However, in a cohort of 230 women who became pregnant despite this advice, 70% progressed to term, only 1 patient relapsed, and there were no maternal deaths (21).

In the United Kingdom, patients remain on urine hCG follow-up for life to confirm that their disease is in remission and are specifically tested 6 and 10 weeks following subsequent pregnancies (1,12). About 2% of low-risk and 5% of high-risk patients relapse and our data suggest that the risk of relapse is higher in patients with low hCG levels at presentation, although the reasons for this are unclear (5,6,20,22).

Management of Specific Complications of Gestational Trophoblastic Disease

Hemorrhage

This usually responds to bed rest and chemotherapy, along with adequate blood transfusion. However, on occasion uterine packs, selective embolization, or laparotomy may be necessary; hysterectomy is rarely required.

Respiratory Failure

This can be multifactorial due to parenchymal tumor deposits and/or tumor, or clot embolization (13). In the majority of patients, respiratory failure can be adequately managed by increasing the inspired oxygen concentration and early chemotherapy. When embolism is suspected, the patient should also be anticoagulated with heparin. The administration of dexamethasone (8 mg, 8 hourly) may prevent deterioration associated with tumor necrosis and edema. If possible, mechanical ventilation should be avoided as the high airway pressures can trigger fatal pulmonary hemorrhage from metastases.

Cerebral Metastases

Chemotherapy in the presence of cerebral metastases may be complicated by intracranial hemorrhage from the tumor and/or increased intracranial pressure. While we have previously aimed to resect accessible solitary metastasis prior to chemotherapy, our recent experience indicates that this is not necessary when patients are commenced on low-dose induction EP chemotherapy (6,23; Figure 24.4). However, should bleeding or uncontrolled raised intracranial pressure ensue then surgery is required. Leaving a skull flap open can be life saving as this leaves space for the brain to expand laterally rather than be forced down through the foramen magnum. Once the disease is under control with chemotherapy, the defect can be repaired. Whole brain radiotherapy adds to toxicity including the risk of long-term memory loss and even more worryingly, the development of fatal multifocal leukoencephalopathy. Moreover, in the Charing Cross experience whole brain radiotherapy does not improve outcomes (23). However, occasionally stereotactic or gamma knife radiotherapy is employed for the treatment of isolated deep-seated lesions that remain after chemotherapy. If multiple tumor deposits are present, prophylactic use of dexamethasone may be useful in preventing cerebral edema due to chemotherapy. The chemotherapy regimen is also modified in patients with overt cerebral metastases (6,20,23). At Charing Cross, these individuals receive intrathecal methotrexate fortnightly with each CO and the dose of methotrexate in EMA is increased to optimize CNS penetration of the cytotoxic agents. In ultra-high-risk patients with liver and brain involvement, IT MTX is given with EP and the MTX dose is increased to 1 g/m^2 within a 1 day EMA in which the second day of dactinomycin and etoposide are omitted. Patients without overt CNS disease but with lung metastases are at high risk of brain metastases, and at our institute receive as prophylaxis three doses of intrathecal methotrexate. This is given at the start of courses of low-risk treatment or with the CO element of high-risk therapy (6,20,23).

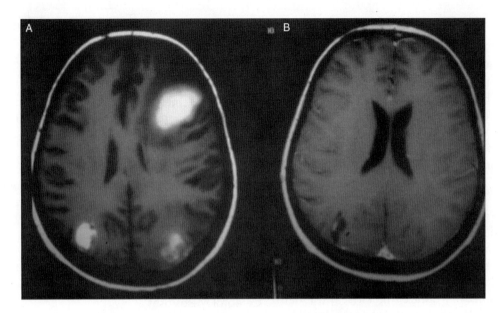

FIGURE 24.4 MRI scan of a patient with choriocarcinoma with (A) brain metastases before and (B) after completion of chemotherapy.

Hepatic Metastases

Historically, the presence of liver metastases has been associated with only a 30% long-term survival rate and when combined with brain involvement, only 10% of patients survive (20). A more recent set of analyses suggests that survival is improving in these patient subgroups probably because of reduced early deaths with the use of low-dose induction EP and through genetic diagnosis, and the exclusion of patients with nongestational tumors (6). Whether the survival of patients with liver metastases is now as good as those without will remain unclear until we have larger patient numbers to study.

Infantile Choriocarcinoma

This is an extremely rare condition with about 50 reported cases worldwide (24). Usually the disease presents within weeks of delivery in the baby first and subsequently may develop in some mothers. Indeed, the disease can present up to 14 months later in the mother so careful hCG monitoring of the mother is important. Since maternal presentation before the infant is also possible, when the disease presents within weeks of birth in the mother, the infant should also have its urinary hCG checked on at least one occasion and repeated if there is any failure to thrive. The outcome in infants with choriocarcinoma is often very poor, possibly due to delayed diagnosis although some have been saved with chemotherapy (24).

Drug Resistant/Relapsed Disease

Approximately 30%–45% of patients become resistant to methotrexate and this is heralded by a plateau or rise in hCG levels (6,25). If this occurs when the hCG is less than 300 IU/L then most patients can be salvaged by switching

to single-agent therapy with actinomycin-D given intravenously daily for 5 days every 2 weeks (Table 24.3; 22). This treatment is sometimes used as a first-line agent in other countries and from nonrandomized data appears to be equally effective to methotrexate. However, it is more toxic inducing alopecia, oral ulceration, nausea, vomiting, and myelosuppression. If the hCG is greater than 300 IU/L when resistance develops then patients are switched to multiagent EMA/CO chemotherapy (Table 24.3; 6,22). In our experience all low-risk patients who develop resistance or relapse can be salvaged with further chemotherapy (EMA/CO or alternative regimens) and thus this group has a close to 100% cure rate (5,6).

Fifteen percent of high-risk patients become resistant and 5% relapse following EMA-CO, and may be salvaged with EP-EMA, or with paclitaxel and cisplatin alternating every 2 weeks with paclitaxel and etoposide (TP-TE; 6,26,27). The TP-TE regimen is much less toxic than EP-EMA, with rates of neutropenia (G3/4) of 42% vs 68%, and renal impairment (G2–4) of 4% vs 41%, respectively, in independent cohort studies (27). A randomized trial is required to directly compare the efficacy and toxicity of the two regimens.

Selected patients may also benefit from high-dose chemotherapy with autologous bone marrow or peripheral stem cell rescue (28,29). In our recent series, 5 of 16 patients treated with high-dose chemotherapy were alive and disease free after 5 years (28 and unpublished data).

A strategy of debulking surgery in an attempt to excise drug-resistant tissue followed by chemotherapy for residual disease can also effectively salvage some patients (30). In this context tumor localization may be aided by whole body CT, MRI, or FDG-PET (31). However, routine excision of postchemotherapy masses in patients with choriocarcinoma who have a normal hCG postchemotherapy does not appear to be beneficial.

Prognosis

All GTN deaths are in high-risk patients, despite salvage rate of greater than 75% in relapsed/resistant patients (6). The current overall 5-year survival rate in high-risk patients is 94%, compared to 86% previously. This improvement has been achieved through a reduction in early deaths (less than 4 weeks of presentation) with the use of induction low-dose EP (etoposide-platinum), prior to EMA/CO chemotherapy to achieve a more gradual reduction in tumor burden without precipitating catastrophic hemorrhage and respiratory failure (6). In addition, the availability of genetic tests have enabled patients with true CCs to be differentiated from uniformly fatal nongestational choriocarcinomas, which historically comprised approximately 5% of patients treated with presumed high-risk GTN (6,14). Drug resistance is currently the main cause of death in high-risk GTN and associated with high hCG levels at presentation, and brain metastases (6). A better understanding of the mechanisms of drug resistance and targeted therapies for these patients is required.

In the long term, EMA/CO therapy also increases the risk of second tumors by 1.3-fold compared to the general population, and may expedite the menopause by an average of 3 years (6,20,32). Low-risk chemotherapy with methotrexate, however, is not associated with any long-term toxicity (22). Importantly neither treatment affects fertility or rates of fetal abnormality in subsequent pregnancies. Currently, twice as many patients receive EMA/CO due to MTX-FA resistance than due to high-risk disease at presentation (6). The development of noncytotoxic strategies to increase the efficacy of MTX-FA has the potential to reduce the number of these young patients exposed to EMA/CO.

Novel Therapies

For those patients with multidrug-resistant and nonresectable disease, a number of new agents also appear to have activity in the disease. These include gemcitabine and pemetrexed in combination with cisplatin or carboplatin (33). Since choriocarcinomas express high levels of folate receptors, folate-conjugated drugs such as EC-145, and the anti-folate receptor antibody farletuzumab represent exciting opportunities for targeted therapy in this disease (34). Indeed, preclinical development of these drugs has frequently been done on choriocarcinoma cell lines (e.g., JEG and JAR cells).

Recent data have also shown that tumor vascularity predicts MTX-FA resistance, and suggests that antiangiogenic drugs such as bevacizumab may be useful (35). Unfortunately, we have thus far not seen any signs of benefit in the 2–3 patients treated with bevacizumab and may be due to the presence of vascular endothelial growth factor (VEGF) independent angiogenic pathways in GTN (36). As some choriocarcinomas overexpress EGFR we have also tried erlotinib also without effect (37). Given that the tumor secretes hCG it is conceivable that anti-hCG targeted therapy might be useful but this remains to be fully explored (38). In addition, a plethora of other new targeted therapies now exist and as we learn more about the biology of multidrug resistant choriocarcinoma, an extended role for these novel agents may be discovered for GTN.

CONCLUSIONS

Choriocarcinoma has transformed from a universally fatal disease to the majority of patients cured with the use of systemic chemotherapy five decades ago. Given the rarity of this disease, the most effective strategy for effective management has been to identify patients with premalignant molar pregnancies, undertake hCG surveillance to identify early the development of GTN, followed by centralized chemotherapy, which is limited to two national centers in the United Kingdom. This strategy has eliminated the need for the majority of patients to undergo additional biopsies beyond the initial histological diagnosis of a molar pregnancy, such that patients today are treated with the more general diagnosis of GTN, rather than being differentiated into invasive mole or choriocarcinoma. Today, with an integrated approach to management the majority of women are cured from their trophoblastic tumors, with their fertility intact.

■ ACKNOWLEDGMENTS

MJS would like to thank the National Commissioning Group and Department of Health for their continuing support of the GTD service. MJS is also supported by the Imperial College Experimental Cancer Medicine Centre grant from Cancer Research UK and the Dept of Health. RA is supported by a Clinician Scientist Fellowship from Cancer Research UK.

■ REFERENCES

1. Seckl MJ, Sebire NJ, Berkowitz RS. Gestational trophoblastic disease. *Lancet.* 2010;376(9742):717–729.
2. Sebire NJ, Foskett M, Fisher RA, Lindsay I, Seckl MJ. Persistent gestational trophoblastic disease is rarely, if ever, derived from non-molar first-trimester miscarriage. *Med Hypotheses.* 2005;64(4):689–693.
3. Sebire NJ, Lindsay I, Fisher RA, Savage P, Seckl MJ. Overdiagnosis of complete and partial hydatidiform mole in tubal ectopic pregnancies. *Int J Gynecol Pathol.* 2005;24(3):260–264.
4. Seckl MJ, Fisher RA, Salerno G, et al. Choriocarcinoma and partial hydatidiform moles. *Lancet.* 2000;356(9223):36–39.

5. Sita-Lumsden A, Short D, Lindsay I, et al. Treatment outcomes for 618 women with gestational trophoblastic tumours following a molar pregnancy at the Charing Cross Hospital, 2000–2009. *Br J Cancer.* 2012;107(11):1810–1814.

6. Alifrangis C, Agarwal R, Short D, et al. EMA/CO for high-risk gestational trophoblastic neoplasia: good outcomes with induction low-dose etoposide-cisplatin and genetic analysis. *J Clin Oncol.* 2013;31(2):280–286.

7. Schmid P, Nagai Y, Agarwal R, et al. Prognostic markers and long-term outcome of placental-site trophoblastic tumours: a retrospective observational study. *Lancet.* 2009;374(9683): 48–55.

8. Paradinas FJ, Fisher RA. Pathology and molecular genetics of trophoblastic disease. *Current Obstet Gynaecol.* 1995;5:6–12.

9. Mitchell H, Bagshawe KD, Newlands ES, Savage P, Seckl MJ. Importance of accurate human chorionic gonadotropin measurement in the treatment of gestational trophoblast disease and testicular cancer. *J Reprod Med.* 2006;51(11):868–870.

10. Bagshawe KD. Risk and prognostic factors in trophoblastic neoplasia. *Cancer.* 1976;38(3):1373–1385.

11. Mitchell H, Seckl MJ. Discrepancies between commercially available immunoassays in the detection of tumour-derived hCG. *Mol Cell Endocrinol.* 2007;260–262:310–313.

12. Sebire NJ, Seckl MJ. Gestational trophoblastic disease: current management of hydatidiform mole. *BMJ.* 2008;337:a1193.

13. Seckl MJ, Rustin GJ, Newlands ES, Gwyther SJ, Bomanji J. Pulmonary embolism, pulmonary hypertension, and choriocarcinoma. *Lancet.* 1991;338(8778):1313–1315.

14. Fisher RA, Savage PM, MacDermott C, et al. The impact of molecular genetic diagnosis on the management of women with hCG-producing malignancies. *Gynecol Oncol.* 2007;107(3):413–419.

15. Fisher RA, Newlands ES. Gestational trophoblastic disease. Molecular and genetic studies. *J Reprod Med.* 1998;43(1):87–97.

16. Fisher RA, Newlands ES, Jeffreys AJ, et al. Gestational and nongestational trophoblastic tumors distinguished by DNA analysis. *Cancer.* 1992;69(3):839–845.

17. Bagshawe KD, Harland S. Immunodiagnosis and monitoring of gonadotrophin-producing metastases in the central nervous system. *Cancer.* 1976;38(1):112–118.

18. FIGO. FIGO staging for gestational trophoblastic neoplasia 2000. *Int J Gynaecol Obstet.* 2002;77(3):285–287.

19. Tidy JA, Rustin GJ, Newlands ES, et al. Presentation and management of choriocarcinoma after nonmolar pregnancy. *Br J Obstet Gynaecol.* 1995;102(9):715–719.

20. Bower M, Newlands ES, Holden L, et al. EMA/CO for high-risk gestational trophoblastic tumors: results from a cohort of 272 patients. *J Clin Oncol.* 1997;15(7):2636–2643.

21. Blagden SP, Foskett MA, Fisher RA, et al. The effect of early pregnancy following chemotherapy on disease relapse and foetal outcome in women treated for gestational trophoblastic tumours. *Br J Cancer.* 2002;86(1):26–30.

22. McNeish IA, Strickland S, Holden L, et al. Low-risk persistent gestational trophoblastic disease: outcome after initial treatment with low-dose methotrexate and folinic acid from 1992 to 2000. *J Clin Oncol.* 2002;20(7):1838–1844.

23. Newlands ES, Holden L, Seckl MJ, McNeish I, Strickland S, Rustin GJ. Management of brain metastases in patients with high-risk gestational trophoblastic tumors. *J Reprod Med.* 2002;47(6):465–471.

24. Sebire NJ, Lindsay I, Fisher RA, Seckl MJ. Intraplacental choriocarcinoma: experience from a tertiary referral center and relationship with infantile choriocarcinoma. *Fetal Pediatr Pathol.* 2005;24(1):21–29.

25. Newlands ES. The management of recurrent and drug-resistant gestational trophoblastic neoplasia (GTN). *Best Pract Res Clin Obstet Gynaecol.* 2003;17(6):905–923.

26. Newlands ES, Mulholland PJ, Holden L, Seckl MJ, Rustin GJ. Etoposide and cisplatin/etoposide, methotrexate, and actinomycin D (EMA) chemotherapy for patients with high-risk gestational trophoblastic tumors refractory to EMA/cyclophosphamide and vincristine chemotherapy and patients presenting with metastatic placental site trophoblastic tumors. *J Clin Oncol.* 2000;18(4):854–859.

27. Wang J, Short D, Sebire NJ, et al. Salvage chemotherapy of relapsed or high-risk gestational trophoblastic neoplasia (GTN) with paclitaxel/cisplatin alternating with paclitaxel/etoposide (TP/TE). *Ann Oncol.* 2008;19(9):1578–1583.

28. El-Helw LM, Seckl MJ, Haynes R, et al. High-dose chemotherapy and peripheral blood stem cell support in refractory gestational trophoblastic neoplasia. *Br J Cancer.* 2005;93(6):620–621.

29. Termrungruanglert W, Kudelka AP, Piamsomboon S, et al. Remission of refractory gestational trophoblastic disease with high-dose paclitaxel. *Anticancer Drugs.* 1996;7(5):503–506.

30. Alifrangis C, Wilkinson MJ, Stefanou DC, Virk JS, Anderson J, Seckl MJ. Role of thoracotomy and metastatectomy in gestational trophoblastic neoplasia: a single center experience. *J Reprod Med.* 2012;57(7–8):350–358.

31. Dose J, Bohuslavizki K, Hüneke B, Lindner C, Jänicke F. Detection of intramural choriocarcinoma of the uterus with 18F-FDG-PET. A case report. *Clin Positron Imaging.* 2000;3(1):37–40.

32. Bower M, Rustin GJ, Newlands ES, et al. Chemotherapy for gestational trophoblastic tumours hastens menopause by 3 years. *Eur J Cancer.* 1998;34(8):1204–1207.

33. Shih IeM. Gestational trophoblastic neoplasia–pathogenesis and potential therapeutic targets. *Lancet Oncol.* 2007;8(7):642–650.

34. Teng L, Xie J, Teng L, Lee RJ. Clinical translation of folate receptor-targeted therapeutics. *Expert Opin Drug Deliv.* 2012;9(8):901–908.

35. Agarwal R, Strickland S, McNeish IA, et al. Doppler ultrasonography of the uterine artery and the response to chemotherapy in patients with gestational trophoblastic tumors. *Clin Cancer Res.* 2002;8(5):1142–1147.

36. Shih IeM. Trophoblastic vasculogenic mimicry in gestational choriocarcinoma. *Mod Pathol.* 2011;24(5):646–652.

37. John M, Rajalekshmy T, Nair B, et al. Expression of epidermal growth factor and its receptor in gestational trophoblastic diseases. *Oncol Rep.* 1997;4(1):177–182.

38. Bagshawe KD, Searle F, Lewis J, Brown P, Keep P. Preliminary therapeutic and localization studies with human chorionic gonadotrophin. *Cancer Res.* 1980;40(8 Pt 2):3016–3017.

25 Placental Site Trophoblastic Tumor

EMILY BERRY

INTRODUCTION

Gestational trophoblastic disease (GTD) encompasses four clinicopathologic forms of growth disturbances of the human placenta: (a) hydatidiform mole (complete and partial); (b) invasive mole; (c) choriocarcinoma; and (d) placental site trophoblastic tumor (PSTT). The term *gestational trophoblastic neoplasia* (GTN) has been applied collectively to the latter three conditions, because the diagnosis and decision to institute treatment are often made without knowledge of the precise histology.

PSTT is a rare manifestation of GTN that may complicate any type of pregnancy and presents in 0.25%–5% of patients with GTD worldwide (1,2). First recognized as a distinct entity in 1976, this uterine tumor was initially named "trophoblastic pseudotumor" to characterize the apparently benign nature of the disease. However, subsequent reports describing aggressive and sometimes fatal outcomes prompted the nomenclature to be changed to PSTT in 1981 (3,4). The disease is unique from other GTDs, and is defined by slow growth, low human chorionic gonadotropin (hCG) serum levels, the late-onset metastatic potential, and most significantly, the relative insensitivity to chemotherapy.

PATHOLOGY

PSTT is biologically different from other forms of GTN in that it represents a neoplastic proliferation of intermediate trophoblast (IT) cells that invade the uterine myometrium at the placental site after a pregnancy. This population of cells has been designated "implantation site IT" because of its resemblance to the trophoblastic cells found at the implantation site. In the implantation site these transformed ITs of PSTT cells are large, polygonal, and often spindle shaped with highly pleomorphic, atypical nuclei that bear little resemblance to other types of trophoblastic cells (5,6). In addition, implantation site ITs infiltrate the endomyometrium and invade blood vessels, features

characteristic of a malignant tumor. As reported by Shih and Kurman (6), these traits can make distinguishing a florid, benign infiltration of the implantation site ("exaggerated placental site") from a PSTT in a specimen of endometrial curettings very difficult.

Pathologic methods used to confirm the diagnosis include immunohistochemical staining of tissue using diluted antibodies for cytokeratin proteins, hCG, and human placental lactogen (hPL). Shih and Kurman (7) reported that positive staining for hPL, alpha-inhibin, and cytokeratin 8/18 (CAM5.2) and negative staining for smooth muscle markers confirm the diagnosis of PSTT. While PSTTs are diffusely (50%–100%) positive for hPL, it is typical to observe only sparse (less than 10%) hCG positivity among tumor cells (8).

In addition, the transformed IT cells of PSTT have a high proliferative activity with an abnormal expression of cell-cycle regulatory molecules, which is not observed in normal IT. This activity is confirmed by the presence of Ki-67, a proliferation marker detected by nuclear labeling in ITs using immunohistochemistry (7). This feature can be exploited in the differential diagnosis of an exaggerated implantation site vs a PSTT, which as noted previously can at times be very difficult in a curettage specimen. The proliferation rate of PSTT as measured by Ki-67 labeling is approximately 14%, which helps to distinguish it from exaggerated placental site reaction that demonstrates no proliferation.

Finally, if mitotic figures are evident, the lesion should be considered a PSTT until proven otherwise. The mitotic rate is variable from less than 1 to greater than 30 mitoses per 10 high-power field (HPF; 9).

CLINICAL PRESENTATION AND DIAGNOSIS

Due to the rarity of this type of tumor, there is little information about its epidemiology and etiology, and few large series on diagnosis and treatment have been published. Risk factors for PSTT are not well understood. The disease is seen mostly in women of reproductive age, although cases have been reported in postmenopausal women. Approximately 53%–78% of PSTT lesions follow a term delivery; the rest arising after abortion or molar pregnancy (10). The time from the index pregnancy to diagnosis is variable and can be up to several years. The differential diagnosis of PSTT includes other forms of GTN, retained products of conception (RPC), uterine arteriovenous malformation (AVM), and the equally rare epithelioid trophoblastic tumor (ETT).

Irregular vaginal bleeding or amenorrhea of varying duration have been the most commonly reported presenting features (75%–92%; 10), but a wide range of other symptoms, often a consequence of metastatic disease, have also been reported including galactorrhea, virilization, nephrotic syndrome, and polycythemia (11). On examination uterine enlargement may be appreciated.

Further evaluation of symptoms often leads to imaging, laboratory investigations, and often an endometrial curettage (dilation and curettage [D&C]). PSTT can also be an incidental finding on a hysterectomy specimen. Most often PSTT is diagnosed when a uterine lesion is seen on imaging and the serum hCG protein is elevated. Due to the lack of syncytiotrophoblast tissue, serum hCG levels are often only modestly elevated in PSTT and correlate neither with the burden nor with malignant behavior, and thus appear to have no predictive value. In addition, the hCG is measured at relatively low levels compared to other forms of GTN. In a review of three large case series, Kim (10) found that serum hCG levels in patients with PSTT tended to be less than 1000 mIU/mL, with the great majority being less than 400 mIU/mL.

In general, while PSTT does produce low levels of serum hPL and this marker may help to distinguish between choriocarcinoma and PSTT, it is not recommended for use as a reliable tumor marker. Likewise, the serum cancer antigen 125 (CA125), found to be elevated in rare cases of PSTT, is not regarded as a useful tumor marker.

Two scenarios that should raise the suspicion for PSTT include low levels of hCG in association with a relatively large tumor or tumor burden and a diagnosis of GTN with an unexpected resistance to chemotherapy, as other forms of GTN are highly chemotherapy sensitive.

The clinical strategy of PSTT is unfortunately individual, but once the diagnosis of PSTT is suspected or established, immediate evaluation for metastases and prognostic factors is crucial. Along with a history and complete physical exam, the following laboratory tests should be obtained: complete blood count including platelets, clotting function studies, serum chemistries including renal and liver function panels, blood type and antibody screen, and determination of quantitative serum hCG levels. Recommended radiographic studies include chest x-ray with CT scan of the chest if x-ray is negative, CT scan of the abdomen and pelvis, pelvic ultrasonography, and CT or MRI of the brain as indicated.

Unlike other forms of malignant GTN, PSTT is often more slow growing, tends to spread locally through the uterus, and can involve lymph nodes (a very rare finding for choriocarcinoma) before metastasizing elsewhere.

In most cases, PSTTs are confined to the uterus. In earlier reports, PSTT presented with metastases in about 10% of cases (12) and metastases develop in an additional 10% of patients during follow-up (13). However, more recent literature suggests that metastases at presentation occur in over 30% and recurrences develop in over 30% of cases (14–16). The most common site of metastasis is lung, but metastases to the brain, liver, spleen, bowel, pancreas, kidney, vagina, and in rare cases retroperitoneal and supraclavicular lymph nodes have been reported.

■ IMAGING

Imaging has many uses in the diagnosis and management of PSTT including evaluating tumor size and detecting metastatic disease. Several imaging modalities have been identified as useful in the evaluation of PSTT but none are specific and thus do not allow definitive distinction from other forms of GTN. PSTT develops from the ITs, a group of cells that diffusely infiltrate the myometrium; therefore, the presence of a discrete mass on imaging may not represent the maximal tumor extension.

Ultrasound

To date, the main role of ultrasound imaging of PSTT has been to aid in diagnosis and to clarify the vascularity of the tumor with the goal of assisting in surgical management.

Transvaginal and transabdominal ultrasonography typically describe a heterogeneous, hyperechoic mass with multiple cystic (vascular) spaces within the myometrium of an enlarged uterus. These features alone do not allow distinction from other forms of GTN, though with the addition of color-flow Doppler imaging both hypervascular and hypovascular forms have been described with or without cystic masses (17,18).

More recently, Zhou et al (19) reported on the ultrasound findings of 14 patients with PSTT and noted that while all lesions were detected by transvaginal ultrasonography, unlike prior studies most lesions were solid with minimal vascularity and borders were often poorly delineated. In general the consensus stands that while ultrasound can aid in the diagnosis of PSTT, the features of this tumor are not specific enough to differentiate them from other forms of GTN, RPC, or AVM.

CT

The role of CT in the management of PSTT is principally in the detection of metastatic disease, which in turn helps assign the stage of disease and guide treatment planning.

MRI

MRI has been reported to allow more accurate tumor localization, clarify vascularity, and demonstrate extension through the myometrium (if present), thus allowing more appropriate surgical planning. As with ultrasound, two different MRI appearances undoubtedly correspond to the hypervascular and relatively hypovascular tumor types. The hypervascular type is described as an isointense mass on T1-weighted imaging and slightly hyperintense on T2, relative to normal myometrium. After the administration of intravenous gadolinium, avid tumor enhancement is shown. The hypovascular tumor type is described as being typically smaller in size, hyperintense to normal myometrium on both T1- and T2-weighted sequences, with some enhancement after gadolinium administration (20,21). However, as with ultrasound, the appearances described are not specific, and do not allow definitive distinction from other forms of GTN.

MRI is also employed to assess pelvic lymph node status, however, this is only relevant in PSTT as the other forms do not tend to metastasize to lymph nodes (22).

Positron Emission Tomography

Imaging with ^{18}F-fluorodeoxyglucose-positron emission tomography (FDG-PET) has proven to be useful for the staging and detection of recurrence in various malignancies. In 2005, Shaw et al (23) described the first reported use of PET imaging for the evaluation of multiple lung nodules in a woman with a new diagnosis of PSTT and a history of pulmonary tuberculosis. The patient had uptake in the uterine tumor but not in the lungs and was treated successfully with hysterectomy with complete response. Likewise, Nieves et al (24) reported on a case of PSTT metastatic to the lung. Disease persistence was detected using FDG-PET imaging, resulting in successful resection of the lesion and a complete response. Chang et al (25) published preliminary results from a small pilot study of gestational trophoblastic tumors (GTTs) that suggest and support the use of PET to identify chemotherapy-resistant lesions that can be removed by surgery, rule out false-positive lesions found by CT scan, define tumor extent more precisely before starting treatment, and confirm complete treatment response in PSTT or recurrent/resistant GTT.

■ STAGING

PSTT is staged according to the revised International Federation of Gynecology and Obstetrics' (FIGO) criteria for GTN as determined in 2000 (Table 25.1; 26). The FIGO stage carries little prognostic significance and is noted but not uniformly used to determine therapy.

■ Table 25.1	FIGO staging of GTN
Stage I	Disease confined to the uterus
Stage II	GTN extends outside the uterus but is limited to the genital structures (adnexa, vagina, broad ligament).
Stage III	GTN extends to the lungs with or without genital tract involvement.
Stage IV	All other metastatic sites.

FIGO, International Federation of Gynecology and Obstetrics; GTN, gestational trophoblastic neoplasia.

While the concurrent FIGO scoring system is routinely used to guide treatment for patients with invasive mole and choriocarcinoma, many studies have shown that this scoring system is not applicable to patients with PSTT and it is therefore not assigned or used to guide therapy. Instead, prognostic factors are used to guide therapy and predict outcomes.

■ PROGNOSTIC FACTORS

With regards to outcomes, various prognostic factors have been proposed to be important, including stage, number of mitoses, depth of myometrial invasion, size of primary tumor, serum hCG level, and duration from the antecedent pregnancy.

Recent literature has consistently found that poor survival was associated with clinical and pathology factors including: interval from previous pregnancy greater than 48 months, FIGO Stage IV disease, antecedent term pregnancy, serum hCG level greater than 1000 IU/L, age older than 35 years, deep myometrial invasion (greater than 1/2), high mitotic rate (greater than 5 per 10 HPF), coagulative necrosis, the presence of tumor cells with clear cytoplasm, and vascular space involvement (1,15,27).

Analysis of a UK-PSTT series has shown that the most important and only factor to remain significant on multivariate analysis was the duration between the antecedent pregnancy and the clinical presentation. In that series, 98% of women were cured if they presented within 4 years, whereas all 13 women presenting beyond this time eventually succumbed to their disease, regardless of disease stage or hCG levels (1). Other series, including two from the United States, found that the interval of greater than 2 years from antecedent pregnancy was the most significant adverse variable for survival (28,29). Feltmate et al (14) recommended that tumors with a mitotic index of greater than 5 mitotic figures/10 HPF were at increased risk of developing recurrence, but it should be noted that there have been several reports of recurrence developing with tumors having less than 2 mitotic figures/10 HPF (30–32).

■ TREATMENT MODALITIES

Although the majority of patients with nonmetastatic PSTT are cured by hysterectomy, a number of cases require aggressive treatment with chemotherapy and/or radiation. The rarity of PSTT along with its unpredictable biological behavior and reduced chemosensitivity means that optimum management is difficult to plan.

Nonmetastatic Disease

The majority of patients with PSTT present with Stage I disease. The current standard management of uterine-confined PSTT is a total hysterectomy with or without bilateral salpingo-oophorectomy. Remission rates of up to 100% have been reported (10). Since adnexal micrometastasis is uncommon (3%; 33), preservation of the ovaries is reasonable.

Although little evidence is available about the optimum extent of surgery needed for patients with Stage I disease, some centers recommend routine bilateral pelvic lymph node sampling (34). Review of the world literature reveals the incidence of lymph node metastases is low (5.9%) and occurs with equal frequency at pelvic and extra-pelvic sites (35). More commonly, PSTT spreads via a hematogenous rather than lymphatic route and in the United States and much of the United Kingdom, pelvic lymphadenectomy is not routinely performed in conjunction with hysterectomy. In terms of the type of hysterectomy, most PSTTs are found in the fundal region, hence radical hysterectomy, as suggested by Saso et al (34), should only be carried out if preoperative imaging suggests disease extension close to the parametria.

In patients who desire future fertility and have good prognostic factors, some investigators argue that hysterectomy may be replaced by focal resection of localized uterine disease or initial combination chemotherapy followed by wedge resection of any residual disease. These approaches are certainly worth considering but are not often successful due to the frequent multifocal nature of the disease and/or positive surgical margins on the resection specimen (1).

The role of postoperative chemotherapy in patients with Stage I or II disease is controversial. Randomized trials have not been done to support the use of chemotherapy and such data are unlikely to be generated in view of the rarity of this disease. Existing studies have yet to define a subset of patients who would benefit from this approach. In view of the poor outcome for patients with recurrent disease, adjuvant chemotherapy is considered for patients with Stage I and II disease who also have risk factors for recurrence (e.g., long interval since antecedent pregnancy, vascular invasion, deep myometrial invasion, serosal involvement, or high mitotic index, or a combination of these factors), or persistently elevated postoperative serum hCG concentration, or both (28,36).

Metastatic Disease

Women with metastatic PSTT at the time of diagnosis are best treated with a multimodal approach including systemic, multiagent, dose-intensive chemotherapy and surgery, and/or radiation for local recurrences or persistent disease as indicated. This approach mimics that of the treatment strategy for the other forms of high-risk metastatic GTN.

The response to chemotherapy in both metastatic and nonmetastatic disease is known to be variable, and the optimum chemotherapy regimen for patients with PSTT remains to be defined. Currently, the clinical impression is that the EMA-EP regimen (etoposide, high-dose methotrexate with folinic acid, actinomycin D, and cisplatin) is a more potent regimen than the EMA-CO regimen (etoposide, high-dose methotrexate with folinic acid, actinomycin D, cyclophosphamide, and vincristine) for metastatic or recurrent PSTT but both have produced complete responses.

Newlands et al in 2000 (37) reported on eight patients treated with the EMA-EP combination and found a 50% complete response rate including a 100% remission in patients whose antecedent pregnancy was less than 24 months prior to diagnosis. Although overall survival in patients with Stage I PSTT approaches 90% after a hysterectomy with or without adjuvant chemotherapy, overall survival is approximately 35%–40% in patients with advanced PSTT.

Metastatic disease is not necessarily a contraindication to surgery. In fact, aggressive surgical management of chemoresistant metastatic disease may be appropriate for those young patients with an otherwise poor prognosis (38). Surgical excision of residual metastatis after treatment with chemotherapy, even in the setting of normalization of serum hCG, is recommended. If viable cancer cells are identified further chemotherapy is recommended to prevent recurrence.

Radiation therapy has been used to good effect in the palliative setting but is not a primary modality of treatment. Prognosis is grave with brain metastasis, but novel treatment such as gamma knife or intrathecal chemotherapy may be of some help.

As stated earlier, PSTT is not a particularly chemosensitive tumor. Large-case series have found anywhere between a 50%–80% rate of persistent or recurrent disease after initial treatment for patients with high risk, Stage III and IV disease. In these patients, long-term disease control is typically achieved with a combination of chemotherapy, surgery, and salvage chemotherapy with on average another two to three multiagent regimens. For second-line chemotherapy, EMA-CO is used for EMA-EP for refractory cases and vice versa; in cisplatin-refractory cases, paclitaxel is added to the regimen as a paclitaxel/cisplatin–paclitaxel/etoposide (TP/TE) regimen. Other commonly used etoposide and platinum-containing regimens include MAE (methotrexate with folinic acid, dactinomycin, and etoposide), CEC (cisplatin, etoposide, and cyclophosphamide), and BEP (bleomycin, etoposide, and cisplatin; 11).

By best estimates, at 10 years, the probability of overall survival for all patients with PTSSs is 70% and the probability of recurrence-free survival is 73%. For patients with Stage I disease, surgery alone is typically sufficient, whereas patients with Stage II, III, and IV disease benefit from combined surgery and chemotherapy. Although most patients with PTSSs can be cured, a substantial number of patients have recurrent disease; for such patients we have shown that the outcome is poor with only 33% achieving long-term remission.

■ SPECIAL ISSUES: FERTILITY PRESERVATION

When PSTT is diagnosed in a woman of childbearing age, the patient's desire for future fertility is a critical issue. Acknowledging that hysterectomy is the preferred treatment option for uterine-confined disease, some centers have studied uterine-conserving surgical procedures in an effort to protect a patient's fertility.

Saso et al (34) described the modified Strausmann procedure (MSP) as an alternative to hysterectomy. This surgical approach consists of temporary arterial occlusion to isolate the uterus, resection of the primary PSTT lesion, followed by uterine reconstruction, and revascularization. Reporting on a series of 5 cases, 4 had close or involved margins and subsequently underwent hysterectomy with no evidence of residual tumor in 2 cases. The authors pointed out the difficulties of assessing margin status intraoperatively with frozen section and the unanticipated occasional multifocal nature of the disease.

Hysteroscopy has been used as both a diagnostic tool (39) and as a means of conservative surgical management of PSTT. Machtinger et al (33) described the first case of hysteroscopic resection of a small (2 × 2 cm) lesion including the underlying myometrium. As surgery alone did not result in normalization of the serum hCG, three cycles of EMA-CO chemotherapy were administered resulting in a normal tumor marker. The authors asserted that this approach might offer a possible treatment option only in highly selected young women (small tumor, confined to the endometrium) who wish to preserve fertility.

Numnum et al (40) described a case of successful conservative management of early stage PSTT with a D&C of the endometrium followed by six cycles of EMA-EP chemotherapy with normalization of the serum hCG after three cycles. The patient remained disease-free for 2 years before successfully delivering a singleton fetus at term after an uncomplicated pregnancy.

More recently, Shen et al (41) described 6 patients with early stage disease treated successfully with a combination of conservative surgical management and multiagent chemotherapy. Surgical management ranged from D&C to tumor resection via hysteroscopic, laparoscopic, and abdominal approaches. The median number of chemotherapy cycles was 5.7 (range 1–14 cycles) and included both intravenous and intra-arterial chemotherapy infused into the uterine arteries. All patients achieved a complete response with a mean follow-up of 47 months (range 10–104 months) and 1 patient has subsequently delivered a term pregnancy.

While these reports are encouraging, conservative management such as localized resection of the tumor should be undertaken with caution and appropriate counseling of the patient, and should be limited to patients of childbearing age with a strong desire to preserve fertility.

■ KEY POINTS

- In a patient with amenorrhea or irregular vaginal bleeding and low-level elevations in the serum hCG, PSTT should be high on the differential diagnosis
- PSTT is confirmed microscopically with the presence of IT cells which express hPL as confirmed by immunohistochemistry
- When PSTT is diagnosed, evaluation for the extent of disease should be undertaken and a clinical stage should be assigned using the FIGO staging system
- The primary choice of treatment for uterine-confined disease (Stage I) is hysterectomy. In cases where fertility preservation is important, localized resection with or without chemotherapy can be considered in patients who lack other risk factors
- Multiagent chemotherapy, preferably with the EMA-EP regimen, is an essential part of treatment of patients with Stage III and IV disease. Rarely is cure achieved in these patients with chemotherapy alone, and surgery and to a lesser extent radiation are used for metastatic lesions.
- Stage IV disease and interval since antecedent pregnancy greater than 24 to 48 months predict poor overall survival

■ REFERENCES

1. Schmid P, Nagai Y, Agarwal R, et al. Prognostic markers and long-term outcome of placental-site trophoblastic tumours: a retrospective observational study. *Lancet.* 2009;374(9683):48–55.
2. Kohorn EI. World-wide results of therapy for gestational trophoblastic disease. *Gynecol Oncol.* 2009;112(Suppl 1):85 (abstr).
3. Kurman RJ, Scully RE, Norris HJ. Trophoblastic pseudotumor of the uterus: an exaggerated form of "syncytial endometritis" simulating a malignant tumor. *Cancer.* 1976;38(3):1214–1226.

4. Scully RE, Young RH. Trophoblastic pseudotumor: a reappraisal. *Am J Surg Pathol.* 1981;5(1):75–76.

5. Shih IM, Seidman JD, Kurman RJ. Placental site nodule and characterization of distinctive types of intermediate trophoblast. *Hum Pathol.* 1999;30(6):687–694.

6. Shih IM, Kurman RJ. The pathology of intermediate trophoblastic tumors and tumor-like lesions. *Int J Gynecol Pathol.* 2001;20(1):31–47.

7. Shih IM, Kurman RJ. Ki-67 labeling index in the differential diagnosis of exaggerated placental site, placental site trophoblastic tumor, and choriocarcinoma: a double immunohistochemical staining technique using Ki-67 and Mel-CAM antibodies. *Hum Pathol.* 1998;29(1):27–33.

8. Kurman RJ. Pathology of trophoblast. *Monogr Pathol.* 1991;(33):195–227.

9. Behtash N, Karimi Zarchi M. Placental site trophoblastic tumor. *J Cancer Res Clin Oncol.* 2008;134(1):1–6.

10. Kim SJ. Placental site trophoblastic tumour. *Best Pract Res Clin Obstet Gynaecol.* 2003;17(6):969–984.

11. Hassadia A, Gillespie A, Tidy J, et al. Placental site trophoblastic tumour: clinical features and management. *Gynecol Oncol.* 2005;99(3):603–607.

12. Larsen LG, Theilade K, Skibsted L, Jacobsen GK. Malignant placental site trophoblastic tumor. A case report and a review of the literature. *APMIS Suppl.* 1991;23:138–145.

13. DiSaia PJ, Creasman WT. Gestational trophoblastic disease. In: DiSaia PJ, Creasman WT, eds. *Clinical Gynecologic Oncology.* 5th ed. St. Louis: Mosby–Year Book, 1997:199–200.

14. Feltmate CM, Genest DR, Wise L, Bernstein MR, Goldstein DP, Berkowitz RS. Placental site trophoblastic tumor: a 17-year experience at the New England Trophoblastic Disease Center. *Gynecol Oncol.* 2001;82(3):415–419.

15. Papadopoulos AJ, Foskett M, Seckl MJ, et al. Twenty-five years' clinical experience with placental site trophoblastic tumors. *J Reprod Med.* 2002;47(6):460–464.

16. Chang YL, Chang TC, Hsueh S, et al. Prognostic factors and treatment for placental site trophoblastic tumor-report of 3 cases and analysis of 88 cases. *Gynecol Oncol.* 1999;73(2):216–222.

17. Sakamoto C, Oikawa K, Kashimura M, Egashira K. Sonographic appearance of placental site trophoblastic tumor. *J Ultrasound Med.* 1990;9(9):533–535.

18. Sumi Y, Ozaki Y, Shindoh N, Katayama H. Placental site trophoblastic tumour: imaging findings. *Radiat Med.* 1999;17(6):427–430.

19. Zhou Y, Lu H, Yu C, Tian Q, Lu W. Sonographic characteristics of placental site trophoblastic tumor. *Ultrasound Obstet Gynecol.* 2012 Jul 17.

20. Hoffman JS, Silverman AD, Gelber J, Cartun R. Placental site trophoblastic tumor: a report of radiologic, surgical, and pathologic methods of evaluating the extent of disease. *Gynecol Oncol.* 1993;50(1):110–114.

21. Brandt KR, Coakley KJ. MR appearance of placental site trophoblastic tumor: a report of three cases. *AJR Am J Roentgenol.* 1998;170(2):485–487.

22. Allen SD, Lim AK, Seckl MJ, Blunt DM, Mitchell AW. Radiology of gestational trophoblastic neoplasia. *Clin Radiol.* 2006;61(4):301–313.

23. Shaw SW, Wang CW, Ma SY, Ng KK, Chang TC. Exclusion of lung metastases in placental site trophoblastic tumor using [18F] fluorodeoxyglucose positron emission tomography: a case report. *Gynecol Oncol.* 2005;99(1):239–242.

24. Nieves L, Hoffman J, Allen G, Currie J, Sorosky JI. Placental-site trophoblastic tumor with PET scan-detected surgically treated lung metastasis. *Int J Clin Oncol.* 2008;13(3):263–265.

25. Chang TC, Yen TC, Li YT, et al. The role of 18F-fluorodeoxyglucose positron emission tomography in gestational trophoblastic tumours: a pilot study. *Eur J Nucl Med Mol Imaging.* 2006;33(2):156–163.

26. FIGO Oncology Committee. FIGO staging for gestational trophoblastic neoplasia 2000. *Int J Gynaecol Obstet.* 2002;77:285–287.

27. Baergen RN, Rutgers JL, Young RH, Osann K, Scully RE. Placental site trophoblastic tumor: A study of 55 cases and review of the literature emphasizing factors of prognostic significance. *Gynecol Oncol.* 2006;100(3):511–520.

28. Hoekstra AV, Keh P, Lurain JR. Placental site trophoblastic tumor: a review of 7 cases and their implications for prognosis and treatment. *J Reprod Med.* 2004;49(6):447–452.

29. Hyman DM, Bakios L, Gualtiere G, et al. Placental site trophoblastic tumor: analysis of presentation, treatment, and outcome. *Gynecol Oncol.* 2013;129(1):58–62.

30. Gloor E, Dialdas J, Hurlimann J, Ribolzi J, Barrelet L. Placental site trophoblastic tumor (trophoblastic pseudotumor) of the uterus with metastases and fatal outcome. Clinical and autopsy observations of a case. *Am J Surg Pathol.* 1983;7(5):483–486.

31. Fukunaga M, Ushigome S. Metastasizing placental site trophoblastic tumor. An immunohistochemical and flow cytometric study of two cases. *Am J Surg Pathol.* 1993;17(10):1003–1010.

32. King LA, Okagaki T, Twiggs LB. Resolution of pulmonary metastases with chemotherapy in a patient with placental site trophoblastic tumor. *Int J Gynecol Cancer.* 1992;2(6):328–331.

33. Machtinger R, Gotlieb WH, Korach J, et al. Placental site trophoblastic tumor: outcome of five cases including fertility preserving management. *Gynecol Oncol.* 2005;96(1):56–61.

34. Saso S, Haddad J, Ellis P, et al. Placental site trophoblastic tumours and the concept of fertility preservation. *BJOG.* 2012;119(3):369–374; discussion 374.

35. Lan C, Li Y, He J, Liu J. Placental site trophoblastic tumor: lymphatic spread and possible target markers. *Gynecol Oncol.* 2010;116(3):430–437.

36. Ajithkumar TV, Abraham EK, Rejnishkumar R, Minimole AL. Placental site trophoblastic tumor. *Obstet Gynecol Surv.* 2003;58(7):484–488.

37. Newlands ES, Mulholland PJ, Holden L, Seckl MJ, Rustin GJ. Etoposide and cisplatin/etoposide, methotrexate, and actinomycin D (EMA) chemotherapy for patients with high-risk gestational trophoblastic tumors refractory to EMA/cyclophosphamide and vincristine chemotherapy and patients presenting with metastatic placental site trophoblastic tumors. *J Clin Oncol.* 2000;18(4):854–859.

38. Dainty LA, Winter WE 3rd, Maxwell GL. The clinical behavior of placental site trophoblastic tumor and contemporary methods of management. *Clin Obstet Gynecol.* 2003;46(3):607–611.

39. Denny LA, Dehaeck K, Nevin J, et al. Placental site trophoblastic tumor: three case reports and literature review. *Gynecol Oncol.* 1995;59(2):300–303.

40. Numnum TM, Kilgore LC, Conner MG, Straughn JM Jr. Fertility sparing therapy in a patient with placental site trophoblastic tumor: a case report. *Gynecol Oncol.* 2006;103(3):1141–1143.

41. Shen X, Xiang Y, Guo L, et al. Fertility-preserving treatment in young patients with placental site trophoblastic tumors. *Int J Gynecol Cancer.* 2012;22(5):869–874.

Future Directions in the Treatment of Gynecologic Cancers

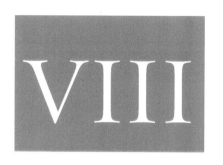

26 Laparoscopy and Robotic-Assisted Surgery in Gynecologic Oncology

FARR R. NEZHAT

EVGENIA POLOSINA

SUSAN S. KHALIL

TAMARA FINGER

JASON STERNCHOS

In the past, laparoscopy has had limited application in gynecologic oncology. It has been used for second-look assessments in ovarian cancer since it was first described in 1973 by Bagley et al (1). However, it was new developments in equipment and instrumentation, such as videolaparoscopy, high-pressure insufflators, and energy sources, in the late 1980s to early 1990s—combined with the work of some of the pioneers of laparoscopic surgery— that made the use of operative laparoscopy in gynecologic oncology feasible (2,3). Over time, the extent of the laparoscopic dissection expanded. The first laparoscopic radical hysterectomy, para-aortic, and pelvic lymphadenectomy were performed by the Nezhats in 1989 and was reported in 1990, 1991, and 1992 (4–6). Dargent and Salvat (7), Querleu et al (8), and Nezhat et al (9) first established the safety and practicability of laparoscopic retroperitoneal and intraperitoneal lymphadenectomy, and radical hysterectomy. In 1996, Amara et al reported the first laparoscopic cytoreductive surgery for advanced ovarian cancer (10). An increasing number of surgeons have since used advanced operative techniques for evaluation and surgical management of gynecologic cancers.

Laparoscopy has the benefit of image magnification to aid in identification of metastatic or recurrent disease, especially in areas such as the upper abdomen, liver and diaphragm surfaces, posterior cul-de-sac, bowel, and mesenteric surfaces. In addition, challenging retroperitoneal spaces of the pelvis, such as the paravesical, pararectal, vesicovaginal, and especially the rectovaginal space, can be accessed laparoscopically. Additional benefits of laparoscopy in gynecologic oncology surgery include limited bleeding from small vessels due to the pressure established by pneumoperitoneum, elimination of large abdominal incisions, shortened hospital stay, and rapid recovery. The ease of recuperation from laparoscopic surgical management thus offers a smooth transition for patients to then undergo planned adjuvant therapies. Postoperative chemotherapy or radiation can be initiated earlier, and radiation complications from bowel adhesions are minimized.

For approximately two decades now, significant progress has been made in advancing the role of laparoscopy in the management of gynecologic malignancy, dealing with key issues such as minimizing radicality of a procedure, management of its complications, disease recurrence, and survival. In fact, laparoscopy is gradually becoming the standard of care for the surgical treatment of majority of the endometrial cancer. Compared to laparotomy, laparoscopy is not only not inferior in terms of survival and recurrence rates, but is associated with significantly less morbidity and improved quality of life (QoL) in the treatment of endometrial cancer (11). As expected, these advanced endoscopic procedures must be carried out by surgeons who have the required skills, contemporary equipment, and trained ancillary staff. Recently, with the introduction of a computer-assisted robotic platform, laparoscopic radical hysterectomy is no longer a procedure limited to surgeons with advanced laparoscopic and vaginal skills (12). Robotic-assisted laparoscopic surgery emerged to overcome the inherent complexity of traditional laparoscopy, while maintaining the benefits of minimally invasive surgery (13).

Robotic-assisted surgery, also known as computer enhanced telesurgery or operative video endoscopy, is the latest innovation and has profoundly revolutionized the concept of minimally invasive surgery in the last three decades.

The Da Vinci robotic platform (Intuitive) was approved by the Food and Drug Administration (FDA) in April 2005 for its use in gynecologic surgery and has multiple applications. In benign gynecology, in urogynecologic procedures, as well as in gynecologic oncology procedures such as radical hysterectomies, pelvic and para-aortic lymphadenectomies, and trachelectomies (14).

The use of laparoscopy, both video-assisted and robotic-assisted, in gynecologic oncology for evaluation and surgical management has increased (Table 26.1).

■ Table 26.1 Comparison of laparotomy, videolaparoscopy, and robotic-assisted videolaparoscopy

Variable	Laparotomy	Videolaparoscopy	Robotic-assisted
Advantages	Dexterity	Well-developed technology	3-D visualization
	Flexibility	Affordable	Increased degrees of motion
	Affordability	Ubiquitous	Improved dexterity over videolaparoscopy
	Ubiquitous	Proven efficacy	Elimination of tremor
			Good geometric accuracy
			Surgeon comfort
Disadvantages	Prone to tremor and fatigue	Loss of haptics	Absence of touch sensation
	Limited geometric accuracy	Loss of 3-D visualization	Expensive
	Longer postoperative course	Limited degrees of motion and dexterity	New technology, unproven benefit
		Amplification of physiologic tremor	Requires additional training and time
			Larger trocar size compared with videolaparoscopy

Adopted from (24).

The da Vinci® Surgical System (Intuitive Surgical, Sunnyvale, CA) is the only actively produced FDA-approved robotic surgical system incorporating an immersive telepresence environment. The setup of this surgical system is based on the principle of robotic telepresence: the main surgeon is seated at a master console away from the operating table, remotely guiding the movements of a patient-side robotic device with a camera arm and two or three operative arms (Figure 26.1). The latest version, the da Vinci® Si model, also supports an assistant surgeon's console. This has meaningful applications in a teaching environment, which does not adversely affect outcomes, as compared to laparoscopic surgery (15; Figure 26.1).

■ OVARIAN TUMORS

The first study to show feasibility of staging in early-stage invasive ovarian cancer was reported in 1994. Querleu and Leblanc (15) reported complete laparoscopic surgical staging procedures for ovarian or fallopian tube cancer. Eight referred patients with ovarian and fallopian tube cancers underwent complete laparoscopic staging after inadequate initial surgical staging. Since this initial series, others have confirmed the feasibility of comprehensive laparoscopic surgical staging of ovarian or fallopian tube cancers (16–19).

Although there is limited published data regarding laparoscopy in advanced ovarian cancer, multiple applications of laparoscopy have thus far emerged in the literature. This includes a triage tool for resectability, primary and secondary cytoreduction, second-look evaluation, and placement of intraperitoneal catheters.

Borderline Ovarian Tumors

Laparoscopic staging in borderline ovarian tumors (BOTs) is increasingly common with advances in endoscopic

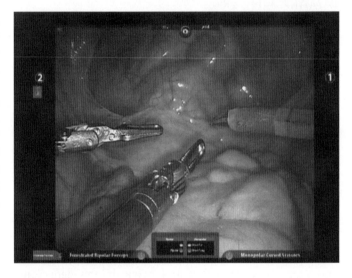

FIGURE 26.1 Robotic laparoscopic instruments: bipolar forceps (left and middle), monopolar electrosurgical scissors (right).

techniques and instruments. To our knowledge, there have not been any studies specifically assessing the application of robotic-assisted surgery in the treatment of BOTs alone. Much of the literature pertaining to robotic-assisted surgery in ovarian cancer is incorporated with other gynecologic malignancies. In one of the first case reports of videolaparoscopic treatment of BOTs (20), Nezhat et al described the surgical staging technique, which included a videolaparoscopic hysterectomy, bilateral adnexectomy, peritoneal sampling, peritoneal cytology, and partial omentectomy. Subsequently, multiple case series studies emerged to further evaluate the clinical outcomes and feasibility of videolaparoscopic treatment of BOTs (22,23,24). In the largest case series to date, 107 patients underwent videolaparoscopic treatment of BOTs. The mean follow-up was 27.5 months with 100% survival and only 4 with evidence of disease (25). A retrospective review was subsequently conducted of 113 patients diagnosed with BOTs, of whom 52 underwent videolaparoscopy and 61 underwent laparotomy. No difference occurred in progression-free survival (PFS) between the two groups with a mean 44-month follow-up (22). The longest documented follow-up (78 months) reports a survival of at least 83% and the remaining patients lost to follow-up (25). A summary of the current literature on videolaparoscopic treatment of BOTs reveals an overall survival of 98%.

Early-Stage Invasive Ovarian Cancer

An estimated 20% of women with epithelial ovarian cancer have early-stage disease at diagnosis. In these patients, complete surgical staging is required to obtain important prognostic information and to plan treatment options.

The first study to show feasibility of videolaparoscopic staging in early-stage invasive ovarian cancer was reported in 1994 (15). This case series included complete pelvic and para-aortic lymph node dissection in 9 patients undergoing restaging procedures for either ovarian or fallopian tube cancers. Since then, several prospective, retrospective, and case series reports have demonstrated the feasibility and safety of a videolaparoscopic approach to the management of early-stage ovarian cancers. Much of the literature pertaining to robotic-assisted surgery in ovarian cancer is incorporated with other gynecologic malignancies. Because of the rarity of early-stage ovarian cancer diagnoses, as well as challenges associated with preoperative diagnoses, a randomized controlled trial has not been feasible. Alternative evaluations of accuracy can be inferred by comparing upstaging rates and nodal yields between laparoscopic and laparotomy cases. In restaging procedures, the current literature suggests the rate of upstaging among complete videolaparoscopic staging procedures ranges from 11% to 19%, while the upstaging rate among patients who had complete laparotomy restaging procedures was reported as 30%–36% (27,28). The feasibility of videolaparoscopic completion of surgical staging in patients with incompletely staged ovarian, fallopian tube, endometrial, and primary peritoneal cancers was shown in Gynecologic Oncology Group (GOG) protocols 9302 and 9402 (78). A total of 84 patients were eligible, of whom 74 had ovarian, fallopian tube, or primary peritoneal cancers. All patients with evidence of metastatic disease or in whom videolaparoscopy was contraindicated were excluded. In all, 58 (69%) patients underwent complete videolaparoscopic staging, confirmed with photographic documentation. Nine (10%) patients were incompletely staged videolaparoscopically because of lack of peritoneal biopsies, cytology, or bilateral lymph nodes. Seventeen patients (20%) required conversion to laparotomy: 13 because of lack of exposure from adhesions, 3 because of complications, and 1 because of metastatic macroscopic disease. Complications associated with videolaparoscopically treated patients included

5 bowel injuries, 1 cystotomy, 1 small bowel obstruction, 1 venotomy, and 2 with extensive blood loss requiring transfusion. In comparing patients treated videolaparoscopically with those treated with laparotomy, the videolaparoscopic group showed a significantly shorter blood loss, hospital stay, and Quetlet index along with comparable nodal yields. In patients undergoing videolaparoscopy, 6 apparent early-stage ovarian cancers were found to have advanced disease. Hospital stay was significantly shorter with videolaparoscopy alone (3 vs 6 days, $P = .04$). The investigators concluded that interval videolaparoscopic staging of gynecologic malignancies can be successfully undertaken in selected patients, but laparotomy for adhesions or metastatic disease and risk of visceral injury should be anticipated (78).

More recently, Nezhat et al (29) published one of the largest retrospective case series of videolaparoscopic staging for apparent early-stage ovarian cancer. Any patient found to have disease beyond the ovary during videolaparoscopic evaluation was excluded. A total of 36 patients who underwent videolaparoscopic staging for apparent early-stage disease were included. Nine patients had been referred for restaging after occult cancer was found on final pathology following cystectomy or adnexectomy. The remaining 27 patients had presented with an adnexal mass. Twenty cases were invasive epithelial tumors, 11 were borderline tumors, and the remaining 5 were nonepithelial tumors (3 granulosa cells, 1 sertoli cell, and 1 dysgerminoma). Of 11 patients who underwent fertility-sparing operations, 6 had borderline tumors, 3 had mucinous carcinomas, and 1 had papillary serous carcinoma. Mean estimated blood loss was 195 mL. There were no major intraoperative complications. Three patients had lymphocele develop: 2 were managed conservatively and 1 required drainage. A mean of 6 peritoneal biopsies as well as 12.2 para-aortic nodes and 14.8 pelvic nodes were obtained. Eighty-three percent of patients underwent omentectomies. Seven patients were upstaged. During a mean follow-up of 55.9 months, 3 patients had recurrences: 2 with borderline tumors in the remaining ovary and 1 with clear cell carcinoma in the pelvis. All 3 recurrences had originally undergone fertility-sparing procedures and had their recurrences subsequently resected with the recurrent clear cell carcinoma managed with adjuvant chemotherapy as well. At the time of publication, all patients were alive with no evidence of disease.

As suggested, these studies support the concept that laparoscopy may offer an advantage in the management of early-stage ovarian cancer by allowing better visualization of difficult areas such as the subdiaphragmatic areas, peritoneal surfaces, obturator spaces, and anterior and posterior cul-de-sacs, as well as magnification and detection of smaller lesions that may be missed on laparotomy. They also suggest superior perioperative outcomes in terms of decreased blood loss, hospital stay, and complication rates while not compromising on accuracy. Thus, comprehensive surgical staging of early-stage ovarian cancer is not only feasible but evidence shows it is at least as safe as laparotomy while offering multiple perioperative and postoperative advantages with comparable recurrence rates and survival outcomes.

Advanced-Stage Invasive Ovarian Cancer

Most patients who are diagnosed with ovarian, fallopian tube, and primary peritoneal epithelial cancer present at advanced stages. Risk factors that contribute to a poor prognosis include the International Federation of Gynecology and Obstetrics (FIGO) stage, volume of residual disease, CA-125 levels, histologic subtype and grade, and other surgical observational factors such as malignant ascites and capsular penetration. The mainstay of treatment for advanced-stage invasive epithelial ovarian cancer is optimal cytoreduction followed by platinum-based combination chemotherapy. Optimal cytoreduction, preferably to microscopic disease, is associated with increased survival (30–33). However, not all patients are able to be optimally cytoreduced at time of initial surgery.

Laparoscopy is an important tool in triaging patients with ovarian cancer and in cytoreductive surgery (Figure 26.2). It also plays a role in placing intraperitoneal ports for the purpose of IP chemotherapy and in second-look procedures. Thus, four applications of laparoscopy in advanced ovarian cancer have emerged thus far in the literature: a triage tool for resectability, placement of intraperitoneal catheters for IP chemotherapy, second-look evaluation, and primary or recurrent cytoreduction in select cases (21,87; Figure 26.2).

Assessment of the Feasibility of Laparoscopic Optimal Cytoreductive Surgery in Ovarian Cancer

Residual disease after surgery is one of the most important prognostic factors for patients with advanced ovarian cancer (34), and the complete excision of all measurable disease has been shown to provide better survival compared with small 1 to 2 cm residual tumor. In fact, a meta-analysis including 6885 patients found that maximal cytoreduction is amongst the most powerful determinants of cohort survival among Stage III and IV ovarian cancer patients. For every 10% increase in maximal cytoreduction in these patients there was an associated 5.5% increase in median survival time. However, depending on individual institutions, surgical skills, and aggressiveness, the percentage of patients with no measurable tumor following debulking surgery ranges from 8% to 85% (30).

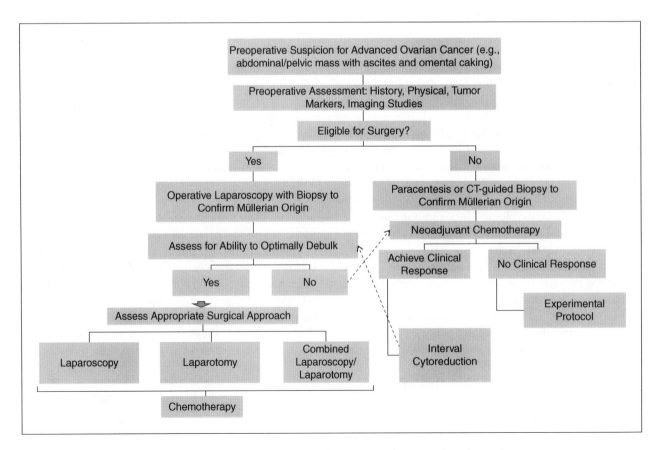

FIGURE 26.2 Treatment algorithm for patients with preoperative suspicion for advanced ovarian cancer.

An accurate and reliable method should be pursued to avoid unnecessary explorative laparotomies and to better select patients for surgical and/or medical specific treatments. Bristow et al (35) elaborated a "predictive index model" based on preoperative CT scanning, which is highly accurate in recognizing patients with advanced epithelial ovarian carcinoma unlikely to undergo optimal primary cytoreductive surgery.

Fagotti et al (36) compared the power of videolaparoscopy with the standard explorative laparotomy in predicting optimal cytoreduction in the same group of advanced ovarian cancer patients. The few well-known indicators of unresectability (i.e., extensive bulky carcinomatosis, agglutinated bowel/mesentery, diaphragm bulky disease, and unresectable upper abdominal metastases) were investigated by videolaparoscopy. The accuracy rate of videolaparoscopy in predicting the laparotomic probability of each one of these parameters ranged from 80% to 100%. In particular, all cases with peritoneal and/or diaphragmatic carcinomatosis, and/or mesentery disease were correctly identified by videolaparoscopy (positive predictive value [PPV] = 100%, 82%, and 100%, respectively), resulting in an overall predictive judgment of unresectability, or negative predictive value (NPV) of 100%. In this context, NPV represents a very important clinical parameter, that is, the rate of inappropriate nonexploration or the ratio of patients thought to have unresectable disease but who will in fact undergo optimal surgery if operated on. This measure corresponds to the false-negative rate and in this study was zero, because in no case was the videolaparoscopic decision changed by the immediately following laparotomy. In this study, an optimal debulking was achievable in 34 of 39 cases (87%) selected as completely resectable by explorative videolaparoscopy. In another series, open videolaparoscopy was used in 285 patients to determine whether the patient could be optimally debulked and they found a 96% accuracy of resectability (37).

Triage of Resectability

One of the first roles of laparoscopy as a triage tool is to rule in or rule out malignancy. Even if malignancy is found, it is not always of primary mullerian origin. Laparoscopy affords the surgeon the opportunity to diagnose a nongynecologic malignancy and to triage/refer the patient accordingly to the appropriate surgeon/oncologist whether the tumor is GI, breast, lung, or of any other primary. However, once a gynecologic malignancy is confirmed the question then becomes whether the tumor can be optimally cytoreduced.

Laparoscopy can be used to identify those patients who are candidates for upfront primary cytoreductive surgery and those patients that might benefit from neoadjuvant chemotherapy (see Figure 26.2) followed by cytoreduction. Thus, laparoscopy is a triage tool in an attempt to increase the rate of patients who can be optimally cytoreduced since these patients have significant survival benefit in the setting of primary advanced-stage ovarian cancer. It can also be used to assess patients with recurrent disease who are candidates for cytoreductive surgery. The sequence of cytoreductive surgery and chemotherapy is determined at the time of diagnostic videolaparoscopy. Once primary mullerian malignancy is confirmed through tissue biopsies, the decision whether the patient can be optimally surgically cytoreduced is then made. If optimal primary cytoreduction can be accomplished then it is immediately performed via laparoscopy (videolaparoscopy or robotic-assisted videolaparoscopy), laparotomy, or a combination of laparoscopy and mini-laparotomy. In this situation, we have achieved the benefits of diagnostic videolaparoscopy for better visualization and assessment of disease in the abdominal-pelvic cavity, especially the upper abdomen, while decreasing the morbidity associated with a large vertical incision. If at the time of initial videolaparoscopy the patient is deemed to likely have a suboptimal cytoreduction due to advanced disease or medical comorbidities, then the decision is made to terminate the procedure after appropriate biopsies are performed and to administer neoadjuvant chemotherapy in a timely fashion. Such patients would then benefit from having only undergone diagnostic videolaparoscopy as opposed to laparotomy because there would be less morbidity, quicker recovery time, and shorter interval to administration of neoadjuvant chemotherapy. Select patients may even begin chemotherapy the day after diagnostic laparoscopy. Neoadjuvant chemotherapy would then be followed by interval cytoreduction either by laparoscopy or by laparotomy based on the response to chemotherapy.

Cytoreductive Surgery for Primary Advanced or Recurrent Ovarian Cancer

There is a paucity of published studies describing laparoscopic debulking of recurrent or primary advanced ovarian cancer. Although there are data to show more favorable perioperative outcomes when comparing a robotic approach to laparotomy for the treatment of endometrial and cervical cancer as well as comparable data to that of a laparoscopic approach (38,71), the evidence in advanced and/or recurrent ovarian cancer is scant. Most of the studies involving advanced/recurrent ovarian cancer describe successful techniques using videolaparoscopy. The first report of successful videolaparoscopic cytoreduction of advanced ovarian cancer was a case series that included 3 patients who all underwent successful total laparoscopic primary or secondary cytoreduction (10).

In a retrospective analysis of a prospective case series, Nezhat et al (39) analyzed their experience with 32 patients with presumed advanced (FIGO Stage IIC or greater) ovarian, fallopian tube, or primary peritoneal cancer who underwent videolaparoscopic triage for resectability. These patients were divided into three groups: (a) diagnostic videolaparoscopy and biopsies; (b) primary cytoreduction and interval debulking via videolaparoscopy; and (c) diagnostic videolaparoscopy followed by primary cytoreduction and debulking via laparotomy. Four of the 32 patients underwent diagnostic videolaparoscopy and biopsies only. Of these, 2 were diagnosed with primary GI malignancies and were referred to medical oncologists, 1 had primary peritoneal cancer but declined debulking due to advanced age and medical comorbidities, and the last 1 was diagnosed with benign disease. Seventeen patients (all greater than Stage IIIA with 2 of them Stage IV), thought to be debulkable videolaparoscopically, underwent primary or interval cytoreduction by videolaparoscopy with no conversions to laparotomy. Fifteen of the 17 patients were optimally debulked to less than 0.5 cm (88.2%). Of note, 9 of 17 patients had upper abdominal disease in addition to pelvic disease. Of these 9 patients, only 1 patient was suboptimally debulked because of her other medical conditions such that she preoperatively declined aggressive management. Eleven of the 32 total patients underwent diagnostic videolaparoscopy followed by primary cytoreduction via laparotomy due to the extent of disease. All 11 patients had greater than Stage IIIB and 8 were optimally debulked to less than 1 cm (72.7%) with 1 to microscopic disease. In the videolaparoscopy group, 9 patients were No Evidence of Disease (NED), 6 were Alive With Disease (AWD), 2 were Died of Disease (DOD), and a 31.7-month median time to recurrence with a 19.7-month mean follow-up time. In the laparotomy group, 3 patients were NED, 5 were AWD, 3 were DOD, and a 21.5-month median time to recurrence with a 25.8-month mean follow-up time. There were no port-site metastases in any of these patients. The authors concluded that in advanced ovarian, fallopian, and primary peritoneal cancer, videolaparoscopy is a technically effective and feasible tool to diagnose, triage, and/or debulk, even with upper abdominal disease, in a well-selected population.

In another retrospective analysis of a prospective case series, Fanning et al (40) evaluated the feasibility and survivability of patients with presumed Stage III/IV primary ovarian cancer undergoing videolaparoscopic-assisted cytoreduction. Twenty-three of the total 25 cases were successfully cytoreduced videolaparoscopically (92%) without conversion to laparotomy. Of the 2 cases converted to laparotomy 1 was converted due to extensive omental disease and the second case due to bulky metastasis surrounding the rectosigmoid. All 25 patients were cytoreduced to less than 2 cm and 36% had no residual disease. Median operative time and blood loss was 2.3 hours and 340 mL, respectively. Median length of stay was 1 day.

Much of the remaining literature involving laparoscopy in the treatment of advanced ovarian cancer involves hand-assisted laparoscopic surgery. However, over the past decade, the use of robotic-assisted laparoscopic surgery for gynecologic malignancies has increased. Recently, Magrina et al (26) compared perioperative and survival outcomes for patients undergoing primary surgical treatment of epithelial ovarian cancer by all three surgical approaches. In their retrospective case-control analysis, they compared 25 patients with ovarian cancer undergoing a robotic-assisted approach to similar patients undergoing a videolaparoscopic approach (27 patients) and laparotomic approach (119 patients). Sixty-percent, 75%, and 87% of the patients in each respective group were found to have FIGO Stage III to Stage IV disease. The remaining patients had FIGO Stage I to Stage II disease. A strength of this study was that patients were also subdivided and compared according to the extent and number of major procedures. The rate of intraoperative complications were similar in all three groups undergoing Type 1 debulking (primary tumor excision defined as routine ovarian cancer staging procedure) and Type 2 debulking (primary tumor excision + one major procedure, i.e., resection of intestines, liver, spleen, or diaphragm). However, in Type 3 debulking (primary tumor excision + two or more major procedures) there were only 2 patients in the robotic-assisted arm (0 complications), no videolaparoscopic patients, and, out of 32 laparotomy patients, 7 (22%) had intraoperative complications. Postoperative complications were similar in all three groups undergoing Type 1 debulking, lower for the robotic-assisted and videolaparoscopy patients undergoing Type 2 debulking, and similar between robotic-assisted and laparotomy patients undergoing Type 3 debulking (no videolaparoscopy patients to compare in this group). Magrina et al concluded that for patients undergoing primary tumor excision of epithelial ovarian cancer alone or with one additional major surgery that robotics and videolaparoscopy is preferable to laparotomy. They also concluded that overall survival is not influenced by the type of surgical approach but by the extent of debulking (complete vs incomplete debulking).

■ CERVICAL CANCER

The radical vaginal hysterectomy (Schauta) was historically associated with a reduction in postoperative morbidity compared with abdominal radical hysterectomy. Dargent is credited with reviving this operation through a combined laparoscopic retroperitoneal lymphadenectomy and radical vaginal hysterectomy. Abu-Rustum (41) summarized 11 reports on 382 laparoscope-assisted radical vaginal hysterectomies (LARVHs) and pelvic and para-aortic lymphadenectomies. The operative time was 225 to 380 minutes with 4 to 5 days of hospital stay. Intra- and postoperative complications included 4%–5% cystotomy, 1%–2% ureteral and 1%–2% vascular injuries, 1%–2% abscess and 1%–2% hematoma formation, and 6%–7%

transfusion. These results appear to be comparable to those of standard laparotomy.

Total laparoscopic radical hysterectomy (TLRH) with pelvic and para-aortic lymph node dissection was first performed in 1989 and reported by Nezhat et al in 1992 (6). Abu-Rustum (41) reviewed eight reports on 146 patients who underwent TLRH with pelvic and para-aortic lymphadenectomy. The mean operative time was 300 minutes with hospital stay of 4 days. Complications included 3%–4% conversion to laparotomy, 2%–3% cystotomy, 2%–3% ureteral injury, and 1%–2% transfusion. It appears that the overall complication rate is acceptable with no compromise in outcome.

Taylor et al performed a retrospective chart review identifying patients with Stage 1A2 and 1B1 cervical cancer who underwent either laparotomy vs laparoscopic radical hysterectomy and pelvic lymph node dissection. They found that laparoscopy is a feasible alternative to laparotomy for early-stage cervical cancer and carries significantly less morbidity (42).

In 2006, Sert and Abeler published on a robotic-assisted laparoscopic radical hysterectomy performed on a patient with Stage IB1 squamous cell carcinoma (43). The same authors published a comparative study looking at the feasibility of robotic-assisted laparoscopic radical hysterectomy and pelvic lymphadenectomy in early cervical cancer patients and compared the results to laparoscopy. The mean operative time was 241 and 300 min in the robotic and laparoscopic groups, respectively. Hospital stay was shorter and blood loss was less in the robotic group; however, the number of lymph nodes, parametrial tissue, and cuff size were similar in both groups (44).

A recent review article by Salicrú et al examined the role of laparoscopic radical hysterectomy in early invasive cervical cancer (45). The laparoscopic approach was associated with less surgical morbidity and with shorter length of hospital stay, although the operation may be longer. Surgical advances including new laparoscopic instrumentation and robotic surgery, may contribute to reducing the duration of the operation and to facilitating learning and teaching of the procedure (45).

Soliman et al compared intraoperative, postoperative, and pathologic outcomes in patients who underwent radical hysterectomy with pelvic lymph node dissection either laparotomy, laparoscopic, or with robotic-assisted laparoscopy. They found that operative time was shorter by laparotomy; however, blood loss was less with laparoscopic and robotic procedures. The robotic arm had the shortest length of stay in comparison to the laparoscopic or laparotomy groups. The pathologic findings were similar in all the groups (46).

Investigators have reported on outcomes with robotic radical hysterectomy for the treatment of cervical carcinoma. Robotic-assisted laparoscopy has been shown to have less blood loss, shorter hospital stay, and fewer complications when compared to laparotomy (47–49). When compared to video-assisted laparoscopy, some studies demonstrate that the robotic approach is associated with comparable blood loss, length of hospital stay, and conversion to laparotomy (50,51). Complication rates with robotic-assisted vs laparoscopic surgery are similar. The most common complications seen with robotic surgeries are lymphocysts/lymphoceles, pelvic infection, and vaginal cuff dehiscence (52). In a meta-analysis of robotic vs videolaparoscopic radical hysterectomy, the percentage of major intraoperative complications were comparable, with more vascular and bladder injury seen during videolaparoscopy, and more nerve injury during robotic radical hysterectomy. The robotic group, however, were found to have a higher number of major postoperative complications than with videolaparoscopy (9.6% vs 5.5%, $P < .05$) including vaginal dehiscence and vaginal cuff, or pelvic abscesses, whereas the videolaparoscopic group had higher rate of fistulas (53). The increase in vaginal cuff dehiscence in the robotic group may be attributable to the extensive use of monopolar and bipolar electrosurgery (54).

Estape et al, on the other hand, demonstrated that the incidence of postoperative complications were less in the robotic group (18.8%) than either the laparoscopic group (23.5%) or the laparotomy group (28.6%; 55). Furthermore, Magrina et al described similar early (less than 6 weeks) major postoperative complications in robotic (7%), videolaparoscopic (6%), and laparotomy (9%) (50).

Fertility-Sparing Procedures

For patients with early-stage cervical cancer desiring fertility-sparing surgery, robotic surgery has been found to play a role. The cervix with adjacent parametrial tissue is resected leaving the uterus in place to allow for childbearing. This is illustrated in several case reports of successful robotic-assisted radical trachelectomies (56–58).

Furthermore; robotic-assisted ovarian transposition has been described in the literature (59).

Advanced or Recurrent Cervical Cancer

There have additionally been reports of robotic-assisted procedures for advanced or recurrent cervical cancer including parametrectomy, pretreatment para-aortic and pelvic lymphadenectomy, anterior pelvic exenteration, and total pelvic exenteration (38).

■ ENDOMETRIAL CANCER

Endometrial cancer is often diagnosed at an early stage and can be successfully treated and often cured with surgery. Traditionally, this surgical approach has been a total abdominal hysterectomy, bilateral salpingo-oophorectomy, cytologic washings, and selective pelvic and para-aortic lymphadenectomy. Though the complication rate of this type of surgery is not extraordinarily high, a significant number of women diagnosed with endometrial cancer also have other comorbidities such as older age, diabetes, hypertension, and obesity. These conditions have been well documented to increase surgical risk and confer a higher perioperative morbidity and mortality. Therefore, the adoption and utilization of minimally invasive surgical techniques to treat this patient population is an attractive option for optimizing patient surgical and oncologic outcomes. Laparoscopy has been used for endometrial cancer in three conditions (a) primary staging in the form of hysterectomy, bilateral salpingo-oophorectomy, lymphadenectomy, and washings, (b) in patients that have undergone a prior hysterectomy and have not been staged, and (c) in the evaluation and management of recurrences.

Laparoscopic Surgical Staging

In 1993, Childers et al was the first to report on laparoscopic lymphadenectomy with laparoscopic assisted vaginal hysterectomy (LAVH) in a series of 59 patients with clinical Stage I disease (60). Lymphadenectomy was performed based on risk factors of tumor grade and depth of invasion. Complications occurred in 5%, including ureteral transection, cystotomy, and development of a pneumothorax in a woman with congenital diaphragm defects. Since the report of this first case series, numerous studies in the literature have subsequently documented the feasibility and safety of laparoscopy for the staging and treatment of endometrial cancer.

A significant portion of the literature recently has focused more on surgical and oncologic outcomes with regard to survival in patients treated by laparoscopy vs laparotomy (see Table 26.4). In a retrospective cohort study by Nezhat et al, 67 patients underwent laparoscopy and 127 underwent laparotomy for clinical Stage I or II endometrial cancer (61). The complication rates between the two groups were comparable. Women undergoing laparoscopy had a shorter hospital stay and less morbidity related to infection. The median follow-up for the laparoscopy and laparotomy group was 36.3 and 29.6 months, respectively. The 2- and 5-year estimated recurrence-free survival (RFS) rates for the laparoscopy and laparotomy groups were 93% vs 91.7% and 88.5% vs 85%, respectively. The 2- and 5-year overall survival rates (100% vs 99.2% and 100% vs 97%) were also similar between the two groups.

Prospective randomized trials comparing laparotomy with laparoscopy for the treatment of endometrial cancer are more limited, especially with regard to survival outcomes. Tozzi et al was the first to report on survival outcomes from a prospective randomized controlled clinical trial of 122 women with endometrial cancer (62). Sixty-three patients were randomized to the laparoscopy arm and 59 to the laparotomy arm. Evaluation of treatment-related morbidity showed a significant reduction in intraoperative complications, such as blood loss (241.3 vs 586.1 mL, $P = .02$) and required transfusions (3 vs 12, $P = .037$). Reductions in mean duration of return of bowel function (2 vs 2.3 days, $P =.02$), and mean length of hospital stay (7.8 vs 11.4 days, $P =.001$) were also seen in the laparoscopic arm when compared to the laparotomy arm. The long-term (greater than 7 days) postoperative complications including wound infections, dehiscence, and hernia formation were significantly higher in the laparotomy group (12% vs 34%, $P =.02$). The conversion rate to laparotomy due to complications was 1.4%. Most importantly, the interim survival analysis revealed no significant difference in overall or disease-free survival (DFS) between the two groups at a median follow-up of 44 months.

Another recent study by Malzoni et al compared total laparoscopic hysterectomy to abdominal hysterectomy, with lymphadenectomy in 159 patients with clinical Stage I endometrial cancer (63). Similar to other studies comparing laparoscopic-assisted vaginal hysterectomy to laparotomy, there was a significantly longer mean operative time in the total laparoscopic arm compared to the laparotomy arm. However, there was less mean operative blood loss, shorter duration of postoperative ileus, and shorter length of hospital stay in the laparoscopic arm. Overall, para-aortic lymph node dissection was performed with a similar frequency between the two groups. The mean number of pelvic and para-aortic lymph nodes removed was not significantly different between the two groups.

After a mean duration of follow-up of 38.5 months (range 2–81 months) the total recurrence rate was approximately 10%. Seven (8.6%) of 81 patients in the laparoscopic group had a recurrence vs 9 (11.5%) of 78 patients of the laparotomy group ($P > .05$).

The GOG has completed a large Phase III randomized study (LAP-2) comparing laparoscopy to laparotomy in patients with clinical stage I or II endometrial carcinoma or sarcoma (64). Nine hundred and twenty patients were randomized to laparotomy and 1696 to laparoscopy. The conversion rate from laparotomy to laparoscopy was 24%, and the majority of these cases were due to poor exposure. Laparoscopy patients had similar rates of intraoperative injuries as laparotomy patients (9.5% vs 7.6%, $P = .11$), fewer postoperative adverse events (27.5% vs 36.9%, $P < .001$), and shorter duration of hospitalization (median 3 vs 4 days, $P < .001$). Recurrence and survival data from the GOG LAP-2 study were published recently. The estimated 5-year recurrence rates were 11.61% and 13.68% for laparoscopy and laparotomy, respectively. The estimated 5-year overall survival was 89.8% for both laparoscopy and laparotomy.

Robotic-Assisted Endometrial Cancer Staging

There have been a number of publications comparing robotic hysterectomy (RH), laparoscopic hysterectomy (LH), and abdominal hysterectomy (AH). Common findings in RH compared with AH include decreased EBL, shorter LOS, and fewer complications (11). With these advantages comes an increase in operative time (ORT). Although the differences between RH and LH are not as distinct, one fairly consistent finding is a lower EBL in RH. Of the three procedures, RH has the fewest complications followed by LH and then AH. In their review Cho and Nezhat (52) analyzed data from 754 procedures. They found complication rates of 10.5% in RH, 12.2% in LH, and 44.6% in AH. Most of the complications in the RH and LH groups relate to trocar sites and the vaginal cuff. Most complications in the AH group have to do with wound infection and bowel dysfunction.

A meta-analysis of the perioperative data for AH, LH, and RH was performed. The data were weighted to account for the variability in sample size. RH had significant benefits over AH in EBL, LOS, lymph node count, and complications. LH had significant benefits over AH in EBL, LOS, and complications. One interesting yet expected finding was the lower conversion rate in RH compared with LH.

Cost

Warren et al (65) conducted a retrospective review with 8061 women in the AH group and 3315 women in the LH group. The overall expenditure for AH was $12,086; the figure for LH was significantly less at $10,868. This study included procedures where patients were kept as inpatients. Sixty percent of video-assisted laparoscopic procedures were performed on an inpatient basis. Under these conditions the expenditure difference was not significant between AH and LH ($12,086 and $11,829, respectively). Their results suggest that LH is most cost effective if performed as an outpatient procedure.

A study by Hilaris et al (66) found a difference in cost attributed to length of stay and the use of disposable instruments. They found that LH with reusable instruments is cheaper in comparison to AH. This difference is mostly attributed to the shorter hospital stay. However, when many disposable instruments (trocars, shears, electrocoagulation devices, uterine manipulators) are used during LH, there may not be a significant difference in cost.

Bijen et al (67) published a review of cost for LH compared with AH. In their review, they introduce two terms: "direct medical cost" and "indirect cost." Direct cost is defined as medical costs related directly to health care (hospital stay, operative procedure, and treatment complications). Indirect costs relate to the impact on society (costs related to the patient's absence from work or normal activities). In their analysis the direct cost of LH was 6.1% higher than that in the AH group. The indirect cost of the LH was 50% of the cost for AH. With these definitions they found that the shorter hospital stay in the LH group compensated for the increased procedure cost. A similar conclusion was reached by Sculpher et al (68) in finding that the most significant variables are the use of disposable instruments and the length of hospital stay.

A discussion of cost would be incomplete without mention of robotics. The Da Vinci system alone costs between $1 million and $2.3 million. This does not include the unique semireusable instruments, the drapes, or the service contract. Although there have been attempts to incorporate robotics into cost analyses comparing the three types of hysterectomies, a comprehensive analysis including the initial cost of the robot, ORT, LOS, and surgical experience has yet to be published (69–76). The maintenance cost alone adds between $100,000 and $180,000 annually. The authors did note that hospital stay is an important factor in cost calculations. Presumably if the incorporation of robotics leads to a shift in hysterectomy to an outpatient procedure, there may be a hospital-wide decrease in cost. As these calculations are currently unavailable, the final question with regard to the cost-effectiveness of the robot for surgical management of endometrial cancer is yet to be answered.

Completion of Staging

Patients who have received a total hysterectomy and found to have a subsequent uterine carcinoma need a reoperation for completion of the staging procedure. Laparoscopy has been evaluated as an effective means to complete surgical staging. Childers et al reported 13 patients in incompletely staged adenocarcinoma of the endometrium who underwent laparoscopic staging (77). All patients had inspection of the entire peritoneal cavity, pelvic washings, and/or pelvic or para-aortic lymphadenectomy, and 2 had their ovaries removed. The average interval between the initial surgery and laparoscopic staging was 47 days. There were no intraoperative complications. The estimated blood loss was less than 50 mL on average and mean hospital stay was 1.5 days. The average number of lymph nodes removed was 17.5. Extrauterine disease was found in 3 patients, 1 with intraperitoneal washings positive for adenocarcinoma, and 2 with pelvic lymph nodes positive for microscopic disease.

The GOG protocol 9402 determined the feasibility of laparoscopically staging in 58 patients with incompletely staged cancers of the uterus, ovary, fallopian tube, and primary peritoneum (78). These patients had a laparoscopic bilateral para-aortic lymphadenectomy. The procedures were individualized based on the extent of the initial surgery and laparotomy was performed for resectable disease. There were initially 95 eligible patients, of whom 9 (10%) women were incompletely staged and 17 patients (20%) underwent a laparotomy. The hospital stay was significantly shorter (3 vs 6 days, P = .4). Of those with a laparoscopy, 6% had bowel complications and 11% was found to have more advanced disease than initially expected. A subgroup analysis of endometrial cancer patients was not performed. These studies conclude that laparoscopy is a safe, effective procedure in patients who require a restaging procedure after an initial surgery, but that laparotomy may result due to adhesions or more advanced disease than expected.

Special Considerations

Obesity

Results from the 2005 to 2006 National Health and Nutrition Examination Survey (NHANES) estimates that 32.7% of U.S. adults are overweight, 34.3% are obese, and 5.9% are extremely obese (79,80). Obesity is related to higher surgical morbidity, including longer operative times, higher blood loss, more postoperative wound complications, and an increased risk of venous thromboembolism. With 68% of patients diagnosed with endometrial cancer meeting the criteria for obesity, the development of a surgical approach that provides comparable staging adequacy with decreased morbidity is essential.

Development of and improvement in technology that utilizes a minimally invasive surgical approach in these patients is of paramount importance. In a retrospective cohort study by Scribner et al, a successful laparoscopic staging procedure was completed in 63.6% of the obese population (81). Obesity was the primary reason in 23.6% of patients for conversion to laparotomy. Eisenhauer et al performed a retrospective analysis comparing surgical outcomes in obese women undergoing surgical staging by laparotomy, laparoscopy, or laparotomy with panniculectomy (82). Both laparotomy with panniculectomy and laparoscopy were associated with higher total lymph node retrieval (P = .002) and decreased incisional complications (P = .002). The median para-aortic lymph node counts were not significant between the three groups.

With the evolution of robotic surgery, many are looking toward this new technology as a means to overcome some of the technical challenges inherent in conventional laparoscopy and the obese patient. Gehrig et al compared TRH with TLH in a retrospective cohort study of 79 obese and morbidly obese patients (83). Complete surgical staging was accomplished in 92% of the robotic patients and in 84% of the laparoscopic cohort. There were no differences between the two groups with regard to laparotomy conversion. For both the obese and morbidly obese patients, robotic surgery was associated with a shorter operative time (189 vs 215 min, P = .0004), less blood loss (50 vs 150 mL, P < .0001), and shorter hospital stay (1.02 vs 1.27 days, P = .0119). There was a significant difference in mean para-aortic (10.3 vs 7.03, P = .01) and total lymph node counts (31.4 vs 24, P = .004) for the two groups. The difference became nonsignificant when only morbidly obese patients were taken into account, suggesting as the authors stated, that robotic technology may not overcome all of the technical difficulties in this patient population.

Elderly

The majority of women diagnosed with endometrial cancer are postmenopausal. Older patients often have comorbidities that place them at increased surgical risk. Therefore, demonstration of the safety of laparoscopy in this patient population has been essential. Scribner et al in a retrospective analysis evaluated a total of 125 women greater than or equal to 65 years of age with clinical Stage I endometrial cancer (84). Laparoscopy was completed in 52/67 (77.6%) attempted procedures. Conversion to laparotomy was secondary to obesity (10.4%), bleeding (6%), intraperitoneal cancer (4.5%), and adhesions (1.5%). Pelvic, common iliac, and para-aortic lymph node counts were similar between the two groups. Although the operative time was significantly longer for the laparoscopic group (236 vs 148 min), there was no increased morbidity attributable to longer duration under anesthesia. They had a shorter length of hospitalization, less estimated blood loss, less postoperative ileus, and less wound complications when compared to the laparotomy group. Quicker recovery times allow elderly patients to maintain their independence and therefore may positively impact their QoL.

Quality of Life Assessment

Zullo et al performed a prospective randomized comparison of QoL as the primary endpoint between laparoscopy and laparotomy for the treatment of early-stage endometrial cancer (85). QoL was assessed by the Italian version of the Short-Form Healthy Survey (SF-36). The baseline QoL at study entry was similar in both treatment groups. At 1, 3, and 6 months from surgery, QoL was significantly higher in the laparoscopy group compared to the laparotomy group. Although QoL was the primary study endpoint, they also noted less intraoperative blood loss, lower drop in hemoglobin levels, less postoperative pain, shorter mean hospitalization, and fewer postoperative complications in the laparoscopy group. The intraoperative complication incidence was similar between the two groups (7.5% vs 7.9%), as was the mean number of pelvic and para-aortic lymph nodes removed.

In the GOG LAP-2 trial, QoL was evaluated in 782 patients. Patient's QoL was assessed using the Functional Assessment of Cancer Therapy-General (FACT-G), a measure of patients' physical, emotional, and social well-being before and after surgery (86). Postsurgical QoL was higher at 1, 3, and 6 weeks postoperatively for patients undergoing laparoscopy. However, observed differences were not significant by 6 months.

■ CONCLUSIONS

The laparoscopic management of several gynecologic malignancies was validated with trials, such as the LAP-2 study that made it acceptable for use with endometrial cancer. These efforts have been further applied to other malignancies, such as with ovarian cancer, often encountered with a challenging presentation. From the first reported laparoscopic cytoreduction for advanced ovarian cancer by Amara et al in 1996, to the debulking of upper abdominal disease, this progress in minimally invasive gynecologic procedures has continued to improve the quality of care and life for these patients (10). Despite periods of doubt in technology, that lead to stagnation, the widespread application of this field and these techniques have challenged the voices of concern from the past while spurring innovative surgical techniques.

This added QoL benefit has not come at the value of quality of care for the patient. The same radical procedures are being performed, but the risk ratio is being decreased with the use of minimally invasive approaches. Not only has minimally invasive surgery helped enhance the QoL for these patients, but also it has garnered greater support for the use of modalities that inflict less on the patient, while conferring the same survival benefits as conventional surgery. This may lead us one day to the ultimate goal, which is the use of noninvasive medical therapy in managing the care of oncology patients.

■ REFERENCES

1. Bagley CM, Young RC, Schein PS, et al. Ovarian cancer metastatic to the diaphragm frequently undiagnosed at laparotomy: a preliminary report. *Am J Obstet Gynecol.* 1973;116:247.
2. Kelley WE Jr. The evolution of laparoscopy and the revolution in surgery in the decade of the 1990s. *JSLS.* 2008;12(4):351–357.
3. Nezhat C, Hood J, Winer W, Nexhat F, Crowgey SR, Garrison CP. Videolaseroscopy and laser laparoscopy in gynaecology. *Br J Hosp Med.* 1987;38(3):219–224.
4. Nezhat C, Nezhat F. *Video Laseroscopy for the Treatment of Upper, Mid, and Lower Peritoneal Cavity Pathology.* Annual Meeting of AAGL, November 1990.
5. Nezhat CR, Nezhat FR, Silfen SL. Videolaseroscopy. The CO2 laser for advanced operative laparoscopy. *Obstet Gynecol Clin North Am.* 1991;18(3):585–604.
6. Nezhat CR, Burrell MO, Nezhat FR, Benigno BB, Welander CE. Laparoscopic radical hysterectomy with paraaortic and pelvic node dissection. *Am J Obstet Gynecol.* 1992;166(3):864–865.
7. Dargent D, Salvat J. *Lienvahissement Ganglionnaire Pelvien.* MEDSI, Paris. 1989.
8. Querleu D, Leblan E, Catelain B. Laparoscopic pelvic lymphadenectomy. *Am J Obstet Gynecol.* 1991;164:579.
9. Nezhat CR, Nezhat FR, Burrell MO, et al. Laparoscopic radical hysterectomy and laparoscopically assisted vaginal radical hysterectomy with pelvic and paraaortic node dissection. *J Gynecol Surg.* 1993;9(2):105–120.
10. Amara DP, Nezhat C, Teng NN, Nezhat F, Nezhat C, Rosati M. Operative laparoscopy in the management of ovarian cancer. *Surg Laparosc Endosc.* 1996;6(1):38–45.
11. Acholonu UC Jr, Chang-Jackson SC, Radjabi AR, Nezhat FR. Laparoscopy for the management of early-stage endometrial cancer: from experimental to standard of care. *J Minim Invasive Gynecol.* 2012;19(4):434–442.
12. Nezhat FR, Datta MS, Liu C, Chuang L, Zakashansky K. Robotic radical hysterectomy versus total laparoscopic radical hysterectomy with pelvic lymphadenectomy for treatment of early cervical cancer. *JSLS.* 2008;12(3):227–237.
13. Nezhat C, Lavie O, Lemyre M, Unal E, Nezhat CH, Nezhat F. Robot-assisted laparoscopic surgery in gynecology: scientific dream or reality? *Fertil Steril.* 2009;91(6):2620–2622.
14. Cho JE, Shamshirsaz AH, Nezhat C, Nezhat C, Nezhat F. New technologies for reproductive medicine: laparoscopy, endoscopy, robotic surgery and gynecology. A review of the literature. *Minerva Ginecol.* 2010;62(2):137–167.
15. Querleu D, LeBlanc E. Laparoscopic infrarenal paraaortic lymph node dissection for restaging of carcinoma of the ovary or fallopian tube. *Cancer.* 1994;73(5):1467–1471.
16. Childers JM, Lang J, Surwit EA, Hatch KD. Laparoscopic surgical staging of ovarian cancer. *Gynecol Oncol.* 1995;59(1):25–33.
17. Spirtos NM, Eisekop SM, Boike G, Schlaerth JB, Cappellari JO. Laparoscopic staging in patients with incompletely staged cancers of the uterus, ovary, fallopian tube, and primary peritoneum: a Gynecologic Oncology Group (GOG) study. *Am J Obstet Gynecol.* 2005;193(5):1645–1649.
18. Tozzi R, Köhler C, Ferrara A, Schneider A. Laparoscopic treatment of early ovarian cancer: surgical and survival outcomes. *Gynecol Oncol.* 2004;93(1):199–203.
19. Tozzi R, Schneider A. Laparoscopic treatment of early ovarian cancer. *Curr Opin Obstet Gynecol.* 2005;17(4):354–358.
20. Nezhat F, Nezhat C, Burrell M. Laparoscopically assisted hysterectomy for the management of a borderline ovarian tumor: a case report, *J Laparoendosc Surg.* 1992;2:167–169.
21. Liu CS, Nagarsheth NP, Nezhat FR. Laparoscopy and ovarian cancer: a paradigm change in the management of ovarian cancer? *J Min Inv Gynecol.* 2009; 16(3):250–262.
22. Romagnolo C, Gadducci A, Sartori E, Zola P, Maggino T. Management of borderline ovarian tumors: results of an Italian multicenter study. *Gynecol Oncol.* 2006;101(2):255–260.
23. Darai E, Teboul J, Fauconnier A, Scoazec JY, Benifla JL, Madelenat P. Management and outcome of borderline ovarian tumors incidentally discovered at or after laparoscopy. *Acta Obstet Gynecol Scand.* 1998;77(4):451–457.
24. Seracchioli R, Venturoli S, Colombo FM, Govoni F, Missiroli S, Bagnoli A. Fertility and tumor recurrence rate after conservative laparoscopic management of young women with early-stage borderline ovarian tumors. *Fertil Steril.* 2001;76:999–1004.
25. Fauvet R, Boccara J, Dufournet C, Poncelet C, Daraï E. Laparoscopic management of borderline ovarian tumors: results of a French multicenter study. *Ann Oncol.* 2005;16:403–410.
26. Magrina JF, Zanagnolo V, Noble BN, Kho RM, Magtibay P. Robotic approach for ovarian cancer: perioperative and survival results and comparison with laparoscopy and laparotomy. *Gynecol Oncol.* 2011;121(1):100–105.
27. Leblanc E, Querleu D, Narducci F, Occelli B, Papageorgiou T, Sonoda Y. Laparoscopic restaging of early stage invasive adnexal tumors: a 10-year experience. *Gynecol Oncol.* 2004;94(3):624–629.
28. Le T, Adolph A, Krepart GV, Lotocki R, Heywood MS. The benefits of comprehensive surgical staging in the management

of early-stage epithelial ovarian carcinoma. *Gynecol Oncol.* 2002;85(2):351–355.

29. Nezhat FR, Ezzati M, Chuang L, Shamshirsaz AA, Rahaman J, Gretz H. Laparoscopic management of early ovarian and fallopian tube cancers: surgical and survival outcome. *Am J Obstet Gynecol.* 2009;200(1):83.e1–83.e6.

30. Bristow RE, Tomacruz RS, Armstrong DK, Trimble EL, Montz FJ. Survival effect of maximal cytoreductive surgery for advanced ovarian carcinoma during the platinum era: a meta-analysis. *J Clin Oncol.* 2002;20(5):1248–1259.

31. Winter WE 3rd, Maxwell GL, Tian C, et al.; Gynecologic Oncology Group Study. Prognostic factors for stage III epithelial ovarian cancer: a Gynecologic Oncology Group study. *J Clin Oncol.* 2007;25(24):3621–3627.

32. Winter WE 3rd, Maxwell GL, Tian C, et al.; Gynecologic Oncology Group. Tumor residual after surgical cytoreduction in prediction of clinical outcome in stage IV epithelial ovarian cancer: a Gynecologic Oncology Group study. *J Clin Oncol.* 2008;26(1):83–89.

33. du Bois A, Reuss A, Pujade-Lauraine E, Harter P, Ray-Coquard I, Pfisterer J. Role of surgical outcome as prognostic factor in advanced epithelial ovarian cancer: a combined exploratory analysis of 3 prospectively randomized phase 3 multicenter trials: by the Arbeitsgemeinschaft Gynaekologische Onkologie Studiengruppe Ovarialkarzinom (AGO-OVAR) and the Groupe d'Investigateurs Nationaux Pour les Etudes des Cancers de l'Ovaire (GINECO). *Cancer.* 2009;115(6):1234–1244.

34. Hoskins WJ, Bundy BN, Thigpen JT, Omura GA. The influence of cytoreductive surgery on recurrence-free interval and survival in small-volume stage III epithelial ovarian cancer: a Gynecologic Oncology Group study. *Gynecol Oncol.* 1992;47(2):159–166.

35. Bristow RE, Duska LR, Lambrou NC, et al. A model for predicting surgical outcome in patients with advanced ovarian carcinoma using computed tomography. *Cancer.* 2000;89(7):1532–1540.

36. Fagotti A, Fanfani F, Ludovisi M, et al. Role of laparoscopy to assess the chance of optimal cytoreductive surgery in advanced ovarian cancer: a pilot study. *Gynecol Oncol.* 2005;96(3):729–735.

37. Vergote I, De Wever I, Tjalma W, Van Gramberen M, Decloedt J, van Dam P. Neoadjuvant chemotherapy or primary debulking surgery in advanced ovarian carcinoma: a retrospective analysis of 285 patients. *Gynecol Oncol.* 1998;71(3):431–436.

38. Yim GW, Kim YT. Robotic surgery in gynecologic cancer. *Curr Opin Obstet Gynecol.* 2012;24(1):14–23.

39. Nezhat FR, DeNoble SM, Liu CS, et al. The safety and efficacy of laparoscopic surgical staging and debulking of apparent advanced stage ovarian, fallopian tube, and primary peritoneal cancers. *JSLS.* 2010;14(2):155–168.

40. Fanning J, Yacoub E, Hojat R. Laparoscopic-assisted cytoreduction for primary advanced ovarian cancer: success, morbidity and survival. *Gynecol Oncol.* 2011;123(1):47–49.

41. Abu-Rustum NR. Laparoscopy 2003: oncologic perspective. *Clin Obstet Gynecol.* 2003;46(1):61–69.

42. Taylor SE, McBee WC Jr, Richard SD, Edwards RP. Radical hysterectomy for early stage cervical cancer: laparoscopy versus laparotomy. *JSLS.* 2011;15(2):213–217.

43. Sert BM, Abeler VM. Robotic-assisted laparoscopic radical hysterectomy (Piver type III) with pelvic node dissection–case report. *Eur J Gynaecol Oncol.* 2006;27(5):531–533.

44. Sert B, Abeler V. Robotic radical hysterectomy in early-stage cervical carcinoma patients, comparing results with total laparoscopic radical hysterectomy cases. The future is now? *Int J Med Robot.* 2007;3(3):224–228.

45. Salicrú S, Gil-Moreno A, Montero A, Roure M, Pérez-Benavente A, Xercavins J. Laparoscopic radical hysterectomy with pelvic lymphadenectomy in early invasive cervical cancer. *J Minim Invasive Gynecol.* 2011;18(5):555–568.

46. Soliman PT, Frumovitz M, Sun CC, et al. Radical hysterectomy: a comparison of surgical approaches after adoption of robotic surgery in gynecologic oncology. *Gynecol Oncol.* 2011;123(2):333–336.

47. Boggess J, Gehrig P, Cantrell L, et al. A Case control study of robotic assisted type III radical hysterectomy with pelvic lymph node dissection compared with open radical hysterectomy. *Am J Obstet Gynecol.* 2008;19:357–359.

48. Lambaudie E, Houvenaeghel G, Walz J, et al. Robot-assisted laparoscopy in gynecologic oncology. *Surg Endosc.* 2008;22(12):2743–2747.

49. Ko EM, Muto MG, Berkowitz RS, Feltmate CM. Robotic versus open radical hysterectomy: a comparative study at a single institution. *Gynecol Oncol.* 2008;111(3):425–430.

50. Magrina JF, Kho RM, Weaver AL, Montero RP, Magtibay PM. Robotic radical hysterectomy: comparison with laparoscopy and lapaprotomy. *Gynecol Oncol.* 2008;109(1):86–91.

51. Nezhat FR, Datta MS, Liu C, Chuang L, Zakashanksy K. Robotic radical hysterectomy versus total laparoscopic radical hysterectomy with pelvic lymphadectomy for treatment of early cervical cancer. *JSLS.* 2008;12:227–237.

52. Cho JE, Nezhat FR. Robotics and gynecologic oncology: review of the literature. *J Minim Invasive Gynecol.* 2009;16(6):669–681.

53. Renato S, Mohamed M, Serena S, et al. Robot-assisted radical hysterectomy for cervical cancer: review of surgical and oncological outcomes. *ISRN Obstet Gynecol.* 2011;2011:872434.

54. Sert MB, Eraker R. Robot-assisted laparoscopic surgery in gynaecological oncology; initial experience at Oslo Radium Hospital and 16 months follow-up. *Int J Med Robot.* 2009;5(4):410–414.

55. Estape R, Lambrou N, Diaz R, Estape E, Dunkin N, Rivera A. A case matched analysis of robotic radical hysterectomy with lymphadenectomy compared with laparoscopy and laparotomy. *Gynecol Oncol.* 2009;113(3):357–361.

56. Persson J, Kannisto P, Bossmar T. Robot-assisted abdominal laparoscopic radical trachelectomy. *Gynecol Oncol.* 2008;111(3):564–567.

57. Chuang LT, Lerner DL, Liu CS, Nezhat FR. Fertility-sparing robotic-assisted radical trachelectomy and bilateral pelvic lymphadenectomy in early-stage cervical cancer. *J Minim Invasive Gynecol.* 2008;15:767–770.

58. Geisler JP, Orr CJ, Manahan KJ. Robotically assisted total laparoscopic radical trachelectomy for fertility sparing in stage IB1 adenosarcoma of the cervix. *J Laparoendosc Adv Surg Tech A.* 2008;18(5):727–729.

59. Molpus KL, Wedergren JS, Carlson MA. Robotically assisted endoscopic ovarian transposition. *JSLS.* 2003;7(1):59–62.

60. Childers JM, Hatch KD, Tran AN, Surwit EA. Laparoscopic para-aortic lymphadenectomy in gynecologic malignancies. *Obstet Gynecol.* 1993;82(5):741–747.

61. Nezhat F, Yadav J, Rahaman J, Gretz H, Cohen C. Analysis of survival after laparoscopic management of endometrial cancer. *J Minim Invasive Gynecol.* 2008;15(2):181–187.

62. Tozzi R, Köhler C, Ferrara A, Schneider A. Laparoscopic treatment of early ovarian cancer: surgical and survival outcomes. *Gynecol Oncol.* 2004;93(1):199–203.

63. Malzoni M, Tinelli R, Cosentino F, Fusco A, Malzoni C. Total laparoscopic radical hysterectomy versus abdominal radical hysterectomy with lymphadenectomy in patients with early cervical cancer: our experience. *Ann Surg Oncol.* 2009;16(5):1316–1323.

64. Walker JL, Piedmonte M, Spirtos N, et al. Phase III trial of laparoscopy vs laparotomy for surgical resection and comprehensive surgical staging of uterine cancer: A Gynecologic Oncology Group (GOG) study founded by NCI. In: *Proceedings from the 37th Annual Meeting of the Society of Gynecologic Oncologists.* March 22–26, 2006. Palm Springs, CA. Abstract 22.

65. Warren L, Ladapo JA, Borah BJ, Gunnarsson CL. Open abdominal versus laparoscopic and vaginal hysterectomy: analysis of a large United States payer measuring quality and cost of care. *J Minim Invasive Gynecol.* 2009;16(5):581–588.

66. Hilaris GE, Tsoubis T, Konstantopoulos V, Pavlakis K. Feasibility, safety, and cost outcomes of laparoscopic management of early endometrial and cervical malignancy. *JSLS.* 2009;13(4):489–495.

67. Bijen CB, Vermeulen KM, Mourits MJ, de Bock GH. Costs and effects of abdominal versus laparoscopic hysterectomy: systematic review of controlled trials. *PLoS ONE.* 2009;4(10):e7340.

68. Sculpher M, Manca A, Abbott J, Fountain J, Mason S, Garry R. Cost effectiveness analysis of laparoscopic hysterectomy compared with standard hysterectomy: results from a randomised trial. *BMJ.* 2004;328(7432):134.

69. Fanning J, Hossler C. Laparoscopic conversion rate for uterine cancer surgical staging. *Obstet Gynecol.* 2010;116(6):1354–1357.

70. Pasic RP, Rizzo JA, Fang H, Ross S, Moore M, Gunnarsson C. Comparing robot-assisted with conventional laparoscopic hysterectomy: impact on cost and clinical outcomes. *J Minim Invasive Gynecol.* 2010;17(6):730–738.

71. Cho JE, Shamshirsaz AH, Nezhat C, Nezhat C, Nezhat F. New technologies for reproductive medicine: laparoscopy, endoscopy, robotic surgery and gynecology. A review of the literature. *Minerva Ginecol.* 2010;62(2):137–167.

72. Holub Z, Jabor A, Bartos P, Eim J, Urbánek S, Pivovarniková R. Laparoscopic surgery for endometrial cancer: long-term results of a multicentric study. *Eur J Gynaecol Oncol.* 2002;23(4):305–310.

73. Litta P, Fracas M, Pozzan C, et al. Laparoscopic management of early stage endometrial cancer. *Eur J Gynaecol Oncol.* 2003;24(1):41–44.

74. Scribner DR Jr, Mannel RS, Walker JL, Johnson GA. Cost analysis of laparoscopy versus laparotomy for early endometrial cancer. *Gynecol Oncol.* 1999;75(3):460–463.

75. Bell MC, Torgerson J, Seshadri-Kreaden U, Suttle AW, Hunt S. Comparison of outcomes and cost for endometrial cancer staging via traditional laparotomy, standard laparoscopy and robotic techniques. *Gynecol Oncol.* 2008;111(3):407–411.

76. Malzoni M, Tinelli R, Cosentino F, et al. Total laparoscopic hysterectomy versus abdominal hysterectomy with lymphadenectomy for early-stage endometrial cancer: a prospective randomized study. *Gynecol Oncol.* 2009;112:126–133.

77. Childers JM, Spirtos NM, Brainard P, Surwit EA. Laparoscopic staging of the patient with incompletely staged early adenocarcinoma of the endometrium. *Obstet Gynecol.* 1994;83(4):597–600.

78. Spirtos NM, Eisekop SM, Boike G, Schlaerth JB, Cappellari JO. Laparoscopic staging in patients with incompletely staged cancers of the uterus, ovary, fallopian tube, and primary peritoneum: a Gynecologic Oncology Group (GOG) study. *Am J Obstet Gynecol.* 2005;193(5):1645–1649.

79. DiSaia PJ, Creasman WT. Adenocarcinoma of the uterus. In: DiSaia PJ, Creasman WT, eds. *Clinical Gynecologic Oncology.* 6th ed. St. Louis: Mosby–Year Book, 2002:137–184.

80. http://www.cdc.gov/nchs/products/pubs/pubd/hestats/overweight/overweight_adult.htm

81. Scribner DR Jr, Walker JL, Johnson GA, McMeekin SD, Gold MA, Mannel RS. Laparoscopic pelvic and paraaortic lymph node dissection: analysis of the first 100 cases. *Gynecol Oncol.* 2001;82(3):498–503.

82. Eisenhauer EL, Wypych KA, Mehrara BJ, et al. Comparing surgical outcomes in obese women undergoing laparotomy, laparoscopy, or laparotomy with panniculectomy for the staging of uterine malignancy. *Ann Surg Oncol.* 2007;14(8):2384–2391.

83. Gehrig PA, Cantrell LA, Shafer A, Abaid LN, Mendivil A, Boggess JF. What is the optimal minimally invasive surgical procedure for endometrial cancer staging in the obese and morbidly obese woman? *Gynecol Oncol.* 2008;111(1):41–45.

84. Scribner DR Jr, Walker JL, Johnson GA, McMeekin DS, Gold MA, Mannel RS. Laparoscopic pelvic and paraaortic lymph node dissection in the obese. *Gynecol Oncol.* 2002;84(3):426–430.

85. Zullo F, Palomba S, Russo T, et al. A prospective randomized comparison between laparoscopic and laparotomic approaches in women with early stage endometrial cancer: a focus on the quality of life. *Am J Obstet Gynecol.* 2005;193(4):1344–1352.

86. Kornblith A, Walker J, Huang H, et al. Quality of life (QOL) of patients in a randomized clinical trial of laparoscopy vs open laparotomy for the surgical resection and staging of uterine cancer: A Gynecologic Oncology Group (GOG) study. In: *Proceedings from the 37th Annual Meeting of the Society of Gynecologic Oncologists*; March 22–26, 2006; Palm Springs, CA. Abstract 22.

87. Nezhat FR, Lavie O. The role of minimally invasive surgery in ovarian cancer. *Int J Gynecol Cancer.* 2013 Jun;23(5):782–783.

27 Innovations in Radiotherapy of Gynecologic Cancers

TYLER M. SEIBERT

DANIEL R. SIMPSON

CATHERYN M. YASHAR

LOREN K. MELL

ARNO J. MUNDT

■ INTRODUCTION

Radiation therapy (RT) has been used in the treatment of gynecologic malignancies for more than a century (1). Over the years, numerous advancements have been made in radiation technologies, which have significantly improved the quality and delivery of treatment. The past 15 years, in particular, have witnessed a series of unprecedented technologic developments, which are being increasingly applied to patients with gynecologic malignancies. The purpose of this chapter is to present three important technologic innovations and review their use in gynecologic cancer patients, namely intensity-modulated RT (IMRT), image-guided RT (IGRT), and stereotactic body RT (SBRT).

■ INTENSITY-MODULATED RADIATION THERAPY

IMRT is an advanced form of three-dimensional conformal RT (3-DCRT) that utilizes sophisticated computerized optimization algorithms to generate dose distributions, which conform the prescription dose to the shape of the target. Such plans significantly reduce the volume of the surrounding normal tissues irradiated to high doses, potentially reducing the risk of untoward sequelae. Highly conformal IMRT plans may also allow the safe delivery of higher more effective doses, thereby improving tumor control rates. First proposed in the 1960s (2), IMRT was not clinically implemented until the 1990s following the development of computerized planning software. Today, IMRT is performed in nearly all radiation centers in the United States (3,4) and is increasingly available at many centers abroad (5–7).

IMRT planning is an *inverse* process whereby the target and the normal tissues are first delineated on a planning CT scan. Specific dose-volume constraints and priorities are then selected and the optimization program generates a treatment plan that best satisfies these goals. This approach is distinguished from the iterative, trial-and-error conventional planning method. An important distinction between the two techniques is whereas conventional approaches result in an acceptable plan, inverse planning generates the optimal one.

During the IMRT optimization process, each treatment beam (typically 5–9) is divided into small "beamlets" whose intensity is individually varied until the desired dose distribution is obtained. The resultant modulated beams are distinguished from the uniform intensity beams used in conventional treatment and are delivered at most centers on linear accelerators equipped with a multileaf collimator (MLC) whose "leaves" move in and out of the beam's path under computer control. The longer the leaves remain open at a particular position, the greater the intensity of radiation. At select centers, IMRT is delivered using customized compensators, volumetric arc therapy, or helical tomotherapy.

When cast into the patient, the resultant modulated beams deposit dose in highly conformal distributions that are nearly always superior to those achieved with conventional planning, particularly in patients with complex target shapes. IMRT plans are also distinguished by rapid dose gradients outside the target, resulting in considerable sparing of neighboring normal tissues. An example of IMRT treatment plan in a gynecology patient undergoing pelvic irradiation is shown in Figure 27.1.

Multiple preclinical studies have been published demonstrating the superiority of IMRT planning over conventional methods in gynecologic cancer patients. In the first published IMRT report, Roeske and coworkers at the University of Chicago compared IMRT and conventional whole pelvic RT plans in 10 gynecology patients (8). The highly conformal IMRT plans provided excellent target coverage while reducing the volume of small bowel irradiated to the prescription dose by a factor of 2 (17.4% vs 33.8%, $P < .001$). Significant reductions were also realized in the volume of bladder (76.6% vs 99.3%, $P < .001$)

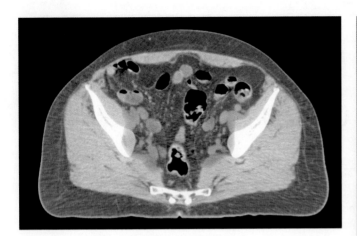

FIGURE 27.1 An example of an intensity-modulated radiation therapy plan in a patient undergoing treatment for endometrial cancer following surgery. The prescription dose is represented by the red region, which conforms to the laterally situated pelvic lymph nodes. Note the sparing of the central normal tissues such as the small bowel and sigmoid colon.

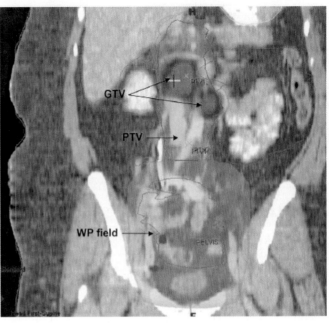

FIGURE 27.2 An example of a simultaneous-integrated boost plan in a cervical cancer patient with bulky para-aortic adenopathy. The gross tumor volume (GTV; red) was escalated, while the para-aortic region (planning target volume [PTV]) was kept at a lower dose level (green). WP, whole pelvic. Reproduced with permission from Ahmed et al (13).

and rectum (57.7% vs 80.3%, $P < .001$) as well. Others have subsequently reported similar benefits in gynecology patients undergoing pelvic (9), extended field (10), pelvic-inguinal (11), and whole abdominal RT (12).

Preclinical studies have also suggested that IMRT may allow the safe delivery of higher than conventional doses in select patients, for example, cervical or endometrial cancer patients with bulky para-aortic lymph nodes (13). In these patients, IMRT plans can be generated that selectively deliver high doses per fraction (e.g., greater than or equal to 2.2 Gy) to the involved nodal sites while simultaneously treating the remainder of the target volume with conventional fraction sizes (1.8–2.0 Gy), an approach known as a "simultaneous integrated boost" (SIB; Figure 27.2). Some investigators have even argued that IMRT planning may provide a means of replacing brachytherapy in gynecologic cancer patients (14,15), although it is unknown whether the doses delivered are truly as biologically effective.

Mundt and colleagues have presented a series of IMRT outcome studies in gynecologic cancer patients focusing on treatment-related toxicities. In their initial series, 40 IMRT patients were compared with a cohort of 35 patients previously treated with conventional RT (16). The two groups were well matched in terms of clinicopathologic and treatment factors. IMRT treatment was associated with fewer grade greater than or equal to 2 (60% vs 91%, $P = .002$) and grade 1 (34% vs 75%, $P = .001$) gastrointestinal (GI) toxicity than conventional RT. Grade 2 genitourinary (GU) toxicity was also less common in the IMRT group (10% vs 20%); however, this difference did not reach statistical significance ($P = .22$). A subsequent report from this group noted lower rates of chronic GI toxicity in the IMRT patients as well (17). Multiple other investigators in the United States and abroad have subsequently reported favorable GI and GU toxicity profiles

in gynecology patients undergoing pelvic RT and/or more comprehensive fields (11,18–22). The recently completed Radiotherapy Oncology Group (RTOG) prospective Phase II trial of adjuvant pelvic IMRT included 58 endometrial cancer patients (23). While a moderately low rate of clinically significant acute GI toxicity was noted (28%), this was not significantly less than that seen in historical controls (40%). However, criticisms of this study include a high rate of plans exceeding the protocol-specified normal tissue constraints and the low rate of grade greater than or equal to 2 sequelae in the historical control group.

To date, outcome studies focusing on tumor control and survival in gynecology patients treated with IMRT are limited. Hasselle et al reported the outcome of 111 cervical cancer patients undergoing IMRT (24). The great majority (86%) received concomitant chemotherapy and were treated with definitive intent. At a median follow-up of 26.6 months, Stage I to Stage IIA patients undergoing definitive treatment had a 3-year overall survival (OS) and cumulative incidence of pelvic failure of 77.4% and 5.3%, respectively. Actuarial 3-year OS for the Stage IIB to Stage IVA and postoperative patients were 61.4% and 100%, respectively. Corresponding cumulative pelvic failure rates were 29.2% and 0%, respectively. Grade 3 or higher chronic toxicity was low (7%). Investigators at Washington University treated 135 cervical cancer patients with IMRT and compared their outcomes with those seen in 317 previously treated conventional RT patients at their institution (25). The two groups were well balanced with great majority of women (89%) received concomitant chemotherapy; however, the median follow-up interval differed between the two groups (IMRT: 22 month, conventional RT: 72 months). Overall, the IMRT patients had a better cause-specific survival (CSS; $P < .0001$) and a trend to a better relapse-free survival (RFS; $P = .07$) than the conventional patients. On multivariate analysis, IMRT was an independent predictor of improved CSS ($P = .0002$). IMRT patients also had a lower rate of grade greater than or equal to 3 GI/GU toxicity (6% vs 17%, $P = .0017$) than conventional patients. Others have reported favorable tumor control rates in cervical (18), endometrial (9), and vulvar (11) cancer patients undergoing IMRT.

A provocative use of IMRT is to spare the bone marrow (BM) in an effort to reduce hematologic toxicity (and thus improve chemotherapy delivery) in gynecology patients receiving concomitant chemoradiotherapy, given the high volume of BM included in conventional RT fields. A reduction of hematologic toxicity was first noted in cervical cancer patients undergoing pelvic IMRT and chemotherapy, despite the fact that their BM was not intentionally spared (26). Mell and coworkers have subsequently shown that inclusion of BM in the IMRT optimization process further reduces the volume of BM irradiated (27). Current work is focused on identifying the critical subregions within the pelvis, that is, active (red) BM sites (see IGRT section below).

At the heart of optimal IMRT, planning is accurate target delineation. Fortunately, in recent years, several target delineation consensus guidelines have been published for cervical cancer patients treated definitively (28) and patients treated adjuvantly (29). Moreover, several investigators have presented detailed outcome studies of treated patients to identify optimal planning constraints for normal tissues (Figure 27.3; 30–32).

It is also imperative that large, sufficiently powered trials are conducted in the coming years evaluating the benefit of IMRT in gynecology patients. Given the high rate of cervical cancer worldwide, these trials should be not only multi-institutional but multinational. Investigators at the University of California San Diego (UCSD) have recently initiated an international co-operative group trial evaluating IMRT in cervical cancer that includes high-volume centers in the United States, Asia, South America, and Europe (33).

■ IMAGE-GUIDED RADIOTHERAPY

IGRT comprises a broad range of technologies that involve the incorporation of imaging into the radiation treatment process. On one hand, IGRT involves the use of sophisticated imaging modalities, for example, positron emission tomography (PET) or MRI, to augment target delineation for treatment planning. However, IGRT also involves a

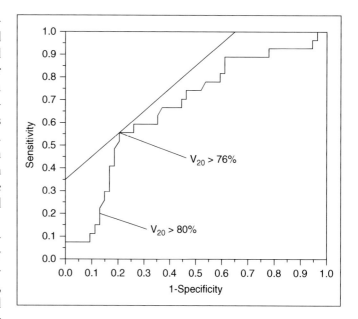

FIGURE 27.3 Normal tissue complication probability modeling for pelvic bone marrow in cervical cancer patients undergoing chemoradiation. This figure illustrates a receiver operating characteristics (ROC) for grade 3 or higher toxicity as a function of the volume of bone marrow receiving 20 Gy or more. Reproduced with permission from Rose et al (30).

number of novel in-room imaging approaches, for example, cone-beam CT (CBCT), to improve treatment delivery.

Conventional RT planning has long been based on two-dimensional (2-D) planar imaging. More recently, however, most centers have adopted CT-based techniques. Increasing attention is now focused on moving beyond CT and exploring more advanced imaging approaches. In a recent survey of practicing radiation oncologists in the United States, 43% of respondents stated that they were currently incorporating more advanced imaging to improve target delineation in their gynecology patients (34). By far, PET was the most common approach incorporated followed by MRI, with less than 5% respondents using other sophisticated imaging. It is not surprising that many physicians utilize PET for target delineation in gynecology patients for it has been shown to be useful in cervical cancer patients, particularly for the delineation of involved para-aortic lymph nodes, allowing these sites to be safely boosted using IMRT (13,35). While MRI is helpful in evaluating disease extent in locally advanced gynecology patients undergoing external beam RT, its true value may be to aid tumor delineation in cervical cancer patients undergoing brachytherapy. MRI-based techniques allow the brachytherapy plan to be tailored to the patient's individual anatomy instead of prescribing dose to standard reference points in the pelvis (Points A and B) as is currently done at most centers worldwide (36). Advanced imaging techniques may also be used to improve the delineation of normal tissues. Investigators at UCSD have explored the role of PET (37) as well as novel MRI sequences (38) to identify hematopoietically active subregions within the pelvic BM (so-called red BM), which can be included as avoidance structures in the IMRT planning process (Figure 27.4).

In-room IGRT approaches are also receiving increasing attention in the radiation oncology community. Initially proposed over 40 years ago, in-room imaging has only recently gained popularity with the increasing availability of multiple commercial systems. Currently, there are four main in-room approaches based on the type of imaging used: ultrasound, video, planar, and volumetric imaging. According to a recent practice survey, 55% of respondents reported using some form of in-room imaging in their gynecology patients, predominantly planar imaging (39). In-room planar images produced using electronic portal imaging devices (EPID) attached to the linear accelerator has long been available in many clinics. Such devices use the megavoltage (MV) treatment beam to generate images. Today, many centers are equipped with kilovoltage (kV) imagers mounted either to the machine gantry or installed in the ceiling and/or floor of the vault, which produce higher quality images with considerably less radiation dose. Both planar-based methods allow patient positioning to be checked and adjustments made

with the patient on the treatment table immediately prior to treatment (Figure 27.5; 40,41).

Several centers are exploring other more sophisticated in-room planar imaging approaches. Yamamoto et al evaluated the potential of delivering a high-dose conformal boost in 10 cervical cancer patients using a real-time tumor-tracking system, consisting of four sets of diagnostic x-ray tubes and imagers (42). The x-ray systems monitor in real-time the location of implanted fiducial markers using motion-tracking software. The beam is then "gated" to irradiate with the position of the markers coincided with their planned position. Others have used the CyberKnife system (Accuray Inc., Sunnyvale, CA) which is equipped with ceiling/floor imagers that monitor the location of implanted fiducial markers in patients undergoing SBRT (see SBRT section below; 43).

Increasing interest is currently focused on volumetric in-room IGRT approaches. Volumetric images are produced using a variety of methods, including in-room CT scanners ("CT-on-rails") or gantry-mounted systems. Gantry-mounted systems consist of an x-ray source and flat-panel detector which obtain planar images at various angles while rotating around the patient. These planar images are then used to generate a volumetric CBCT

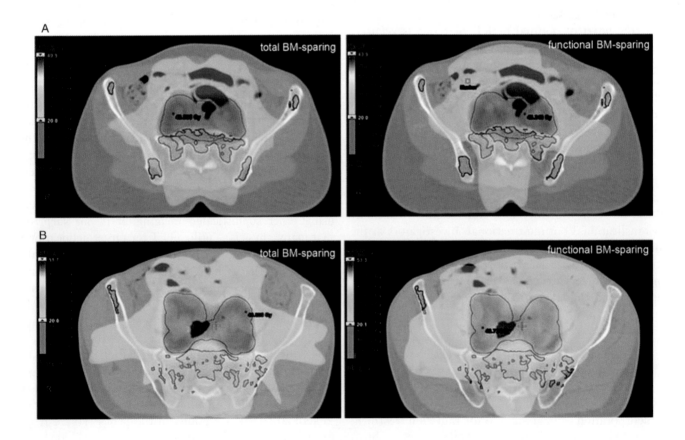

FIGURE 27.4 Axial views of the pelvis showing isodose regions greater than 20 Gy in (A) a cervical cancer patient and (B) an anal cancer patient. Functional bone marrow (BM) volume is shown in red. The dosimetry results from the total BM-sparing and functional BM-sparing intensity modulated radiation therapy are compared. Reproduced with permission from Liang et al (38).

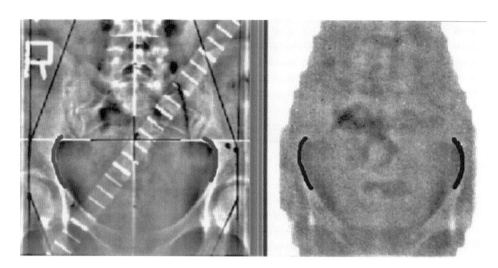

FIGURE 27.5 In-room image-guided radiotherapy (IGRT) using planar imaging in a patient with cervical cancer undergoing whole pelvic radiotherapy. In the left image, the reference image is shown with a manually drawn contour (gray in this black-and-white image). In the right image, an electronic portal imaging-device (EPID) image is shown in which a similar structure is contoured (black). Reproduced with permission from Stroom et al (41).

image. These scans are currently used at many centers to adjust patient positioning based on bone and soft tissue landmarks (44).

While current IGRT approaches focus on improving target delineation and patient positioning, a potential future use of IGRT is adaptive IGRT, whereby the treatment plan is *adapted* to changes in the tumor occurring during treatment. Currently, RT plans are based on simulation (static) images obtained prior to treatment and are then delivered daily over multiple weeks. It has been shown that cervical cancers rapidly regress during treatment and that adapting to such changes may potentially improve the treatment plan. van de Bunt and colleagues re-planned patients with intact cervical cancer undergoing RT after 30 Gy based on repeat MRI (45). Re-planning was found to significantly improve rectal sparing for all patients. Small bowel sparing was also improved in women with bulky disease. Several groups are now exploring whether adaptive RT could be based on in-room volumetric imaging, potentially with re-planning performed "on-line" perhaps even as frequently as daily with the patient on the treatment table. However, on-line re-planning requires a number of time-consuming steps to be rapidly performed including image reconstruction, image deformation, and re-optimization. Fortunately, novel high-speed computer-based approaches using graphics processing unit (GPU) technologies allow the entire re-planning process (which may currently take hours) to be completed within seconds (46,47). Nevertheless, technical barriers are only one hurdle to overcome. Even if one *can* adapt treatment, the question remains whether one *should* do so. It is possible that adapting treatment as a tumor regresses may help minimize RT-related toxicities (by reducing dose to healthy nearby normal tissues) but may also adversely impact on tumor control (by under-dosing the target). It is

imperative that adaptive IGRT techniques be evaluated on carefully designed prospective clinical trials before they are introduced into the clinic.

■ STEREOTACTIC BODY RADIOTHERAPY

SBRT is an advanced form of radiation delivery whereby high doses of radiation are administered in 1 to 5 fractions with high precision to small targets throughout the body. While it is unclear how "high" these doses must be to qualify as SBRT, most investigators utilize at least 5 to 7 Gy per fraction. Of note, more aggressive regimens are commonly used in select sites, for example, 18 Gy × 1 fraction (spine tumors) and 20 Gy × 3 fractions (lung tumors).

Initially developed for the treatment of intracranial tumors, stereotactic treatment was expanded to extracranial sites in the early 1990s. In the first published SBRT series, Blomgren and colleagues treated 42 tumors in multiple sites throughout the body with minimum doses of 7.7 to 30 Gy delivered in 1 to 4 fractions and reported an overall local control of 80% (48). More recently, high control rates have been reported in the treatment of metastatic tumors to the liver (49) and spine (50). Promising results have also been presented using SBRT to primary tumors including lung (51) and prostate (52) cancer. Initially performed using bulky immobilization devices equipped with external coordinate systems allowing stereotactic setup and tumor localization, SBRT is performed today using in-room planar/volumetric imaging obviating the need for stereotactic systems.

Multiple centers throughout the United States and abroad have begun treating patients with SBRT. In a recent survey of practicing radiation oncologists in this country, 63.9% of respondents reported using SBRT, with the majority having adopted it only since 2008 and two-thirds of nonusers planning to implement it in the near future (53). Despite this growing enthusiasm, SBRT is rarely used today in gynecologic cancers. In fact, *none* of the respondents in the national survey reported having treated a gynecology patient. However, it is likely that its use in these patients will grow in the coming years.

One potential indication of SBRT in gynecologic cancer patients is the treatment of involved lymph nodes, particularly in the para-aortic region (54). Choi and colleagues used SBRT to treat isolated para-aortic node metastases in 30 women with uterine or cervical cancer (Figure 27.6; 43). Patients received a total dose of 33 to 45 Gy delivered over 3 fractions using the CyberKnife system together with concurrent chemotherapy. All patients had fiducial markers implanted near the tumors prior to treatment that were tracked during treatment. At a median follow-up of 15 months, the 4-year actuarial local control was 67.4%. Of note, women with a target size less than or equal to 17 cc and those with tumors achieving a complete response on follow-up PET had a local control rate of 100% and 90.9%, respectively. Toxicity was low, with only 6 patients developing a grade greater than or equal to Grade 3 (5 of which were hematologic). Only 1 patient developed a severe late toxicity (ureteral stricture).

Another possible indication for SBRT in gynecologic cancer patients is as an alternative to brachytherapy, particularly in women who refuse or are unable to undergo brachytherapy. In 2005, Mollà and colleagues reported their experience using SBRT in place of brachytherapy in 16 women with either endometrial (9 patients) or cervical (7 patients) cancer (55). Patients were given either 20 Gy in 5 fractions for intact disease or 14 Gy in 2 fractions in lieu of postoperative brachytherapy. SBRT was performed with the Novalis System (BrainLAB AG, Feldkirchen, Germany). Of these 16 patients, only 1 had failed locally. There was also a single case of Grade 3 toxicity (rectal bleeding, beginning 18 months after SBRT), which occurred in a previously irradiated patient.

■ CONCLUSIONS

Recent technological advancements afford possibilities for improvement of the radiotherapeutic treatment of gynecologic cancers by facilitating the delivery of higher radiation doses to target volumes while minimizing the volume of normal tissues irradiated and thus the risk of significant acute and chronic sequelae. IMRT is the most mature of these recent technologic developments. However, increasingly sophisticated IMRT approaches continue to be introduced and tested. IGRT, arguably the oldest of these novel approaches, may not only help improve current treatment planning and delivery but may one day help transform the RT treatment process from a static to a dynamic one, whereby treatment plans are adapted to changes in the tumor during treatment, potentially as frequently as every day with the patient on the treatment table. Finally, although currently rarely used in gynecologic cancers, it is likely that SBRT, which is rapidly being adopted throughout the radiation oncology community, will be increasingly used in gynecologic cancers. It is hoped that as these and other novel technologies are introduced to the clinic. Well-designed prospective clinical trials will be conducted evaluating the potential benefits and risks of these approaches.

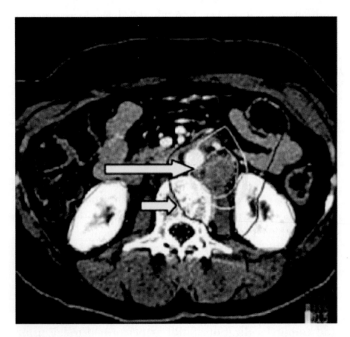

FIGURE 27.6 Stereotactic body radiotherapy (SBRT) treatment plan in a cervical cancer patient with a recurrent para-aortic lymph node. The radiation dose was prescribed to cover the involved lymph node plus a 2-mm margin (sky-blue line indicated by long arrow). The outermost line is the 30% dose line (blue line indicated by a short arrow). Reproduced with permission from Choi et al (43).

■ REFERENCES

1. Cleaves M. Radium: with a preliminary note on radium rays in the treatment of cancer. *Med Rec.* 1903;64:1719–1723.
2. Takahashi, S. Conformation radiotherapy. Rotation techniques as applied to radiography and radiotherapy of cancer. *Acta Radiol Diagn (Stockh).* 1965;Suppl 242:1+.
3. Mell, LK, Roeske, JC, Mundt, AJ. A survey of intensity-modulated radiation therapy use in the United States. *Cancer.* 2003;98(1):204–211.
4. Mell, LK, Mehrotra, AK, Mundt, AJ. Intensity-modulated radiation therapy use in the U.S. *Cancer.* 2005;104(6):1296–1303.
5. Teshima T, Numasaki H, Shibuya H, et al. Japanese society of therapeutic radiology and oncology database committee. Japanese structure survey of radiation oncology in 2007 based on

institutional stratification of patterns of care study. *Int J Radiat Oncol Biol Phys.* 2010;78(5):1483–1493.

6. Yin W, Chen B, Tian F, Yu Y, Kong FM. (2008). The growth of radiation oncology in mainland China during the last 10 years. *Int J Radiat Oncol Biol Phys.* 2008;70(3):795–798.

7. Chauvet B, Bolla M, Alies-Patin A, et al. (2009). [French radiotherapy database: results of a survey of French radiation oncology centers in 2007]. *Cancer Radiother.* 2009;13(6–7):466–470.

8. Roeske JC, Lujan A, Rotmensch J, Waggoner SE, Yamada D, Mundt AJ. Intensity-modulated whole pelvic radiation therapy in patients with gynecologic malignancies. *Int J Radiat Oncol Biol Phys.* 2000;48(5):1613–1621.

9. Beriwal S, Jain SK, Heron DE, et al. (2006). Clinical outcome with adjuvant treatment of endometrial carcinoma using intensity-modulated radiation therapy. *Gynecol Oncol.* 2006;102(2):195–199.

10. Portelance L, Chao KS, Grigsby PW, Bennet H, Low D. Intensity-modulated radiation therapy (IMRT) reduces small bowel, rectum, and bladder doses in patients with cervical cancer receiving pelvic and para-aortic irradiation. *Int J Radiat Oncol Biol Phys.* 2001;51(1):261–266.

11. Beriwal S, Heron DE, Kim H, et al. (2006). Intensity-modulated radiotherapy for the treatment of vulvar carcinoma: a comparative dosimetric study with early clinical outcome. *Int J Radiat Oncol Biol Phys.* 2006;64(5):1395–1400.

12. Hong L, Alektiar K, Chui C, et al. (2002). IMRT of large fields: whole-abdomen irradiation. *Int J Radiat Oncol Biol Phys.* 2002;54(1):278–289.

13. Ahmed RS, Kim RY, Duan J, Meleth S, De Los Santos JF, Fiveash JB. IMRT dose escalation for positive para-aortic lymph nodes in patients with locally advanced cervical cancer while reducing dose to bone marrow and other organs at risk. *Int J Radiat Oncol Biol Phys.* 2004:60(2):505–512.

14. Guerrero M, Li XA, Ma L, Linder J, Deyoung C, Erickson B. Simultaneous integrated intensity-modulated radiotherapy boost for locally advanced gynecological cancer: radiobiological and dosimetric considerations. *Int J Radiat Oncol Biol Phys.* 2005;62(3):933–939.

15. Low DA, Grigsby PW, Dempsey JF, et al. (2002). Applicator-guided intensity-modulated radiation therapy. *Int J Radiat Oncol Biol Phys.* 2002;52(5):1400–1406.

16. Mundt AJ, Lujan AE, Rotmensch J, et al. (2002). Intensity-modulated whole pelvic radiotherapy in women with gynecologic malignancies. *Int J Radiat Oncol Biol Phys.* 2002;52(5):1330–1337.

17. Mundt AJ, Mell LK, Roeske JC. Preliminary analysis of chronic gastrointestinal toxicity in gynecology patients treated with intensity-modulated whole pelvic radiation therapy. *Int J Radiat Oncol Biol Phys.* 2003;56(5):1354–1360.

18. Chen MF, Tseng CJ, Tseng CC, Kuo YC, Yu CY, Chen WC. (2007). Clinical outcome in posthysterectomy cervical cancer patients treated with concurrent Cisplatin and intensity-modulated pelvic radiotherapy: comparison with conventional radiotherapy. *Int J Radiat Oncol Biol Phys.* 2007;67(5):1438–1444.

19. Hsieh CH, Wei MC, Lee HY, et al. (2009). Whole pelvic helical tomotherapy for locally advanced cervical cancer: technical implementation of IMRT with helical tomotherapy. *Radiat Oncol.* 2009;4:62.

20. Zhou Q, Tang Y, Shu XL, Liu L. [Preliminary study of intensity-modulated radiation therapy for recurrent cervical cancer]. *Zhonghua Fu Chan Ke Za Zhi.* 2007;42(11):730–732.

21. Salama JK, Mundt AJ, Roeske J, Mehta N. (2006). Preliminary outcome and toxicity report of extended-field, intensity-modulated radiation therapy for gynecologic malignancies. *Int J Radiat Oncol Biol Phys.* 2006;65(4):1170–1176.

22. Gerszten K, Colonello K, Heron DE, et al. Feasibility of concurrent cisplatin and extended field radiation therapy (EFRT) using intensity-modulated radiotherapy (IMRT) for carcinoma of the cervix. *Gynecol Oncol.* 2006;102(2):182–188.

23. Jhingran A, Winter K, Portelance L, et al. A phase II study of intensity modulated radiation therapy to the pelvis for postoperative patients with endometrial carcinoma: radiation therapy oncology group trial 0418. *Int J Radiat Oncol Biol Phys.* 2012;84(1):e23–e28.

24. Hasselle MD, Rose BS, Kochanski JD, et al. Clinical outcomes of intensity-modulated pelvic radiation therapy for carcinoma of the cervix. *Int J Radiat Oncol Biol Phys.* 2011;80(5):1436–1445.

25. Kidd EA, Siegel BA, Dehdashti F, et al. Clinical outcomes of definitive intensity-modulated radiation therapy with fluorodeoxyglucose-positron emission tomography simulation in patients with locally advanced cervical cancer. *Int J Radiat Oncol Biol Phys.* 2010;77(4):1085–1091.

26. Brixey CJ, Roeske JC, Lujan AE, Yamada SD, Rotmensch J, Mundt AJ. Impact of intensity-modulated radiotherapy on acute hematologic toxicity in women with gynecologic malignancies. *Int J Radiat Oncol Biol Phys.* 2002;54(5):1388–1396.

27. Mell LK, Kochanski JD, Roeske JC, et al. Dosimetric predictors of acute hematologic toxicity in cervical cancer patients treated with concurrent cisplatin and intensity-modulated pelvic radiotherapy. *Int J Radiat Oncol Biol Phys.* 2006;66(5):1356–1365.

28. Lim K, Small W, Portelance L, et al. Gyn IMRT Consortium. Consensus guidelines for delineation of clinical target volume for intensity-modulated pelvic radiotherapy for the definitive treatment of cervix cancer. *Int J Radiat Oncol Biol Phys.* 2011;79(2):348–355.

29. Small W, Mell LK, Anderson P, et al. Consensus guidelines for delineation of clinical target volume for intensity-modulated pelvic radiotherapy in postoperative treatment of endometrial and cervical cancer. *Int J Radiat Oncol Biol Phys.* 2008;71(2):428–434.

30. Rose BS, Aydogan B, Liang Y, et al. Normal tissue complication probability modeling of acute hematologic toxicity in cervical cancer patients treated with chemoradiotherapy. *Int J Radiat Oncol Biol Phys.* 2011;79(3):800–807.

31. Roeske JC, Bonta D, Mell LK, Lujan AE, Mundt AJ. A dosimetric analysis of acute gastrointestinal toxicity in women receiving intensity-modulated whole-pelvic radiation therapy. *Radiother Oncol.* 2003;69(2):201–207.

32. Simpson DR, Song WY, Moiseenko V, et al. Normal tissue complication probability analysis of acute gastrointestinal toxicity in cervical cancer patients undergoing intensity modulated radiation therapy and concurrent cisplatin. *Int J Radiat Oncol Biol Phys.* 2012;83(1):e81–e86.

33. International Radiotherapy Technologies and Oncology Consortium (IRTOC). *International evaluation of radiotherapy technology effectiveness in cervical cancer (INTERTECC): a phase II/III clinical trial of IMRT with concurrent cisplatin for stage I-IVA cervical carcinoma.* Available at: http://radonc.ucsd.edu/research/irtoc/Pages/trials.aspx. Accessed August 23, 2012.

34. Simpson DR, Lawson JD, Nath SK, Rose BS, Mundt AJ, Mell LK. Utilization of advanced imaging technologies for target delineation in radiation oncology. *J Am Coll Radiol.* 2009;6(12):876–883.

35. Esthappan J, Mutic S, Malyapa RS, et al. Treatment planning guidelines regarding the use of CT/PET-guided IMRT for cervical carcinoma with positive paraaortic lymph nodes. *Int J Radiat Oncol Biol Phys.* 2004;58(4):1289–1297.

36. Pötter R, Haie-Meder C, Van Limbergen E, et al. GEC ESTRO Working Group. Recommendations from gynaecological (GYN) GEC ESTRO working group (II): concepts and terms in 3D image-based treatment planning in cervix cancer brachytherapy-3D dose volume parameters and aspects of 3D image-based anatomy, radiation physics, radiobiology. *Radiother Oncol.* 2006;78(1):67–77.

37. Rose BS, Liang Y, Lau SK, et al. Correlation between radiation dose to ^{18}F-FDG-PET defined active bone marrow subregions and acute hematologic toxicity in cervical cancer patients treated with chemoradiotherapy. *Int J Radiat Oncol Biol Phys.* 2012;83(4):1185–1191.

38. Liang Y, Bydder M, Yashar CM, et al. Prospective study of functional bone marrow-sparing intensity modulated radiation

therapy with concurrent chemotherapy for pelvic malignancies. *Int J Radiat Oncol Biol Phys.* 2013;85(2):406–414.

39. Simpson DR, Lawson JD, Nath SK, Rose BS, Mundt AJ, Mell LK. A survey of image-guided radiation therapy use in the United States. *Cancer.* 2010;116(16):3953–3960.

40. Sorcini B, Tilikidis A. Clinical application of image-guided radiotherapy, IGRT (on the Varian OBI platform). *Cancer Radiother.* 2006;10(5):252–257.

41. Stroom JC, Olofsen-van Acht MJ, Quint S, et al. On-line set-up corrections during radiotherapy of patients with gynecologic tumors. *Int J Radiat Oncol Biol Phys.* 2000;46(2):499–506.

42. Yamamoto R, Yonesaka A, Nishioka S, et al. High dose three-dimensional conformal boost (3DCB) using an orthogonal diagnostic X-ray set-up for patients with gynecological malignancy: a new application of real-time tumor-tracking system. *Radiother Oncol.* 2004;73(2):219–222.

43. Choi CW, Cho CK, Yoo SY, et al. Image-guided stereotactic body radiation therapy in patients with isolated para-aortic lymph node metastases from uterine cervical and corpus cancer. *Int J Radiat Oncol Biol Phys.* 2009;74(1):147–153.

44. McBain CA, Henry AM, Sykes J, et al. X-ray volumetric imaging in image-guided radiotherapy: the new standard in on-treatment imaging. *Int J Radiat Oncol Biol Phys.* 2006;64(2):625–634.

45. van de Bunt L, van der Heide UA, Ketelaars M, et al. Conventional, conformal, and intensity-modulated radiation therapy treatment planning of external beam radiotherapy for cervical cancer: the impact of tumor regression. *Int J Radiat Oncol Biol Phys.* 2006;64:189–196.

46. Jia X, Gu X, Graves YJ, Folkerts M, Jiang SB. GPU-based fast Monte Carlo simulation for radiotherapy dose calculation. *Phys Med Biol.* 2011;56(22):7017–7031.

47. Gu X, Jelen U, Li J, Jia X, Jiang SB. (2011). A GPU-based finite-size pencil beam algorithm with 3D-density correction for radiotherapy dose calculation. *Phys Med Biol.* 2011;56(11):3337–3350.

48. Blomgren H, Lax I, Näslund I, Svanström R. Stereotactic high dose fraction radiation therapy of extracranial tumors using an accelerator. Clinical experience of the first thirty-one patients. *Acta Oncol.* 1995;34(6):861–870.

49. Katz AW, Carey-Sampson M, Muhs AG, Milano MT, Schell MC, Okunieff P. Hypofractionated stereotactic body radiation therapy (SBRT) for limited hepatic metastases. *Int J Radiat Oncol Biol Phys.* 2007;67(3):793–798.

50. Gerszten PC, Burton, SA, Ozhasoglu C, Welch WC. Radiosurgery for spinal metastases: clinical experience in 500 cases from a single institution. *Spine.* 2007;32(2):193–199.

51. Timmerman R, Paulus R, Galvin J, et al. Stereotactic body radiation therapy for inoperable early stage lung cancer. *JAMA.* 2010;303(11):1070–1076.

52. King CR, Brooks JD, Gill H, Presti JC. Long-term outcomes from a prospective trial of stereotactic body radiotherapy for low-risk prostate cancer. *Int J Radiat Oncol Biol Phys.* 2012;82(2):877–882.

53. Pan H, Simpson DR, Mell LK, Mundt AJ, Lawson JD. A survey of stereotactic body radiotherapy use in the United States. *Cancer.* 2011;117(19):4566–4572.

54. Higginson DS, Morris DE, Jones EL, Clarke-Pearson D, Varia MA. Stereotactic body radiotherapy (SBRT): technological innovation and application in gynecologic oncology. *Gynecol Oncol.* 2011;120(3):404–412.

55. Mollà M, Escude L, Nouet P, et al. Fractionated stereotactic radiotherapy boost for gynecologic tumors: an alternative to brachytherapy? *Int J Radiat Oncol Biol Phys.* 2005;62(1):118–124.

28 PARP Inhibitors in Gynecologic Malignancies

LESLIE BRADFORD

ALLISON AMBROSIO

MICHAEL J. BIRRER

Ovarian cancer accounts for 140,000 deaths annually world-wide and is the leading cause of gynecologic cancer-related mortality in the United States (1,2). Approximately 10% of ovarian cancers occur on a hereditary basis and are associated with mutations *BRCA1* or *BRCA2* (3).These tumor suppressor genes play a crucial role in double-stranded DNA repair and the homologous recombination (HR) pathway. This process also relies on the enzyme poly (adenosine) diphosphate [ADP]-ribose (PARP) that is important for the repair of single stranded breaks. This has led to targeting HR-deficient tumors in *BRCA*-mutation carrying patient populations using a new class of drugs called PARP inhibitors.

■ MECHANISMS OF DNA REPAIR

The development of targeted therapies has resulted in a dramatic change in oncology care over the last decade. One approach has been to target activated pathways (resulting from gene amplification or mutation). Conversely, another approach has been to target defects within a tumor cell resulting from inactivation of growth inhibitor genes (tumor suppressor genes). The latter has been more difficult given the recessive nature of tumor suppressor genes. However, a potentially successful example is the targeting of defects in DNA repair. *BRCA1* and *BRCA2* are tumor suppressor genes whose deficiency results in an inability to repair double-strand breaks (DSBs) in DNA via HR (4,5). Preclinical models have demonstrated that *BRCA*-deficient cells experiencing a DNA DSB undergo cell death. There is a salvage pathway that repairs DSBs called nonhomologous end joining (NHEJ), which simply ligates the DNA ends together. This process is inefficient and results in a high number of mutations. The cell either survives with DNA mutations or undergoes cell death. Clinically, this translates to an increased risk of hereditary breast and ovarian cancer in *BRCA1*- and *BRCA2*-deficient patients (6). This DNA repair defect can be therapeutically exploited. By blocking the enzyme PARP, which normally repairs single-strand breaks (SSBs), SSBs accumulate in DNA. At the time of fork replication, these SSBs are then converted to DSBs leading to the events described above.

PARP1 and PARP2

PARP is a family of nuclear proteins (17 members) involved in DNA repair. The best characterized member of this family is PARP1, which is involved in base-excision repair. Specifically, it functions to repair DNA that has been damaged by radiation or alkylating agents. Once a SSB has occurred, PARP1 binds to the strand break and starts to synthesize poly (ADP-ribose) (PAR) on acceptor repairs. Subsequently, PARP1 loses its affinity for DNA; however, DNA repair proteins are recruited to the damaged DNA (7; Figure 28.1)

PARP1 is also involved in double-strand DNA breaks (DSB). In this case, it attaches to the DNA protein kinase catalytic subunit and recruits other enzymes involved in DSB repair, including ataxia telangiectasia mutated (ATM), MRE11, and topoisomerase I (Figure 28.1).

As noted above, the HR system functions to repair DSB. When DNA damage occurs, ATM mobilizes many proteins, notably products of the tumor suppressor genes *BRCA1* and *BRCA2*, such as RAD51, a recombination enzyme. These products are carried to the DSB site for error-free DNA repair. If there is a defect in *BRCA1* or *BRCA2*, DSB occurs via an error-prone mechanism (a nonhomologous end-joining repair system), which carries an increased risk of chromosomal alterations (8).

Synthetic Lethality

The success of PARP inhibition relies on the concept of *synthetic lethality*. First described in 1946 by Dobzhansky, *synthetic lethality* occurs when a mutation in one of two genes has no effect individually, yet the combination of mutations results in cell death (9). The success of PARP1 inhibition with regard to cytotoxic effects of *BRCA1*- and *BRCA2*-deficient cells is a result of both a lack of SSB repair by PARP1 and the lack of DSB repair because of *BRCA*

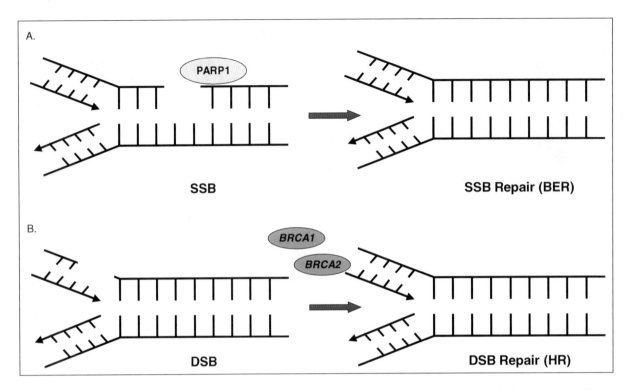

FIGURE 28.1   DNA repair mechanisms. (A) PARP1 is crucial for the repair of single-strand breaks (SSB), especially by the process of base-excision repair (BER). PARP1 detects and binds SSBs, thus initiating the process. (B) *BRCA1* and *BRCA2* are crucial for the repair of double-strand breaks (DSBs) in DNA and collapsed replication forks. This is accomplished by homologous recombination (HR). PARP, poly (adenosine) diphosphate [ADP]-ribose.

mutations and resultant HR dysfunction (Figure 28.2). In 1997, Hartwell et al first suggested that this concept could be further applied to cancer therapeutics (10). The advantages of synthetic lethality include the therapeutic window between normal cells and the cancer cells with less toxic side effects from a cytotoxic chemotherapy regimen.

BRCAness

Although mutations in *BRCA1* and *BRCA2* are rare in sporadic cancers, deficiency in other genes that are involved in the complex pathway of HR may confer such tumors with sensitivity to PARP inhibitors. This concept, referred to as *BRCAness*, suggests that PARP inhibitors may have a clinical effect beyond *BRCA*-deficient tumors, to tumors with any degree of HR dysfunction (11). It has been hypothesized that mutation or methylation of genes involved in the Faconi DNA repair pathway could produce HR deficiency and sensitivity to PARP inhibitors. Aberrant methylation of the *BRCA1* promoter has been described in 11%–14% of sporadic breast cancers and in an even higher percentage, 5%–31% of sporadic ovarian cancers (12).

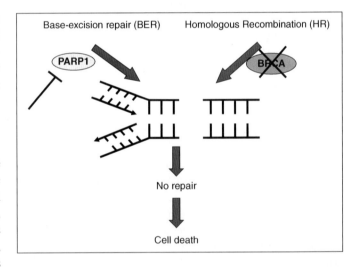

FIGURE 28.2   Cells with *BRCA* mutation and PARP1 inhibition: Synthetic lethality arises when a combination of mutations in two or more genes leads to cell death, whereas a mutation in only one of these genes does not. A cancer cell with mutations in the *BRCA* gene has a limited capacity for repairing damaged DNA, but can still remain viable. If another route of DNA repair is also inhibited, such as base-excision repair (BER) by the PARP1 enzyme, the cancer cell loses an important fail-safe and is more likely to die. PARP, poly (adenosine) diphosphate [ADP]-ribose.

■ CLINICAL DEVELOPMENT OF PARP INHIBITORS

The first PARP inhibitor to be identified was Nicotinamide (13). Several third-generation PARP inhibitors are currently being tested in clinical trials for safety and efficacy. Prior to 2005, PARP inhibitors were used as chemosensitizing agents in clinical trials. After 2005, trials began to focus on patient populations of *BRCA1* and *BRCA2* mutation carriers. The first Phase I study, presented at the 2007

American Society of Clinical Oncology (ASCO) meeting, focused on patients with hereditary cancers related to *BRCA* mutations (14,15). Since then, the concept of "BRCAness" and its clinical relevance in triple-negative breast cancers has become a target of much investigation (16). The initial excitement surrounding PARP inhibition has been somewhat dampened with reports that iniparib may not inhibit PARP (49), negative results from a Phase III trial in triple-negative breast cancer (16), no PFS difference in a randomized trial (Kaye Doxil study), and no significant improvement in overall survival noted in maintenance chemotherapy studies with olaparib (17,18).

Summary of Preclinical Data

BRCA1 and *BRCA2* mutant cells demonstrate marked sensitivity of PARP inhibitors in both in vitro and in vivo studies (4,5,10,19,20). Farmer et al (5), for instance, demonstrated that *BRCA*-deficient cells were dramatically (100–1000 fold) more sensitive to PARP inhibition compared to wild-type cell lines.

PARP1 inhibitors may also exhibit an effect in tumor cells with PTEN deficiency. Preclinical studies have demonstrated that sensitivity of human tumor cells to cisplatin administered with a PARP1 inhibitor vs paclitaxel with a PARP1 inhibitor was higher in PTEN-deficient cells compared to wild type because of HR defects. This was subsequently confirmed in in vivo models and suggests a potential role of PARP inhibition with PI3K/AKT inhibitors (21).

Clinical Data

PARP inhibitors were initially thought to be a potentially beneficial treatment specifically for tumors with germline *BRCA* mutations. Mounting evidence of frequent somatic deficiency in the *BRCA* pathway led to reconsideration of this therapeutic approach. Hennessy et al, for instance, analyzed 235 cases of epithelial ovarian cancer. They found that among the 44 *BRCA1/2* mutations detected, at least 43% of the *BRCA1* mutations and 29% of the *BRCA2* mutations were somatic (22). More recently, analysis of serous epithelial ovarian cancer through the Cancer Genome Atlas found that a combination of somatic and germline events led to *BRCA1/2* mutations in 22% of cases. The high frequency of other related mutations, such as *EMSY*, *PTEN*, *PAD51C*, and *ATM* suggests that about 50% of serous epithelial ovarian cancer cases have disruption of the HR pathway and may, in turn, be susceptible to PARP inhibitor therapy (23). In fact, a majority of ongoing and completed clinical trials include patients with a sporadic component (Table 28.1)

Monotherapy

In the first proof-of-concept study, olaparib (AZD2281) was studied in *BRCA* mutation carriers with ovarian cancer

(15). Olaparib was initially given at a dose of 10 mg, once daily, for 2 of every 3 weeks. This dose was subsequently increased to 60 mg or more, twice daily, given continuously in 4-week cycles. Sixty patients with a variety of solid tumor types were enrolled. PARP inhibition by more than 90%, as compared with the value at baseline, was observed in cells from patients treated with 60 mg or more of olaparib twice daily. Overall, 28% of patients demonstrated an objective response by Response Evaluation Criteria in Solid Tumors (RECIST) criteria with a median duration of 7 months. Importantly, antitumor activity was demonstrated at doses well below the maximum-tolerated dose with the occurrence of mild gastrointestinal symptoms and fatigue (15).

The subsequent expansion cohort from this study included a total of 50 *BRCA1* and *BRCA2* mutation-carrying patients who were treated with olaparib 200 mg PO BID. Of the cohort, 13 were platinum-sensitive, 24 platinum-resistant, and 13 platinum-refractory. Objective response rates by RECIST were 46%, 33%, and 0%, respectively (24). This trial confirmed the antitumor activity of olaparib in both platinum-sensitive and platinum-resistant patient populations and its apparent lack of activity in refractory patients.

A Phase II trial of olaparib was performed as an international collaboration known as ICEBERG (International Collaborative Expertise for BRCA Education and Research Through Genetics). The study included women who were *BRCA* mutation carriers with recurrent ovarian, fallopian, and primary peritoneal carcinoma. The trial design consisted of two dose cohorts: 100 mg twice daily (the dose at which responses were first seen in the Phase I trial) and 400 mg twice daily (the maximum-tolerated dose in the Phase I trial). Overall response ranged from 13% in the low-dose group to 33% in the high-dose group. As demonstrated in the Phase I trial, common toxicities included mild fatigue, nausea, and anemia (25).

An additional Phase II trial with olaparib was performed in Canada. This included women with platinum-sensitive recurrent, high-grade serous, or undifferentiated sporadic epithelial ovarian cancer, *BRCA*-deficient epithelial ovarian, fallopian, or primary peritoneal cancer, and triple-negative breast cancer (26). Among 91 patients enrolled, 64 with epithelial ovarian cancer were treated. The majority (47 of 64 patients) had sporadic disease. Among the 17 mutation carriers, 65% had *BRCA1* mutations and 29% had *BRCA2* mutations. The objective response rate was 41% in mutation carriers and 24% in patients with sporadic ovarian cancer, a notable difference from the dose-escalation portion of the Phase I trial, where no responses were seen in nonmutation carriers. This study further confirmed that any degree of HR dysregulation within a tumor, or *BRCA*ness, may result in an improved response to therapy with a PARP inhibitor.

Currently, there are multiple ongoing trials of PARP inhibitors as monotherapy, including olaparib, veliparib,

■ **Table 28.1**   Clinical trials of PARP inhibitors in epithelial ovarian cancer

Identifier	PARP Inhibitor	Phase of Development	Study Design	Patient Population	Findings
Completed Trials					
NCT00516373	Olaparib	I	Dose escalation	Recurrent EOC with expansion cohort of *BRCA*-deficient EOC, FTC, or PPC	MTD 400 mg BID; clinical benefit rate 46% in expansion cohort
NCT00494442 ICEBERG 2	Olaparib	II	Two-arm randomization; 100 mg BID vs 400 mg BID	Recurrent, *BRCA*-deficient EOC, FTC, PPC	RR of 13% (100 mg BID) vs 33% (400 mg BID)
NCT00679783	Olaparib	II		Recurrent, *BRCA*-deficient EOC, FTC, PPC, or sporadic, high-grade serous EOC	RR 41% in *BRCA*-deficient EOC RR 24% in sporadic EOC
NCT00526617	Veliparib + Temozolomide	I		*BRCA*-deficient EOC, FTC, PPC	n/a
Ongoing Clinical Trials					
NCT01445418	Olaparib + Carboplatin	I		Recurrent, *BRCA*-deficient or sporadic EOC, FTC, PPC	
NCT01237067	Olaparib + Carboplatin	I	Sequencing study	Recurrent EOC, FTC, PPC, cervical or uterine cancer	Hypothesizes that Carboplatin prior to Olaparib administration is more effective than Olaparib prior to Carboplatin administration
NCT00516724	Olaparib + Carboplatin; Olaparib + Paclitaxel; Olaparib + Carboplatin + Paclitaxel	I	Three arm	Advanced EOC	
NCT00647062	Olaparib + Carboplatin	I	With maintenance Olaparib until progression	*BRCA*-deficient or sporadic, serous ECO with expansion cohort of BRCA-deficient EOC	Olaparib 400 mg BID Carboplatin AUC 5 CBR of 83%
NCT01116648	Olaparib + Cediranib	I		Recurrent serous EOC, FTC, PPC	RR 56%
NCT01116648	Olaparib + Cediranib; Olaparib alone	II	Two-arm randomization	Recurrent serous EOC, FTC, PPC	
NCT00749502	MK4827	I		Expansion cohorts of: Recurrent, platinum-resistant EOC, FTC, PPC Recurrent, platinum-sensitive EOC, FTC, PPC Recurrent endometrial cancer	10 of 12 patients with PR had sporadic EOC
NCT01227941	MK4827 + PLD	I		Expansion cohort of recurrent, platinum-resistant EOC, FTC, PPC	Study terminated

(Continued)

■ **Table 28.1** Clinical trials of PARP inhibitors in epithelial ovarian cancer *(Continued)*					
Identifier	**PARP Inhibitor**	**Phase of Development**	**Study Design**	**Patient Population**	**Findings**
NCT00892736	Veliparib	I	Continuous dosing	Recurrent, *BRCA*-deficient or sporadic, platinum-resistant EOC, FTC, PPC	
NCT00576654	Veliparib + Ironotecan	I		Recurrent cancer	7 of 32 patients enrolled have EOC CBR of 61%
NCT01145430	Veliparib + PLD	I		Recurrent EOC, FTC, PPC	
NCT01233505	Veliparib + Oxaliplatin + Capecitibine	I		*BRCA*-deficient EOC, FTC, PPC; mucinous EOC	Suspended
NCT00535119	Veliparib + Carboplatin + Paclitaxel	I	Stratified by *BRCA* mutation status	*BRCA*-deficient or sporadic EOC, FTC, PPC; recurrent gynecologic cancer	
NCT01366144	Veliparib + Carboplatin + Paclitaxel	I		Recurrent gynecologic cancer	
NCT00989651 GOG 9923	Veliparib + Carboplatin + Paclitaxel + Bevacizumab	I		Newly diagnosed, stage II-IV EOC, FTC, PPC	
NCT01459380 GOG 9927	Veliparib + Carboplatin + PLD	I		Recurrent, platinum-sensitive EOC, FTC, PPC	
NCT01012817	Veliparib + Topotecan	I/II	Phase II expansion cohort	Recurrent EOC or PPC	
NCT00677079	Iniparib	II		Recurrent, *BRCA*-deficient EOC, FTC, PPC	
NCT01033123	Iniparib + Carboplatin; Gemcitabine			Recurrent, platinum-sensitive EOC, FTC, PPC	12 of 17 patients with confirmed response
NCT01033292	Iniparib + Carboplatin; Gemcitabine			Recurrent, platinum-resistant EOC, FTC, PPC	6 of 19 patients with confirmed response
NCT01078662	Olaparib	II		Recurrent *BRCA*-deficient EOC	
NCT00753545	Olaparib; Placebo	II	Olaparib maintenance 400 mg BID	Recurrent, platinum-sensitive EOC	Median PFS 8.4 months (Olaparib) vs 4.8 months (placebo)
NCT00628251 ICEBERG 3	Olaparib 200 mg BID; Olaparib 400 mg BID; PLD	II		Recurrent *BRCA*-deficient EOC	Median PFS of 6.5 vs 8.8 vs 7.1 months RR of 25 vs 31 vs 18%
NCT01081951	Carboplatin + Paclitaxel +/– Olaparib	II		Recurrent, platinum-sensitive EOC	
NCT01113957	Veliparib + Temozolomide; PLD	II	PLD crossover allowed	Recurrent, serous EOC, FTC, PPC	
NCT01306032	Metronomic Cyclophosphamide +/– Veliparib	II		Recurrent, *BRCA*-deficient or sporadic EOC, FTC, PPC	
NCT00664781	AGO14699	II		Recurrent *BRCA*-deficient EOC and breast cancer	RR 5% and CBR 32% in EOC and breast cancer combined

BID, twice daily; CBR, clinical benefit rate; EOC, epithelial ovarian cancer; FTC, fallopian tube cancer; MTD, maximum-tolerated dose; PFS, progression-free survival; PLD, pegylated liposomal doxorubicin; PPC, primary peritoneal cancer; RR, response rate.

iniparib, MK4827, and AGO14699. Preliminary results from a Phase I of MK4827 indicate a partial response among 10 of 12 patients. Of those with stable disease, half are *BRCA*-deficient and the other patients have sporadic disease (27). The Phase II of AGO14699 included women with *BRCA*-deficient ovarian (24 of 41 patients enrolled) or breast cancer. While the overall response rate was low across the entire cohort (5%), stable disease contributed to a clinical benefit rate of 32% (28).

Given the initial activity of PARP1 inhibitors in early phase trials, single-agent randomized trials were conducted in both the recurrent and maintenance situations. A three-arm study of olaparib at different dosages (200 mg twice daily and 400 mg twice daily) compared to liposomal doxorubicin demonstrated response rates of 31%, 25%, and 18%, respectively; however, progression-free survival (PFS) was similar across the three groups (8.8, 6.5, and 7.1 months, respectively; 29). The toxicity of olaparib, including at a higher dosage, was acceptable. In a second randomized Phase II trial, olaparib administered at 400 mg twice daily maintenance therapy was compared with placebo in a cohort of women with recurrent, platinum-sensitive, serous epithelial ovarian cancer who had demonstrated partial or complete response to platinum therapy (30). Preliminary findings include a statistically significant improvement in PFS from 4.8 to 8.4 months. Final analysis of the data confirmed a benefit with regard to PFS (8.4 vs 4.8 months, Hazard Ratio 0.35; 95% confidence interval [CI], 0/25–0.49, $P < .001$); however, there was no statistically significant difference in overall survival (17).

Combination Regimens

Preclinical studies have demonstrated that *BRCA*-deficient cells have an increased sensitivity to platinum-based chemotherapy (31,32). This is consistent with clinical experiences that women with *BRCA1*- and *BRCA2*-associated ovarian cancer had a more favorable response to platinum-based chemotherapy regimens and improved overall survival (33,34).

This effect can be explained by the mechanism of action of each of these classes of chemotherapeutics. Platinum compounds, such as cisplatin and carboplatin, form adducts with guanine bases of DNA, thus producing DNA crosslinks. Nucleotide excision repair (NER) plays a major role in repairing these platinum-induced crosslinks (35). Excision of these crosslinks by NER is followed by gap filling of SSBs. There is increasing evidence that HR is also needed to repair platinum-induced DNA damage, both with regard to SSBs and DSBs (36,37). It therefore appears that overlapping mechanisms of action provide PARP inhibitors and platinum compounds share a spectrum of therapeutic efficacy against *BRCA*-associated ovarian cancer, forming the basis for many of the combination trials that will be reviewed herein.

The further potentiation of DNA-damage from cytotoxic agents provides the rationale for studying PARP1 inhibitors in combination with traditional, cytotoxic chemotherapy, namely platinum agents. In general, such combinations also result in greater potentiation of myelosuppressive effects with resultant dose reductions or delays in treatment (38). This is seen more commonly with olaparib than with iniparib (BSI201).

Preliminary results from a Phase I study of olaparib and carboplatin with maintenance olaparib until progression demonstrated an impressive 83% clinical benefit rate in patients with recurrent epithelial ovarian cancer (39).

The most promising combination appears to be the combination of iniparib with gemcitabine and carboplatin. This regimen has been particularly successful in triple-negative breast cancer (16). In a study of 41 patients with platinum-sensitive, high-grade ovarian cancer, iniparib (administered as 5–6 mg/kg on days 1, 4, 8, and 11 every 3 weeks) with gemcitabine (1000 mg/m², days 1 and 8) and carboplatin (area under the curve [AUC] 4, day 1) demonstrated an overall response rate of 64%. The response rate in the *BRCA*-mutated population was less than in the wild-type population (60% vs 71%, respectively). The PFS was 9.5 months. There was notable toxicity with 42% of patients experiencing Grades 3 to 4 thrombocytopenia, 59% with Grades 3 to 4 neutropenia, and 41% of patients requiring dose reductions (40).

This same regimen was studied in 34 platinum-resistant patients. The overall response rate was 25%. Patients with *BRCA*-mutations had a better response rate (50%) compared to those with wild-type *BRCA*. Nevertheless, this study confirmed the activity of combination therapy with PARP inhibitors in tumors without *BRCA* mutations but with HR dysfunction. With regard to toxicity, a large percentage of patients experienced fatigue (71%, only 6% Grades 3–4). Other toxicities included Grades 3 to 4 thrombocytopenia (26%), neutropenia (46%), dose reductions (85%), and dose delays (27%; 41).

Maintenance Therapy

The rationale for studying PARP inhibitors as maintenance therapy for ovarian cancer derives from the observation that a large number of sporadic high-grade serous ovarian cancer demonstrate HR dysfunction. These tumors are predicted to be responsive to PARP inhibitors and demonstrate repeated responses to treatment with platinum-based regimens likely also due to an intrinsic weakness in DNA repair.

As discussed previously, a large randomized Phase II of olaparib as maintenance therapy demonstrated an improvement in PFS, but not overall survival (17). Toxicity was moderate in the olaparib group, with about half of patients requiring modifications to their treatment.

Efficacy in Non-*BRCA* Mutants

As discussed earlier, certain tumors demonstrated dysfunctional HR, either through germ line or acquired somatic defects in the HR pathway. This phenomenon has been termed "BRCAness" and such tumors appear to respond more robustly to PARP inhibition. The first proof-of-concept data was provided by Gelmon et al, who demonstrated that women with recurrent, sporadic, high-grade epithelial ovarian cancer had an objective response rate to single-agent olaparib of 24% (26).

Resistance

As with most cancer therapeutics, resistance is likely to develop. It has been suggested that prior exposure and resistance to platinum agents may lead to resistance to PARP inhibitors (42). There have been reported documented reports of resistance to PARP inhibitors. Although the mechanism remains unknown, it has been shown that those patients carrying *BRCA* mutations may subsequently develop a secondary mutation that restores *BRCA* function (43–46). For platinum refractory patients the trial by Fong et al showed no responses to olaparib (24). This is consistent with the molecular characterization of these tumors that appear substantially different from other ovarian cancers. It is worth noting, however, that patients who failed to respond to olaparib may subsequently respond to platinum-based chemotherapy (47).

■ CHALLENGES WITH FUTURE DRUG DEVELOPMENT AND TRIALS

The initial Phase II of iniparib in triple-negative breast cancer brought a wave of excitement and active development of PARP inhibitors. Subsequent reports that iniparib does not inhibit PARP, as well as additional negative trials with other PARP inhibitors has lessened some of the excitement regarding drug development. Combination trials remain an area of interest and potential promise, yet challenges remain. While preclinical data suggest that sequential administration of traditional chemotherapy followed by PARP inhibition may be most effective (39,48) in clinical trials, however, it has not yet been demonstrated whether treatment with traditional cytotoxic chemotherapy and a PARP inhibitor has additive or synergistic effects. Likewise, questions regarding the dose, duration, sequence (sequential or concurrent administration), and differences among specific PARP inhibitors remain.

Although dose has been explored both in preclinical models and trial, the specific dose and optimal degree of enzyme inhibition remains undetermined. Likewise, the most effective duration of treatment remains to be defined. There are theoretic issues of continuous vs intermittent inhibition with regard to effectiveness and toxicity. Long-term exposure to a DNA repair inhibitor may increase the risk of secondary malignancies especially leukemia. With regard to sequencing of administration, preclinical evidence suggests that administering olaparib before carboplatin diminishes DNA damage. It is hypothesized that PARP inhibition preceding cytotoxic chemotherapy enhances alternative DNA repair pathways and recovery from chemotherapy (48). Finally, a challenge lies in comparing one PARP inhibitor to another. In vitro data suggest that iniparib may employ a different mechanism of action compared to that of olaparib and veliparib (49). Namely, it appears that olaparib and veliparib employ PARP1 and PARP2, whereas iniparib likely inhibits PARP5 and PARP6. The clinical implications of these findings are not yet clear and are undergoing active research.

In summary, PARP inhibitors have demonstrated impressive activity in epithelial ovarian, fallopian, and primary peritoneal carcinomas, both in the Phase I and Phase II setting. Responses have been noted in both *BRCA*-deficient and sporadic tumors as well as platinum-sensitive and resistant patient populations. PARP inhibitors appear to be well tolerated as monotherapy as well as in combination with traditional cytotoxic chemotherapy.

Perhaps most importantly, the evolution of PARP inhibition as treatment for ovarian cancer is an example of rational drug development. It began as a therapeutic aimed at germ line *BRCA*-mutated malignancies and has since expanded to include tumors with somatic mutations in *BRCA1* and *BRCA2*, as well as tumors that demonstrate dysfunction of the HR pathway. As such, our approach to treating ovarian cancer will need to evolve to better recognize the incredible heterogeneity, both with regard to histology and molecular pathways, displayed by these tumors.

■ REFERENCES

1. Jemal A, Siegel R, Xu J, Ward E. Cancer statistics, 2010. *CA Cancer J Clin*. 2010;60(5):277–300.
2. Ferlay J, Autier P, Boniol M, Heanue M, Colombet M, Boyle P. Estimates of the cancer incidence and mortality in Europe in 2006. *Ann Oncol*. 2007;18(3):581–592.
3. Boyd J, Sonoda Y, Federici MG, et al. Clinicopathologic features of BRCA-linked and sporadic ovarian cancer. *JAMA*. 2000;283(17):2260–2265.
4. Bryant HE, Schultz N, Thomas HD, et al. Specific killing of BRCA2-deficient tumours with inhibitors of poly(ADP-ribose) polymerase. *Nature*. 2005;434(7035):913–917.
5. Farmer H, McCabe N, Lord CJ, et al. Targeting the DNA repair defect in BRCA mutant cells as a therapeutic strategy. *Nature*. 2005;434(7035):917–921.
6. Wooster R, Weber BL. Breast and ovarian cancer. *N Engl J Med*. 2003;348(23):2339–2347.
7. Rouleau M, Patel A, Hendzel MJ, Kaufmann SH, Poirier GG. PARP inhibition: PARP1 and beyond. *Nat Rev Cancer*. 2010;10(4):293–301.

8. Sessa C. Update on PARP1 inhibitors in ovarian cancer. *Ann Oncol*. 2001;22 (Supp. 8):viii72–viii76.

9. Dobzhansky T. Genetics of natural populations; recombination and variability in populations of Drosophila pseudoobscura. *Genetics*. 1946;31:269–290.

10. Hartwell LH, Szankasi P, Roberts CJ, Murray AW, Friend SH. Integrating genetic approaches into the discovery of anticancer drugs. *Science*. 1997;278(5340):1064–1068.

11. Konstantinopoulos PA, Spentzos D, Karlan BY, et al. Gene expression profile of BRCAness that correlates with responsiveness to chemotherapy and with outcome in patients with epithelial ovarian cancer. *J Clin Oncol*. 2010;28(22):3555–3561.

12. Turner N, Tutt A, Ashworth A. Hallmarks of 'BRCAness' in sporadic cancers. *Nat Rev Cancer*. 2004;4(10):814–819.

13. Clark JB, Ferris GM, Pinder S. Inhibition of nuclear NAD nucleosidase and poly ADP-ribose polymerase activity from rat liver by nicotinamide and 5'-methyl nicotinamide. *Biochim Biophys Acta*. 1971;238(1):82–85.

14. Yap TA, Boss DS, Fong PC, et al. First in human phase I pharmacokinetic (PK) and pharmacodynamic (PD) study of KU-0059436 (Ku), a small molecule inhibitor of poly ADP-ribose polymerase (PARP) in cancer patients (p), including BRCA1/2 mutation carriers. *J Clin Oncol*. 2007;25:3529.

15. Fong PC, Boss DS, Yap TA, et al. Inhibition of poly(ADP-ribose) polymerase in tumors from BRCA mutation carriers. *N Engl J Med*. 2009;361(2):123–134.

16. O'Shaughnessy J, Osborne C, Pippen JE, et al. Iniparib plus chemotherapy in metastatic triple-negative breast cancer. *N Engl J Med*. 2011;364(3):205–214.

17. Ledermann J, Harter P, Gourley C, et al. Olaparib maintenance therapy in platinum-sensitive relapsed ovarian cancer. *N Engl J Med*. 2012;366(15):1382–1392.

18. Oza, AM. Olaparib plus paclitaxel plus carboplatin (P/C) followed by olaparib maintenance treatment in patients (pts) with platinum-sensitive recurrent serous ovarian cancer (PSRSOC): A randomized, open-label phase II study. *J Clin Oncol*. 2012;30(Suppl; Abstr 5001).

19. McCabe N, Turner NC, Lord CJ, et al. Deficiency in the repair of DNA damage by homologous recombination and sensitivity to poly(ADP-ribose) polymerase inhibition. *Cancer Res*. 2006;66(16):8109–8115.

20. Hay T, Matthews JR, Pietzka L, et al. Poly(ADP-ribose) polymerase-1 inhibitor treatment regresses autochthonous BRCA2/p53-mutant mammary tumors *in vivo* and delays tumor relapse in combination with carboplatin. *Cancer Res*. 2009;69(9):3850–3855.

21. Mendes-Pereira AM, Martin SA, Brough R, et al. Synthetic lethal targeting of PTEN mutant cells with PARP inhibitors. *EMBO Mol Med*. 2009;1(6–7):315–322.

22. Hennessy BT, Timms KM, Carey MS, et al. Somatic mutations in BRCA1 and BRCA2 could expand the number of patients that benefit from poly (ADP ribose) polymerase inhibitors in ovarian cancer. *J Clin Oncol*. 2010;28(22):3570–3576.

23. Cancer Genome Atlas Research Network. Integrated genomic analyses of ovarian carcinoma. *Nature*. 2011;474;609–615.

24. Fong PC, Yap TA, Boss DS, et al. Poly(ADP)-ribose polymerase inhibition: frequent durable responses in BRCA carrier ovarian cancer correlating with platinum-free interval. *J Clin Oncol*. 2010;28(15):2512–2519.

25. Audeh MW, Carmichael J, Penson RT, et al. Oral poly(ADP-ribose) polymerase inhibitor olaparib in patients with BRCA1 or BRCA2 mutations and recurrent ovarian cancer: a proof-of-concept trial. *Lancet*. 2010;376(9737):245–251.

26. Gelmon KA, Tischkowitz M, Mackay H, et al. Olaparib in patients with recurrent high-grade serous or poorly differentiated ovarian carcinoma or triple-negative breast cancer: a phase 2, multicentre, open-label, non-randomised study. *Lancet Oncol*. 2011;12(9):852–861.

27. Schelman WR, Sandhu SK, Moreno Garcia V, et al. First-in-human trial of poly(ADP-ribose) polymerase (PARP) inhibitor MK-4827 in advanced ovarian cancer patients with antitumor activity in BRCA-deficient tumors and sporadic ovarian cancers (SOC). *J Clin Oncol*. 2011;29(Suppl): abstract 3102.

28. Drew Y, Ledermann JA, Jones A, et al. Phase II trial of the poly(ADP-ribose) polymerase (PARP) inhibitor AG-014699 in BRCA 1 and 2 mutated, advanced ovarian and/or locally advanced or metastatic breast cancer. *J Clin Oncol*. 2011;29(Suppl):abstract 3104.

29. Kaye S, Kaufmann B, Lubinsky J, et al. Phase II study of the oral PARP inhibitor Olaparib (AZD2281) versus liposomal doxorubicin in ovarian cancer patients with BRCA1 and/or BRCA2 mutations. *Ann Oncol*. 2010;21(Supp 8):vii304 (Abstract 3725).

30. Ledermann JA, Harter P, Gourley C, et al. Phase II randomized placebo-controlled study of olaparib (AZD2281) in patients with platinum-sensitive relapsed serous ovarian cancer (PSRSOC). *J Clin Oncol*. 2011;29(Suppl): abstract 5003.

31. Bhattacharyya A, Ear US, Koller BH, Weichselbaum RR, Bishop DK. The breast cancer susceptibility gene BRCA1 is required for subnuclear assembly of Rad51 and survival following treatment with the DNA cross-linking agent cisplatin. *J Biol Chem*. 2000;275(31):23899–23903.

32. Sgagias MK, Wagner KU, Hamik B, et al. Brca1-deficient murine mammary epithelial cells have increased sensitivity to CDDP and MMS. *Cell Cycle*. 2004;3(11):1451–1456.

33. Tan DS, Rothermundt C, Thomas K, et al. "BRCAness" syndrome in ovarian cancer: a case-control study describing the clinical features and outcome of patients with epithelial ovarian cancer associated with BRCA1 and BRCA2 mutations. *J Clin Oncol*. 2008;26(34):5530–5536.

34. Bolton KL, Chenevix-Trench G, Goh C, et al.; EMBRACE; kConFab Investigators; Cancer Genome Atlas Research Network. Association between BRCA1 and BRCA2 mutations and survival in women with invasive epithelial ovarian cancer. *JAMA*. 2012;307(4):382–390.

35. Sibghat-Ullah, Husain I, Carlton W, Sancar A. Human nucleotide excision repair in vitro: repair of pyrimidine dimers, psoralen and cisplatin adducts by HeLa cell-free extract. *Nucleic Acids Res*. 1989;17:4471–4484.

36. Zdraveski ZZ, Mello JA, Marinus MG, et al. Multiple pathways of recombination define cellular responses to cisplatin. *Chem Biol*. 2000;7:39–50.

37. Lin ZP, Lee Y, Lin F, et al. Reduced level of ribonucleotide reductase R2 subunits increases dependence on homologous recombination repair of cisplatin-induced DNA damage. *Mol Pharmacol*. 2011;80(6):1000–1012.

38. Plummer R, Jones C, Middleton M, et al. Phase I study of the poly(ADP-ribose) polymerase inhibitor, AG014699, in combination with temozolomide in patients with advanced solid tumors. *Clin Cancer Res*. 2008;14(23):7917–7923.

39. Lee J, Squires J, Hays JL, et al. A pharmacokinetics/pharmacodynamics study of sequence specificity of the PARP inhibitor olaparib with carboplatin in refractory/recurrent women's cancers: NCT01237067. *J Clin Oncol*. 2011;29(Suppl):abstract TPS158.

40. Penson RT. A phase II trial of iniparib (BSI201) in combination with gemcitabine/carboplatin (GC) in patients with platinum sensitive recurrent ovarian cancer. *J Clin Oncol*. 2011; 29(Suppl):333s (Abstr 5004).

41. Birrer MJ. A phase II trial of iniparib (BSI201) in combination with gemcitabine/carboplatin (GC) in patients with platinum resistant recurrent ovarian cancer. *J Clin Oncol*. 2011;(Suppl):(Abstr 5005).

42. Javle M, Curtin NJ. The potential for poly(ADP-ribose) polymerase inhibitors in cancer therapy. *Therapeutic Advances in Medical Oncology*. 2011;3:257–267.

43. Sakai W, Swisher EM, Karlan BY, et al. Secondary mutations as a mechanism of cisplatin resistance in BRCA2-mutated cancers. *Nature*. 2008;451(7182):1116–1120.

44. Swisher EM, Sakai W, Karlan BY, Wurz K, Urban N, Taniguchi T. Secondary BRCA1 mutations in BRCA1-mutated ovarian carcinomas with platinum resistance. *Cancer Res.* 2008;68(8): 2581–2586.

45. Sakai W, Swisher EM, Jacquemont C, et al. Functional restoration of BRCA2 protein by secondary BRCA2 mutations in BRCA2-mutated ovarian carcinoma. *Cancer Res.* 2009;69(16):6381–6386.

46. Norquist B, Wurz KA, Pennil CC, et al. Secondary somatic mutations restoring BRCA1/2 predict chemotherapy resistance in hereditary ovarian carcinomas. *J Clin Oncol.* 2011;29(22): 3008–3015.

47. Ang J, Yap TA, Fong P, et al. Preliminary experience with the use of chemotherapy (CT)following treatment with olaparib, a poly(ADP-ribose) polymerase inhibitor (PARPi), in patients with BRCA1/2-deficient ovarian cancer (BDOC). *J Clin Oncol.* 2010;28(Suppl 15s):abstract 5041.

48. Hays JL, Kim G, Mariani J, et al. Sequence specific effects on DNA and cell damage with the PARP inhibitor olaparib (AZD2281) and carboplatin. *J Clin Oncol.* 2011;29(Suppl):abstract 5025.

49. Ji J, Lee MP, Kadota M, et al. Pharmacodynamic and pathway analysis of three presumed inhibitors of poly(ADP-ribose) polymerase: ABT-888, AZD2281, and BSI201. *Cancer Res.* 2011;71(Suppl 1):abstract 4526.

29 Hormonal Treatment in Gynecologic Oncology

ASHLEY FORD HAGGERTY

CHRISTINA S. CHU

Hormonal therapy has been studied for the treatment of both primary and recurrent cancer, either in addition to chemotherapy or as a primary treatment. While hysterectomy and bilateral salpingo-oophorectomy is the mainstay of treatment for both endometrial and ovarian cancer (OC), new research has demonstrated that conservative therapy with hormonal treatment may be considered in well-selected subsets of patients.

■ PROGESTERONE THERAPY FOR EARLY ENDOMETRIAL CANCER

In the normal menstrual cycle, estrogen is responsible for the growth of the endometrial glandular epithelium while progesterone inhibits this endometrial proliferation, leading to stromal decidualization and cellular differentiation. It is well known that for normal endometrial growth to occurs the ratio of estrogen to progesterone must be maintained in a balanced cycle, as an excess in estrogen or a loss of the suppressive effect of progesterone leads to pathology such as hyperplasia and cancer. Approximately 80% of all endometrial cancers (ECs) are classified as Type I carcinoma and are related to excess estrogen exposure (1).

Progesterone acts on the endometrium by binding to progesterone receptors (PR), leading to stimulation of multiple signaling pathways, which are subsequently modulated by a variety of factors including micro (mi)RNAs, epigenetic factors, and downregulation of genes (eg, integrins and K-cadherin) resulting in apoptosis (1). Improved response rates and trends toward increased survival have been noted in patients based on tumor expression of PR, with recurrence shown to be increased in patients with PR-negative tumors (2). Though earlier studies showed improved clinical outcome based on receptor status, newer data examining the locations and subtypes of PRs make these associations less clear.

A variety of drugs and dosing options are available for progesterone therapy, including oral progesterone (those most commonly used include medroxyprogesterone acetate [MPA] and megestrol acetate [MA]), injectable and implantable forms, and the newer intrauterine delivery (IUD) system (3,4; Table 29.1). Primary treatment with progesterone has been clearly demonstrated to be effective in the treatment of endometrial hyperplasia (5–7). Since the 1960s, investigators have also attempted to evaluate progestins for use in primary treatment for EC. Studies have documented complete response (CR) rates ranging from 50% to 70% (1,8). Both oral and intrauterine progesterones directly alter the endometrial architecture (8,9). In two large systematic reviews, 214 patients with Stage IA EC were treated with various progesterones between 1966 and 2007. While 23% did not respond, 51%–72% of patients achieved a CR, though 19%–24% eventually recurred (10,11). The most recent systematic review published in 2012 identified 38 studies in which 280 women with early EC were treated with either oral or intrauterine progesterone. Overall, the initial response rate was 74.6% with a CR rate of 48.2%, over a median follow-up of 39 months. Again, 35.4% of patients recurred and persistent disease was noted in 25.4% (12).

Though no randomized clinical trials comparing hormonal treatment to traditional surgery have been performed, several prospective preclinical and Phase I/II trials have evaluated the use of progestin as primary therapy (13–15). Although the majority of patients with EC are postmenopausal women, almost 10% of those affected are under the age of 45, and 70% of these women are nulliparous at the time of diagnosis (16). Hysterectomy for treatment of EC in this younger population significantly affects a patient's fertility options and may result in loss of ovarian function if bilateral salpingo-oophorectomy is performed. Thus, early studies of primary hormonal therapy have mainly focused on subsets of patients, both likely to benefit from nonsurgical options and to respond to progesterone. These include patients with tumors of endometrioid histology and young women who desire fertility-preservation (17). Two small prospective studies investigated oral progesterone in women younger than 40 with Stage IA EC and demonstrated a high rate of response (13,17). Twenty-two

■ **Table 29.1** Hormonal treatment options for early endometrial cancer

Hormone Type	Dose Range	Reported Response Rates (%)	References
Oral MPA	250–1500 mg/day	8%–78%	8–14,16–18,21,24
Oral MA	80–160 mg/day	33%–100%	3,6,8,10,11–14,16,18,20,22
Hydroxyprogesterone caproate	200–250 mg/day	7%–18%	13,20
LNG-IUD	52 mg Device	25%–100%	9,11,14,15,18–24

LNG-IUD, Levonorgestrel intrauterine device; MA, megestrol acetate; MPA, medroxyprogesterone acetate

women were treated for 26 weeks with oral MPA followed by cyclic estrogen-progestin therapy for 6 months; 55% (12/22) demonstrated CR, however 47% eventually recurred (13). Another study included 9 women under the age of 40 with early EC who received oral MPA for 6 months and demonstrated a 78% overall response rate, with 2 women experiencing recurrence (17).

Several other recent retrospective reports in the literature have examined the use of the progestin levonorgestrel intrauterine device (LNG-IUD) as primary treatment for EC, particularly as a fertility-preserving option. The LNG-IUD is a 19-nortestosterone derivative, which has been shown to have a profound local progestational effect on the endometrium, with few systemic side effects. This T-shaped device contains a total of 52 mg of LNG, released at an initial rate of 20 mcg daily and declining progressively to half of that dose by the end of its 5-year therapeutic life (3). Success has been variable, with CR rates ranging from 25% to 75% in Grade 1, Stage I disease (9,14,15,18–22). The LNG-IUD may also be an attractive treatment option for women who are deemed to be poor surgical candidates, as high doses of progesterone are delivered directly to the site of pathology with minimal side effects (15). In addition, higher local concentrations of progesterone may be achieved within the endometrium compared to oral therapy (3). The largest study reported to date evaluated 12 women deemed to have excessive surgical risk, who underwent dilation and curettage (D&C) and placement of a progesterone IUD for Grade 1, clinical Stage I disease. After serial endometrial sampling for 1 year, 6 women were reported to have negative histology (16). The overall effectiveness as reported in the literature of treatment in women who are poor surgical candidates with early well-differentiated cancer ranges from 58% to 100% (15,18,19,23,24).

■ THERAPY FOR ADVANCED AND RECURRENT ENDOMETRIAL CANCER

A variety of investigators have evaluated the use of progesterone in women with advanced or recurrent EC.

Early studies utilized oral progestins (MPA, MA, and hydroxyprogesterone acetate) with response rates as high as 56% (25–27); however, later multicenter trials were only able to demonstrate response rates of 15%–20% (8,28). Progesterone is less efficacious with more aggressive tumors, as advanced and recurrent EC is more frequently Type II and less hormonally responsive compared to early stage disease that is predominately Type I, with higher reported overall response rates of 50%–70% (8). Additionally, higher doses of progesterone have not been shown to correlate with improved outcome: Thigpen et al evaluated progestin doses of 200 mg vs 1000 mg per day in an attempt to overcome resistance due to presumed PR downregulation, but only achieved a 10% response rate (28).

Although progestational agents are the most often studied and utilized for hormonal treatment of EC, other hormonal therapies have been studied. A significant portion of ECs express estrogen receptors (ER; 29). Tamoxifen is a selective ER modulator that exerts its antiestrogenic effect through competitive binding to ER on cancer cells. Studies have combined tamoxifen with weekly oral progesterone demonstrating response rates ranging from 27% to 33% (29,30). Leslie et al utilized fulvestrant, a pure estrogen antagonist with high affinity for ER, but demonstrated only minimal effect in recurrent disease (31).

There is no accepted consensus as to the optimal patient, drug, route, dose, or duration of therapy. Although the majority of women in the literature treated with progesterone have a documented response within 12 weeks, time to response has varied from 4 to 60 weeks (10,16), with a minimum accepted treatment length of 6 months. Patients should undergo frequent histologic evaluation of the endometrium with either endometrial biopsy or D&C. Routine sampling should continue after conclusion of treatment, as studies have demonstrated a high risk of recurrence, even in patients with complete pathologic response. For the nonresponder, options include increasing the dose/potency of progesterone or counseling for definitive surgical management. For women who elect for fertility-sparing therapy, pregnancy rates range from 32% to 100% in patients attempting to conceive after treatment

(12,17,18,32,33). Hysterectomy should be readdressed at completion of childbearing. Clear disadvantages for conservative management exist, including the limitation of imaging to assess myometrial invasion, the 22% rate of extrauterine spread in clinical early stage disease, and the risk of synchronous OC, with a rate of up to 19% in one retrospective study (34).

■ HORMONAL THERAPY OF OVARIAN CANCER

Epidemiologic studies suggest that steroid hormones also play a role in the development of OC. Progesterone and gonadotropin-releasing hormone (GnRH) may protect against development of cancer, while estrogens, androgens, and gonadotropins may play a causative role. Estrogen is theorized to have a causative role in OC due to ovulation-induced trauma to the ovarian surface epithelium and resultant genetic instability of the cell layer. ER is also expressed in OC, with higher levels in serous and endometrioid types, as well as specific isoforms expressed only in certain subtypes (i.e., only ERβ in clear cell and mucinous tumors; 30,33). Multiple in vitro and preclinical studies have identified several hormonal therapies with potential for treatment of recurrent or refractory OC (Table 29.2), with few side effects, including estrogens, aromatase, gonadotropins, anti-androgens, and progesterone (35).

Tamoxifen has been shown to have minimal side effects with modest efficacy and may be considered in heavily pretreated patients with recurrent disease and poor performance status (36). Tamoxifen has been used in several small clinical trials in patients with advanced disease, with a resultant CR of 9%–13%, stable disease

■ Table 29.2 Experimental hormonal treatments for ovarian cancer

Hormonal Treatment Type	Medications Studied	Reported Response Rates (%)	References
Estrogens	Tamoxifen	9%–42%	35–44
Aromatase	Letrozol		
	Anastrazole	0%–42%	35,46
	Exemestane		
Gonadotropins agonists	Leuprolide acetate		
	Goserelin	0%–22%	
	Triptorelin		35,47,49,50–53
Gonadotropin antagonists	Cetrorelix	18%	
Anti-androgens	Danazol	4%–6%	35,54
	Flutamide		
Progesterones	MPA	2%–5%	35,57,58
	MA		

MA, megestrol acetate; MPA, medroxyprogesterone acetate

(SD) in up to 38%, and 42% greater than or equal to 12-month progression-free survival (35–39). Tamoxifen has also been studied in combination with platinum-based chemotherapy as well as with a GnRH analogue but with inconsistent results (40–44). More research is warranted to evaluate the relationship of ER status and concomitant chemotherapy (45), since ER status, as in breast cancer, is the most promising predictor for response to tamoxifen.

Aromatase, which converts androstenedione to estrone in adipose and the skin, contributes to circulating levels of estrogen and its expression has been identified in malignant ovarian epithelial cells. Aromatase inhibitors block aromatization to estrogen and competitively bind ER (35). There have been several Phase II trials evaluating letrozol, anastrazole, or exemestane, which have demonstrated CR rates of 0%–35%, partial response rates of 0%–16%, and SD rates of 19%–42% (35,46).

The "gonadotropin hypothesis" considers excessive stimulation of ovarian tissue by gonadotropins as a cause of OC. The underlying basis of this theory includes the protective effects of pregnancy and oral contraceptive use, which suppress gonadotropins, and the increased risk of OC in women with increasing levels of circulating luteinizing hormone and follicle-stimulating hormone, such as in menopause and polycystic ovarian syndrome (35). GnRH1 receptors have been discovered in 80% of epithelial OC (EOC) (47). Twelve clinical trials have evaluated GnRH agonists, including leuprolide acetate, goserelin, and triptorelin, in 369 patients with refractory or recurrent EOC with a range of CR of 0%–3%, partial response of 0%–22%, and SD in the range 3%–70% (35). Additionally, smaller studies demonstrated increased efficacy specifically in recurrent granulosa cell tumors and low-grade EOC (48). GnRH agonists have also been used as additive to first-line platinum-based chemotherapy (49–52). Only one trial demonstrated a higher CR rate but with no survival benefit. These negative findings are thought to be due to neutralizing effects of chemotherapy and the protective effect on tumor cells afforded by the anti-apoptotic activity of the GnRH agonist (52). However, a GnRH antagonist, cetrorelix, was well-tolerated in 17 patients with refractory OC and resulted in an 18% partial response rate and a 35% SD rate for 12 months (53).

The effectiveness of anti-androgen therapy has also been evaluated, after data demonstrated that patients with endometriosis treated with danazol had a 3.2-fold increased risk of developing OC, and that postmenopausal women with OC had higher circulating levels of androstenedione and dehydroepiandrosterone (35), though results are disappointing. Androgen receptors are expressed in up to 90% of EOC; however, their role in causation is still under investigation (54). Flutamide, an androgen receptor inhibitor, was evaluated in two small Phase II trials with response rates of 4.3%–6.3% and SD in 1%–28% (55,56). Newer in vitro studies have shown promise in abiraterone, a CYP17 inhibitor that suppresses generation of estrogens and androgens, which has been efficacious in hormone-resistant prostate and breast cancer (54).

Progesterone plays a protective role in OC, with lower incidence rates seen among women with higher circulating levels, such as those with twin pregnancies, increased parity, and use of oral contraceptives employing higher potency progestins. Progesterone inhibits proliferation of ovarian surface epithelial cells, causing apoptosis and decreased tumor invasion. PR expression in EOC ranges from 26% to 49%, with highest levels of expression noted in endometrioid tumors (64%–91%), conferring a more favorable prognosis (35). A meta-analysis of 13 trials including 432 patients treated with MPA or MA, calculated a CR of 2.3%, partial response of 4.9%, and SD in 10.9% (35). In vitro, progesterone has been demonstrated to reverse paclitaxel multidrug resistance; however, this finding was not replicated in clinical trials (57). RU486 (mifepristone), a synthetic antiprogestin that competitively inhibits PR, was shown in vitro to inhibit cancer cell growth. The follow-up in vivo studies demonstrated that RU486 reversed platinum resistance and when studied in 34 patients, found an overall response rate of 25.6%, with a CR of 8.8% (58).

Other hormonal pathways have been assessed by in vitro studies for a role in treatment of OC, including anti-Mullerian hormone, prolactin, and growth hormone (59–61). Although OC is influenced by hormonal relationships, it is still unclear which hormone-regulated mechanisms are involved in tumorigenesis. The estimated overall response rates to hormonal therapy in recurrent OC is only 10% (35); however, the favorable side effect profile may make this an option for selected patients.

■ CONCLUSIONS

Since the 1960s, investigators have evaluated the use of hormonal therapy for primary and recurrent cancer. Recently, however, utilizing the research from in vitro and translational studies, rapid advancements have been made in the hormonal therapy of gynecologic cancers. These experimental treatments have included novel combinations of hormones and have taken advantage of new technology that enables the identification and location of specific hormonal receptors for targeted therapy. Future studies will continue to advance the use of hormones with minimal side effects to treat both primary and recurrent disease in gynecologic oncology.

■ REFERENCES

1. Yang S, Thiel KW, Leslie KK. Progesterone: the ultimate endometrial tumor suppressor. *Trends Endocrinol Metab.* 2011;22(4):145–152.

2. Jongen V, Briët J, de Jong R, et al. Expression of estrogen receptor-alpha and -beta and progesterone receptor-A and -B in a large cohort of patients with endometrioid endometrial cancer. *Gynecol Oncol.* 2009;112(3):537–542.

3. Rodriguez MI, Warden M, Darney PD. Intrauterine progestins, progesterone antagonists, and receptor modulators: a review of gynecologic applications. *Am J Obstet Gynecol.* 2010;202(5):420–428.

4. Speroff L, Darney PF. *A Clinical Guide for Contraception.* Philadelphia, PA: Lippincott Williams & Wilkins; 2005.

5. Inki P. Long-term use of the levonorgestrel-releasing intrauterine system. *Contraception.* 2007;75(6 Suppl):S161–S166.

6. Wildemeersch D, Dhont M. Treatment of nonatypical and atypical endometrial hyperplasia with a levonorgestrel-releasing intrauterine system. *Am J Obstet Gynecol.* 2003;188(5):1297–1298.

7. Varma R, Soneja H, Bhatia K, et al. The effectiveness of a levonorgestrel-releasing intrauterine system (LNG-IUS) in the treatment of endometrial hyperplasia–a long-term follow-up study. *Eur J Obstet Gynecol Reprod Biol.* 2008;139(2):169–175.

8. Kim JJ, Chapman-Davis E. Role of progesterone in endometrial cancer. *Semin Reprod Med.* 2010;28(1):81–90.

9. Wheeler DT, Bristow RE, Kurman RJ. Histologic alterations in endometrial hyperplasia and well-differentiated carcinoma treated with progestins. *Am J Surg Pathol.* 2007;31(7):988–998.

10. Ramirez PT, Frumovitz M, Bodurka DC, Sun CC, Levenback C. Hormonal therapy for the management of grade 1 endometrial adenocarcinoma: a literature review. *Gynecol Oncol.* 2004;95(1):133–138.

11. Chiva L, Lapuente F, González-Cortijo L, et al. Sparing fertility in young patients with endometrial cancer. *Gynecol Oncol.* 2008;111(2 Suppl):S101–S104.

12. Gunderson CC, Fader AN, Carson KA, Bristow RE. Oncologic and reproductive outcomes with progestin therapy in women with endometrial hyperplasia and grade 1 adenocarcinoma: a systematic review. *Gynecol Oncol.* 2012;125(2):477–482.

13. Ushijima K, Yahata H, Yoshikawa H, et al. Multicenter phase II study of fertility-sparing treatment with medroxyprogesterone acetate for endometrial carcinoma and atypical hyperplasia in young women. *J Clin Oncol.* 2007;25(19):2798–2803.

14. Kim YB, Holschneider CH, Ghosh K, Nieberg RK, Montz FJ. Progestin alone as primary treatment of endometrial carcinoma in premenopausal women. Report of seven cases and review of the literature. *Cancer.* 1997;79(2):320–327.

15. Montz FJ, Bristow RE, Bovicelli A, Tomacruz R, Kurman RJ. Intrauterine progesterone treatment of early endometrial cancer. *Am J Obstet Gynecol.* 2002;186(4):651–657.

16. Shah MM, Wright JD. Management of endometrial cancer in young women. *Clin Obstet Gynecol.* 2011;54(2):219–225.

17. Yamazawa K, Hirai M, Fujito A, et al. Fertility-preserving treatment with progestin, and pathological criteria to predict responses, in young women with endometrial cancer. *Hum Reprod.* 2007;22(7):1953–1958.

18. Laurelli G, Di Vagno G, Scaffa C, Losito S, Del Giudice M, Greggi S. Conservative treatment of early endometrial cancer: preliminary results of a pilot study. *Gynecol Oncol.* 2011;120(1):43–46.

19. Dhar KK, NeedhiRajan T, Koslowski M, Woolas RP. Is levonorgestrel intrauterine system effective for treatment of early endometrial cancer? Report of four cases and review of the literature. *Gynecol Oncol.* 2005;97(3):924–927.

20. Signorelli M, Caspani G, Bonazzi C, Chiappa V, Perego P, Mangioni C. Fertility-sparing treatment in young women with endometrial cancer or atypical complex hyperplasia: a prospective single-institution experience of 21 cases. *BJOG.* 2009;116(1):114–118.

21. Wang CB, Wang CJ, Huang HJ, et al. Fertility-preserving treatment in young patients with endometrial adenocarcinoma. *Cancer.* 2002;94(8):2192–2198.

22. Niwa K, Tagami K, Lian Z, Onogi K, Mori H, Tamaya T. Outcome of fertility-preserving treatment in young women with endometrial carcinomas. *BJOG.* 2005;112(3):317–320.

23. Tjalma W, Janssens D, Wildemeersch D, Colpaert C, Watty K. Conservative management of atypical endometrial hyperplasia

and early invasive carcinoma with intrauterine levonorgestrel: a progesterone receptor study. *Eur J Cancer Suppl.* 2004;2:93–94.

24. Cade T, Quinn A, Rome R, Neesham D. Progestin treatment options for early endometrial cancer. *Br J Obstet Gynaecol.* 2010;117:879–884.

25. Reifenstein EC Jr. The treatment of advanced endometrial cancer with hydroxyprogesterone caproate. *Gynecol Oncol.* 1974;2(2–3):377–414.

26. Piver MS, Barlow JJ, Lurain JR, Blumenson LE. Medroxyprogesterone acetate (Depo-Provera) vs. hydroxyprogesterone caproate (Delalutin) in women with metastatic endometrial adenocarcinoma. *Cancer.* 1980;45(2):268–272.

27. Thigpen JT, Brady MF, Alvarez RD, et al. Oral medroxyprogesterone acetate in the treatment of advanced or recurrent endometrial carcinoma: a dose-response study by the Gynecologic Oncology Group. *J Clin Oncol.* 1999;17(6):1736–1744.

28. Decruze SB, Green JA. Hormone therapy in advanced and recurrent endometrial cancer: a systematic review. *Int J Gynecol Cancer.* 2007;17(5):964–978.

29. Singh M, Zaino RJ, Filiaci VJ, Leslie KK. Relationship of estrogen and progesterone receptors to clinical outcome in metastatic endometrial carcinoma: a Gynecologic Oncology Group study. *Gynecol Oncol.* 2007;106(2):325–333.

30. Thigpen T, Brady MF, Homesley HD, Soper JT, Bell J. Tamoxifen in the treatment of advanced or recurrent endometrial carcinoma: a Gynecologic Oncology Group study. *J Clin Oncol.* 2001;19(2):364–367.

31. Leslie KK, Stein MP, Kumar NS, et al. Progesterone receptor isoform identification and subcellular localization in endometrial cancer. *Gynecol Oncol.* 2005;96(1):32–41.

32. Lowe MP, Cooper BC, Sood AK, Davis WA, Syrop CH, Sorosky JI. Implementation of assisted reproductive technologies following conservative management of FIGO grade I endometrial adenocarcinoma and/or complex hyperplasia with atypia. *Gynecol Oncol.* 2003;91(3):569–572.

33. Zheng H, Kavanagh JJ, Hu W, Liao Q, Fu S. Hormonal therapy in ovarian cancer. *Int J Gynecol Cancer.* 2007;17(2):325–338.

34. Soliman PT, Oh JC, Schmeler KM, et al. Risk factors for young premenopausal women with endometrial cancer. *Obstet Gynecol.* 2005;105(3):575–580.

35. Yang S, Thiel KW, De Geest K, Leslie KK. Endometrial cancer: reviving progesterone therapy in the molecular age. *Discov Med.* 2011;12(64):205–212.

36. Williams CJ. Tamoxifen for relapse of ovarian cancer. *Cochrane Database Syst Rev.* 2001:CD001034.

37. Perez-Gracia JL, Carrasco EM. Tamoxifen therapy for ovarian cancer in the adjuvant and advanced settings: systematic review of the literature and implications for future research. *Gynecol Oncol.* 2002;84(2):201–209.

38. Markman M, Webster K, Zanotti K, Rohl J, Belinson J. Use of tamoxifen in asymptomatic patients with recurrent small-volume ovarian cancer. *Gynecol Oncol.* 2004;93(2):390–393.

39. Markman M, Webster K, Zanotti K, Peterson G, Kulp B, Belinson J. Phase 2 trial of carboplatin plus tamoxifen in platinum-resistant ovarian cancer and primary carcinoma of the peritoneum. *Gynecol Oncol.* 2004;94(2):404–408.

40. Benedetti Panici P, Greggi S, Amoroso M, et al. A combination of platinum and tamoxifen in advanced ovarian cancer failing platinum-based chemotherapy: results of a Phase II study. *Int J Gynecol Cancer.* 2001;11(6):438–444.

41. Schwartz PE, Chambers JT, Kohorn EI, et al. Tamoxifen in combination with cytotoxic chemotherapy in advanced epithelial ovarian cancer. A prospective randomized trial. *Cancer.* 1989;63(6):1074–1078.

42. Hasan J, Ton N, Mullamitha S, et al. Phase II trial of tamoxifen and goserelin in recurrent epithelial ovarian cancer. *Br J Cancer.* 2005;93(6):647–651.

43. Hofstra LS, Mourits MJ, de Vries EG, Mulder NH, Willemse PH. Combined treatment with goserelin and tamoxifen in patients with advanced chemotherapy resistant ovarian cancer. *Anticancer Res.* 1999;19(4C):3627–3630.

44. Hatch KD, Beecham JB, Blessing JA, Creasman WT. Responsiveness of patients with advanced ovarian carcinoma to tamoxifen. A Gynecologic Oncology Group study of second-line therapy in 105 patients. *Cancer.* 1991;68(2):269–271.

45. Li YF, Hu W, Fu SQ, Li JD, Liu JH, Kavanagh JJ. Aromatase inhibitors in ovarian cancer: is there a role? *Int J Gynecol Cancer.* 2008;18(4):600–614.

46. Völker P, Gründker C, Schmidt O, Schulz KD, Emons G. Expression of receptors for luteinizing hormone-releasing hormone in human ovarian and endometrial cancers: frequency, autoregulation, and correlation with direct antiproliferative activity of luteinizing hormone-releasing hormone analogues. *Am J Obstet Gynecol.* 2002;186(2):171–179.

47. Kavanagh JJ, Roberts W, Townsend P, Hewitt S. Leuprolide acetate in the treatment of refractory or persistent epithelial ovarian cancer. *J Clin Oncol.* 1989;7(1):115–118.

48. Emons G, Ortmann O, Teichert HM, et al. Luteinizing hormone-releasing hormone agonist triptorelin in combination with cytotoxic chemotherapy in patients with advanced ovarian carcinoma. A prospective double blind randomized trial. Decapeptyl Ovarian Cancer Study Group. *Cancer.* 1996;78(7):1452–1460.

49. Medl M, Peters-Engel C, Fuchs G, Leodolter S. Triptorelin (D-Trp-6-LHRH) in combination with carboplatin-containing polychemotherapy for advanced ovarian cancer: a pilot study. *Anticancer Res.* 1993;13(6B):2373–2376.

50. Falkson CI, Falkson HC, Falkson G. Cisplatin versus cisplatin plus D-Trp-6-LHRH in the treatment of ovarian cancer: a pilot trial to investigate the effect of the addition of a GnRH analogue to cisplatin. *Oncology.* 1996;53(4):313–317.

51. Rzepka-Górska I, Chudecka-Glaz A, Kosmider M, Malecha J. GnRH analogues as an adjuvant therapy for ovarian cancer patients. *Int J Gynaecol Obstet.* 2003;81(2):199–205.

52. Verschraegen CF, Westphalen S, Hu W, et al. Phase II study of cetrorelix, a luteinizing hormone-releasing hormone antagonist in patients with platinum-resistant ovarian cancer. *Gynecol Oncol.* 2003;90(3):552–559.

53. Papadatos-Pastos D, Dedes KJ, de Bono JS, Kaye SB. Revisiting the role of antiandrogen strategies in ovarian cancer. *Oncologist.* 2011;16(10):1413–1421.

54. Tumolo S, Rao BR, van der Burg ME, Guastalla JP, Renard J, Vermorken JB. Phase II trial of flutamide in advanced ovarian cancer: an EORTC Gynaecological Cancer Cooperative Group study. *Eur J Cancer.* 1994;30A(7):911–914.

55. Vassilomanolakis M, Koumakis G, Barbounis V, Hajichristou H, Tsousis S, Efremidis A. A phase II study of flutamide in ovarian cancer. *Oncology.* 1997;54(3):199–202.

56. Markman M, Kennedy A, Webster K, Kulp B, Peterson G, Belinson J. Phase I trial of paclitaxel plus megestrol acetate in patients with paclitaxel-refractory ovarian cancer. *Clin Cancer Res.* 2000;6(11):4201–4204.

57. Rocereto TF, Saul HM, Aikins JA Jr, Paulson J. Phase II study of mifepristone (RU486) in refractory ovarian cancer. *Gynecol Oncol.* 2000;77(3):429–432.

58. Anttonen M, Färkkilä A, Tauriala H, et al. Anti-Müllerian hormone inhibits growth of AMH type II receptor-positive human ovarian granulosa cell tumor cells by activating apoptosis. *Lab Invest.* 2011;91(11):1605–1614.

59. Tan D, Chen KE, Khoo T, Walker AM. Prolactin increases survival and migration of ovarian cancer cells: importance of prolactin receptor type and therapeutic potential of S179D and G129R receptor antagonists. *Cancer Lett.* 2011;310(1):101–108.

60. Papadia A, Schally AV, Halmos G, et al. Growth hormone-releasing hormone antagonists inhibit growth of human ovarian cancer. *Horm Metab Res.* 2011;43(11):816–820.

61. MacLaughlin DT, Donahoe PK. Müllerian inhibiting substance/anti-Müllerian hormone: a potential therapeutic agent for human ovarian and other cancers. *Future Oncol.* 2010 Mar;6(3):391–405.

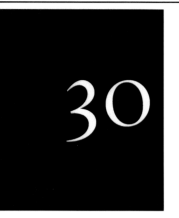

30 Genomic and Proteomic Biomarkers for Ovarian Cancer Screening, Prognosis, and Individualization of Chemotherapy

SAYEEMA DAUDI

HEIDI GODOY

KUNLE ODUNSI

■ INTRODUCTION

Epithelial ovarian cancer (EOC) represents the most lethal gynecologic malignancy in women. Within the United States alone, the annual incidence remains elevated at 21,880 cases and 13,850 women are estimated to have died of ovarian cancer in 2010 (1). Despite considerable efforts directed at early detection, there are currently no cost-effective screening strategies (2). The majority of women present with disseminated disease at initial diagnosis and carry a 5-year overall survival (OS) of 10%–30% (3). In contrast, fewer than 20% of women present with Stage I ovarian carcinoma, are confined to the ovaries at diagnosis, and carry a 5-year survival rate in excess of 90% (4). Patients with advanced-stage disease will have a relapsing and remitting course with a 2-year median survival after a recurrence (5–7). Better insights into our fundamental understanding of disease onset and progression at the molecular level are required to improve early disease detection and to develop effective, targeted screening and treatment strategies.

In consideration of the current diagnostic limitation of identifying early-stage ovarian cancer, new approaches for the molecular diagnosis of ovarian cancer have been introduced. An ideal screening modality for the early detection of ovarian carcinoma has yet to be identified. In order for an effective screening strategy, a sufficient interval must exist between the development of early-stage carcinoma and metastasis to permit screening at practical intervals. In addition to ease of access and a cost-effective approach, early detection of ovarian cancer requires a high sensitivity and a particularly high specificity to attain an acceptable positive predictive value.

■ CANCER GENOMICS

The World Health Organization (WHO) has introduced a new classification of ovarian carcinomas and divides it into the following histological subtypes: (a) high-grade serous, (b) low-grade serous, (c) endometrioid, (d) mucinous, and (e) clear cell carcinoma. These subtypes might reflect the etiologies involved in the dysregulation and activation of cellular pathways and therefore account for the different clinical behaviors of ovarian carcinoma. The latest discoveries have allowed for these heterogeneous histological patterns to be distinguished by protein and gene analysis. This gene expression profiling proves to be a useful prognostic tool, predicting chemotherapy sensitivity and a tailored cancer therapy (8–10).

Microarray profiling has allowed for the comprehensive genetic profiling of cancer through the study of many thousands of genes simultaneously (11–16). The resultant identification of molecular signatures, which permit the classification of histologic tumor subtypes, predict clinical end points, identify the genetic expression of the cellular environment and in turn the functional status of the cellular tissue, with final revelation into the drug resistance involved with ovarian carcinogenesis (17–21). An important consideration during analysis of gene expression profiles is that only a small proportion of the genome represents the actual expressed genes in any given cell type. An even smaller number of these genes may be susceptible to the consequences of carcinogenic events, which tend to accumulate vast genetic mutations or loci with genetic amplification. In turn, only a small subset of these genes may be the precursor to protein products that regulate the cellular pathways of proliferation, differentiation, and apoptosis, all of which are the perceived basic factors driving carcinogenesis. An important goal in the molecular profiling of cancer is to identify these specific, infrequent, but deadly genetic derangements and thus the causally important proteins.

■ BIOMEDICAL GENOMIC TECHNIQUES

A comprehensive description of the genomic techniques is beyond the scope of this review; however, it remains difficult to follow the clinical logic without a clear understanding of the fundamental principles. A number of methods have been developed for quantitative measurement of the DNA copy number changes in cancer genomes. These methods include digital karyotyping and microarray-based techniques of single-nucleotide polymorphism (SNP) array, comparative genomic hybridization, and oligonucleotide microarray analysis.

Laser Capture Microdissection

As a large number of genes tend to be analyzed in microarray assays, the risk of erroneous clinical associations remains high. Additionally, the genetic and proteomic analysis of a pure and native cellular environment is important to determine accurate clinical end points. The most current personalized investigative studies are migrating from the use of tissue culture cells to the identification of pertinent genes and proteins from changes visualized in actual diseased human tissue. The diseased cells in a tissue block may constitute a tiny proportion of the entire analyzed sample, especially in the premalignant tissue population. To avoid analysis of contaminated cellular tissue, some studies use tissue culture to grow the cellular fraction of interest. A barrier to using these types of cultured tissue for analysis is that the cultured cells may become altered during the culturing process. Ultimately, the genetic and protein expression pattern does not represent the true molecular events taking place in the native tissues from which they were derived. This challenge can be overcome by new techniques using tissue microdissection. The method of laser capture microdissection (LCM) has been developed as a dependable method in the procurement of pure, native cell populations from the heterogeneous diseased tissue taken from paraffin-embedded or fresh-frozen tissue specimens, and/or normal control specimens (22–24). The advantage in this type of technique is to fully preserve the natural cellular state and obtain an accurate representation of the genetic and proteomic expression profiles. In this way, the individualized gene expression profile can be generated for each histologic subcategory for EOC and correlated to the genetic signature and then further with the etiology and response to treatment (Figures 30.1 and 30.2; 25,26).

Digital Karyotyping

Digital karyotyping counts the sequence tags from specific loci distributed throughout the human genome and provides a digital analysis to precisely locate amplified and deleted chromosomal regions (27,28).

cDNA-Microarray Analysis

Gene expression analysis can be accomplished by a transcription profiling microarray. A DNA-microarray chip and an RNA sample (either total RNA or enriched messenger RNA [mRNA] are the important materials involved in a DNA-microarray assay. The DNA-microarray chip is composed of a chemically coated (nylon, silicon, or nitrocellulose membrane) glass matrix. These microdissected tissue samples from the previously described LCM technology can supply RNA specimens, which are amplified and subsequently converted to cDNA. These polynucleotides are attached to the DNA-microarray chip by high-speed robotic machinery or photolithography. The polynucleotides are made from complementary DNA (cDNA microarrays, 500–5000 base pairs [bps]), or shorter oligodeoxynucleotide sequences (25–50 bps, oligonucleotide microarrays; 29). The microarray chips, containing cDNA and complementary RNA, are then labeled with a fluorescent or radioactive probe for control and study subjects. The intensity of the emitted fluorescence signals for each spot on the microarray chip correlates to a specific expression pattern, called a gene signature. These gene signatures are associated with specific clinical data points, such as patient survival and chemotherapy response.

Based on this rationale, researchers have used these new technologies to survey many genetic panels for the purpose of accurate tumor classification based on tissue histology for individual patients, which then leads to a specific individualized prediction on treatment response to various agents, with the final goal being a well-designed patient-tailored treatment plan based on each patient's affected, expressed genetic profile.

Comparative Genomic Hybridization

Comparative Genomic Hybridization (CGH) has been developed as a whole genome assay to detect gains and losses of the gene copy number. This assay has successfully identified several chromosome regions in ovarian carcinoma with an abnormal gene copy number. In turn various abnormal chromosome regions and their associated altered genes have been identified. With the use of proteomic technology, the specific protein expression profile and associated clinical effect can be effectively determined.

MicroRNA Profiling

Another method to detect gene expression and post-translational modification of protein expression is found through microRNA (miRNA) technology. The miRNAs are 19 to 24 nucleotides long and do not encode proteins. These miRNA strands silence target mRNAs, leading to an inhibition of translation. Screening for miRNA expression levels is routinely performed using array technologies to obtain a miRNome profile and confirmation using

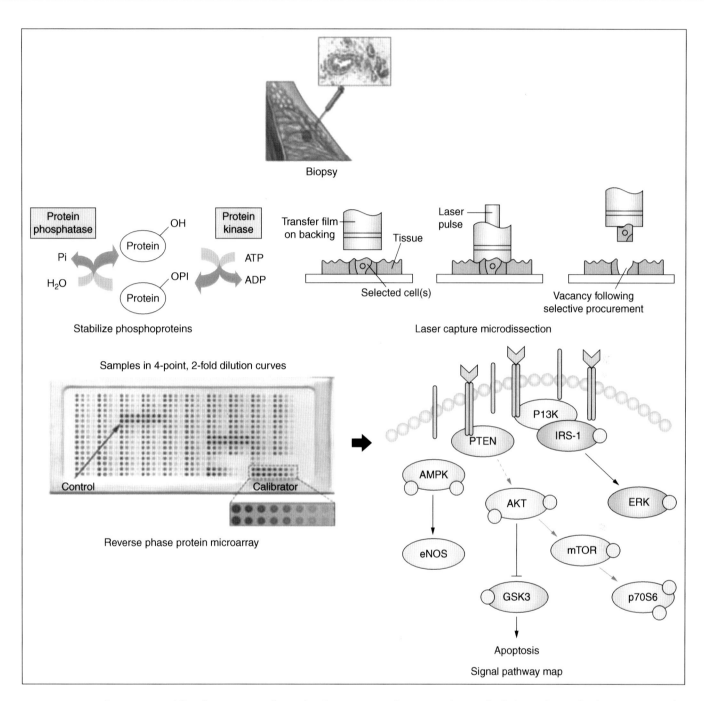

FIGURE 30.1 Proteomics workflow for mapping cell-signaling kinase activity. Biopsy samples are divided into aliquots for diagnosis or translational research. Protein conformation and enzymatic activity are retained if the tissue is frozen or fixed in a solution that blocks both phosphatase and kinase activity. Tissues contain heterogeneous cellular populations (e.g., epithelium, cancer cells, fibroblasts, endothelium, and immune cells). Laser capture microdissection (LCM), using a stained tissue section under direct microscopic visualization, is used to procure pure cell populations. LCM directly procures the subpopulation of cells selected for study, while leaving behind all of the contaminating cells. A stained section of the heterogeneous tissue is mounted on a glass microscope slide and viewed under high magnification. The experimenter selects the individual cell(s) to be studied via a computer screen. A stationary near-IR (infrared) laser mounted in the optical axis of the microscope stage is used for melting a thermolabile polymer film, which is mounted on the bottom surface of an optical-quality plastic cap. The polymer melts only in the vicinity of the laser pulse, forming a polymer-cell composite. When the polymer cap is lifted from the tissue section, only the desired cells for study are excised from the heterogeneous cellular population. Using appropriate buffers, the cellular constituents are solubilized and printed in a multiplexed, reverse phase protein microarray format. Proteins from all subcellular locations can be mapped based on activity level, thus generating a cell-signaling profile of a specific cellular population. Adapted from Mueller et al (25).

techniques, such as Northern blotting. This technique can provide the analysis of all known miRNAs similar to that for mRNA profiling. miRNAs have demonstrated differential expression in a range of various tissue specimens and can therefore be correlated to disease outcome. A study analyzing miRNA signatures in a range of tumor types suggested that the expression pattern of a relatively small number of miRNAs was more accurate than cDNA

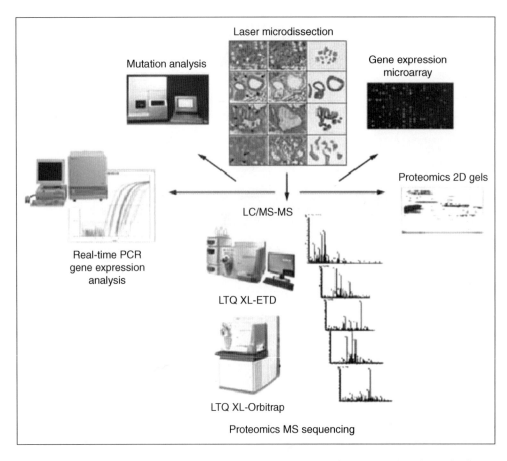

FIGURE 30.2 Applications of laser capture microdissection to genomic and proteomic discovery and analysis of cell type-specific molecular changes. The extracted proteins, DNA, or RNA can be analyzed by any method that has sufficient sensitivity. Examples include gene-associated somatic mutation analysis of tumor etiology and progression (upper left), gene expression measurement by real-time polymerase chain reaction (PCR) (middle left), or transcript arrays (upper right), proteomic fractionization of proteins by two-dimensional (2D) gels (middle right), and protein sequencing by mass spectrometry (MS) (lower) such as LC/MS-MS, liquid chromatography/mass spectrometry or LTQ-XL-ETD, electron transfer dissociation. Adapted from Devita et al (26).

arrays in classifying human cancers (30). Several studies support the use of miRNA profiling as providing significant contribution to the diagnosis of ovarian carcinoma and its effective prognosis.

■ **TRANSCRIPTIONAL PROFILING PREDICTS THE CLINICAL BEHAVIOR OF EPITHELIAL OVARIAN CANCER**

Ovarian carcinoma is known for its clinical heterogeneity (31), whereby, patients with histologically similar tumors, particularly within the more common serous cancers, exhibit a wide range of clinical prognosis. Two separate and quite distinct subgroups of serous cancer have been recently recognized (32,33).

Type I low-grade serous carcinomas are more common and tend to carry specific molecular pathogenesis, such as mutations in *KRAS* and *BRAF* (33). These carcinomas are found to arise from the epithelial surface of the ovary and follow a step-wise progression through microinvasive tumors, to borderline tumors, and ultimately to fulminant invasive disease (34).

Type 2 high-grade serous carcinomas disseminate rapidly and tend to arise from the fimbrial end of the fallopian tube (35,36). These carcinomas carry the *BRCA1/2* gene mutations and *p53* gene mutation have been seen to occur early in the disease process (36–38). Type 2 serous carcinomas demonstrate a better response to platinum-based chemotherapy (39).

These various outcomes suggest biologic subtypes in the basic mechanics of the disease. This histologic heterogeneity of ovarian carcinoma and the poor understanding of its origin further complicate biomarker discovery, making it implausible to efficiently detect all ovarian carcinoma subtypes from a single biomarker. Instead, a panel of biomarkers unique to a stage and subtype of EOC will ultimately prove to be the clinically practical choice.

Until the advent of DNA-microarray technology, evaluation of this cellular mechanics were considered one factor at a time, allowing for the identification of *TP53*, *MYC*, *ABC* transporters, *BCL2*, and *BRCA* genes (40). However, none of these altered genes reliably allowed for a prediction in therapeutic response and overall prognosis. Efforts at gene recognition have shifted to microarray analysis as the multifactorial nature of these genes has been clearly and repeatedly observed.

Transcriptional Profiling of Ovarian Cancer Histologic Subtypes

Investigators have now focused their studies on developing vast cDNA/RNA gene microarrays in which patterns of gene expression in EOC as compared to normal ovarian tissue have been identified. This analysis has identified several genes, with their respective protein products that are differentially expressed in EOC. Additionally, several studies have focused on the alterations demonstrated in the DNA copy number (41–43). These studies indicate that EOC display more diffuse chromosomal gene alterations than other histologic and graded ovarian carcinomas. Any variation to these patterns have been correlated with changes in histologic subcategories and, therefore, clinical tumor response with specific treatment regimens. Array-based technology has shown that the different histological subtypes of ovarian carcinoma are distinguishable based on their overall genetic expression profiles. In the following section, a summary of the major molecular alterations classifying each of the main histologic subtypes of EOC will be presented (Table 30.1; 37,44–46).

A common finding among several recent studies allows for support on the ability to distinguish between low-grade serous ovarian carcinoma from high-grade carcinoma based on the gene expression profiles (42,45,47–50). A number of genes shown to be differentially expressed in EOC are known to be involved in many important cellular mechanisms including cell-cycle regulation, apoptosis, tumor invasion, and control of local immunity (47,51).

Using oligonucleotide microarray analysis, Schwartz et al studied 113 patients with EOC and demonstrated that mucinous and clear cell EOCs could be distinguished from serous EOC based on genetic profiles. In this study, endometrioid EOCs showed significant gene expression overlap with other histologic subtypes of ovarian carcinoma, suggesting underlying shared mechanisms involved in this carcinogenesis (44).

Zorn et al used cDNA-microarray analysis to compare the genetic expression signatures for ovarian, uterine, and renal clear cell adenocarcinomas (46). Despite the various origins of disease, these carcinomas were shown to express a similar genetic profile. These results indicate that agents proven to be successful in other carcinomas, such as tyrosine kinase inhibitors (sunitinib and sorafenib), may be a focus of novel therapeutic potential in gynecologic clear cell adenocarcinomas.

Berchuck et al published their data regarding prediction of optimal vs suboptimal cytoreduction of advanced-stage serous ovarian cancer with the use of microarray technology (52). This group used Affymetrix U133A GeneChip microarrays to detect genes differentially expressed in optimally debulked advanced EOC compared to suboptimally debulked disease. A 32-gene profile was created from the leading 120 differentially expressed genes identified from the commercial microarray. This genetic signature successfully predicted the debulking status in 72.7% of advanced EOC and 60% of early-stage EOC seen in an independent validation set. These findings suggest that molecular differences do exist between optimally and suboptimally debulked EOC. As with many studies in genomic analysis, their small sample size continues to be a limitation and precludes any definite conclusion. This type of multigenic predictive model could potentially allow for a clinical prediction of the likelihood of optimal tumor debulking from inspection of the tumor biopsy and therefore potentially end the debate regarding neoadjuvant chemotherapy as compared to an initial attempt at aggressive debulking.

Transcriptional Profiling for Clinical Prognosis

Despite the frequent initial favorable response to chemotherapy, the poor prognosis of advanced-stage EOC is well known. The classic prognostic criteria of age, International Federation of Gynecology and Obstetrics (FIGO) stage, histopathologic tumor classification, pathologic grade of differentiation and debulking status are insufficient to accurately predict the survival of an individual patient (53). There remains an obvious need for improvement of these clinical criteria. Early identification of the approximately 80% of patients who will die from disease progression despite the standard frontline therapy is critical in impacting the progression-free survival (PFS) and most importantly, the OS in EOC. New genetic profile data attempt to guide initial therapeutic choices, instead of the standard frontline therapy in those identified as nonresponders. Some genetic studies have also reported on the prediction of survival in EOCs.

Several well-designed studies have recognized specific clinical outcomes in EOC, based on genetic microarray analysis (Table 30.2; 52,54–61). The clinical and surgical prognostic factors have been well established, including the above mentioned classic features (53), but also the quantity of residual disease after tumor cytoreduction (62,63), and the response of the serum CA125 during adjuvant frontline chemotherapy (66). Many other parameters have been studied as putative prognostic tools, such as BRCA status, EGF receptors, p53, and BCL-2; nevertheless no established clinical impact has been determined. As in the case of many genetic expression studies, the limitation of clinical extrapolation continues secondary to the inconsistent data analysis techniques, coupled with resultant nonoverlapping genetic signatures.

Lancaster et al described a series of 31 advanced-stage serous carcinomas, in which there were 14 long-term survivors (defined as survival for greater than 7 years after diagnosis) and 17 short-term survivors (defined as death

■ Table 30.1 Gene expression profiling studies related to histologic subtype in epithelial ovarian carcinoma

Reference	Tumor Characteristics	Number Samples in Validation Set	Technical Validation	Microarray Platform	Gene Signature	Summary of Findings
Jazaeri et al (2002) (37)	61 samples 30%BRCA1 26%BRCA2	10	rt-PCR	Custom 7651 cDNA	110 53	110 gene signature separates BRCA1 and BRCA2-associated ovarian carcinomas 53 gene signature separates BRCA1 and sporadic ovarian carcinomas
Schwartz et al (2002) (44)	113 samples 47% Serous 29% Endometrioid 9% Mucinous 7% Clear Cell 85% Mixed	31	rt-PCR Immunohistochemistry Principal Component Analysis Leave-1-out Cross Validation	HumanGeneFL ~7000 Oligos[a]	73	Separates clear cell EOC From serous EOC
Lu et al (2004) (45)	42 samples 40% Serous 21% Endometrioid 21% Mucinous 17% Clear Cell	42	rt-PCR Immunohistochemistry	U95Av2 ~41,441 Oligos[a]	86	Combination of HE4, CA-125, MUC1 separates the EOC subtypes
Zorn et al (2005) (46)	44 samples 55% Serous 25% Endometrioid 20% Clear Cell	75	rt-PCR Immunohistochemistry Leave-1-out Cross Validation	Custom 11,000 cDNA	43	Cluster analysis separates clear cell carcinomas from other epithelial ovarian cancer subtypes 43 gene signature separates epithelial ovarian cancer from normal ovarian epithelium

[a]According to the sequences listed in GenBank.
EOC, epithelial ovarian cancer; rt-PCR, reverse transcription-polymerase chain reaction.

■ Table 30.2 Gene expression profiling studies related to clinical outcome in epithelial ovarian carcinoma

Reference	Tumor Characteristics	Number Samples in Validation Set	Technical Validation	Microarray Platform	Gene Signature	Summary of Findings
Berchuck et al (2005) (54)	**54[b] samples** 100% Serous 83% FIGO III/IV	11[c] 68[d]	rt-PCR Tree Analysis Linear Discriminant Analysis	U133A ~22,000 Oligos[a]	186	Prediction of overall survival <3 years vs >7 years
Bild et al (2006) (55)	**145 samples** Varied History 100% FIGO III/IV	NA	NA	U133A ~22,000 Oligos[a]	Co-activation of SRC and βcatenin oncogenic pathways	Prediction of overall survival 29 vs 91 months
Bonome et al (2008) (56)	**95 samples** 100% Serous 100% FIGO III	90 29[e]	Leave-1-out Cross Validation	U133A ~22,000 Oligos[a]	No robust signature in optimally debulked 572 gene signature in suboptimally debulked	Prediction of overall survival
Hartmann et al (2005) (57)	**51 samples** 87% Serous 97% FIGO III/IV	28	NA	Custom ~21,600 cDNA	14	Prediction of recurrence <21 vs >21 months
Lancaster et al (2004) (58)	**31 samples** 100% Serous 100% FIGO III/IV	NA	NA	HumanGeneFL ~7000 Oligos[a]	43	Prediction of overall survival <2 vs >7 years
Partheen et al (2006) (59)	**54 samples** 100% Serous 100% FIGO III	NA	NA	Custom ~27,000 cDNA	204	Prediction of overall survival death from disease vs >5 years
Spentzos et al (2004) (61)	**34 samples** 91% Serous 96% FIGO III/IV	34	Leave-1-out Cross Validation	U95Av2 ~12,600 Oligos[a]	115	Prediction of PFS: Early relapse (<26 months) vs late relapse (>58 months) Prediction of overall survival: <30 months vs median "not yet reached"

[a]Affymetrix, Santa Clara, CA. [b]Patients with advanced-stage EOC. [c]Patients with early-stage EOC. [d]Patients from Spentzos et al (61). [e]Patients from Berchuck et al (54).
EOC, epithelial ovarian cancer; FIGO, International Federation of Gynecology and Obstetrics; PFS, progression-free survival.

less than 2 years after diagnosis; 58). A unique profile of 43 genes distinctly identified the two groups independently. Many of the identified genes in the specific cluster were associated with immune response, suggesting that immune function influences ovarian cancer progression.

Spentzos et al studied genetic profile expression using oligonucleotide microarrays (Affymetrix U95A2 arrays), which represent 12,625 genes from 68 patients with EOC; 91% of the tumor samples were obtained at the time of a debulking procedure from serous carcinoma. Their group discovered a prognostic 115-gene signature referred to as the Ovarian Cancer Prognostic Profile (OCPP; 61). This OCPP was able to predict OS (as median OS of "not yet reached" vs 30 months, respectively; log-rank, $P = .004$) and progression-free interval. The long-term survival in the favorable group reached a plateau of approximately 70%. The OCPP retained independent prognostic power when multivariate analysis was applied to include known risk factors, such as FIGO staging, grade of differentiation, success of cytoreduction, and age. Additionally, genes such as estrogen receptor binding site associated antigen-9 were overexpressed in the favorable prognosis group. Genes encoding for angiogenesis-related proteins, such as vascular endothelial growth factor (VEGF)-C, tyrosine kinases receptors, such as platelet-derived growth factor receptor, mesenchymal markers, such as fibronectin and vimentin, and proinvasive enzymes, such as plasminogen activator inhibitor Type 1 were overexpressed in the unfavorable group. This study, not only identified genetic signatures, but also tumor specific pertinent genes, which may be the focus of future studies.

Berchuck et al went on to describe a 186-gene expression profile as a prognostic factor using a sample set of 65 serous EOCs, which were collected from 24 patients having Stage III/IV EOC and demonstrating an OS of greater than 7 years (long-term survivors), 30 samples from Stage III/IV EOC with an OS of less than 3 years (short-term survivors), and a "control" group of 11 patients from Stage I/II EOC (early stage; 54). A microarray expression pattern using the short- and long-term survivors, were placed on an Affymetrix U133A 2.0 array (with more than 14,500 established genes). Using a Kaplan–Meier plot for survival, significant differences ($P = .0074$) were shown to exist between long- and short-term survivors as compared to the early-stage group, with 85% accuracy. A distinct expression profile model had been developed for each category and this allowed the investigators to draw important conclusions and classify all early-stage patients as long-term survivors. This implies a shared biologic subclassification into a favorable prognostic group between these early-stage patients and long-term survivors. The prognostic value of this resultant gene signature was confirmed with external validation using the above-mentioned independent set of 68 patients reported by Spentzos et al earlier that year. The authors further went on to validate this study using an independent set of patient samples from three separate

institutions (65). In this study, their group was also able to show a 3-fold difference in expression in the *MAL* gene between short- and long-term survivors and a greater than 20-fold difference between short-term survivors and early-stage carcinomas. Immunohistochemical stains of *MAL* indicated a higher level of expression to be associated with a shorter survival. The *MAL* gene is therefore an important target for the focus of future studies.

Hartmann et al created cDNA microarrays from 79 patients with EOC to develop a genetic signature, which recognized women at high risk for recurrence after receiving frontline adjuvant chemotherapy in the treatment of EOC. These investigators identified a 14-gene expression signature that allowed for a distinction between early recurrence (less than 21 months) and late recurrence (greater than 21 months; 57). The 21-month cutoff was chosen based on the median value of time to progression for all patients.

Partheen et al screened 54 patients with Stage III serous ovarian carcinoma, including 20 long-term survivors (defined as greater than 5 years after diagnosis) and 34 patients who died from their disease (59). Thirteen tumors were identified by whole genome hierarchical clustering, to include 12 long-term survivors. However, the other 8 long-term survivors were distributed across all remaining clusters.

Bonome et al have studied a large relevant series of 185 Stage III, high-grade, serous ovarian carcinomas treated with cytoreductive surgery (90 patients were optimally debulked and 95 patients were suboptimally debulked) and platinum-based adjuvant therapy (54). A distinct molecular signature was unable to be identified in the optimally debulked patients. On the other hand, a 572-gene signature was identified within the suboptimally debulked tumors. Several of the genes that were overexpressed in tumors with a poor prognosis, were directly related to pathways modulating cellular proliferation, chemoresistance, and apoptosis.

Results from expression array analysis have shown a similar pattern of abnormalities in poorly differentiated Stage I and Stage III EOCs, consistent with the possibility that Stage I ovarian cancer is, in fact, the precursor of advanced-stage disease (60).

Microarrays Predict Chemotherapy Response in Epithelial Ovarian Cancer

Several groups have identified patterns of gene expression that predict a response to chemotherapeutic agents in EOC, and in turn to prognosis. Six studies based on microarray technology have identified genetic profiles involved in predicting a response to frontline platinum and taxane chemotherapy in EOC. These have been summarized in Table 30.3 (66–71). A limitation to the interpretation of these studies continues to be the definition by which a response to therapy is established as either clinical or pathologic.

■ Table 30.3 Gene expression profiling studies predict chemotherapy response in epithelial ovarian carcinoma

Reference	Tumor Characteristics	Number Samples in Validation Set	Technical Validation	Microarray Platform	Gene Signature	Summary of Findings
Selvanayagam et al (2004) (66)	8 samples 20% Serous 100% FIGO III/IV	NA	NA	Custom ~10,700 cDNA	Clustering analysis distinguished resistant from sensitive tumors	Prediction of PFS: Relapse or Progression (< 6 months) vs late relapse (>6 months)
Bernardini et al (2005) (67)	22 samples 100% Serous 100% FIGO III/IV	10	rt-PCR Leave-1-out Cross Validation	Custom 19,200 cDNA	22	Prediction of PFS: Relapse or Progression (<6 months) vs late relapse (>6 months)
Dressman et al (2007) (68)	83 samples 100% Serous 100% FIGO III/IV	36	Robust Multi-Array Analysis	U133A ~22,000 Oligos[a]	1727	Prediction of complete clinical response
Helleman et al (2006) (69)	24 samples 58% Serous 82% FIGO IIB to IV	72	rt-PCR Leave-1-out Cross Validation	Custom ~18,000 cDNA	69	Prediction of complete clinical response
Jazaeri et al (2005) (70)	45 samples 83% Serous 100% FIGO IIC to IV	NA	rt-PCR Leave-1-out Cross Validation Immunohistochemistry	Custom 40,000 cDNA to compare primary chemosensitive and chemoresistant tumors 7600 cDNA to compare post-chemotherapy and primary tumors	85	Prediction of PFS: Early Relapse (< 6 months) vs late relapse) (> 13 months)
Spentzos et al (2004) (71)	24 samples 92% Serous 95% FIGO III/IV	36	Leave-1-out Cross Validation	U95Av2 ~12,600 Oligos[a]	93	Prediction of complete pathologic response based on second look procedure

[a]Affymetrix, Santa Clara, CA.
FIGO, International Federation of Gynecology and Obstetrics; PFS, progression-free survival.

This makes direct comparison of the genetic signatures identified by various investigators difficult.

Selvanayagam et al, created a custom 10,000-gene cDNA microarray to compare the expression profiles of 4 resistant tumors after platinum-based chemotherapy and an equivalent group of platinum-sensitive tumors (66). Tumor resistance was defined as a progression or relapse within 6 months after the end of chemotherapy. A total of 300 genes were differentially expressed and clearly distinguished resistant tumors from sensitive tumors. Important genes were identified as the focus of future research. This remains a landmark study in that it is the leading research to propose the potential of gene expression profiles derived from a primary tumor to predict a treatment response.

Jazaeri et al identified two cDNA microarrays, which compared the expression profiles of 21 pretreatment chemosensitive tumors with those of 24 pretreatment chemoresistant tumors (70). In this study, chemosensitive tumors were defined as those with a complete response to chemotherapy with a progression-free interval of at least 13 months. Conversely, chemoresistance was defined as those with residual disease after chemotherapy or a complete response to chemotherapy and then a subsequent relapse less than 6 months after initiation of chemotherapy. A total of 85 genes were differentially expressed between the two groups, with a less than or equal to a 2-fold difference between the mean expression levels. These 85 genes may represent those specific genes involved in chemoresistance. These investigators proposed that a small proportion of tumor cells will express these chemoresistant genes, and will potentially be left over after frontline treatment with platinum/taxane. This would explain the small magnitude of difference in gene expression among the sensitive and resistant groups. A predictive model of response to chemotherapy yielded a rate of accurate prediction of 77.8%. As a secondary part of this study, a 7585-gene microarray was next used to compare the 45 pretreatment samples with 15 posttreatment samples collected during interval or second-look procedures. Fewer and smaller differences were noted in gene expression levels of primary chemoresistant samples and posttreatment samples from primary chemosensitive samples and posttreatment samples. Proliferation genes were found to be underexpressed in posttreatment samples that sustain the theory of a decreased proliferation environment leading to the development of chemoresistance.

Bernardini et al compared 22 serous ovarian carcinomas including 8 resistant and 14 sensitive tumors to chemotherapy (67). Resistance was defined according to the extent of decrease in CA125 levels after platinum/taxane-based frontline chemotherapy. As part of this study, a 22-gene model was found to predict tumor resistance with 100% accuracy.

Independent validation of the predictive gene signature was not used in any of the prior studies. As an improvement to study design, Spentzos et al, identified a 93-gene signature, termed the Chemotherapy Response Profile (CRP), which allowed for a prediction of a complete pathologic response at second-look laparoscopy/laparotomy (SLL) with a 91% accuracy (71). This group used a set of 24 patients with EOC, who underwent SLL after completion of their frontline platinum/taxane-based chemotherapy, and those with the presence of residual disease at SLL were defined to have chemoresistance. This patient set was validated against a second set of 36 patients who had not undergone SLL. The CRP was able to differentiate those with favorable survival (median, not yet reached) over the patients with an unfavorable prognosis (median, 41 months). These genes identified in the CRP included pro-apoptotic BAX, which grants sensitivity to taxane therapy (70,71). The limitation of the CRP genetic signatures having no overlap with the OCPP genetic signature was once again demonstrated in this study. However, importantly, both genetic signatures indicated clear prognostic significance. The distinction has been attributed to these studies using different clinical end points (OCPP used survival, while CRP used chemoresistance) and these correspond to separate molecular processes.

In patients with EOC, Helleman et al discovered and validated a set of 9 genes that independently predicted resistance to platinum-based chemotherapy (69). In this study, patients with response to chemotherapy or stable disease (responders to chemotherapy) were compared to patients with progressive disease on chemotherapy (nonresponders). Twenty-four specimens including 19 responders and 5 nonresponders were examined using 18K cDNA microarrays and identified 69 differentially expressed genes, from which this 9-gene model was determined. This 9-gene predictor was validated by an independent set of 72 tumors (63 responders and 9 nonresponders), with a sensitivity of 89% and a specificity of 59%.

By far, one of the largest studies performed to date has been established by Dressman et al (68). Dressman used a set of 83 patients with Stage III/IV serous ovarian carcinoma to create a gene expression model that predicts a complete clinical response after platinum-based chemotherapy (assessed by clinical, radiographic, and serum CA125 level criteria). A 1727-gene model was identified that predicted the probability of response with 84% accuracy in the sample set and 78% accuracy in the validation set of 36 independent tumors. Additionally, by taking advantage of genetic profiles highlighted in previous work by Bild et al (55,74), these researchers were able to identify important oncogenic pathways in these patients and in 12 previously identified commercial ovarian carcinoma cell lines. These genetic expression patterns specifically identified the SRC and Rb/E2F pathways to be active in patients with platinum-resistant carcinomas. This has in turn allowed for possible patient-centered therapeutic response, as studies have focused to identify agents that may selectively inhibit these pathways during in vitro analysis, resulting in sensitivity to previously resistant platinum agents. This remains a hallmark study in that the authors have successfully identified genetic profiles capable of predicting platinum resistance with a significant degree of accuracy. It also has highlighted a critical oncogenic pathway, which may be a potential target for targeted therapy. Both aspects of this classic study clearly indicate a potential for genetic profiling to be an important focus of personalized oncologic therapy.

A significant focus of current genomic research remains the issue of resistance to chemotherapeutic agents. Despite a large collection of differentially expressed genetic profiles that have been identified, few have been validated in human correlation studies. The identified gene families of metallothioneins, gap junction genes, cell-cycle regulation genes, and Fanconi Anemia DNA-repair genes have been found to be upregulated in platinum-resistant cell lines. Conversely, genes from the ATP-binding subfamily, cell-cycle regulation, sterol metabolism, and topoisomerases are often upregulated in taxol-resistant cell lines. Table 30.4 summarizes important functional genes involved in platinum and taxane resistance, which have been validated to some degree in the clinical setting (70,174–180).

These and many similar trials indicate how microarray technology may allow for future individualized patient therapy. Genetic signatures identified in patients early in their tumor course may allow for a clinical decision tree based on classification from genetic profiles into long- or short-term survivors. In those individuals identified as short-term survivors, genetic signatures may identify other more effective frontline chemotherapeutic agents, or identify specific biologically involved oncogenic pathways, which in turn may lead to individualized therapy.

Microarray to Predict the Early Detection of Epithelial Ovarian Cancer

Genetic profiles are a continued focus in the identification of differentially upregulated genes specific to ovarian carcinoma and further to determine the associated encoded protein biomarkers, which may be revealed in the serum of patients affected with early-stage ovarian carcinoma.

Meinhold-Heerlein et al identified differentially expressed genes using oligonucleotide microarrays to highlight 275 protein biomarkers (181). These proteins were tested against 67 affected patients and control specimens. Osteopontin, kallikrein-10, and matrix metalloproteinase-7, when used with the CA125 assay demonstrated sensitivity and specificity values of 96%–98.7% and 99.7%–100%, respectively, for distinguishing patients with early-stage disease from the control specimens. Other markers, such as, prostanin, whey

acidic protein HE4, epithelial cell adhesion molecule, and brain creatine kinase have been identified in similar microarray studies and have been validated in small patient sets.

The limitations of these studies continue to rest in the clinical and practical application of these biomarkers. As with many diverse study designs, the methods by which the control samples were obtained vary from whole ovary samples, ovarian surface epithelim (OSE), OSE exposed to short-term culture, or immortalized OSE cells. All of these methods can alter the biochemical pathways within the cellular mechanics and ultimately change the expressed genes and associated biomarkers. As previously discussed, the protocols used in tissue processing can result in contaminated tissue specimens and may allow for variation in the genetic expression profiles. This would directly confound any microarray analysis study. Additionally, many of these studies analyze small sample sizes, which ultimately lead to bias in the results.

■ FOCAL GENETIC LOCI

The genetic loci identified in many recent studies promise both biologic and clinical significance. The functional effects of gene amplification and overexpression are currently in the youth of discovery. Table 30.4 summarizes the upregulated genes associated with ovarian carcinogenesis.

CTNNB1

CTNNB1 has been found to be mutated primarily in endometrioid ovarian carcinomas (EndoOC) over other histologic subtypes (144). CTNNB1, which encodes beta-catenin, has been responsible for cellular dysregulation in 16%–38% of EndoOC. The classic Wnt/beta-catenin (Wnt/β-cat) signaling pathway is vital to cellular fate and survival. Wu et al studied 72 EndoOCs in a mouse model (145), and discovered that mutations in the Wnt/β-cat signaling pathway were associated with mutations known to inactivate the P13K/Pten signaling pathway in low-grade and low-stage tumors. Conclusions can therefore be drawn regarding these altered pathways to be particularly characteristic in this type of EndoOC.

Despite, the association of the Wnt/β-cat signaling pathway with low grade and early-stage tumors, Bild et al has shown genetic profiles that identify an associated poor prognosis (74). The authors used cell lines to identify gene expression signatures that reflect the activation status of oncogenic pathways, specifically the SRC and Wnt/β-cat signaling pathway. These signature profiles were then applied to a series of 145 Stage III/IV ovarian carcinomas. The investigators concluded that a co-activation of the

■ **Table 30.4**   Significant amplified genes associated with ovarian carcinoma

Gene	Associated Protein	Biological Function	Clinical Application	Potential Targeted Therapy	References
Mesothelin	Mesothelin	Cell surface marker	Prolonged overall survival	M912	(50,75–78)
NOTCH3	Notch3	Signaling receptor	Tumor recurrence	γ-Secretase inhibitor	(79–81)
NF-κB	NF-κB1 NF-κB2	Signal transduction	Poor progression-free survival	PS1145	(82–88,91)
Fatty Acid Synthase	Fatty acid synthase	Fatty acid metabolism	Poor overall survival	C93	(89–90,92–98))
MUC4	Mucin-4	Signal transduction	No significant association	Humanized Muc4 mAb	(99–104)
Claudin	Claudin3 Claudin4 Claudin7	Tight junction proteins	Poor overall survival	*Clostridium perfringens* enterotoxin	(105–109)
Folate Receptor-α	Folic acid receptor	Mediates cellular uptake of folate	Cell surface target	MORAb-003 BGC 945	(110–113)
Osteopontin	Osteopontin	Cell survival Cell invasion	Serum marker	hu1A12	(114–120)
Apo-E	Apoprotein-E	Cell survival	Prolonged overall survival	NA	(121–123)
Kallikrein	Kallikrein	Protease	Poor progression-free survival Poor overall survival Chemoresistance	NA	(125–135)
BRCA	Brca	Signal transduction	Poor overall survival	NA	(136–138)
HLA-G	HLA-G	Immune evasion Immune suppression	Susceptible marker for chemotherapy	NA	(139–143)
CTNNB1	β-Catenin	Cell survival	Poor overall survival	NA	(144–145)
TP53	p53	Cell survival	Present in high-grade carcinoma	NA	(38,146–151)
KRAS BRAF	NA	Signal transduction	Serous tumor initiation	NA	(152–156)
PIK3CA	PI3K	Signal transduction	Tumor invasion Chemoresistance	NA	(157–161)
CCNE1	Cyclin E	Genetic instability	Poor overall survival	NA	(162–166)
RSF1 (HBXAP)	Rsf-1	Chromatin remodeling	Poor overall survival	NA	(167–168)
NACC1	NAC1	Transcription mediation	Poor progression-free survival	NA	(169–173)

SRC and Wnt/β-cat signaling pathway clearly identifies a patient subset with poor survival (median survival of 29 vs 91 months).

PTEN

Inactivating mutations of the tumor suppressor gene *PTEN* have been reported in 14%–21% of EndoOC. These *PTEN* mutations have been shown to be quite rare in other ovarian histologic subtypes (182). The inactivation of *PTEN* contributes to the activation of the P13K/Pten signaling pathway, which has been implicated in tumor propagation and chemoresistance in ovarian carcinoma.

TP53

TP53 has been found to be mutated in at least 50% of high-grade serous carcinomas (38,146–148,151). Leitao et al has demonstrated an overexpression of p53 and a mutation of *TP53* in much more than 50% of Stage I serous carcinomas. This indicates that the *TP53* mutation is an early event in the carcinogenesis of high-grade serous carcinomas (150). Furthermore, genomic profiling, using whole genome oligonucleotide microarrays of a cisplatin-sensitive ovarian cancer cell line and its resistant derivative, has demonstrated the *TP53* signaling pathway as critical in the development of cellular resistance (175).

The EndoOCs share many genetic features with its uterine equivalent. Indeed, *TP53* mutations have been found to be common in both ovarian and uterine endometrioid carcinomas. These mutations have been reported in more than 60% of EndoOCs (147). Additionally, in this study, Kolasa et al displayed the lack of Wnt/β-cat or P13K/Pten signaling pathway defects in these high grade tumors, which concurrently demonstrated the *TP53* mutation. Conclusions can then be drawn suggesting that the *TP53* mutation acts distinct from the *PTEN* and *CTNNB1* mutation, which are primarily involved in low-grade tumors.

In a classic study performed by Wu et al, oligonucleotide microarrays were used to analyze the global gene expression in 41 serous, 37 endometrioid, 13 mucinous, and 8 clear cell ovarian carcinomas (145), a substantial overlap between the expression profiles of endometrioid and serous ovarian carcinomas were demonstrated. Endometrioid tumors with mutated gene expression profiles similar to serous carcinomas were usually high grade and harbored the *TP53* mutation. Expression profiles of endometrioid tumors distinct from serous carcinomas tended to be low-grade and harbored mutations of *CTNNB1*, *PTEN*, and *PIK3CA*. These molecular findings support the division of endometrioid and serous carcinomas into two major subtypes, based primarily on cellular grading. Shared genetic alterations of *TP53*, for example, may be responsible for similarities in the gene expression profiles between high-grade endometrioid and serous carcinomas. Conversely, the *TP53* mutation in clear cell carcinomas is generally found to be low in frequency.

KRAS and BRAF

Activating mutations of *KRAS* and one of its downstream effectors, *BRAF*, are found to be present in over half of the low-grade serous ovarian carcinomas, in 75% of mucinous ovarian carcinomas, but not in EndoOC and the more common high-grade serous carcinomas (152–156). Mutations in these genetic loci lead to the activation of the MAPK signaling pathway. The Ras/Ref/MEK/MAPK signaling pathway has been well established, through molecular genetic studies, to be important in the pathogenesis of low-grade serous ovarian carcinomas. Mutation in the *KRAS* and *BRAF* genes have been shown to be early events associated with the transformation of serous cystadenomas into serous tumors.

Based on SNP array analysis and DNA copy number alterations, Nakayama et al identified these next gene loci (*CCNEI* [cyclin E1], *AKT2, NOTCH3, RSF1,* and *PIK3CA*) to be present in the frequently amplified chromosomal regions of purified ovarian tumor specimens (41).

PIK3CA

The amplification *PIK3CA*, which codes for the protein PI3K, has been shown to be involved in the dysregulation of the PI3K/Pten signaling pathway. The ultimate effect of this alteration leads to tumor invasion and chemoresistance in ovarian carcinoma (157,160). *PIK3CA* mutations have been identified in 20%–25% of endometrioid and clear cell ovarian carcinomas, but in only 2% of serous ovarian carcinomas (158,161). Biomarkers including the X-Linked Inhibitor of Apoptosis Protein (XIAP) have been implicated in this involved pathway (159).

Cyclin E1

CNE1 gene amplification contributes to the propagation of ovarian carcinoma and genetic instability (162,166). This effect has been especially seen in the presence of *TP53* genetic mutations (165). Additionally, the *CCNE1* gene encodes for low molecular weight cyclin E, which has been implicated in a poor clinical prognosis for ovarian carcinoma (163,164).

RSF1

The *RSF1* gene has been shown to be involved in chromatin remodeling and encodes for the Rsf-1 protein. The overexpression of Rsf-1 has been implicated in tumor cellular proliferation, while its knockdown has been shown to inhibit ovarian carcinoma tumorigenesis (168). In this study, Shih Ie et al were able to demonstrate that patients with *RSF1* gene amplification or Rsf-1 overexpression displayed a negative impact on OS than those without these genetic alterations. This study went on to describe an association with carboplatin and taxol resistance in vitro, when the Rsf-1 protein was overexpressed. This may explain the ultimate clinical effect of poor prognosis with Rsf-1 overexpression.

NOTCH3

Several studies using various genomic techniques have contributed to support the association regarding the *NOTCH3* amplification with EOC (79–81). Inactivation of Notch3 in cell lines that overexpress this protein has been shown to suppress cellular proliferation and induce apoptosis, but not in those with minimal Notch3 expression. This supports the claim that Notch3 is required for the growth and propagation of Notch3 expressed EOCs. This may allow for a potential therapeutic avenue and the focus of future study.

BRCA

Recent data indicate that *BRCA1* and *BRCA2* genes may be inactivated in ovarian carcinoma and particularly in EOC, through mechanisms aside from gene mutation (137). Hypermethylation of the *BRCA1* promoter along with a loss of the Brca1 protein expression has been observed in

15%–31% of sporadic ovarian carcinomas, in a population based study of 110 women (136). Additionally, EOC with both genetic and epigenetic inactivation of *BRCA1* have been shown to display different molecular changes involving the PI3K/Pten signaling pathway from each other (138). In this study, EOC with *BRCA1* mutations generally show a decreased *PTEN* mRNA level, while those with epigenetic loss of *BRCA1* showed copy number gains of *PIK3CA*.

Wilms' Tumor-1

The *Wilms' Tumor-1 (WT1)* gene encodes for a protein involved in the development of the genitourinary system. Acs et al has demonstrated specific expression of *WT1* in EOC as compared to the other histologic types of ovarian carcinoma (183).

Hepatocyte Nuclear Factor-1beta

A number of genes have been reported to be preferentially expressed in clear cell ovarian carcinomas, among them is *HNF-1β* (44,46,49,50,184). The *Hepatocyte Nuclear Factor-1beta (HNF-1β)* gene expresses a protein crucial to upregulating glucose/glycogen metabolism, in various body tissues. Knockdown of *HNF-1β* expression in clear cell ovarian carcinoma cells induces apoptosis, implicating *HNF-1β* to be essential for cellular survival of tumor cells.

MUC2, MUC3, MUC17, CDX1, and CDX2

Based on gene expression profiling, the pattern of gene expression in mucinous ovarian carcinomas has been shown to be clearly discernible from serous, endometrioid, and clear cell ovarian carcinomas (44,185). Specifically *MUC2*, *MUC3*, and *MUC17* genes are characteristic of mucinous carcinomas, regardless of their tissue origin. Intestinal type differentiation is seen in many mucinous tumors and is expressed by the *CDX1* and *CDX2* genes (caudal type homeobox transcription factors). These genes were also shown to be preferentially expressed in mucinous ovarian carcinomas.

■ FROM GENOMICS TO PROTEOMICS

Proteomic-based technology, which allows for an examination of the expressed proteins within a tissue specimen, accompanies genomic technology to allow for a better understanding of the distinct pathogenic pathways and ultimate biomarkers involved in tumorigenesis. Gene mutations, leading to changes in gene transcription and translation, with subsequent functional cellular protein production (the proteome) are well served as potential biomarkers for early EOC detection, identification

of recurrence, and treatment modification (186). In the same manner, environmental factors also, to some extent, contribute to tumor pathogenesis. Additionally, pharmacologic treatment modalities intervening in the disease process do so by interacting at the protein level. These effects cannot be assessed by examination of the genome alone. The potential targets of proteomics can be focused on the identification of novel protein and peptide modifications, the demonstration of clustering expression patterns of known proteins, or the quantification of expression levels of proteins and their various posttranslational modifications. Ultimately, the application of proteomics to the development and validation of screening prognostic biomarkers remains a focus of current investigations. Furthermore, proteomic technology allows for the identification of biomarker panels to predict the behavior of cancer during the development, progression, or treatment of carcinogenesis. The discovery of molecular targets or target pathways is currently under way.

Proteomic Biomarkers for Ovarian Cancer: Screening, Prognosis, and Personalized Chemotherapy

The goal to improve upon early screening technologies and to provide more targeted treatments in EOC has directed the field of high-throughput techniques over the past decade. The use of proteomics for early-stage detection of ovarian cancer, potential prognostication, and tailoring of chemotherapy regimens has become a reality of this "new" science in the past decade.

The approaches used in proteomics to detect clinical biomarkers typically involve a broad spectrum of samples and large amounts of chemical information on the protein level as compared to other biomic studies. In this manner, proteomic profiling has emerged as a fundamental instrument for the study of ovarian carcinoma at a molecular level. Proteomics has allowed for the examination of treatment effect and for the discovery of new biomarkers.

The vast milieu of proteins available for analysis, the wide range in concentration, molecular size, polarization, and ionization of proteins within tissue and blood, makes for a complicated investigation (186). An extensive array of mass spectrometry instruments must be employed, as there is no discrete tool that is able to satisfy all the requirements for the growing field of proteomics (187). These factors make the identification of a novel biomarker through proteomic technology all the more challenging.

Most proteomic studies have used blood specimens as the preliminary material for examination of the proteomic milieu. Blood specimens are ideal secondary to the ease of access and its ability to be distributed throughout the tissue microenvironment. Venous blood flows through the tumor and acquires cellular debris and products of secreted proteins. A wealth of information is harbored in the blood and other bodily fluids, which can provide information into the molecular aberrancies causing malignancies and ultimately contribute to the discovery of biomarkers.

Numerous analytical impediments have become obvious, primarily, compendiums of the plasma proteome have shown that more than 95% of the total protein concentration results from a few highly abundant proteins, such as immunoglobulins, albumin, and coagulation proteins (188). These highly abundant proteins complicate the detection of low abundant proteins, which could be the pertinent biomarker of interest. For this reason, investigators have turned their attention to profiling other body fluids including urine, ascites, and saliva.

Quantification of proteins by mass spectrometry is currently the most popular technique, as mass spectrometry has the ability to identify a large number of novel proteins as potential biomarkers. These proteomic methods for the discovery of biomarkers continue to encompass a broad spectrum and involve an extensive protein profile content as compared to other forms of biomic studies to date (189).

■ BIOMARKERS

A practical biomarker has been established to be a measurable and easily assessable biological substance providing diagnostic, prognostic, or treatment-directed information determined to guide patient care. An extensive list of serum markers have been evaluated alone and in combination with CA125 by a multitude of investigators. Some of the most promising markers include: Human Epididymis Protein-4 (HE4), Mesothelin, Kallikrein(s), Osteopontin, COX-2, IGFBP-5, Apolipoprotein-E, VEGF (75,76,114,117,121,130,132,133,135,190–197). Proteomic approaches to identify these markers have used a variety of techniques from enzyme-linked immunosorbent assay (ELISA) to mass spectrometry. We will discuss some of the most promising biomarkers for the detection of early-stage EOC, recurrence of EOC, and sensitivity to chemotherapeutic agents identified through proteomics. However, this is not intended to be a complete review of ovarian cancer biomarkers.

■ PROTEOMIC TECHNIQUES

Proteomics continues to show promise for the detection of specific protein biomarkers to diagnose early disease. Due to the difficult nature of proteome and biomarker discovery efforts, investigators have applied their entire arsenal of proteomic tools and the various approaches have been described generally as follows: (a) Examine the pattern of peaks on mass spectrometry. (b) Identify a limited number of critical markers by various proteomic analyses, so as to allow further study by more conventional techniques (198).

Many difficulties inherent to the discovery of candidate proteomes in biomarker studies and in clinical trials continue to contribute to the impractical screening of EOC. Current studies lack the specific population size to detect statistically significant differences. These challenges call to standardize experiments across institutions and continue to thwart investigative efforts in the discovery of clinically relevant proteins released from the EOC tumor.

A number of techniques allow for the recognition of proteins produced during a particular disease process, which can then assist in early disease diagnosis.

Protein Separation

2D-Polyacrylamide Gel Electrophoresis (2D-PAGE) has classically been the gold-standard discovery-based tool used in proteomic technology. A major limitation in this technique has been the ability to identify only a small percentage of the entire proteome. Recently, newer technology, such as Multi-Dimensional Liquid Chromatography for the display of particular proteomic patterns, are being used to access the less accessible regions of the proteome. These approaches enable the assessment of changes to intact molecules including glycosylation, phosphorylation, and other posttranslational modifications. Nevertheless, 2D-PAGE remains a standard and reliable separation technique, especially for the larger-molecular mass region of the proteome. In 2D-PAGE, proteins are separated based on charge and molecular mass. The tissue or serum samples are denatured into the polypeptide subunits, which are separated by isoelectric focusing, based on an immobilized pH gradient within the polyacrylamide gel strips. Next the proteins are separated based on molecular size after transfer of the polypeptide subunits to a separate polyacrylamide gel. These techniques gain sensitivity for specific protein molecules by the use of immunoblotting. In this manner, multiple forms of individual proteins can be readily visualized.

Protein Identification and Characterization

Specialized software has been developed to properly analyze the 2D-gel electrophoresis images, with accurate comparisons, both within the laboratory, but also to comprehensive proteome databases via the Internet. Using these methods, the differences in isolated protein concentrations, between healthy and diseased samples can be disclosed. Proteins of interest can then be identified using a combination of highly sensitive mass spectrometric (MS) methods. These MS techniques prove to be indispensable, as they require less protein material and have higher throughput than the classic sequencing methods.

In Surface-Enhanced Laser Desorption/Ionization-Time of Flight (SELDI-TOF) or, the Matrix-Assisted Laser Desorption/TOF (MALDI-TOF), the protein subunits are ionized by electrospray ionization and the mass of ions are measured by various coupled analyzers (199). MALDI-TOF uses a matrix that traps a subset of proteins in the sample, which is subsequently ionized and analyzed by TOF. Conversely, SELDI-TOF uses a commercial chip customized with specific bait molecules that either chemically binds protein samples using cationic or hydrophobic interactions, or use an antibody to which samples bind followed by a matrix to facilitate ionization. The time required for the ions to reach the detector plate is a function of the mass-to-charge ratio, which is unique to each individual peptide or protein. In this manner, these TOF analyzers measure the time for ions to travel from the source to the detector and assist in protein identification (200). The masses of peptides can then be measured by MS to produce a peptide mass fingerprint. The peptide mass fingerprint can be compared to peptide signatures predicted from the theoretical protein sequences found within international proteomic databases, thus allowing for protein identification. MALDI-TOF and SELDI-TOF are widely used in proteomics as highly sensitive techniques to identify proteome signatures with their posttranslational modifications.

Protein Microarray

Classically, candidate biomarkers were identified using crude discovery techniques such as semi-quantitative immunoblotting, immunohistochemical staining, in situ hybridization, ELISAs, and western blot analysis of known proteins. These methods lend to labor intensive, time consuming techniques, which are often reliant on subjective analysis. The recent use of protein microarray technology has allowed the quantification of multiple data points, including the expression levels of important proteins and their activated peptide molecules. These molecules compose the critical signaling junctures involved in cancer proliferation, survival, and angiogenesis (201).

There are two separate types of protein microarray techniques: (a) Forward Phase Protein Array (FPPA) and (b) Reverse Phase Protein Array (RPPA). In the FPPA, an antibody is immobilized on a matrix in an array, after which the sample of interest is incubated with this matrix. Each spot on this array corresponds to a different bait protein. In the RPPA format, an unknown sample is applied to an array, after which the array is incubated with antibodies, so as to detect the defined protein. This technique has undergone specific revision and optimization and therefore has become a popular method of analysis (201,202).

Whole body protein arrays (WBPA) using the RPPA technique has taken proteomic technology to a new level. WBPA incorporates LCM-procured normal and diseased cell populations derived from patient-based tissue specimens to determine organ-specific antigens. In this manner, WBPA becomes directly applicable to the identification and characterization of potential targets for T-cell–mediated vaccines. The ideal vaccine should have abundance of protein expression in cancer cells, but a low protein expression in normal tissue. WBPA provides a high-throughput method to screen and prioritize potential vaccine candidates, through the identification of ideal vaccine targets by highly specific probes to the immobilized cancer cell proteins.

■ POSTTRANSCRIPTIONAL PROFILING TO PREDICT THE CLINICAL BEHAVIOR OF EOC

Proteomic Signature to Predict the Presence of EOC

In 2002, Petricoin et al described and outlined the development of a new model for the diagnosis of disease based on pattern analysis of serum proteomic profiles. SELDI-TOF technology was used to evaluate high-volume mass spectral patterns from high-throughput mass spectrometry. This technique was able to discern 117 healthy women from patients with ovarian cancer using a clustering algorithm (203). This represents a novel approach to the identification of proteins as potential biomarkers; however, criticism of his data remains, as there were relatively few early-stage patients and investigators have had difficulty reproducing the initial results. It is speculated that markers identified by proteomics have been normal serum proteins that have undergone posttranslational modification in the tumor microenvironment or due to proteases released by the tumor.

A large Gynecologic Oncology Group trial (GOG-220), has been designed to generate and validate a proteomic signature profile that can diagnose ovarian carcinoma in the setting of a pelvic mass. At this point, serum samples have been collected from greater than 2000 women prior to surgical intervention in the clinical scenario of a pelvic mass and the laboratory analysis is scheduled to start. The primary objective of this study has been to create a protein pattern signature to differentiate malignant ovarian disease from benign or from a non-ovarian malignancy in presurgical specimens using MS and complex analytical bioinformatics. Secondary objectives include the differential analysis of early vs late stage disease, histologic differentiation, prediction of postoperative residual disease, and prognostic outcome.

Posttranscriptional Profiling of Ovarian Cancer Histologic Subtypes

Köbel et al has retrospectively studied 21 candidate tissue biomarkers with tissue microarray immunohistochemical analysis, in a group of 500 women with an optimal cytoreductive procedure (204). Expression analysis of these data demonstrated 10 of the 21 proteins were differentially expressed within a given subtype and were consistently expressed across the various stages of carcinomatosis. In comparison, 20 of the 21 proteins studied were differentially expressed across subtypes, suggesting that distinct biochemical events are more associated with the histologic subtype as opposed to the stage of carcinomatosis. Thus, the early and advanced-stage EOCs differ mainly based on the histologic subtype, while within a particular subtype there is no difference of protein expression between early and advanced-stage tumors. Schwartz et al and Zorn et al were described previously to have shown similar differentiation on a molecular and genetic level among women with the same stage and histologic type of ovarian carcinoma (44,46).

These studies may explain the different responses that patients demonstrate to chemotherapy and the different survival outcomes. Future study designs should, therefore, take into account the distinct expression profiles of each histologic subtype. The lumping of EOC subtypes in the current studies leads to abhorrent conclusions and can conceal many important discoveries. Clearly, further adequately powered studies and expert subtyping of cohorts are required to validate the discovery and development of subtype-specific biomarkers. A shift in the design of current biomarker investigations and in clinical trials is necessary to incorporate the consideration of histologic subtypes as distinct disease processes, so as to allow for this move toward subtype-specific management of EOC. At this point, further determination regarding the approach to treatment remains necessary.

Proteomic Techniques to Predict Chemotherapy Response in Epithelial Ovarian Cancer

Posadas et al applied the RPPA technique to evaluate biochemical signaling events of the targeting agents imatinib (Gleevac) and gefitinib in recurrent and advanced ovarian carcinoma via separate clinical Phase II trials (205,206). Neither agent demonstrated sufficient clinical activity to warrant further trials or to allow assessment of the relationship between target modulation and outcome. The RPPA did, however, demonstrate the presence of the target and the ability of the agent to inhibit the target in the tumor. The authors determine that modulation of these targets was insufficient to impact tumor injury with single agent therapy.

Posadas et al then carried these trials one step further, by designing a Phase I clinical trial and subsequently a Phase II trial to assess the combination of bevacizumab, a monoclonal antibody against vascular endothelial growth factor and sorafenib, a receptor tyrosine kinase inhibitor of raf kinase and vascular endothelial growth factor receptor 2. The main hypothesis entails a coupling inhibition of the downstream signaling and upstream events would lead to an effective disruption of the survival pathways in both the cancer cell and the relatively uninvolved cells present in the tumor microenvironment. This Phase I trial enrolled patients with recurrent ovarian carcinoma and demonstrated 43% of the patients (6 out of 13) to have a partial response to treatment (207). The RPPA analysis of the Phase I and II trials is ongoing in regards to an assessment of the protein array patterns of expression for the critical proteins that confer sensitivity or resistance to bevacizumab used in combination with sorafenib.

Predict the Early Detection of EOC

In 2003, Kozak et al, identified three panels of protein signatures, which were differentially expressed in EOC patients as compared to healthy patients or those with early-stage EOC (208). Later, this group successfully identified these differentially expressed proteins as Apolipoproptein A1 (AA1), Hemoglobin, Transthyretin (TTR), and Transferrin (209). Zhang et al reported similar proteins, specifically AA1 and TTR to be differentially expressed in patients with early-stage EOC and were able to apply this as an independent validation set (210).

Most of the novel biomarkers discovered to date are acute phase proteins, which are not linked to a specific disease process. It remains an imperative part of proteomic studies specifically focusing on the optimization potential biomarkers for the early diagnosis of EOC, to be combined with and compared with CA125 assay sensitivity and specificity. This will allow for a practical application of the novel biomarker into the clinical setting.

■ CONCLUSIONS

For over a decade now, DNA microarrays have amplified the search of molecular and phenotypic correlations in cancer research. This microarray technology has the potential to significantly affect treatment decision making in EOC. Despite the lack of supportive data, this has led to the initiation of "personalized medical therapy" in the form of novel commercial genetic marker assays. The small sample size and the lack of independent validation continue to raise concerns over the reliability and clinical application of the results (211). The appropriate caution must be maintained until the data in the gynecologic oncology field become adequately validated. Validation of genomic and proteomic investigations rely on the crucial collaboration of national and international multidisciplinary teams consisting of basic scientists and clinicians.

The use of expression microarray in routine clinical practice has been appropriately applied with significant consideration in that quality control mechanisms are still necessary (18,211). Additionally, larger studies with appropriate clinical designs, adjustment for known predictors and proper validation, continue to be necessary. Based on these findings, a set of usable guidelines, Minimum Information about A Microarray Experiment (MIAME), for statistical analysis and reporting of clinical microarray studies were created (212,213). These guidelines were designed to provide assurance regarding microarray data and that results derived from its analysis can be independently verified. As an extension to these guidelines, making the data publicly available will simplify analysis and interpretation of the results, assisting in the validation of these investigations.

A difficulty that remains is that transcript information cannot provide direct profiling of the activated signal pathway proteins that constitute the actual drug targets. As RNA transcripts do not correlate with functional post-translational events such as phosphorylation or protein–protein interactions, there is little connection between the synthetic proteins and the cellular drug targets. This functional liaison will become available as genomic and proteomic technologies become integrated (19,214). The efficient and standardized use of genomics and proteomics technologies will ultimately contribute to dramatic changes in the approach to treating ovarian carcinoma. It is in these future studies, where ultimately, personalized cancer diagnostics and individualized therapies will be developed.

Summary

- Genetic profiles that distinguish between the histologic subtypes of epithelial ovarian carcinoma have been clearly identified. Prognostic implication has also been correlated to each subtype in regards to OS.
- Gene signatures identified in microarray analysis can predict clinical outcome (initial surgical outcomes and survival) and response to first-line platinum-based chemotherapy in epithelial ovarian carcinoma.
- Microarray technology has identified many genes and in turn their associated signaling pathways involved in the tumor propagation of epithelial ovarian carcinoma.
- Several genes that may be implicated in the development of frontline chemotherapy resistance have been identified. Few have been validated with clinical correlation.
- Proteomics is the study of protein expression in body fluids, including: blood, plasma, serum, urine, saliva, sweat.
- Mass-spectrometry-based programs are the key to high throughput proteomics
- CA125 remains the most sensitive and specific marker when evaluated alone. However, many biomarkers may be added to CA125 to identify a composite marker with greater sensitivity and specificity.
- Other tissues may provide useful information including urine and ascites. Ascites fluid may provide information on sensitivity to chemotherapies and possibly offer tools to prognosticate.

■ REFERENCES

1. Jemal A, Siegel R, Xu J, Ward E. Cancer statistics, 2010. *CA Cancer J Clin.* 2010;60(5):277–300.
2. Paley PJ. Ovarian cancer screening: are we making any progress? *Curr Opin Oncol.* 2001;13(5):399–402.
3. Fishman DA, Bozorgi K. The scientific basis of early detection of epithelial ovarian cancer: the National Ovarian Cancer Early Detection Program (NOCEDP). *Cancer Treat Res.* 2002;107:3–28.
4. Engel J, Eckel R, Schubert-Fritschle G, et al. Moderate progress for ovarian cancer in the last 20 years: prolongation of survival, but no improvement in the cure rate. *Eur J Cancer.* 2002;38(18):2435–2445.
5. Ozols RF. Challenges for chemotherapy in ovarian cancer. *Ann Oncol.* 2006;17(Suppl 5):v181–v187.
6. Ozols RF. Systemic therapy for ovarian cancer: current status and new treatments. *Semin Oncol.* 2006;33(2 Suppl 6):S3–S11.
7. Agarwal R, Linch M, Kaye SB. Novel therapeutic agents in ovarian cancer. *Eur J Surg Oncol.* 2006;32(8):875–886.
8. Pepe MS, Etzioni R, Feng Z, et al. Phases of biomarker development for early detection of cancer. *J Natl Cancer Inst.* 2001;93(14):1054–1061.
9. Ludwig JA, Weinstein JN. Biomarkers in cancer staging, prognosis and treatment selection. *Nat Rev Cancer.* 2005;5(11):845–856.
10. Ozols RF, Bookman MA, Connolly DC, et al. Focus on epithelial ovarian cancer. *Cancer Cell.* 2004;5(1):19–24.
11. Golub TR. Genome-wide views of cancer. *N Engl J Med.* 2001;344(8):601–602.
12. Golub TR. Genomic approaches to the pathogenesis of hematologic malignancy. *Curr Opin Hematol.* 2001;8(4):252–261.
13. Golub TR, Slonim DK, Tamayo P, et al. Molecular classification of cancer: class discovery and class prediction by gene expression monitoring. *Science.* 1999;286(5439):531–537.
14. Elvidge G. Microarray expression technology: from start to finish. *Pharmacogenomics.* 2006;7(1):123–134.
15. Tefferi A, Bolander ME, Ansell SM, Wieben ED, Spelsberg TC. Primer on medical genomics. Part III: Microarray experiments and data analysis. *Mayo Clin Proc.* 2002;77(9):927–940.
16. Iyer VR, Eisen MB, Ross DT, et al. The transcriptional program in the response of human fibroblasts to serum. *Science.* 1999;283(5398):83–87.
17. Simon R. Roadmap for developing and validating therapeutically relevant genomic classifiers. *J Clin Oncol.* 2005;23(29):7332–7341.
18. Ntzani EE, Ioannidis JP. Predictive ability of DNA microarrays for cancer outcomes and correlates: an empirical assessment. *Lancet.* 2003;362(9394):1439–1444.
19. Carr KM, Rosenblatt K, Petricoin EF, Liotta LA. Genomic and proteomic approaches for studying human cancer: prospects for true patient-tailored therapy. *Hum Genomics.* 2004;1(2):134–140.
20. Chung CH, Levy S, Chaurand P, Carbone DP. Genomics and proteomics: emerging technologies in clinical cancer research. *Crit Rev Oncol Hematol.* 2007;61(1):1–25.

21. Quackenbush J. Extracting biology from high-dimensional biological data. *J Exp Biol.* 2007;210(Pt 9):1507–1517.
22. Emmert-Buck MR, Bonner RF, Smith PD, et al. Laser capture microdissection. *Science.* 1996;274(5289):998–1001.
23. Espina V, Heiby M, Pierobon M, Liotta LA. Laser capture microdissection technology. *Expert Rev Mol Diagn.* 2007;7(5):647–657.
24. Rodriguez AS, Espina BH, Espina V, Liotta LA. Automated laser capture microdissection for tissue proteomics. *Methods Mol Biol.* 2008;441:71–90.
25. Mueller C, Liotta LA, Espina V. Reverse phase protein microarrays advance to use in clinical trials. *Mol Oncol.* 2010;4(6):461–481.
26. DeVita, VT, Lawrence, TS, Rosenberg, SA. *Devita, Hellman & Rosenberg's Cancer: Principles & Practice of Oncology.* Wolters Kluwer/Lippincott Williams & Wilkins; 2011.
27. Wang TL, Maierhofer C, Speicher MR, et al. Digital karyotyping. *Proc Natl Acad Sci USA.* 2002;99(25):16156–16161.
28. Leary RJ, Cummins J, Wang TL, Velculescu VE. Digital karyotyping. *Nat Protoc.* 2007;2(8):1973–1986.
29. Ramaswamy S, Golub TR. DNA microarrays in clinical oncology. *J Clin Oncol.* 2002;20(7):1932–1941.
30. Lu J, Getz G, Miska EA, et al. MicroRNA expression profiles classify human cancers. *Nature.* 2005;435(7043):834–838.
31. Gilks CB. Subclassification of ovarian surface epithelial tumors based on correlation of histologic and molecular pathologic data. *Int J Gynecol Pathol.* 2004;23(3):200–205.
32. Dehari R, Kurman RJ, Logani S, Shih IeM. The development of high-grade serous carcinoma from atypical proliferative (borderline) serous tumors and low-grade micropapillary serous carcinoma: a morphologic and molecular genetic analysis. *Am J Surg Pathol.* 2007;31(7):1007–1012.
33. Kurman RJ, Shih IeM. Pathogenesis of ovarian cancer: lessons from morphology and molecular biology and their clinical implications. *Int J Gynecol Pathol.* 2008;27(2):151–160.
34. Auersperg N, Wong AS, Choi KC, Kang SK, Leung PC. Ovarian surface epithelium: biology, endocrinology, and pathology. *Endocr Rev.* 2001;22(2):255–288.
35. Kindelberger DW, Lee Y, Miron A, et al. Intraepithelial carcinoma of the fimbria and pelvic serous carcinoma: Evidence for a causal relationship. *Am J Surg Pathol.* 2007;31(2):161–169.
36. Lee Y, Miron A, Drapkin R, et al. A candidate precursor to serous carcinoma that originates in the distal fallopian tube. *J Pathol.* 2007;211(1):26–35.
37. Jazaeri AA, Yee CJ, Sotiriou C, Brantley KR, Boyd J, Liu ET. Gene expression profiles of BRCA1-linked, BRCA2-linked, and sporadic ovarian cancers. *J Natl Cancer Inst.* 2002;94(13):990–1000.
38. Singer G, Stöhr R, Cope L, et al. Patterns of p53 mutations separate ovarian serous borderline tumors and low- and high-grade carcinomas and provide support for a new model of ovarian carcinogenesis: a mutational analysis with immunohistochemical correlation. *Am J Surg Pathol.* 2005;29(2):218–224.
39. Cass I, Baldwin RL, Varkey T, Moslehi R, Narod SA, Karlan BY. Improved survival in women with BRCA-associated ovarian carcinoma. *Cancer.* 2003;97(9):2187–2195.
40. Gadducci A, Cosio S, Tana R, Genazzani AR. Serum and tissue biomarkers as predictive and prognostic variables in epithelial ovarian cancer. *Crit Rev Oncol Hematol.* 2009;69(1):12–27.
41. Nakayama K, Nakayama N, Jinawath N, et al. Amplicon profiles in ovarian serous carcinomas. *Int J Cancer.* 2007;120(12):2613–2617.
42. Meinhold-Heerlein I, Bauerschlag D, Hilpert F, et al. Molecular and prognostic distinction between serous ovarian carcinomas of varying grade and malignant potential. *Oncogene.* 2005;24(6):1053–1065.
43. Mayr D, Kanitz V, Anderegg B, et al. Analysis of gene amplification and prognostic markers in ovarian cancer using comparative genomic hybridization for microarrays and immunohistochemical analysis for tissue microarrays. *Am J Clin Pathol.* 2006;126(1):101–109.
44. Schwartz DR, Kardia SL, Shedden KA, et al. Gene expression in ovarian cancer reflects both morphology and biological behavior, distinguishing clear cell from other poor-prognosis ovarian carcinomas. *Cancer Res.* 2002;62(16):4722–4729.
45. Lu KH, Patterson AP, Wang L, et al. Selection of potential markers for epithelial ovarian cancer with gene expression arrays and recursive descent partition analysis. *Clin Cancer Res.* 2004;10(10):3291–3300.
46. Zorn KK, Bonome T, Gangi L, et al. Gene expression profiles of serous, endometrioid, and clear cell subtypes of ovarian and endometrial cancer. *Clin Cancer Res.* 2005;11(18):6422–6430.
47. Bonome T, Lee JY, Park DC, et al. Expression profiling of serous low malignant potential, low-grade, and high-grade tumors of the ovary. *Cancer Res.* 2005;65(22):10602–10612.
48. Gilks CB, Vanderhyden BC, Zhu S, van de Rijn M, Longacre TA. Distinction between serous tumors of low malignant potential and serous carcinomas based on global mRNA expression profiling. *Gynecol Oncol.* 2005;96(3):684–694.
49. Hough CD, Cho KR, Zonderman AB, Schwartz DR, Morin PJ. Coordinately up-regulated genes in ovarian cancer. *Cancer Res.* 2001;61(10):3869–3876.
50. Hough CD, Sherman-Baust CA, Pizer ES, et al. Large-scale serial analysis of gene expression reveals genes differentially expressed in ovarian cancer. *Cancer Res.* 2000;60(22):6281–6287.
51. Landen CN Jr, Birrer MJ, Sood AK. Early events in the pathogenesis of epithelial ovarian cancer. *J Clin Oncol.* 2008;26(6):995–1005.
52. Berchuck A, Iversen ES, Lancaster JM, et al. Prediction of optimal versus suboptimal cytoreduction of advanced-stage serous ovarian cancer with the use of microarrays. *Am J Obstet Gynecol.* 2004;190(4):910–925.
53. Holschneider CH, Berek JS. Ovarian cancer: epidemiology, biology, and prognostic factors. *Semin Surg Oncol.* 2000;19(1):3–10.
54. Berchuck A, Iversen ES, Lancaster JM, et al. Patterns of gene expression that characterize long-term survival in advanced stage serous ovarian cancers. *Clin Cancer Res.* 2005;11(10):3686–3696.
55. Bild AH, Yao G, Chang JT, et al. Oncogenic pathway signatures in human cancers as a guide to targeted therapies. *Nature.* 2006;439(7074):353–357.
56. Bonome T, Levine DA, Shih J, et al. A gene signature predicting for survival in suboptimally debulked patients with ovarian cancer. *Cancer Res.* 2008;68(13):5478–5486.
57. Hartmann LC, Lu KH, Linette GP, et al. Gene expression profiles predict early relapse in ovarian cancer after platinum-paclitaxel chemotherapy. *Clin Cancer Res.* 2005;11(6):2149–2155.
58. Lancaster JM, Dressman HK, Whitaker RS, et al. Gene expression patterns that characterize advanced stage serous ovarian cancers. *J Soc Gynecol Investig.* 2004;11(1):51–59.
59. Partheen K, Levan K, Osterberg L, Horvath G. Expression analysis of stage III serous ovarian adenocarcinoma distinguishes a sub-group of survivors. *Eur J Cancer.* 2006;42(16):2846–2854.
60. Shridhar V, Lee J, Pandita A, et al. Genetic analysis of early- versus late-stage ovarian tumors. *Cancer Res.* 2001;61(15):5895–5904.
61. Spentzos D, Levine DA, Ramoni MF, et al. Gene expression signature with independent prognostic significance in epithelial ovarian cancer. *J Clin Oncol.* 2004;22(23):4700–4710.
62. Chi DS, Eisenhauer EL, Lang J, et al. What is the optimal goal of primary cytoreductive surgery for bulky stage IIIC epithelial ovarian carcinoma (EOC)? *Gynecol Oncol.* 2006;103(2):559–564.
63. Aletti GD, Dowdy SC, Gostout BS, et al. Aggressive surgical effort and improved survival in advanced-stage ovarian cancer. *Obstet Gynecol.* 2006;107(1):77–85.
64. Tate S, Hirai Y, Takeshima N, Hasumi K. CA125 regression during neoadjuvant chemotherapy as an independent prognostic factor for survival in patients with advanced ovarian serous adenocarcinoma. *Gynecol Oncol.* 2005;96(1):143–149.
65. Berchuck A, Iversen ES, Luo J, et al. Microarray analysis of early stage serous ovarian cancers shows profiles predictive of favorable outcome. *Clin Cancer Res.* 2009;15(7):2448–2455.

66. Selvanayagam ZE, Cheung TH, Wei N, et al. Prediction of chemotherapeutic response in ovarian cancer with DNA microarray expression profiling. *Cancer Genet Cytogenet.* 2004;154(1):63–66.

67. Bernardini M, Lee CH, Beheshti B, et al. High-resolution mapping of genomic imbalance and identification of gene expression profiles associated with differential chemotherapy response in serous epithelial ovarian cancer. *Neoplasia.* 2005;7(6):603–613.

68. Dressman HK, Berchuck A, Chan G, et al. An integrated genomic-based approach to individualized treatment of patients with advanced-stage ovarian cancer. *J Clin Oncol.* 2007;25(5):517–525.

69. Helleman J, Jansen MP, Span PN, et al. Molecular profiling of platinum resistant ovarian cancer. *Int J Cancer.* 2006;118(8):1963–1971.

70. Jazaeri AA, Awtrey CS, Chandramouli GV, et al. Gene expression profiles associated with response to chemotherapy in epithelial ovarian cancers. *Clin Cancer Res.* 2005;11(17):6300–6310.

71. Spentzos D, Levine DA, Kolia S, et al. Unique gene expression profile based on pathologic response in epithelial ovarian cancer. *J Clin Oncol.* 2005;23(31):7911–7918.

72. Strobel T, Swanson L, Korsmeyer S, Cannistra SA. BAX enhances paclitaxel-induced apoptosis through a p53-independent pathway. *Proc Natl Acad Sci USA.* 1996;93(24):14094–14099.

73. Strobel T, Kraeft SK, Chen LB, Cannistra SA. BAX expression is associated with enhanced intracellular accumulation of paclitaxel: a novel role for BAX during chemotherapy-induced cell death. *Cancer Res.* 1998;58(21):4776–4781.

74. Bild AH, Potti A, Nevins JR. Linking oncogenic pathways with therapeutic opportunities. *Nat Rev Cancer.* 2006;6(9):735–741.

75. Huang CY, Cheng WF, Lee CN, et al. Serum mesothelin in epithelial ovarian carcinoma: a new screening marker and prognostic factor. *Anticancer Res.* 2006;26(6C):4721–4728.

76. Yen MJ, Hsu CY, Mao TL, et al. Diffuse mesothelin expression correlates with prolonged patient survival in ovarian serous carcinoma. *Clin Cancer Res.* 2006;12(3 Pt 1):827–831.

77. Chang K, Pastan I. Molecular cloning of mesothelin, a differentiation antigen present on mesothelium, mesotheliomas, and ovarian cancers. *Proc Natl Acad Sci USA.* 1996;93(1):136–140.

78. Ordóñez NG. Application of mesothelin immunostaining in tumor diagnosis. *Am J Surg Pathol.* 2003;27(11):1418–1428.

79. Park JT, Li M, Nakayama K, et al. Notch3 gene amplification in ovarian cancer. *Cancer Res.* 2006;66(12):6312–6318.

80. Shih IeM, Wang TL. Notch signaling, gamma-secretase inhibitors, and cancer therapy. *Cancer Res.* 2007;67(5):1879–1882.

81. Nickoloff, BJ, Osborne BA, Miele L. Notch signaling as a therapeutic target in cancer: a new approach to the development of cell fate modifying agents. *Oncogene.* 2003;22(42):6598–6608.

82. Pahl HL. Activators and target genes of Rel/NF-kappaB transcription factors. *Oncogene.* 1999;18(49):6853–6866.

83. Perkins ND. Post-translational modifications regulating the activity and function of the nuclear factor kappa B pathway. *Oncogene.* 2006;25(51):6717–6730.

84. Bassères DS, Baldwin AS. Nuclear factor-kappaB and inhibitor of kappaB kinase pathways in oncogenic initiation and progression. *Oncogene.* 2006;25(51):6817–6830.

85. Tang G, Minemoto Y, Dibling B, et al. Inhibition of JNK activation through NF-kappaB target genes. *Nature.* 2001;414(6861):313–317.

86. Chen C, Edelstein LC, Gélinas C. The Rel/NF-kappaB family directly activates expression of the apoptosis inhibitor Bcl-x(L). *Mol Cell Biol.* 2000;20(8):2687–2695.

87. Mabuchi S, Ohmichi M, Nishio Y, et al. Inhibition of inhibitor of nuclear factor-kappaB phosphorylation increases the efficacy of paclitaxel in *in vitro* and *in vivo* ovarian cancer models. *Clin Cancer Res.* 2004;10(22):7645–7654.

88. Mabuchi S, Ohmichi M, Nishio Y, et al. Inhibition of NFkappaB increases the efficacy of cisplatin in *in vitro* and *in vivo* ovarian cancer models. *J Biol Chem.* 2004;279(22):23477–23485.

89. Gansler TS, Hardman W 3rd, Hunt DA, Schaffel S, Hennigar RA. Increased expression of fatty acid synthase (OA-519) in ovarian neoplasms predicts shorter survival. *Hum Pathol.* 1997;28(6):686–692.

90. Grunt TW, Wagner R, Grusch M, et al. Interaction between fatty acid synthase- and ErbB-systems in ovarian cancer cells. *Biochem Biophys Res Commun.* 2009;385(3):454–459.

91. Kleinberg L, Dong HP, Holth A, et al. Cleaved caspase-3 and nuclear factor-kappaB p65 are prognostic factors in metastatic serous ovarian carcinoma. *Hum Pathol.* 2009;40(6):795–806.

92. Kuhajda FP. Fatty acid synthase and cancer: new application of an old pathway. *Cancer Res.* 2006;66(12):5977–5980.

93. Kuhajda FP, Jenner K, Wood FD, et al. Fatty acid synthesis: a potential selective target for antineoplastic therapy. *Proc Natl Acad Sci USA.* 1994;91(14):6379–6383.

94. Menendez JA, Lupu R. Fatty acid synthase and the lipogenic phenotype in cancer pathogenesis. *Nat Rev Cancer.* 2007;7(10):763–777.

95. Menendez JA, Vellon L, Mehmi I, et al. Inhibition of fatty acid synthase (FAS) suppresses HER2/neu (erbB-2) oncogene overexpression in cancer cells. *Proc Natl Acad Sci USA.* 2004;101(29):10715–10720.

96. Pizer ES, Wood FD, Heine HS, Romantsev FE, Pasternack GR, Kuhajda FP. Inhibition of fatty acid synthesis delays disease progression in a xenograft model of ovarian cancer. *Cancer Res.* 1996;56(6):1189–1193.

97. Wang HQ, Altomare DA, Skele KL, et al. Positive feedback regulation between AKT activation and fatty acid synthase expression in ovarian carcinoma cells. *Oncogene.* 2005;24(22):3574–3582.

98. Zhou W, Han WF, Landree LE, et al. Fatty acid synthase inhibition activates AMP-activated protein kinase in SKOV3 human ovarian cancer cells. *Cancer Res.* 2007;67(7):2964–2971.

99. Bafna S, Singh AP, Moniaux N, Eudy JD, Meza JL, Batra SK. MUC4, a multifunctional transmembrane glycoprotein, induces oncogenic transformation of NIH3T3 mouse fibroblast cells. *Cancer Res.* 2008;68(22):9231–9238.

100. Davidson B, Baekelandt M, Shih IeM. MUC4 is upregulated in ovarian carcinoma effusions and differentiates carcinoma cells from mesothelial cells. *Diagn Cytopathol.* 2007;35(12):756–760.

101. Ponnusamy MP, Singh AP, Jain M, Chakraborty S, Moniaux N, Batra SK. MUC4 activates HER2 signalling and enhances the motility of human ovarian cancer cells. *Br J Cancer.* 2008;99(3):520–526.

102. Singh AP, Chaturvedi P, Batra SK. Emerging roles of MUC4 in cancer: a novel target for diagnosis and therapy. *Cancer Res.* 2007;67(2):433–436.

103. Theodoropoulos G, Carraway CA, Carraway KL. MUC4 involvement in ErbB2/ErbB3 phosphorylation and signaling in response to airway cell mechanical injury. *J Cell Biochem.* 2009;107(1):112–122.

104. Workman HC, Sweeney C, Carraway KL 3rd. The membrane mucin Muc4 inhibits apoptosis induced by multiple insults via ErbB2-dependent and ErbB2-independent mechanisms. *Cancer Res.* 2009;69(7):2845–2852.

105. Agarwal R, D'Souza T, Morin PJ. Claudin-3 and claudin-4 expression in ovarian epithelial cells enhances invasion and is associated with increased matrix metalloproteinase-2 activity. *Cancer Res.* 2005;65(16):7378–7385.

106. Kleinberg L, Holth A, Trope CG, Reich R, Davidson B. Claudin upregulation in ovarian carcinoma effusions is associated with poor survival. *Hum Pathol.* 2008;39(5):747–757.

107. Morin PJ. Claudin proteins in human cancer: promising new targets for diagnosis and therapy. *Cancer Res.* 2005;65(21):9603–9606.

108. Rangel LB, Agarwal R, D'Souza T, et al. Tight junction proteins claudin-3 and claudin-4 are frequently overexpressed in ovarian cancer but not in ovarian cystadenomas. *Clin Cancer Res.* 2003;9(7):2567–2575.

109. Santin AD, Cané S, Bellone S, et al. Treatment of chemotherapy-resistant human ovarian cancer xenografts in C.B-17/SCID mice

by intraperitoneal administration of Clostridium perfringens enterotoxin. *Cancer Res.* 2005;65(10):4334–4342.

110. Basal E, Eghbali-Fatourechi GZ, Kalli KR, et al. Functional folate receptor alpha is elevated in the blood of ovarian cancer patients. *PLoS ONE.* 2009;4(7):e6292.

111. Gibbs DD, Theti DS, Wood N, et al. BGC 945, a novel tumor-selective thymidylate synthase inhibitor targeted to alpha-folate receptor-overexpressing tumors. *Cancer Res.* 2005;65(24):11721–11728.

112. Kalli KR. MORAb-003, a fully humanized monoclonal antibody against the folate receptor alpha, for the potential treatment of epithelial ovarian cancer. *Curr Opin Investig Drugs.* 2007;8(12):1067–1073.

113. Kalli KR, Oberg AL, Keeney GL, et al. Folate receptor alpha as a tumor target in epithelial ovarian cancer. *Gynecol Oncol.* 2008;108(3):619–626.

114. Brakora KA, Lee H, Yusuf R, et al. Utility of osteopontin as a biomarker in recurrent epithelial ovarian cancer. *Gynecol Oncol.* 2004;93(2):361–365.

115. Dai J, Peng L, Fan K, et al. Osteopontin induces angiogenesis through activation of PI3K/AKT and ERK1/2 in endothelial cells. *Oncogene.* 2009;28(38):3412–3422.

116. Kim HJ, Lee HJ, Jun JI, et al. Intracellular cleavage of osteopontin by caspase-8 modulates hypoxia/reoxygenation cell death through p53. *Proc Natl Acad Sci USA.* 2009;106(36):15326–15331.

117. Kim JH, Skates SJ, Uede T, et al. Osteopontin as a potential diagnostic biomarker for ovarian cancer. *JAMA.* 2002; 287(13):1671–1679.

118. Rosen DG, Wang L, Atkinson JN, et al. Potential markers that complement expression of CA125 in epithelial ovarian cancer. *Gynecol Oncol.* 2005;99(2):267–277.

119. Song G, Cai QF, Mao YB, Ming YL, Bao SD, Ouyang GL. Osteopontin promotes ovarian cancer progression and cell survival and increases HIF-1alpha expression through the PI3-K/Akt pathway. *Cancer Sci.* 2008;99(10):1901–1907.

120. Visintin I, Feng Z, Longton G, et al. Diagnostic markers for early detection of ovarian cancer. *Clin Cancer Res.* 2008;14(4):1065–1072.

121. Chen YC, Pohl G, Wang TL, et al. Apolipoprotein E is required for cell proliferation and survival in ovarian cancer. *Cancer Res.* 2005;65(1):331–337.

122. Ho YY, Deckelbaum RJ, Chen Y, Vogel T, Talmage DA. Apolipoprotein E inhibits serum-stimulated cell proliferation and enhances serum-independent cell proliferation. *J Biol Chem.* 2001;276(46):43455–43462.

123. Mahley RW, Rall SC Jr. Apolipoprotein E: far more than a lipid transport protein. *Annu Rev Genomics Hum Genet.* 2000;1:507–537.

124. Davidson B, Xi Z, Klokk TI, et al. Kallikrein 4 expression is upregulated in epithelial ovarian carcinoma cells in effusions. *Am J Clin Pathol.* 2005;123(3):360–368.

125. Diamandis EP, Scorilas A, Fracchioli S, et al. Human kallikrein 6 (hK6): a new potential serum biomarker for diagnosis and prognosis of ovarian carcinoma. *J Clin Oncol.* 2003;21(6):1035–1043.

126. Ghosh MC, Grass L, Soosaipillai A, Sotiropoulou G, Diamandis EP. Human kallikrein 6 degrades extracellular matrix proteins and may enhance the metastatic potential of tumour cells. *Tumour Biol.* 2004;25(4):193–199.

127. Kapadia C, Ghosh MC, Grass L, Diamandis EP. Human kallikrein 13 involvement in extracellular matrix degradation. *Biochem Biophys Res Commun.* 2004;323(3):1084–1090.

128. Kuk C, Kulasingam V, Gunawardana CG, Smith CR, Batruch I, Diamandis EP. Mining the ovarian cancer ascites proteome for potential ovarian cancer biomarkers. *Mol Cell Proteomics.* 2009;8(4):661–669.

129. Luo LY, Katsaros D, Scorilas A, et al. The serum concentration of human kallikrein 10 represents a novel biomarker for ovarian cancer diagnosis and prognosis. *Cancer Res.* 2003;63(4): 807–811.

130. Magklara A, Mellati AA, Wasney GA, et al. Characterization of the enzymatic activity of human kallikrein 6: Autoactivation, substrate specificity, and regulation by inhibitors. *Biochem Biophys Res Commun.* 2003;307(4):948–955.

131. Michael IP, Sotiropoulou G, Pampalakis G, et al. Biochemical and enzymatic characterization of human kallikrein 5 (hK5), a novel serine protease potentially involved in cancer progression. *J Biol Chem.* 2005;280(15):14628–14635.

132. Shan SJ, Scorilas A, Katsaros D, Diamandis EP. Transcriptional upregulation of human tissue kallikrein 6 in ovarian cancer: clinical and mechanistic aspects. *Br J Cancer.* 2007;96(2):362–372.

133. Shih IeM, Salani R, Fiegl M, et al. Ovarian cancer specific kallikrein profile in effusions. *Gynecol Oncol.* 2007;105(2):501–507.

134. Xi Z, Kaern J, Davidson B, et al. Kallikrein 4 is associated with paclitaxel resistance in ovarian cancer. *Gynecol Oncol.* 2004;94(1):80–85.

135. Yousef GM, Polymeris ME, Yacoub GM, et al. Parallel overexpression of seven kallikrein genes in ovarian cancer. *Cancer Res.* 2003;63(9):2223–2227.

136. Baldwin RL, Nemeth E, Tran H, et al. BRCA1 promoter region hypermethylation in ovarian carcinoma: a population-based study. *Cancer Res.* 2000;60(19):5329–5333.

137. Cannistra SA. BRCA-1 in sporadic epithelial ovarian cancer: lessons learned from the genetics of hereditary disease. *Clin Cancer Res.* 2007;13(24):7225–7227.

138. Press JZ, De Luca A, Boyd N, et al. Ovarian carcinomas with genetic and epigenetic BRCA1 loss have distinct molecular abnormalities. *BMC Cancer.* 2008;8:17.

139. Davidson B, Elstrand MB, McMaster MT, et al. HLA-G expression in effusions is a possible marker of tumor susceptibility to chemotherapy in ovarian carcinoma. *Gynecol Oncol.* 2005;96(1):42–47.

140. Fons P, Chabot S, Cartwright JE, et al. Soluble HLA-G1 inhibits angiogenesis through an apoptotic pathway and by direct binding to CD160 receptor expressed by endothelial cells. *Blood.* 2006;108(8):2608–2615.

141. Rebmann V, Busemann A, Lindemann M, Grosse-Wilde H. Detection of HLA-G5 secreting cells. *Hum Immunol.* 2003; 64(11):1017–1024.

142. Sheu JJ, Shih IeM. Clinical and biological significance of HLA-G expression in ovarian cancer. *Semin Cancer Biol.* 2007; 17(6):436–443.

143. Singer G, Rebmann V, Chen YC, et al. HLA-G is a potential tumor marker in malignant ascites. *Clin Cancer Res.* 2003; 9(12):4460–4464.

144. Wright K, Wilson P, Morland S, et al. beta-catenin mutation and expression analysis in ovarian cancer: exon 3 mutations and nuclear translocation in 16% of endometrioid tumours. *Int J Cancer.* 1999;82(5):625–629.

145. Wu R, Hendrix-Lucas N, Kuick R, et al. Mouse model of human ovarian endometrioid adenocarcinoma based on somatic defects in the Wnt/beta-catenin and PI3K/Pten signaling pathways. *Cancer Cell.* 2007;11(4):321–333.

146. Chan WY, Cheung KK, Schorge JO, et al. Bcl-2 and p53 protein expression, apoptosis, and p53 mutation in human epithelial ovarian cancers. *Am J Pathol.* 2000;156(2):409–417.

147. Kolasa IK, Rembiszewska A, Janiec-Jankowska A, et al. PTEN mutation, expression and LOH at its locus in ovarian carcinomas. Relation to TP53, K-RAS and BRCA1 mutations. *Gynecol Oncol.* 2006;103(2):692–697.

148. Kupryjanczyk J, Szymanska T, Madry R, et al. Evaluation of clinical significance of TP53, BCL-2, BAX and MEK1 expression in 229 ovarian carcinomas treated with platinum-based regimen. *Br J Cancer.* 2003;88(6):848–854.

149. Kupryjanczyk J, Thor AD, Beauchamp R, et al. p53 gene mutations and protein accumulation in human ovarian cancer. *Proc Natl Acad Sci USA.* 1993;90(11):4961–4965.

150. Leitao MM, Soslow RA, Baergen RN, Olvera N, Arroyo C, Boyd J. Mutation and expression of the TP53 gene in early

stage epithelial ovarian carcinoma. *Gynecol Oncol.* 2004;93(2): 301–306.

151. Wen WH, Reles A, Runnebaum IB, et al. p53 mutations and expression in ovarian cancers: correlation with overall survival. *Int J Gynecol Pathol.* 1999;18(1):29–41.

152. Caduff RF, Svoboda-Newman SM, Bartos RE, Ferguson AW, Frank TS. Comparative analysis of histologic homologues of endometrial and ovarian carcinoma. *Am J Surg Pathol.* 1998;22(3):319–326.

153. Enomoto T, Weghorst CM, Inoue M, Tanizawa O, Rice JM. K-ras activation occurs frequently in mucinous adenocarcinomas and rarely in other common epithelial tumors of the human ovary. *Am J Pathol.* 1991;139(4):777–785.

154. Ichikawa Y, Nishida M, Suzuki H, et al. Mutation of K-ras protooncogene is associated with histological subtypes in human mucinous ovarian tumors. *Cancer Res.* 1994;54(1):33–35.

155. Mayr D, Hirschmann A, Löhrs U, Diebold J. KRAS and BRAF mutations in ovarian tumors: a comprehensive study of invasive carcinomas, borderline tumors and extraovarian implants. *Gynecol Oncol.* 2006;103(3):883–887.

156. Singer G, Oldt R 3rd, Cohen Y, et al. Mutations in BRAF and KRAS characterize the development of low-grade ovarian serous carcinoma. *J Natl Cancer Inst.* 2003;95(6):484–486.

157. Arboleda MJ, Lyons JF, Kabbinavar FF, et al. Overexpression of AKT2/protein kinase Bbeta leads to up-regulation of beta1 integrins, increased invasion, and metastasis of human breast and ovarian cancer cells. *Cancer Res.* 2003;63(1):196–206.

158. Campbell IG, Russell SE, Choong DY, et al. Mutation of the PIK3CA gene in ovarian and breast cancer. *Cancer Res.* 2004;64(21):7678–7681.

159. Dan HC, Sun M, Kaneko S, et al. Akt phosphorylation and stabilization of X-linked inhibitor of apoptosis protein (XIAP). *J Biol Chem.* 2004;279(7):5405–5412.

160. Meng Q, Xia C, Fang J, Rojanasakul Y, Jiang BH. Role of PI3K and AKT specific isoforms in ovarian cancer cell migration, invasion and proliferation through the p70S6K1 pathway. *Cell Signal.* 2006;18(12):2262–2271.

161. Nakayama K, Nakayama N, Kurman RJ, et al. Sequence mutations and amplification of PIK3CA and AKT2 genes in purified ovarian serous neoplasms. *Cancer Biol Ther.* 2006;5(7):779–785.

162. Bedrosian I, Lu KH, Verschraegen C, Keyomarsi K. Cyclin E deregulation alters the biologic properties of ovarian cancer cells. *Oncogene.* 2004;23(15):2648–2657.

163. Davidson B, Skrede M, Silins I, Shih IeM, Trope CG, Flørenes VA. Low-molecular weight forms of cyclin E differentiate ovarian carcinoma from cells of mesothelial origin and are associated with poor survival in ovarian carcinoma. *Cancer.* 2007;110(6):1264–1271.

164. Farley J, Smith LM, Darcy KM, et al.; Gynecologic Oncology Group. Cyclin E expression is a significant predictor of survival in advanced, suboptimally debulked ovarian epithelial cancers: a Gynecologic Oncology Group study. *Cancer Res.* 2003;63(6):1235–1241.

165. Minella AC, Swanger J, Bryant E, Welcker M, Hwang H, Clurman BE. p53 and p21 form an inducible barrier that protects cells against cyclin E-cdk2 deregulation. *Curr Biol.* 2002;12(21):1817–1827.

166. Spruck CH, Won KA, Reed SI. Deregulated cyclin E induces chromosome instability. *Nature.* 1999;401(6750):297–300.

167. Choi JH, Sheu JJ, Guan B, et al. Functional analysis of 11q13.5 amplicon identifies Rsf-1 (HBXAP) as a gene involved in paclitaxel resistance in ovarian cancer. *Cancer Res.* 2009;69(4):1407–1415.

168. Shih IeM, Sheu JJ, Santillan A, et al. Amplification of a chromatin remodeling gene, Rsf-1/HBXAP, in ovarian carcinoma. *Proc Natl Acad Sci USA.* 2005;102(39):14004–14009.

169. Davidson B, Berner A, Trope' CG, Wang TL, Shih IeM. Expression and clinical role of the bric-a-brac tramtrack broad complex/poxvirus and zinc protein NAC-1 in ovarian carcinoma effusions. *Hum Pathol.* 2007;38(7):1030–1036.

170. Ishibashi M, Nakayama K, Yeasmin S, et al. A BTB/POZ gene, NAC-1, a tumor recurrence-associated gene, as a potential

target for Taxol resistance in ovarian cancer. *Clin Cancer Res.* 2008;14(10):3149–3155.

171. Jinawath N, Vasoontara C, Yap KL, et al. NAC-1, a potential stem cell pluripotency factor, contributes to paclitaxel resistance in ovarian cancer through inactivating Gadd45 pathway. *Oncogene.* 2009;28(18):1941–1948.

172. Nakayama K, Nakayama N, Davidson B, et al. A BTB/POZ protein, NAC-1, is related to tumor recurrence and is essential for tumor growth and survival. *Proc Natl Acad Sci USA.* 2006;103(49):18739–18744.

173. Nakayama K, Nakayama N, Wang TL, Shih IeM. NAC-1 controls cell growth and survival by repressing transcription of Gadd45GIP1, a candidate tumor suppressor. *Cancer Res.* 2007;67(17):8058–8064.

174. Goto T, Takano M, Sakamoto M, et al. Gene expression profiles with cDNA microarray reveal RhoGDI as a predictive marker for paclitaxel resistance in ovarian cancers. *Oncol Rep.* 2006;15(5):1265–1271.

175. Li J, Wood WH 3rd, Becker KG, Weeraratna AT, Morin PJ. Gene expression response to cisplatin treatment in drug-sensitive and drug-resistant ovarian cancer cells. *Oncogene.* 2007;26(20):2860–2872.

176. Macleod K, Mullen P, Sewell J, et al. Altered ErbB receptor signaling and gene expression in cisplatin-resistant ovarian cancer. *Cancer Res.* 2005;65(15):6789–6800.

177. Roberts D, Schick J, Conway S, et al. Identification of genes associated with platinum drug sensitivity and resistance in human ovarian cancer cells. *Br J Cancer.* 2005;92(6):1149–1158.

178. Kim JS, Baek SJ, Sali T, Eling TE. The conventional nonsteroidal anti-inflammatory drug sulindac sulfide arrests ovarian cancer cell growth via the expression of NAG-1/MIC-1/GDF-15. *Mol Cancer Ther.* 2005;4(3):487–493.

179. Cheng TC, Manorek G, Samimi G, Lin X, Berry CC, Howell SB. Identification of genes whose expression is associated with cisplatin resistance in human ovarian carcinoma cells. *Cancer Chemother Pharmacol.* 2006;58(3):384–395.

180. Samimi G, Manorek G, Castel R, et al. cDNA microarray-based identification of genes and pathways associated with oxaliplatin resistance. *Cancer Chemother Pharmacol.* 2005;55(1):1–11.

181. Meinhold-Heerlein I, Bauerschlag D, Zhou Y, et al. An integrated clinical-genomics approach identifies a candidate multi-analyte blood test for serous ovarian cancer. *Clin Cancer Res.* 2007;13(2 Pt 1):458–466.

182. Obata K, Morland SJ, Watson RH, et al. Frequent PTEN/MMAC mutations in endometrioid but not serous or mucinous epithelial ovarian tumors. *Cancer Res.* 1998;58(10):2095–2097.

183. Acs G, Pasha T, Zhang PJ. WT1 is differentially expressed in serous, endometrioid, clear cell, and mucinous carcinomas of the peritoneum, fallopian tube, ovary, and endometrium. *Int J Gynecol Pathol.* 2004;23(2):110–118.

184. Tsuchiya A, Sakamoto M, Yasuda J, et al. Expression profiling in ovarian clear cell carcinoma: identification of hepatocyte nuclear factor-1 beta as a molecular marker and a possible molecular target for therapy of ovarian clear cell carcinoma. *Am J Pathol.* 2003;163(6):2503–2512.

185. Heinzelmann-Schwarz VA, Gardiner-Garden M, Henshall SM, et al. A distinct molecular profile associated with mucinous epithelial ovarian cancer. *Br J Cancer.* 2006;94(6):904–913.

186. Sidransky D. Emerging molecular markers of cancer. *Nat Rev Cancer.* 2002;2(3):210–219.

187. Schuchardt S, Sickmann A. Protein identification using mass spectrometry: a method overview. *EXS.* 2007;97:141–170.

188. Cadron I, Van Gorp T, Timmerman D, Amant F, Waelkens E, Vergote I. Application of proteomics in ovarian cancer: which sample should be used? *Gynecol Oncol.* 2009;115(3):497–503.

189. Hanash S. Disease proteomics. *Nature.* 2003;422(6928):226–232.

190. Drapkin R, von Horsten HH, Lin Y, et al. Human epididymis protein 4 (HE4) is a secreted glycoprotein that is overexpressed by serous and endometrioid ovarian carcinomas. *Cancer Res.* 2005;65(6):2162–2169.

191. Collins Y, Tan DF, Pejovic T, et al. Identification of differentially expressed genes in clinically distinct groups of serous ovarian carcinomas using cDNA microarray. *Int J Mol Med.* 2004;14(1):43–53.

192. Hefler LA, Zeillinger R, Grimm C, et al. Preoperative serum vascular endothelial growth factor as a prognostic parameter in ovarian cancer. *Gynecol Oncol.* 2006;103(2):512–517.

193. Hellström I, Raycraft J, Hayden-Ledbetter M, et al. The HE4 (WFDC2) protein is a biomarker for ovarian carcinoma. *Cancer Res.* 2003;63(13):3695–3700.

194. Rudlowski C, Pickart AK, Fuhljahn C, et al. Prognostic significance of vascular endothelial growth factor expression in ovarian cancer patients: a long-term follow-up. *Int J Gynecol Cancer.* 2006;16 Suppl 1:183–189.

195. Shah CA, Lowe KA, Paley P, et al. Influence of ovarian cancer risk status on the diagnostic performance of the serum biomarkers mesothelin, HE4, and CA125. *Cancer Epidemiol Biomarkers Prev.* 2009;18(5):1365–1372.

196. Welsh JB, Zarrinkar PP, Sapinoso LM, et al. Analysis of gene expression profiles in normal and neoplastic ovarian tissue samples identifies candidate molecular markers of epithelial ovarian cancer. *Proc Natl Acad Sci USA.* 2001;98(3):1176–1181.

197. Zheng Y, Katsaros D, Shan SJ, et al. A multiparametric panel for ovarian cancer diagnosis, prognosis, and response to chemotherapy. *Clin Cancer Res.* 2007;13(23):6984–6992.

198. Bast RC Jr, Badgwell D, Lu Z, et al. New tumor markers: CA125 and beyond. *Int J Gynecol Cancer.* 2005;15 Suppl 3:274–281.

199. Aebersold R, Mann M. Mass spectrometry-based proteomics. *Nature.* 2003;422(6928):198–207.

200. Koomen J, Hawke D, Kobayashi R. Developing an understanding of proteomics: an introduction to biological mass spectrometry. *Cancer Invest.* 2005;23(1):47–59.

201. Sheehan KM, Calvert VS, Kay EW, et al. Use of reverse phase protein microarrays and reference standard development for molecular network analysis of metastatic ovarian carcinoma. *Mol Cell Proteomics.* 2005;4(4):346–355.

202. Winters M, Dabir B, Yu M, Kohn EC. Constitution and quantity of lysis buffer alters outcome of reverse phase protein microarrays. *Proteomics.* 2007;7(22):4066–4068.

203. Petricoin EF, Ardekani AM, Hitt BA, et al. Use of proteomic patterns in serum to identify ovarian cancer. *Lancet.* 2002;359(9306):572–577.

204. Köbel M, Kalloger SE, Boyd N, et al. Ovarian carcinoma subtypes are different diseases: implications for biomarker studies. *PLoS Med.* 2008;5(12):e232.

205. Posadas EM, Kwitkowski V, Kotz HL, et al. A prospective analysis of imatinib-induced c-KIT modulation in ovarian cancer: a phase II clinical study with proteomic profiling. *Cancer.* 2007;110(2):309–317.

206. Posadas EM, Liel MS, Kwitkowski V, et al. A phase II and pharmacodynamic study of gefitinib in patients with refractory or recurrent epithelial ovarian cancer. *Cancer.* 2007;109(7):1323–1330.

207. Azad NS, Posadas EM, Kwitkowski VE, et al. Combination targeted therapy with sorafenib and bevacizumab results in enhanced toxicity and antitumor activity. *J Clin Oncol.* 2008;26(22):3709–3714.

208. Kozak KR, Amneus MW, Pusey SM, et al. Identification of biomarkers for ovarian cancer using strong anion-exchange ProteinChips: potential use in diagnosis and prognosis. *Proc Natl Acad Sci USA.* 2003;100(21):12343–12348.

209. Kozak KR, Su F, Whitelegge JP, Faull K, Reddy S, Farias-Eisner R. Characterization of serum biomarkers for detection of early stage ovarian cancer. *Proteomics.* 2005;5(17):4589–4596.

210. Zhang Z, Bast RC Jr, Yu Y, et al. Three biomarkers identified from serum proteomic analysis for the detection of early stage ovarian cancer. *Cancer Res.* 2004;64(16):5882–5890.

211. Dupuy A, Simon RM. Critical review of published microarray studies for cancer outcome and guidelines on statistical analysis and reporting. *J Natl Cancer Inst.* 2007;99(2):147–157.

212. Knudsen TB, Daston GP; Teratology Society. MIAME guidelines. *Reprod Toxicol.* 2005;19(3):263.

213. Brazma A, Hingamp P, Quackenbush J, et al. Minimum information about a microarray experiment (MIAME)-toward standards for microarray data. *Nat Genet.* 2001;29(4):365–371.

214. Hancock W, Apffel A, Chakel J, et al. Integrated genomic/proteomic analysis. *Anal Chem.* 1999;71(21):742A–748A.

31

Incorporating Translational Research Into Gynecologic Cancers While Balancing the Focus of Personalized Medicine

SETSUKO K. CHAMBERS

KEITH A. JOINER

■ DEFINING TRANSLATIONAL RESEARCH

Focus on and investment in translational research is a current national priority. The term "translational research" originally spanned the spectrum from basic discovery to experiments with human cell lines in vitro, preclinical in vivo models, human tissue correlation studies, drug or technologic discovery, to early phase clinical trials. The definition is broadened to include population science with epidemiologic studies, leading to intervention studies. It can be bidirectional; from bench to bedside, or proceed in a reverse direction with findings at the bedside leading to mechanistic insights discovered in the laboratory. Prevention, risk, detection, therapeutic, or survivorship endpoints are among those being studied.

The NCI SPORE (Specialized Program of Research Excellence) uses the following definition of translational research in its guidelines: "Translational research uses knowledge of human biology to develop and test the feasibility of cancer-relevant interventions in humans and/or determines the biological basis for observations made in individuals with cancer or in populations at risk for cancer." The term "interventions" is used in its broadest sense.

More specific definitions are in use for the broader spectrum of translational research, which vary somewhat nationally. Briefly:

T1 First in-human, proof-of-concept research/move basic discovery to candidate health application.

T2 Definitive clinical trials to change standard of care/ assesses T1 data for development of evidence-based guidelines.

T3 Practice-based research/moves T2 into practice through delivery and dissemination.

T4 Population-based research/evaluates the results of this application in populations—for instance, feasibility, cost effectiveness. These definitions significantly broaden original definitions of translational research.

This national priority on translational research has recently reached new heights as technologic advances in genome sequencing have become more feasible at an individual level. The plethora of data that has begun to emerge, the scope and extent of which will only continue to amplify, has led to many questions about how best to apply the information to patients.

This chapter will first serve as an overview of some examples of major advances in this area pertaining to gynecologic oncology; we do not intend on being comprehensive. We then examine some of the current opportunities and challenges in the area of translational research as it applies to personalized medicine.

■ GENOMIC ANALYSIS OF EPITHELIAL OVARIAN CANCER

The Cancer Genome Atlas Project has been completed and epithelial ovarian cancer was one of the focus disease sites. Hence, this cancer with a high mortality has been intensively and comprehensively studied by this project as well as others (1–5). The levels of investigation include analysis of genome sequence, promoter methylation and DNA copy number, mRNA, and microRNA (miRNA) expression profiling. Among the high-grade serous subtype, collectively the findings show: almost all have loss of p53 function; approximately 50% of tumors show a defective homologous recombination or *BRCA* pathway. Over 90% of tumors show loss of the *OPCML* tumor suppressor pathway that leads to activation of several receptor tyrosine kinases. What is clear is that there is very significant genomic complexity with high copy number variations and a high mutation rate compared to other cancers studied. Not unexpectedly, high-grade serous ovarian carcinomas share similar genomic abnormalities, as does the basal, or triple negative form of breast cancer (6). In general, among ovarian cancers, most single tumor types, with some exceptions, have been found to contain many different mutations and driver genes. We also know that different pathways are activated to drive proliferation, invasion, metastasis, resistance, and toxicity. In epithelial ovarian cancer, such complexity added to the finding of predominance of the role of tumor suppressors, rather than activating oncogenes, leads to challenges in the therapeutic application of these findings to patients.

■ SOME EXAMPLES OF PROGRESS FROM TRANSLATIONAL RESEARCH IN GYNECOLOGIC CANCER, MAINLY OVARIAN CANCER

1. We have clearly learned from large-scale integrated genomic analyses, as well as other studies, that epithelial ovarian cancer can be more precisely divided into molecular categories rather than the traditional histologic subtypes. The latter categories largely did not translate into a difference in treatment, with mucinous ovarian carcinoma treated the same as serous carcinoma; and high-grade serous carcinoma treated the same as low-grade serous carcinoma. Our understanding of the molecular abnormalities and pathways associated with these cancers has significantly increased. Currently, in ongoing clinical trials, patients are being triaged to different treatments, using molecular categories. But since the category of epithelial ovarian cancers is now being divided into several molecularly distinct categories, accruals can be difficult to achieve with small numbers within certain categories potentially limiting their prioritization for clinical trials.

2. The BRCAness or homologous recombination defects found in approximately half of epithelial ovarian cancers is one of the more exciting and translatable findings arising from these genomic analyses. This brings to the forefront the potential therapeutic impact of the poly (ADP-ribose) polymerase (PARP) inhibitors, drugs that are not yet routinely available but are under testing in clinical trials. The frequency of this finding opens up relevant studies to patients who do not carry a germline BRCA mutation. The finding also explains the high responses seen in both germline BRCA positive and BRCA negative recurrent ovarian cancer patients with the PARP inhibitor olaparib (7). Progression-free, but not overall, survival advantage was demonstrated when olaparib was used as a form of consolidation therapy in platinum-sensitive ovarian cancer, a finding that was observed in the presence or absence of germline BRCA mutation (8).

3. An important area of progress comes from research that shows that the majority of high-grade serous carcinoma, at least in the women at high risk for this disease, initiates in the fallopian tube rather than the ovary (9,10). A molecular signature likely underlies a precursor (serous tubal intraepithelial carcinoma) in the fallopian tube mucosa (11,12). This translates into proposals of different surgical management schemes, such as removal of the tube alone in premenopausal high-risk women, allowing them to retain ovarian function with attendant quality of life. These data also contribute to the several reasons for continued failure of various ovarian cancer screening programs directed toward imaging of the ovaries, to reliably detect epithelial ovarian cancer at an early stage, or to reduce mortality (13–16).

4. Continued progress in the search for ovarian, tubal, or peritoneal cancer susceptibility genes is demonstrated. While women who carry the BRCA1 or BRCA2 germline mutations account for approximately 10% of all ovarian cancer cases, it is predicted that they account for less than half the excess familial risk. Thus, we are aware that there exist other yet to be identified susceptibility alleles for this disease, which are likely to confer moderate- to low-penetrance susceptibility. A genome-wide association study comparing cases to controls has identified a new susceptibility locus on 9p22.2 containing 12 single-nucleotide polymorphisms (SNPs) significantly associated with risk. Validation was performed of the most significant SNP, which was found to have the strongest association with risk for the serous subtype (17). A focused study of germline mutations was also carried out, using massively parallel sequencing, demonstrating that 24% of unselected ovarian, fallopian tube, and peritoneal carcinoma cases had loss-of-function mutations in a total of 12 genes, including BRCA1 and BRCA2 (18). Over 30% of cases with germline mutations had no family history of breast or ovarian cancer. The implications of findings in these two studies relate to population genetic testing.

5. As stated above, among ovarian cancers, there are a few exceptions to the finding that there exist multiple molecular drivers within a single tumor type. In contrast to epithelial ovarian cancers, including the high-grade serous carcinoma subtype, the granulosa cell tumors of the ovary constitute such an exception. Initiated on the basis of whole-transcriptome sequencing, extended to a cohort of adult granulosa cell tumors of the ovary, the finding that over 90% of these tumors contained a single point mutation in the FOXL2 gene suggested that this one pathway could represent a critical driver in the development of these tumors (19). Among other genes, the ovarian specific aromatase gene promoter has been shown to

be a direct target of this mutation containing *FOXL2* transcription factor (20). This finding suggests that this mutation enhances the transcription of aromatase and may render the tumor more sensitive to aromatase inhibitors. To date, only sporadic case reports are available on the therapeutic use of aromatase inhibitors in granulosa cell tumors (21).

6. An epic step forward in translational research in gynecologic oncology is in the development and implementation of the human papillomavirus (HPV) vaccine to prevent cervical cancer. HPV DNA and its link to development of cervical cancer has long been recognized. Several vaccines have been tested, first in girls, then in the last couple of years in boys. When given to unvaccinated females, studies show a greater than 90% efficacy in the prevention of high-grade CIN including adenocarcinoma in situ, with a lesser effect still evident in females who had evidence of prior infection with the vaccine-relevant HPV subtype. In males, there is high efficacy of the vaccine against genital warts and, in relevant populations, anal intraepithelial neoplasia. The vaccine is currently recommended by the Advisory Committee on Immunization Practices, for both female and male adolescents. There remain substantial barriers to access, however, both in the United States and worldwide (22,23). Several cost-effectiveness studies, critical in particular to global health application, have been performed (16,24). Questions that also remain to be answered are the duration of vaccine efficacy and effect of vaccine on reduction of cervical cancer (16).

■ BIOSPECIMEN SCIENCE IS CRITICAL TO SUCCESS OF TRANSLATIONAL RESEARCH AND PERSONALIZED MEDICINE

Tumor banks are a cornerstone of translational research and considerable experience with tumor banks has spawned the development and evolution of Biospecimen Science (25). Standards for strict quality control of the tissue/biological specimen processing and of the annotation are now in place, although not yet uniformly implemented nationally for many reasons. These standards have resulted from experience with misleading tumor profiling results which could not be validated. The creation, maintenance, and quality assurance of a large-scale annotated biorepository, with informatics capability and potentially time-saving automated equipment and alternative storage models, are extremely costly. But the clear overall direction is to create such standardized biorepositories in order to provide the best quality molecular correlative data to contribute to databases of very large populations of the

future. Some leaders believe that whole genome characterization will become a routine part of cancer pathology. Such databases would include clinical factors such as reproductive, behavioral, environmental, and other phenotypic factors, as well as disease, treatment, response, survival, to add to the genotypic factors. This type of database can then be probed for many associations including those with disease or with wellness and response to interventions in subsets of patients. There would be sufficient power for analysis of even small subsets, data that can then be tested prospectively.

■ BIOMARKERS AND TARGETED THERAPY—AN EXAMPLE OF THE COMPLEXITY WHEN TRYING TO IMPLEMENT PERSONALIZED MEDICINE

The plethora of molecular information from profiling of patient samples has also led to stricter guidelines for their reporting and definitions of validated "biomarkers." Again, these guidelines have resulted from the inability to validate initial reports of a "promising" marker. The number of validated, clinically useful, markers still remains small (26). The markers can derive from many sources, including tumor samples, patient imaging, blood/urine nucleic acids or proteins, circulating blood cells, and/or typing of DNA (genotyping), RNA, and/or miRNAs. Biomarkers have been defined as prognostic (provide information about the patient's outcome, regardless of therapy), predictive (can be used in advance of therapy to estimate response or survival to specific treatment compared to another treatment), pharmacodynamic (marker changes after treatment are associated with target modulation by a specific agent), or surrogate (marker substitutes for a clinical endpoint) markers (27). The information may lead to reverse translational investigation of the biology underlying the specific findings.

That a single marker is overexpressed in a tumor sample does not necessarily indicate that application of a targeted therapy directed toward the pathway implied by the marker will result in a response or survival advantage. Targeted therapy is complicated. As described above, the majority of tumors have multiple interconnecting and redundant activated molecular pathways. In our Phase II study of bevacizumab (targeted to vascular endothelial growth factor [VEGF]) and erlotinib (targeted to EGFR) in recurrent epithelial ovarian cancer patients, our findings suggest that those tumors that have elevated VEGF are more, not less, likely to be resistant to this targeted therapy (28). In general, targeted therapy will have more success in the rarer tumors or some hematologic malignancies where the genomic complexity is less and where there may be a dominant driver pathway aberration.

There are several examples of successful targeted therapy targeting oncogenes in nongynecologic cancers. In patients with advanced non-small-cell lung cancer and with confirmed activating mutation in EGFR, erlotinib was shown in a randomized Phase III study compared to chemotherapy, to significantly improve progression-free survival (PFS) by nearly 9 months, while having significantly less toxicity (29). Studies of erlotinib in ovarian cancer in general have not been limited to patients with activated EGFR mutations and the activity was only modest (30). In amplified or highly overexpressed *HER2*-positive breast cancer, trastuzumab added to adjuvant chemotherapy significantly improved disease-free survival (DFS) and decreased mortality (31). While results of studies of anti-*HER2* agents in *HER2*-overexpressed epithelial ovarian cancer have been disappointing, recent evidence points to *HER2* amplification in the subset of mucinous ovarian carcinomas with pilot data suggesting response from trastuzumab, which needs validation in a clinical trial (32).

At the same time, there are also clear examples of success with a targeted agent in one tumor type harboring the target, which is not seen when other tumor types also harboring the same target, are studied with the same agent. Targeting activating *BRAF* oncoprotein mutation in melanoma with vemurafenib is highly effective while treatment with vemurafenib in colon cancer patients harboring the same mutation was disappointing. Studies find that *BRAF* inhibition in these colon tumors results in rapid feedback activation of the EGFR pathway, which supports continued proliferation (33).

■ EXPANDING THE VIEW

We have discussed examples of the application of molecular information to the diagnosis, treatment, risk assessment, and prevention of gynecologic cancers. Doing so conforms with the current understanding of translational medicine. We now describe a more global view of translational medicine and some of the less commonly discussed or recognized contributions toward health. In particular, we explore the relationship between translational medicine and personalized medicine. The latter term, like the moniker translational medicine, is now commonplace. Yet the use of the term and its application to any specific situation vary widely, and tend to undervalue the full potential. Confounding the issue, personalized medicine is variably used interchangeably with the terms precision medicine, prospective health care, wellness care, and even patient-centered care, which tends to obfuscate the fundamental difference between health care and health promotion.

Individuals value health. Health care (or medical care or application of translational medicine to care) is only valued by consumers in so far as they promote health, by preventing, diagnosing, or treating disease. Note the use of the term consumer. Synonyms, including consumer and customer, connote an individual who is not necessarily ill, and is seeking the best approach to remain (or become) healthy. To wit, a consumer would far prefer that translational medicine and personalized medicine be used to maintain their healthy, cancer-free state in the first place, rather than only when they become a patient because a gynecologic cancer has been diagnosed. The latter application of translational/personalized medicine not only short-changes the power and potential of the concept, but also substantially undervalues the enormous increases in understanding, at a scientific level, of preventable or manageable risk factors for gynecologic cancer.

The fullest and richest application of personalized medicine includes, for individuals at any age, but certainly no later than puberty, a health risk analysis, which is then used to construct a personalized health plan for the individual. This risk analysis, which comprises a large database, includes, in addition to a full health profile, a determination of genetic, environmental, and lifestyle factors that modulate the risk for gynecologic cancers. This plan is updated on a regular basis, as necessitated by changes in any of the above factors. Incorporating into the plan a discussion with the consumer about the influence of obesity, high-fat diet, a sedentary lifestyle, hormonal exposure, reproductive factors, sexual activity, smoking, alcohol, and more, is just as essential as determining genetic risk factors, based on sophisticated new technologies. Importantly, the molecular understanding of risk factors such as hormonal therapy to gynecologic cancers is every bit as sophisticated as defining genetic predispositions, or molecular profiling of tumors, yet does not typically receive the fanfare of the latter.

To maximize the likelihood of success, the personalized health plan should be "co-created" between the provider and the consumer. A health plan that is prescribed by the provider without adequately embracing the family, social, environmental, financial, and emotional circumstances of the consumer is unlikely to be effective. A very common and difficult issue is weight control. Consumers need a health plan that fits with their activities of daily living and takes into account individual and highly personal attitudes about weight and weight management, personal finances, work obligations, family, social and cultural pressures, and more. Motivational interviewing is one approach to development of a plan that incorporates those elements.

We end by providing a specific example of the broad (but admittedly not currently comprehensive) application of translational/personalized medicine by gynecologic oncologists to the adult population.

The University of Arizona Cancer Center multidisciplinary High-Risk Clinic opened in 2004 for the care of women at risk for breast and ovarian cancers. Here we concentrate on potentially modifiable health behavioral factors such as physical activity and diet for risk reduction, in addition to other risk reduction and early detection modalities along with genetic counseling and testing. Large-scale prospective intervention studies have shown the benefit of low-fat dietary pattern on both risk for breast cancer and relapse-free survival (RFS) in women with breast cancer (34,35). Moreover, the Women's Health Initiative study also showed a reduction in ovarian cancer risk from a low-fat diet (34). The University of Arizona faculty has been instrumental in these studies. They have also helped advance achievement of significant and sustained change in health behaviors in at-risk populations by applying the use of a telephone counseling strategy, resulting in adherence to study intervention (36,37). This strategy has also been more cost-effective than standard dietician-based in-person counseling approaches. The mechanisms for a benefit from a low-fat, more plant-based eating pattern include reduction in: immunomodulation and inflammation including prostaglandins, oxidative stress, levels of hormonal exposure, and insulin-adiposity interactions. Diet-related epigenetic effects on gene (perhaps even miRNA) expression may also modulate carcinogenesis (38). The role of physical activity has also been studied in reduction of ovarian cancer risk and while the studies are not entirely consistent, in general it appears that moderate activity may be preferable to vigorous physical activity.

Among women who have already developed ovarian cancer, to date there has been no prospective intervention study of effect of low-fat diet or exercise on their outcome. A recent meta-analysis suggested little relationship between obesity and ovarian cancer survival (39). To that end, the Gynecologic Oncology Group (GOG) has opened a large-scale national trial (GOG-0225) led by University of Arizona Cancer Center faculty to prospectively examine, in a randomized fashion, the role of dietary and physical activity lifestyle change in women with ovarian cancer who are disease-free, on PFS. Quality of life will also be measured and molecular correlative studies performed.

■ REFERENCES

1. The Cancer Genome Atlas Research Network. Integrated genomic analyses of ovarian carcinoma. *Nature.* 2011;474:609–615.
2. Press JZ, De Luca A, Boyd N, et al. Integrated genomic analyses of ovarian carcinoma. *BMC Cancer.* 2008;8:17.
3. Ahmed AA, Etermadmoghadam D, Temple J, et al. Driver mutations in TP53 are ubiquitous in high grade serous carcinoma of the ovary. *J Pathol.* 2010;221:49–56.
4. McKie AB, Vaughan S, Zanini E, et al. The OPCML tumor suppressor functions as a cell surface repressor-adaptor, negatively regulating receptor tyrosine kinases in epithelial ovarian cancer. *Cancer Discov.* 2012;2:156.
5. Landen CN, Birrer MJ, Sood AK. Early events in the pathogenesis of epithelial ovarian cancer. *J Clin Onc.* 2008;26: 1995–1005.
6. The Cancer Genome Atlas Network. Comprehensive molecular portraits of human breast tumours. *Nature.* 2012;490:61–70.

7. Gelmon KA, Tischkowitz M, Mackay H, et al. Olaparib in patients with recurrent high-grade serous or poorly differentiated ovarian carcinoma or triple-negative breast cancer: a phase 2, multicentre, open-label, non-randomised study. *Lancet Oncol.* 2011;12:852–861.
8. Ledermann J, Harter P, Gourley C, et al. Olaparib maintenance therapy in platinum-sensitive relapsed ovarian cancer. *N Engl J Med.* 2012;366:1382–1392.
9. Callahan MJ, Crum CP, Medeiros F, et al. Primary fallopian tube malignancies in BRCA-positive women undergoing surgery for ovarian cancer risk reduction. *J Clin Oncol.* 2007;25: 3985–3990.
10. Kindelberger DW, Lee Y, Miron A, et al. Intraepithelial carcinoma of the fimbria and pelvic serous carcinoma: Evidence for a causal relationship. *Am J Surg Pathol.* 2007;31:161–169.
11. Lee Y, Niron A, Drapkin R, et al. A candidate precursor to serous carcinoma that originates in the distal fallopian tube. *J Pathol.* 2007;211:26–35.
12. Kuhn E, Kurman RJ, Vang R, et al. TP53 mutations in serous tubal intraepithelial carcinoma and concurrent pelvic high-grade serous carcinoma—evidence supporting the clonal relationship of the two lesions. *J Pathol.* 2012;226:421–426.
13. Menon U, Gentry-Maharaj A, Hallett R et al. Sensitivity and specificity of multimodal and ultrasound screening for ovarian cancer, and stage distribution of detected cancers: results of the prevalence screen of the UK Collaborative Trial of Ovarian Cancer Screening (UKCTOCS). *Lancet Oncol.* 2009;10: 327–340.
14. Partridge E, Kreimer AR, Greenlee RT, et al. Results from four rounds of ovarian cancer screening in a randomized trial. *Obstet Gynecol.* 2009;113:775–782.
15. Buys SS, Partridge E, Black A, et al. Effect of screening on ovarian cancer mortality: the Prostate, Lung, Colorectal and Ovarian (PLCO) Cancer Screening Randomized Controlled Trial. *JAMA.* 2011;305:2295–2303.
16. Kulasingam S, Havrilesky L. Health economics of screening for gynaecological cancers. *Best Pract Res Clin Obstet Gynaecol.* 2012;26:163–173.
17. Song H, Ramus SJ, Tyrer J, et al. A genome-wide association study identifies a new ovarian cancer susceptibility locus on 9p22.2. *Nat Genet.* 2009;41:996–1001.
18. Walsh T, Casadei S, Lee MK, et al. Mutations in 12 genes for inherited ovarian, fallopian tube, and peritoneal carcinoma identified by massively parallel sequencing. *Proc Natl Acad Sci USA.* 2011;108:18032–18037.
19. Shah SP, Kobel M, Senz J, et al. Mutation of FOXL2 in granulosa-cell tumors of the ovary. *N Engl J Med.* 2009;360:2719–2729.
20. Fleming NI, Knower KC, Lazarus KA, et al. Aromatase is a direct target of FOXL2: C134W in granulosa cell tumors via a single highly conserved binding site in the ovarian specific promoter. *PLoS ONE.* 2010;5:e14389.
21. Alhilli MM, Long HJ, Podratz KC, et al. Aromatase inhibitors in the treatment of recurrent ovarian granulosa cell tumors: brief report and review of the literature. *J Obstet Gynecol Res.* 2011;38:340–344.
22. Downs LS, Scarini I, Einstein MH et al. Overcoming the barriers to HPV vaccination in high-risk populations in the US. *Gynecol Oncol.* 2010;117:486–490.
23. Lowy DR, Schiller JT. Reducing HPV-associated cancer globally. *Cancer Prev Res.* 2012;5:18–23.
24. Seto K, Marra F, Raymakers A, et al. The cost effectiveness of human papillomavirus vaccines: a systematic review. *Drugs.* 2012;72:715–743.
25. Vaught JB, Henderson MK, Compton CC. Biospecimens and biorepositories: from afterthought to science. *Cancer Epid Biomarkers Prev.* 2012;21:253–255.
26. McShane LM, Altman DG, Sauerbrei W, et al. Reporting recommendations for tumor marker prognostic studies (REMARK). *J Natl Cancer Inst.* 2005;97:1180–1184.

27. Jain RK, Duda DG, Willett CG, et al. Biomarkers of response and resistance to antiangiogenic therapy. *Nature Rev Clin Oncol.* 2009;6:327–338.

28. Chambers SK, Clouser MC, Baker AF, et al. Overexpression of tumor vascular endothelial growth factor A may portend an increased likelihood of progression in a phase II trial of bevacizumab and erlotinib in resistant ovarian cancer. *Clin Cancer Res.* 2010;16:5320–5328.

29. Zhou C, Wu Y-L, Chen G, et al. Erlotinib versus chemotherapy as first-line treatment for patients with advanced EGFR mutation-positive non-small-cell lung cancer (OPTIMAL, CTONG-0802): a multicentre, open-label, randomised, phase 3 study. *Lancet Oncol.* 2011;12:735–742.

30. Palayekar MJ, Herzog TJ. The emerging role of epidermal growth factor receptor inhibitors in ovarian cancer. *Int J Gynecol Cancer.* 2008;18:879–890.

31. Romond EH, Perez EA, Bryant J, et al. Trastuzumab plus adjuvant chemotherapy for operable HER2-positive breast cancer. *N Engl J Med.* 2005;353:1673–1684.

32. McAlpine JN, Weigand KC, Vang R, et al. HER2 overexpression and amplification is present in a subset of ovarian mucinous carcinomas and can be targeted with trastuzumab therapy. *BMC Cancer.* 2009;9:433.

33. Prahallad A, Sun C, Huang S, et al. Unresponsiveness of colon cancer to BRAF(V600E) inhibition through feedback activation of EGFR. *Nature.* 2012;483:100–103.

34. Prentice RL, Thomson CA, Cann BJ, et al. Low-fat dietary pattern and cancer incidence in the Women's Health Initiative Dietary Modification Randomized Controlled Trial. *J Natl Cancer Inst.* 2007;99:1534–1543.

35. Chlebowski RT, Blackburn GL, Thomson CA, et al. Dietary fat reduction and breast cancer outcome: interim efficacy results from the Women's Intervention Nutrition Study. *J Natl Cancer Inst.* 2006;98:1767–1776.

36. Pierce JP, Newman VA, Flatt SW, et al. Telephone counseling intervention increases intakes of micronutrient- and phytochemical-rich vegetables, fruit and fiber in breast cancer survivors. *J Nutr.* 2004;134:452–458.

37. Pierce JP, Natarajan L, Sun S, et al. Increases in plasma carotenoid concentrations in response to a major dietary change in the women's healthy eating and living study. *Cancer Epid Biomarkers Prev.* 2006;15:1886–1892.

38. Rose SA, Dwyer J, Umer A, et al. Introduction: diet, epigenetic events and cancer prevention. *Nutr Rev.* 2008;66:S1–S6.

39. Protani MM, Nagle CM, Webb PM. Obesity and ovarian cancer survival: a systematic review and meta-analysis. *Cancer Prev Res.* 2012;5:901–910.

32 Integrative Medicine in Gynecologic Oncology

AMY STENSON

TANJA PEJOVIC

■ DEFINITION AND HISTORY

Integrative medicine is defined as "the practice of medicine that reaffirms the importance of the relationship between practitioner and patient, focuses on the whole person, is informed by evidence, and makes use of all appropriate therapeutic approaches, health care professionals, and disciplines to achieve optimal health and healing (1). Integrative oncology applies that philosophy to the complex care of patients with cancer in an effort to encompass both conventional therapy (surgical, chemotherapy, molecular, and radiotherapy) and complementary or alternative approaches with the intent of optimizing treatment and increasing quality of life (2). Integrative oncology seeks to treat the whole person and emphasizes awareness and sensitivity to the mental, emotional, and spiritual needs of the patient (3). The Society for Integrative Oncology (SIO) is an international organization dedicated to these pursuits. SIO has assembled panels of experts to help health care professionals make evidence-based decisions. Practice guidelines have been developed, are continuously updated, and are available on the SIO website (www.integrativeOnc.org; 4).

A distinction should be made between "complementary" and "alternative" therapies. While alternative therapies are promoted as a substitution for mainstream care and generally do not have scientific foundations, complementary medicine seeks unconventional treatment modalities with known efficacy. Complementary therapies are typically combined with standard oncologic care to enhance treatment effectiveness, increase overall wellness, or decrease the adverse side effects of conventional therapy.

■ EPIDEMIOLOGY

Complementary and alternative medicine (CAM) use in oncology is common. Patients may seek these therapies to augment or replace traditional treatments.

The National Center for Health Statistics has conducted surveys to assess the use of CAM in the United States. Among U.S. adults surveyed (n = 31,044), 50% used some form of CAM and an additional 25% used prayer to improve their health (5). Studies of CAM use in cancer patients reveal that a large proportion of patients use some form of complementary or alternative therapy (studies range from 10%–80% depending on the definition of CAM), with the majority using it in addition to traditional therapy. A recent study of patients undergoing radiation showed that 38% used CAM, that they on average spent about $300/month, and that only 40% discussed its use with their health care provider (HCP; 6). Another study reported CAM initiation rates of about 50% after a cancer diagnosis; and that rates of use were higher among females and patients with higher education levels (7). In 2002, a study of women with gynecologic cancer showed that while nearly half (49.6%) used CAM, only a quarter of those patients discussed this with their physician (8). Women in this study reported improved psychosocial well-being, increased hope, and optimism as being the more important benefits of CAM therapies. Surveys have demonstrated that cancer patients do not rely on HCPs for CAM information, but rather seek this information from friends, media, and the Internet (9,10). It is therefore difficult for them to discern the level of evidence that exist to support a given therapy.

Cancer patients are often reluctant to discuss the use of CAM with HCP. Patients may believe their HCP will object or be indifferent to the use of CAM, or consider that the HCP may not be knowledgeable in these areas. This perception leads to a gap in communication and trust between the patient and their HCP, which can result in dangerous alternative therapy use or unpredictable side effects. It is important for HCPs to remain open to the use of CAM, to inquire about its use on a routine basis, and to obtain a basic working knowledge of what the most common CAM therapies entail in order to provide instructive guidance to patients regarding these issues. Patients supported by their HCPs in the exploration of CAM therapies are less likely to pursue dangerous or unproven alternatives and are more likely to adhere to evidence-based therapies (4). It is therefore recommended that HCPs inquire about

CAM as a routine evaluation of cancer patients and that they provide guidance about the advantages and limitations of different complementary therapies in an evidence-based, patient-centered manner.

In this chapter, we will focus on the integrative use of complementary therapies to promote health and healing for patients with gynecologic cancer. There are limited data in this arena and great need for further investigation. Recommendations will be made based on the limited data that exist, extrapolation from other fields, and experience of the authors. It is also useful to consider the risk of potential harm vs the probability that something might be helpful. It is of primary importance to "do no harm" by assessing the safety of a proposed intervention, even if the efficacy is unknown. If deemed safe, then a discussion can be held regarding likely benefit to the patient and the financial implications of the therapy.

■ MASSAGE THERAPY

Massage involves manual manipulation of soft tissues to promote relaxation, relieve tension, and enhance well-being. In cancer patients, it has been shown to reduce anxiety, pain, fatigue, and distress (11,12). It may also play a role in control of nausea (13,14). There are a variety of massage techniques described including Swedish, Thai, shiatsu, aromatherapy, reflexology, and acupressure. Other bodywork techniques address posture and movement. A well-accepted practice in the care of breast cancer patients involves manual lymph drainage to decrease edema. For cancer patients, massage therapy may help alleviate anxiety or pain and may be recommended as part of holistic cancer care. The addition of aromatherapy has been associated with improved anxiety and mood for up to 6 weeks after the session (15). In patients with ovarian cancer, regular massage use has been associated with reduced feelings of hopelessness (16).

Massage therapy is generally safe when performed by trained therapists. For any cancer patient, care should be taken to avoid deep or intense pressure near cancer lesions, enlarged lymph nodes, radiation fields, medical devices, or in patients with a bleeding tendency. Vigorous lower limb massage should be avoided in patients with deep venous thrombosis (17).

■ MIND–BODY MEDICINE

There is an innate belief that what we think and feel can influence our health and healing. Chronic stress has been shown to have negative health consequences and may play a role in disease progression and overall mortality (18,19). The psychological and social impacts of stress are significant, leading to increased suffering from anxiety, depression, or other emotional problems. Mind–body medicine aims to address these issues and restore control to the patient. Meditation, hypnosis, relaxation techniques, cognitive-behavioral therapy, biofeedback, guided imagery, yoga, and Tai Chi are some examples of mind–body medicine that are becoming part of an integrative approach to care (20). Mindfulness-based stress reduction has been associated with improved mood- and stress-related symptoms for up to 6 months postintervention (21). Limited data also suggest improved immune function (increased NK cell cytotoxicity, decreased inflammation and cortisol levels; 22). Yoga has been shown to improve sleep quality, increase emotional well-being, decrease anxiety, and diminish chemotherapy-associated nausea (23–25). Tai Chi has been associated with increased aerobic function, strength, self-esteem, flexibility, and quality of life for patients with breast cancer (26,27). Relaxation techniques can significantly decrease stress, anger, fatigue, and anxiety without side effects (28). Given the safety, demonstrated efficacy, and acceptability of these modalities they may be widely recommended to patients undergoing treatment for cancer.

■ MUSIC THERAPY

Music therapy is usually geared to a patient's specific situation and experience with music. It can involve listening to, creating, or talking about music with a trained music therapist. A variety of music therapy interventions have been shown to have beneficial effects on anxiety, pain, mood, and quality of life. Music therapy has also been documented to be associated with small reductions in pulse, respiratory rate, and blood pressure (29). In one study, patients participating in music therapy showed increased relaxation and energy as well as increased salivary Immunoglobulin A (IgA), and lower cortisol levels (30). Another benefit has been an improved ability to communicate feelings such as fear or sadness, and to manage stress (31). Additionally, some benefit of music therapy on the quality of life for people in end-of-life care has been suggested (32). Given the safety of music, it may be recommended for cancer patients to alleviate symptoms and improve quality of life.

■ PHYSICAL ACTIVITY

The positive effects of exercise on overall health have been well documented. A recent Cochrane database review demonstrated the positive effects of exercise among cancer patient undergoing active treatment at 12 weeks and 6 months after program initiation (33). A wide variety of exercise modalities were evaluated and included walking, cycling, resistance training, strength training, yoga, and qigong. Beneficial effects included improved overall health-related quality of life, decreased anxiety, depression and fatigue, and improved sleep, emotional well-being, physical functioning, and mood. The review also suggested that moderate to vigorous intensity programs have more pronounced effects than mild-intensity programs. A similar review analyzed the effect of exercise for cancer survivors and also demonstrated improved self-esteem and positive effects on emotional well-being, sexuality, sleep patterns, social functioning, anxiety, fatigue, and pain (34).

Further research is needed to evaluate the effects of exercise by cancer type and treatment modality. Additional investigation should be promoted to identify the appropriate intensity, duration, and type of exercise to optimize outcomes. Given the complexity of cancer care and the variation in patient preferences, it is reasonable to individualize exercise programs to meet the needs and desires of each patient. A major goal of any program will be to ensure that the patient is motivated to continue to participate and has the support needed to do so. Adjustments should be made for patients during adjuvant therapy including reducing the duration or intensity of the program as needed. After treatment one of two general public health guidelines can be followed: (a) 20 minutes of vigorous exercise at least 3 days/week or (b) 30 minutes of moderate intensity exercise on more than 5 days/week (35).

Energy Therapy

Examples of energy therapies are Reiki, healing touch, polarity therapy, and qigong. Energy therapy is thought to exert its effect through manipulation of a patient's bioenergy and may involve light touch, mind–body interaction, and positive expectations. Healing touch has even demonstrated benefits for patients without physical contact. These therapies may alleviate stress, enhance relaxation, and provide a sense of protection or safety to patients. Commonly reported effects are relaxation and calming (36). A recent Cochrane review showed a modest effect in pain relief (37). Certification is available for HCPs on healing touch after participation in an educational program (38). Bioelectromagnetic therapies have not been shown to be helpful for control of cancer symptoms, progression, or in the treatment of menopausal symptoms (39).

Acupuncture

Acupuncture originated from traditional Chinese medicine and employs the use of needle, heat, or pressure stimulation to specific points on the body to regulate the flow of "qi" (vital energy). It has been shown to effectively treat both acute and chronic pain; studies have demonstrated efficacy of acupuncture for headaches, postoperative pain, and cancer-related pain (40–42). Benefits of acupuncture

for cancer-related pain clearly outweigh risks and this modality can be recommended for patients.

Acupuncture has also been shown to safely reduce chemotherapy-related nausea and vomiting and may be as effective as antiemetic medications (43,44). A study of patients with ovarian cancer in 2009 evaluated the role of combining vitamin B6 and acupuncture treatment to relieve nausea and vomiting, showing significant synergistic benefit of this treatment in decreasing nausea and vomiting (45). A recent review further advocated acupuncture's benefits for the treatment of postoperative gastroparesis, opioid-induced constipation, opioid-induced pruritus, chemotherapy-induced neuropathy, and joint or neck pain related to cancer treatment (46). In patients with gynecologic malignancy undergoing chemotherapy, acupuncture has been shown to mitigate the effects of chemotherapy on white blood cell values and suggests a myeloprotective effect of acupuncture (47).

In the United States, acupuncture needles are regulated as medical devices and must be sterile, single use, filiform, and very thin (28–40 gauge). It is considered very safe when performed by well-trained practitioners. Minor adverse events, such as minor pain or bleeding, occur in less than 0.05% of patients (48). However, care should be taken in patients with bleeding tendency and some believe it should be avoided at tumor sites (4).

■ NUTRITION

It is well known that a healthy diet plays an important role in reducing the risk of cancer. It has also been well documented that a patient's nutritional status is an important influence on healing from surgery in patients with gynecologic malignancy (49). Patients will often seek to optimize their own health and wellness through attention to nutrition after a cancer diagnosis is made. The U.S. Department of Agriculture recommends that half of the diet should be fruits and vegetables (preferable fresh), a quarter come from whole grains, and the other quarter lean protein sources such as seafood, legumes, poultry, eggs, or red-meat sources.

The American Institute on Cancer Prevention and the World Cancer Research Fund have made the following recommendations regarding lifestyle choices and cancer prevention in a recent document (50):

1. Be as lean as possible without becoming underweight
2. Be physically active for at least 30 minutes every day
3. Avoid sugary drinks and limit consumption of energy-dense foods.
4. Eat a variety of vegetables, fruits, whole grains, and legumes
5. Limit consumption of red meats and avoid processed meats

6. Limit alcoholic beverages to 2 per day (men) and 1 per day (women)
7. Limit consumption of salty foods
8. Do not use supplements to prevent cancer
9. Mothers should breastfeed exclusively for 6 months if possible
10. After treatment, cancer survivors should follow nutritional recommendations for cancer prevention

Many malignancies are associated with obesity (e.g., endometrial, breast) and there is some evidence that a diet high in saturated fat may elevate that risk (51). In addition, it is thought that glucose regulation and elevated insulin levels may play a role in the development of cancer. It has been shown that for women with endometrial cancer, there was an increase in all cause and cancer-related mortality for obese women (52). Type 2 diabetes is also associated with the development of endometrial cancer (53).

■ DIETARY SUPPLEMENTS

Although many patients take dietary supplements to augment outcomes during cancer treatment, there is very little strong scientific evidence to support this practice to prevent cancer recurrence. Most of the literature regarding the role of supplements in prevention and treatment of cancer in women is available for breast cancer. Far less is known about potential benefits of supplements in women with gynecologic cancers.

Ovarian Cancer

Oxidative damage can transform normal to malignant cells. There is a lot of popular and other press that boosts the use of antioxidants to counteract tissue damage and decrease cancer risk. In some cases mega-doses of vitamin A, beta-carotene, and vitamin C are recommended. The evidence for this practice is very weak; however, antioxidant intake from dietary sources might be of benefit. For example, there is some evidence a diet rich in carotenoids, including beta-carotene and especially alpha-carotene, can decrease the risk of ovarian cancer in postmenopausal women (54).

Women who regularly consume tea, including green tea or black tea, appear to have a significantly lower risk of developing ovarian cancer compared to women who seldom drink tea (55,56). In one prospective population study, women who consume two or more cups of tea daily have a 46% lower risk of ovarian cancer compared to women who do not regularly consume tea (56). There also appears to be a trend that suggests higher consumption of tea or longer duration of use further reduces the risk of ovarian cancer. Green tea is not fermented, to differ from black tea, and it usually contains a greater amount of the natural constituents of tea leaves. One of the constituents of tea, epigallocatechin gallate (EGCG), is a polyphenolic compound thought to have several anticancer properties. EGCG is an antioxidant and free radical scavenger. There is also some evidence that it might induce certain enzymes that detoxify carcinogens and possibly decrease new blood vessel growth (angiogenesis) in tumors (57). There is no evidence for benefit of consuming green tea tablets or pills.

Cervical Dysplasia

Green tea as an oral or topical preparation seems to reduce cervical dysplasia caused by human papillomavirus (HPV) infection (58). In addition treatment with indole-3-carbinol for 12 weeks led to complete regression of CIN in 45%–50% of patients with Stage II and Stage III CIN. Lower doses of 200 mg per day seem to be just as effective as higher doses of 400 mg per day (59). The evidence for the role of beta-all-trans-retinoic acid for mild or moderate intraepithelial cervical neoplasia is considered insufficient.

Endometrial Cancer

There is some evidence that women who regularly consume approximately 2 servings per week of fatty fish have a reduced risk for endometrial cancer (60). The evidence for the role of lignans including flaxseed and increased soy intake in decreasing uterine cancer risk is insufficient (61,62).

■ POSTTREATMENT SEXUAL DYSFUNCTION AND MENOPAUSAL SYMPTOMS

Women with gynecologic cancer are a particularly vulnerable group that may greatly benefit from a comprehensive integrated gynecologic cancer program. With improvement in early detection and therapy for gynecologic cancer, long-term survival is common. Women with gynecologic cancer not only face the treatment side effects of general chemotherapy and radiation but because of the location of disease and the effect that treatment has on the sexual and reproductive organs, women often deal with issues surrounding sexuality, intimacy, and self-image. Treatment of gynecologic malignancy with surgery, chemotherapy, and/or pelvic radiation has profound effects on the female reproductive system. Optimal cancer treatment often results in removal or radiation of the ovaries, uterus, pelvic lymph nodes, vagina, and vulva. Pelvic surgery has the potential to result in vaginal shortening, scarring, or postoperative pain. Pelvic radiation can lead to significant scarring of the vagina, making penetrative intercourse uncomfortable and in some cases impossible. These changes result in an immense impact on the quality of life in patients with all gynecologic cancers (63).

In addition, removal of the ovaries as part of the treatment recommendations for most types of gynecologic cancer results in the rapid onset of menopausal symptoms. Decreased levels of estrogen and possibly minor circulating androgens may lead to decreased libido, atrophy of the vagina, and/or painful intercourse. Some women also experience changes in overall mood and energy levels. Changes in sexuality have been reported in several studies in different populations of women receiving radiation treatment, surgery, chemotherapy, and immunotherapy (64). Systemic chemotherapy and radical pelvic surgery have been reported to have the greatest impact on sexual functioning (65).

Additionally, evidence is emerging that cancer survivors suffer cognitive impairment as a result of chemotherapy. Such cognitive impairments are often referred to as "chemo brain" or "chemo fog" (66). These studies have concluded that there is evidence for cognitive changes associated with cancer and cancer treatments and that cognitive deficits are diffuse, and involve the domains of attention and concentration, verbal and visual memory, and processing speed (66).

However, cognition assessment has never been performed in women treated for gynecologic cancers. These women are affected not only by the chemotherapy treatment, but, in majority of cases, also by hormonal changes of menopause. For example Shaywitz et al using MRI showed improved activation in the inferior parietal lobule during storage of verbal material when postmenopausal women were treated with supplemental estrogen (67).

Interventions to Improve Sexuality and Intimacy

Hormone replacement therapy (HRT) for women with treatment-induced menopausal symptoms has the potential to significantly improve quality of life. When there is a need to avoid estrogen or progesterone (e.g., ER/PR positive tumor histology) there are several alternatives available. Gabapentin (600–2400 mg/day) has been shown to significantly decrease the intensity and frequency of hot flushes (68–70). Most common side effects reported were somnolence or dizziness and these improved after 2 weeks of therapy. Selective serotonin reuptake inhibitor (SSRI) and serotonin–norepinephrine reuptake inhibitor (SNRI) have also been shown to diminish the symptoms of menopause (71); however, relapse is common when use is discontinued and women may experience side effects such as decreased libido (72). For women with hypoactive sexual desire disorder, transdermal testosterone has been shown to be safe and effective and may be considered (73,74).

Women frequently seek alternative therapies to ameliorate the symptoms of menopause. Phytoestrogens are most commonly used (e.g., red clover extract, soy products); however, a large meta-analysis concluded that they are ineffective (75). Black cohosh appears to be safe, have the biggest benefit in improving the symptoms of menopause, and evidence supports its use (76). For mood-related symptoms, consideration can be given to the use of St John's wort (76).

Although gynecologic cancer therapies frequently have a significant impact on sexuality, intimacy, and quality of life, very little data exist regarding these issues (77). Further research and focus on this area is imperative. For women with complaints of dyspareunia, vaginal pain, or discomfort, the use of vaginal dilators, pelvic physical therapy, topical emollients, topical estrogens, and topical anesthetics may improve sexual function for some patients and exploration into these areas should be encouraged (78). Nightly application of 4%–5% lidocaine solution has been shown to decrease dyspareunia in patients with vulvar vestibulitis (79). This may also be applied before or after intercourse as needed. For women with vaginal shortening or constriction, use of dilators and/or physical therapy may help to regain sexual function (80). Psychosocial counseling regarding body image, sexuality, health, and relationships may be considered an important part of holistic healing for patients recovering from gynecologic cancer.

■ POTENTIAL RISKS OF COMPLEMENTARY MEDICINE

Potential risks of any complementary or alternative therapy should be considered in patients recovering from cancer. Unfortunately, there is a lack of quality control for supplements, making it difficult to assess content safety (81). Some botanical supplements may interact with prescription medications, chemotherapy, or radiation resulting in decreased efficacy or increased toxicity (82,83). Another consideration is the costs of CAM therapies, which can be substantial for some patients who are paying out of pocket. It is important to inquire about CAM use, to discuss these issues openly and honestly with patients, and apply both common sense and the best scientific evidence available to assess the risk/benefit ratio on a case-by-case basis.

■ CONCLUSIONS

The use of CAM for patients with gynecologic cancer is common and should be discussed with patients as part of an integrative and holistic approach to treatment. Attention to nutrition, exercise, and stress management is likely to result in improved wellness, quality of life, and in some cases prognosis. Mind–body approaches such as meditation, yoga, Tai Chi, music therapy, relaxation techniques, and massage have been shown to decrease stress/anxiety/anger, improve mood, decrease treatment side effects, increase quality of life, and may augment immune function. There is some evidence that green tea can prevent and/or augment resolution of gynecologic cancer or precancers. The impact of gynecologic cancer treatment on sexuality, intimacy, and menopausal symptoms is significant. Approaches to ameliorate these impacts include the use of HRT, gabapentin, SSRI/SNRIs, black cohosh, pelvic physical therapy, vaginal dilators, topical anesthetics, and psychosocial counseling. Complementary therapies are recommended as part of the holistic care of patients with gynecologic cancer and are likely to improve the quality of life and outcomes for patients undergoing treatment.

■ REFERENCES

1. Kligler B, Maizes V, Schachter S, et al.; Education Working Group, Consortium of Academic Health Centers for Integrative Medicine. Core competencies in integrative medicine for medical school curricula: a proposal. *Acad Med.* 2004;79(6): 521–531.

2. Sagar SM. The integrative oncology supplement–a paradigm for both patient care and communication. *Curr Oncol.* 2008;15(4):166–167.

3. Remen RN. Practicing a medicine of the whole person: an opportunity for healing. *Hematol Oncol Clin North Am.* 2008;22(4):767–773, x.

4. Deng GE, Frenkel M, Cohen L, et al.; Society for Integrative Oncology. Evidence-based clinical practice guidelines for integrative oncology: complementary therapies and botanicals. *J Soc Integr Oncol.* 2009;7(3):85–120.

5. Barnes PM, Powell-Griner E, McFann K, Nahin RL. Complementary and alternative medicine use among adults: United States, 2002. *Adv Data.* 2004:1–19.

6. Gillett J, Ientile C, Hiscock J, Plank A, Martin JM. Complementary and alternative medicine use in radiotherapy: what are patients using? *J Altern Complement Med.* 2012;18(11):1014–1020.

7. Vapiwala N, Mick R, Hampshire MK, Metz JM, DeNittis AS. Patient initiation of complementary and alternative medical therapies (CAM) following cancer diagnosis. *Cancer J.* 2006;12(6):467–474.

8. Swisher EM, Cohn DE, Goff BA, et al. Use of complementary and alternative medicine among women with gynecologic cancers. *Gynecol Oncol.* 2002;84(3):363–367.

9. Hyodo I, Amano N, Eguchi K, et al. Nationwide survey on complementary and alternative medicine in cancer patients in Japan. *J Clin Oncol.* 2005;23(12):2645–2654.

10. Molassiotis A, Fernadez-Ortega P, Pud D, et al. Use of complementary and alternative medicine in cancer patients: a European survey. *Ann Oncol.* 2005;16(4):655–663.

11. Ahles TA, Tope DM, Pinkson B, et al. Massage therapy for patients undergoing autologous bone marrow transplantation. *J Pain Symptom Manage.* 1999;18(3):157–163.

12. Grealish L, Lomasney A, Whiteman B. Foot massage. A nursing intervention to modify the distressing symptoms of pain and nausea in patients hospitalized with cancer. *Cancer Nurs.* 2000;23(3):237–243.

13. Mehling WE, Jacobs B, Acree M, et al. Symptom management with massage and acupuncture in postoperative cancer patients: a randomized controlled trial. *J Pain Symptom Manage.* 2007;33(3):258–266.

14. Billhult A, Bergbom I, Stener-Victorin E. Massage relieves nausea in women with breast cancer who are undergoing chemotherapy. *J Altern Complement Med.* 2007;13(1):53–57.

15. Wilkinson SM, Love SB, Westcombe AM, et al. Effectiveness of aromatherapy massage in the management of anxiety and depression in patients with cancer: a multicenter randomized controlled trial. *J Clin Oncol.* 2007;25(5):532–539.

16. Gross AH, Cromwell J, Fonteyn M, Matulonis UA, Hayman LL. Hopelessness and complementary therapy use in patients with ovarian cancer. *Cancer Nurs.* 2013 Jul-Aug;36(4):256–264.

17. Jabr FI. Massive pulmonary emboli after legs massage. *Am J Phys Med Rehabil.* 2007;86(8):691.

18. Antoni MH, Lutgendorf SK, Cole SW, et al. The influence of bio-behavioural factors on tumour biology: pathways and mechanisms. *Nat Rev Cancer.* 2006;6(3):240–248.

19. Glaser R, Kiecolt-Glaser JK. Stress-induced immune dysfunction: implications for health. *Nat Rev Immunol.* 2005;5(3):243–251.

20. Astin JA. Mind-body therapies for the management of pain. *Clin J Pain.* 2004;20(1):27–32.

21. Carlson LE, Ursuliak Z, Goodey E, Angen M, Speca M. The effects of a mindfulness meditation-based stress reduction program on mood and symptoms of stress in cancer outpatients: 6-month follow-up. *Support Care Cancer.* 2001;9(2):112–123.

22. Witek-Janusek L, Albuquerque K, Chroniak KR, Chroniak C, Durazo-Arvizu R, Mathews HL. Effect of mindfulness based stress reduction on immune function, quality of life and coping in women newly diagnosed with early stage breast cancer. *Brain Behav Immun.* 2008;22(6):969–981.

23. Cohen L, Warneke C, Fouladi RT, Rodriguez MA, Chaoul-Reich A. Psychological adjustment and sleep quality in a randomized trial of the effects of a Tibetan yoga intervention in patients with lymphoma. *Cancer.* 2004;100(10):2253–2260.

24. Moadel AB, Shah C, Wylie-Rosett J, et al. Randomized controlled trial of yoga among a multiethnic sample of breast cancer patients: effects on quality of life. *J Clin Oncol.* 2007;25(28):4387–4395.

25. Raghavendra RM, Nagarathna R, Nagendra HR, et al. Effects of an integrated yoga programme on chemotherapy-induced nausea and emesis in breast cancer patients. *Eur J Cancer Care (Engl).* 2007;16(6):462–474.

26. Mustian KM, Katula JA, Zhao H. A pilot study to assess the influence of tai chi chuan on functional capacity among breast cancer survivors. *J Support Oncol.* 2006;4(3):139–145.

27. Mustian KM, Katula JA, Gill DL, Roscoe JA, Lang D, Murphy K. Tai Chi Chuan, health-related quality of life and self-esteem: a randomized trial with breast cancer survivors. *Support Care Cancer.* 2004;12(12):871–876.

28. Decker TW, Cline-Elsen J, Gallagher M. Relaxation therapy as an adjunct in radiation oncology. *J Clin Psychol.* 1992; 48(3):388–393.

29. Bradt J, Goodill SW, Dileo C. Dance/movement therapy for improving psychological and physical outcomes in cancer patients. *Cochrane Database Syst Rev.* 2011;(10):CD007103.

30. Burns SJ, Harbuz MS, Hucklebridge F, Bunt L. A pilot study into the therapeutic effects of music therapy at a cancer help center. *Altern Ther Health Med.* 2001;7(1):48–56.

31. Richardson MM, Babiak-Vazquez AE, Frenkel MA. Music therapy in a comprehensive cancer center. *J Soc Integr Oncol.* 2008;6(2):76–81.

32. Bradt J, Dileo C. Music therapy for end-of-life care. *Cochrane Database Syst Rev.* CD007169.

33. Mishra SI, Scherer RW, Snyder C, Geigle PM, Berlanstein DR, Topaloglu O. Exercise interventions on health-related quality of life for people with cancer during active treatment. *Cochrane Database Syst Rev.* 2012;8:CD008465.

34. Mishra SI, Scherer RW, Geigle PM, et al. Exercise interventions on health-related quality of life for cancer survivors. *Cochrane Database Syst Rev.* 8:CD007566.

35. Doyle C, Kushi LH, Byers T, et al.; 2006 Nutrition, Physical Activity and Cancer Survivorship Advisory Committee; American Cancer Society. Nutrition and physical activity during and after cancer treatment: an American Cancer Society guide for informed choices. *CA Cancer J Clin.* 2006;56(6):323–353.

36. Cook CA, Guerrerio JF, Slater VE. Healing touch and quality of life in women receiving radiation treatment for cancer: a randomized controlled trial. *Altern Ther Health Med.* 2004;10(3):34–41.

37. So PS, Jiang Y, Qin Y. Touch therapies for pain relief in adults. *Cochrane Database Syst Rev.* 2008:CD006535.

38. Engebretson J, Wardell DW. Energy-based modalities. *Nurs Clin North Am.* 2007;42(2):243–259, vi.

39. Carpenter JS, Neal JG. Other complementary and alternative medicine modalities: acupuncture, magnets, reflexology, and homeopathy. *Am J Med.* 2005;118 Suppl 12B:109–117.

40. Melchart D, Linde K, Fischer P, et al. Acupuncture for recurrent headaches: a systematic review of randomized controlled trials. *Cephalalgia.* 1999;19(9):779–786; discussion 765.

41. Alimi D, Rubino C, Pichard-Léandri E, Fermand-Brulé S, Dubreuil-Lemaire ML, Hill C. Analgesic effect of auricular acupuncture for cancer pain: a randomized, blinded, controlled trial. *J Clin Oncol.* 2003;21(22):4120–4126.

42. Crew KD, Capodice JL, Greenlee H, et al. Pilot study of acupuncture for the treatment of joint symptoms related to adjuvant aromatase inhibitor therapy in postmenopausal breast cancer patients. *J Cancer Surviv.* 2007;1(4):283–291.

43. Ezzo JM, Richardson MA, Vickers A, et al. Acupuncture-point stimulation for chemotherapy-induced nausea or vomiting. *Cochrane Database Syst Rev.* 2006:CD002285.

44. Lee A, Fan LT. Stimulation of the wrist acupuncture point P6 for preventing postoperative nausea and vomiting. *Cochrane Database Syst Rev.* 2009:CD003281.

45. You Q, Yu H, Wu D, Zhang Y, Zheng J, Peng C. Vitamin B6 points PC6 injection during acupuncture can relieve nausea and vomiting in patients with ovarian cancer. *Int J Gynecol Cancer.* 2009;19(4):567–571.

46. Lu W, Rosenthal DS. Acupuncture for cancer pain and related symptoms. *Curr Pain Headache Rep.* 2013;17(3):321.

47. Lu W, Matulonis UA, Doherty-Gilman A, et al. Acupuncture for chemotherapy-induced neutropenia in patients with gynecologic malignancies: a pilot randomized, sham-controlled clinical trial. *J Altern Complement Med.* 2009;15(7):745–753.

48. Melchart D, Weidenhammer W, Streng A, et al. Prospective investigation of adverse effects of acupuncture in 97 733 patients. *Arch Intern Med.* 2004;164(1):104–105.

49. Kathiresan AS, Brookfield KF, Schuman SI, Lucci JA 3rd. Malnutrition as a predictor of poor postoperative outcomes in gynecologic cancer patients. *Arch Gynecol Obstet.* 2011;284(2):445–451.

50. Wiseman M. The second World Cancer Research Fund/American Institute for Cancer Research expert report. Food, nutrition, physical activity, and the prevention of cancer: a global perspective. *Proc Nutr Soc.* 2008;67(3):253–256.

51. Lindemann K, Vatten LJ, Ellstrøm-Engh M, Eskild A. Body mass, diabetes and smoking, and endometrial cancer risk: a follow-up study. *Br J Cancer.* 2008;98(9):1582–1585.

52. Chia VM, Newcomb PA, Trentham-Dietz A, Hampton JM. Obesity, diabetes, and other factors in relation to survival after endometrial cancer diagnosis. *Int J Gynecol Cancer.* 2007;17(2):441–446.

53. Saltzman BS, Doherty JA, Hill DA, et al. Diabetes and endometrial cancer: an evaluation of the modifying effects of other known risk factors. *Am J Epidemiol.* 2008;167(5):607–614.

54. Cramer DW, Kuper H, Harlow BL, Titus-Ernstoff L. Carotenoids, antioxidants and ovarian cancer risk in pre- and postmenopausal women. *Int J Cancer.* 2001;94(1):128–134.

55. Zhang M, Binns CW, Lee AH. Tea consumption and ovarian cancer risk: a case-control study in China. *Cancer Epidemiol Biomarkers Prev.* 2002;11(8):713–718.

56. Larsson SC, Wolk A. Tea consumption and ovarian cancer risk in a population-based cohort. *Arch Intern Med.* 2005;165(22):2683–2686.

57. Gupta S, Saha B, Giri AK. Comparative antimutagenic and anticlastogenic effects of green tea and black tea: a review. *Mutat Res.* 2002;512(1):37–65.

58. Ahn WS, Yoo J, Huh SW, et al. Protective effects of green tea extracts (polyphenon E and EGCG) on human cervical lesions. *Eur J Cancer Prev.* 2003;12(5):383–390.

59. Bell MC, Crowley-Nowick P, Bradlow HL, et al. Placebo-controlled trial of indole-3-carbinol in the treatment of CIN. *Gynecol Oncol.* 2000;78(2):123–129.

60. Terry PD, Rohan TE, Wolk A. Intakes of fish and marine fatty acids and the risks of cancers of the breast and prostate and of other hormone-related cancers: a review of the epidemiologic evidence. *Am J Clin Nutr.* 2003;77(3):532–543.

61. Zeleniuch-Jacquotte A, Lundin E, Micheli A, et al. Circulating enterolactone and risk of endometrial cancer. *Int J Cancer.* 2006;119(10):2376–2381.

62. Goodman MT, Wilkens LR, Hankin JH, Lyu LC, Wu AH, Kolonel LN. Association of soy and fiber consumption with the risk of endometrial cancer. *Am J Epidemiol.* 1997;146(4):294–306.

63. Juraskova I, Butow P, Robertson R, Sharpe L, McLeod C, Hacker N. Post-treatment sexual adjustment following cervical and endometrial cancer: a qualitative insight. *Psychooncology.* 2003;12(3):267–279.

64. Wilmoth MC, Botchway P. Psychosexual implications of breast and gynecologic cancer. *Cancer Invest.* 1999;17(8):631–636.

65. Young-McCaughan S. Sexual functioning in women with breast cancer after treatment with adjuvant therapy. *Cancer Nurs.* 1996;19(4):308–319.

66. Ahles TA, Saykin AJ, Furstenberg CT, et al. Neuropsychologic impact of standard-dose systemic chemotherapy in long-term survivors of breast cancer and lymphoma. *J Clin Oncol.* 2002;20(2):485–493.

67. Shaywitz SE, Shaywitz BA, Pugh KR, et al. Effect of estrogen on brain activation patterns in postmenopausal women during working memory tasks. *JAMA.* 1999;281(13):1197–1202.

68. Hayes LP, Carroll DG, Kelley KW. Use of gabapentin for the management of natural or surgical menopausal hot flashes. *Ann Pharmacother.* 2011;45(3):388–394.

69. Butt DA, Lock M, Lewis JE, Ross S, Moineddin R. Gabapentin for the treatment of menopausal hot flashes: a randomized controlled trial. *Menopause.* 2008;15(2):310–318.

70. Pandya KJ, Morrow GR, Roscoe JA, et al. Gabapentin for hot flashes in 420 women with breast cancer: a randomised double-blind placebo-controlled trial. *Lancet.* 2005;366(9488):818–824.

71. Freeman EW, Guthrie KA, Caan B, et al. Efficacy of escitalopram for hot flashes in healthy menopausal women: a randomized controlled trial. *JAMA.* 2011;305(3):267–274.

72. Joffe H, Guthrie KA, Larson J, et al. Relapse of vasomotor symptoms after discontinuation of the selective serotonin reuptake inhibitor escitalopram: results from the menopause strategies: finding lasting answers for symptoms and health research network. *Menopause.* 2013;20(3):261–268.

73. Krapf JM, Simon JA. The role of testosterone in the management of hypoactive sexual desire disorder in postmenopausal women. *Maturitas.* 2009;63(3):213–219.

74. Davis SR, Braunstein GD. Efficacy and safety of testosterone in the management of hypoactive sexual desire disorder in postmenopausal women. *J Sex Med.* 2012;9(4):1134–1148.

75. Pitkin J. Alternative and complementary therapies for the menopause. *Menopause Int.* 2012;18(1):20–27.

76. Geller SE, Studee L. Botanical and dietary supplements for menopausal symptoms: what works, what does not. *J Womens Health (Larchmt).* 2005;14(7):634–649.

77. Carter J, Stabile C, Gunn A, Sonoda Y. The physical consequences of gynecologic cancer surgery and their impact on sexual,

emotional, and quality of life issues. *J Sex Med.* 2013;10 Suppl 1:21–34.

78. Goetsch MF. Unprovoked vestibular burning in late estrogen-deprived menopause: a case series. *J Low Genit Tract Dis.* 2012;16(4):442–446.

79. Zolnoun DA, Hartmann KE, Steege JF. Overnight 5% lidocaine ointment for treatment of vulvar vestibulitis. *Obstet Gynecol.* 2003;102(1):84–87.

80. Yang EJ, Lim JY, Rah UW, Kim YB. Effect of a pelvic floor muscle training program on gynecologic cancer survivors with pelvic floor dysfunction: a randomized controlled trial. *Gynecol Oncol.* 2012;125(3):705–711.

81. Sovak M, Seligson AL, Konas M, et al. Herbal composition PC-SPES for management of prostate cancer: identification of active principles. *J Natl Cancer Inst.* 2002;94(17):1275–1281.

82. Beijnen JH, Schellens JH. Drug interactions in oncology. *Lancet Oncol.* 2004;5(8):489–496.

83. Sparreboom A, Cox MC, Acharya MR, Figg WD. Herbal remedies in the United States: potential adverse interactions with anti-cancer agents. *J Clin Oncol.* 2004;22(12):2489–2503.

33 *Multidisciplinary Palliative Care*

PAUL BASCOM

■ INTRODUCTION

Despite the considerable advances in the treatment of gynecological cancers, there are many patients for whom treatment ultimately fails to forestall the progression of their disease. For patients whose disease cannot be cured or even controlled, palliative care is indicated. This chapter will highlight some principles of palliative care useful in the management of gynecological cancer patients, whose disease and symptom burden are no longer responsive to treatment.

■ DEFINITIONS

The word "palliative" stems from the Latin root *pallium,* which means "shield or cloak." Palliative care can be understood as care that shields a patient from the burdens of an advancing cancer. The word palliative can have quite distinct connotations, depending on the clinical circumstance in which it is employed and on the understanding of the person employing the term:

Palliative Versus Curative

In the realm of cancer treatment, the term palliative is used in contrast to the word "curative," specifically in terms of the goal of therapy. When it is determined that a cancer cannot be cured, the goal of therapy is said to be palliative. Palliative surgery, palliative chemotherapy, palliative radiation therapy—all refer to those treatments that are employed when cure is no longer the goal. These palliative treatments carry the expectation of modifying the course of the disease with response or remission and/or of prolonging life, though without the hope of cure.

Palliative/Disease Modifying Versus Palliative/ Limited to Control of Symptoms

In the realm of palliative care, the term palliative carries a much more focused clinical connotation. Typically,

palliative care refers to the managing the myriad of physical, psychological, social, and spiritual needs of the patient with progressive illness, without the expectation of altering the underlying course of the disease. For the purposes of this chapter, palliative will be used to describe this latter clinical scenario.

Generalized Palliative Care Versus Specialized Palliative Care

The term "generalized palliative care" describes a set of knowledge and skills that should be part of the armamentarium of any physician or institution caring for patients with advanced cancer. "Specialized palliative care" describes the distinct medical subspecialty and dedicated palliative care teams that have emerged over the last 2 decades, teams that provide a level of care beyond what would be expected of a generalist cancer physician. For the purposes of this chapter, "palliative care" will refer to the involvement of specialized palliative care teams. However, the basic principles of palliative care discussed herein can be employed by any physician caring for patients with advancing cancer.

Multidisciplinary Palliative Care

By definition, palliative care is multidisciplinary in nature and provided by a team, rather than by a single individual. Formal palliative care teams often include physicians, nurse practitioners, clinical nurse specialists, social workers, pharmacists, and chaplains. The scope of palliative care is broad and encompasses the physical, psychological, social, and spiritual dimensions of patient needs. Generalized palliative care is provided also by individual practitioners working in collaboration with other professionals at their institution, though without the formal affiliations that define a palliative care team. While each member of the team brings a special set of skills to each patient's care, also there can and should be substantial overlap. Physicians need some familiarity with counseling and other social work interventions, for example, while social workers ought to have some basic knowledge of pain assessment.

■ SCOPE OF SERVICE

Generally speaking, palliative care interventions can be separated into the domains of goal setting, symptom control, care coordination/discharge planning, and care in the last days of life (1). While diseases sometimes may be similar, patients can be quite unique in the particulars of their social situations, psychological make-ups, spiritual beliefs, and approaches to decision making. Specific guidelines or treatment protocols for palliative care will never be able to encompass this variability. Instead, this chapter will provide some important principles to keep in mind when caring for a patient who needs palliative care.

■ GOALS OF CARE

Perhaps the single most important domain of palliative care is that of clarifying goals of care. The typical goal of most medical treatment is to eliminate or control the underlying disease. That is what most patients "want" as well—to get better, to make their disease go away. As long as there is disease-directed therapy that carries a reasonable promise of forestalling death, or even of a cure, most patients will choose disease-directed therapy.

Palliative care often involves guiding patients and families to different goals when forestalling death for a while is no longer possible. Clarification of goals of care becomes necessary when treatments for the disease are no longer available or, at times, are no longer desired. This can happen a few weeks after diagnosis, or sometimes years. Once the goal of living longer has been let go, patients and families will be free to explore the many achievable goals available to them such as good symptom control, time at home with family, and peaceful dying in a location of their choosing. Attention to a realistic evaluation of disease status and the likely benefits of further treatment is essential and fundamental to good palliative care. Without a degree of certainty on the part of the physician that ongoing treatment is more likely harmful than beneficial, no patient should be expected to shift her goals away from disease-modifying treatment.

There are two fundamental skills needed to successfully guide patients toward wise decisions about goals of care. The first skill is the ability to accurately assess the chances of response to treatment. The usually comes a time in a disease trajectory where treatment is more likely to shorten life that prolong it (2). The second skill is to learn to accurately prognosticate about when death is nearing. The second fundamental skill is the ability to communicate these clinical realities in a direct, understandable, and compassionate manner to the patient and her family.

■ PROGNOSTICATION

Central to the process of guiding patients and families to explore other goals is the need for their physician to accurately assess prognosis. Studies have shown that physicians are poor at making accurate prognoses. In a study, upon referral to hospice, physicians routinely overestimated prognosis by a factor of 5 (3). This may represent lack of clinical knowledge, lack of understanding of the importance of accurate prognosis, cultural prejudices, or at times the fundamental uncertainty of a clinical course. There is some evidence that palliative care can provide a measure of increased accuracy in prognosis (4).

Prognostication can be challenging. Patients whose cancers share the same site of origin and stage may have a quite different illness trajectory. Average survival rates provide information about the average patient, yet do not account for the range of possible outcomes. In a study of surgical outcomes in the treatment of bowel obstruction for ovarian cancer, the median survival was 90 days, but the range spanned from less than 1 day to 6 years (5).

Two cases of ovarian cancer described below were identical at presentation yet had vastly different outcomes, thus highlighting this variability.

Case 1

A 70-year-old woman presented to her physician with abdominal swelling that had developed over the previous 4 weeks. Physical examination revealed cachexia and an abdominal fluid wave. Ultrasound demonstrated a large ovarian mass and moderate ascites. Diagnostic and therapeutic paracentesis confirmed the diagnosis of stage 3 ovarian cancer. Chemotherapy was initiated. Within a week of initial chemotherapy, the patient had experienced a steady decline and had become bedbound. Physical examination revealed rapid reaccumulation of ascites and an ECOG score of 4. Palliative care was consulted to help clarify goals of care, to manage the symptoms of impending death, and to provide emotional support for the family. Within a few days, the patient died in the hospital of rapidly advancing disease.

Case 2

A 70-year-old woman presented to her physician with abdominal swelling that had developed over the previous 4 weeks. Physical exam revealed a well-appearing woman with an abdominal fluid wave. Ultrasound demonstrated a large ovarian mass and moderate ascites. Diagnostic and therapeutic paracentesis confirmed the diagnosis of stage 3 ovarian cancer. Chemotherapy was initiated. The patient had a complete disease response with prompt improvement in symptoms. She required no further paracentesis. Over the ensuing years, when disease progression was noted, second- and third-line chemotherapeutic regimens were successful at restoring control of her disease. Six years later, palliative care was consulted when symptoms of partial small bowel obstruction developed and the options for chemotherapy had been exhausted. Palliative care helped to manage the nausea associated with the obstruction and to create a plan for care at home in the last weeks of the patient's life.

■ SHARING BAD NEWS

Once the physician is confident that the patient's disease is advancing and that there are no available treatments, the next fundamental and essential step is to share that information with the patient and the family. This information must be provided with skill and compassion. This information will force the patient to confront the reality and perhaps immediacy of dying. Some level of emotional distress is unavoidable. Even the most compassionate physician cannot make the news of one's death "okay." Importantly, patients and families cannot make informed and wise decisions about their goals and options without passing through some level of distress. Without confronting the reality of dying, patients will continue to make decisions for treatment based on their desire "not to die."

Doctors understandably prefer to avoid difficult conversations. It is always easier to avoid issues of mortality, and to instead recommend some treatment that "might" work. It is also easier for the physician to move responsibility for treatment decisions onto the patient. When the patient "refuses treatment," this shifts the responsibility for the decision onto the patient, and makes things less distressing for the physician. However, most patients, when given a choice between dying and not dying, will choose "not dying." To have a productive conversation with patients and their families about changing goals of care means ensuring that patients understand that "not dying" is no longer one of the options.

Communicating effectively with patients near the end of life is a skill that can be learned. Oncotalk is a National Cancer Institute-funded training program developed at the University of Washington that includes videos and other instructional aids to improve communication skills. Distilled to a couple of essential principles, the Oncotalk founders describe the twin goals of recognition and guidance as being particularly important in achieving effective and compassionate communication. Distilled to its essence, the training asks physician to reflect on their conversation with the patients and their families, asking themselves: "Have I demonstrated that I recognize the patient's experience hearing the news?" and "Have I provided guidance to the next steps?" (6).

■ SETTING ALTERNATIVE GOALS

Once the immediate emotional distress of accepting that one is dying of cancer has passed, many patients may feel relief and a heightened sense of emotional comfort. Studies of early palliative care consultation in patients with metastatic lung cancer demonstrated prompt improvement in quality of life, specifically in the domains of depression and emotional well-being (7). The reasons for this are still speculative. One possibility is that the palliative care intervention allowed patients to pivot from the inevitably elusive goal of avoiding dying to more achievable goals.

■ SYMPTOM CONTROL

Good control of physical symptoms is fundamental to palliative care, and begins with a comprehensive and accurate assessment of the source of the symptoms. Physical examination, radiographs, and laboratory tests can help illuminate what might be causing the symptom. At times, this may point to interventions that can alter the underlying condition. The best symptom relief is achieved by alleviation of the underlying condition. Many times, however, the underlying condition will prove inalterable, and pharmacological and nonpharmacological treatments will be the only remedies.

Ultimately, the patient's self-report of what they experience is the gold standard for symptom assessment. Clinical data only serve to direct what interventions might be useful for a specific symptom. Additionally, the patient is the only one who can determine when symptom control is adequate. For many patients, even a high of symptom burden is tolerable. For others, even modest symptoms are more than they can tolerate.

■ PAIN

Pain can be divided into several basic categories: visceral pain, somatic pain, and neuropathic pain. Patients with ovarian cancers will experience visceral pain from intra-abdominal spread of cancer. Patients with vulvar and cervical cancers may have more somatic pain from local spread of disease and direct extension into somatic tissues. Neuropathic pain can also occur from direct extension of cervical cancer into local nerves, or as a late complication of some chemotherapeutic regimens. In general, visceral pain is less severe and more responsive to opiate analgesics.

In contrast to the acute and transitory nature of postoperative pain, the pain associated with palliative care will likely be chronic and progressive. Thus, pain treatment also will require a sustained effort over time, with frequent need to adjust and alter the treatment regimen.

Pain Treatment

Opiate analgesics are the gold standard of pain relief in palliative care. Mild pain may respond to nonopiate analgesics such as acetaminophen. However, there is no reason to delay or avoid using the opiate analgesics due to misguided fears about side effects or addiction. The opiate analgesics have been utilized by physicians since antiquity. The modern era of opiate analgesics began in the early 1800s with the discovery that morphine was the active ingredient in opium. All subsequent developments in opiate analgesic therapy have only been minor alterations to this basic theme.

Opiates have been misclassified as weak or strong. Strength is a function of dose. All opiates or their synthetic cousins, the opioids, are weak or strong depending on how much is administered. In addition to the gold standard of morphine, a naturally occurring opiate, there are the semisynthetic opiates derived from natural opium. These have all been in use since the 1920s. They include hydromorphone, oxycodone, hydrocodone, and oxymorphone. Some patients have preferences, and selection of which agent to use depends more on preference and availability than on pharmacology. Oxycodone is available as an IV formulation in Europe but not in the United States. Fentanyl, a synthetic opioid, is preferred by some patients. Fentanyl is necessary for those patients who are intolerant to standard opiates or who require transdermal administration due to inability to take oral preparations.

Dosing

The correct dose provides acceptable pain relief without intolerable side effects. The variability in dose can be extraordinary, even within the same disease state. Some patients may require only 10 mg of oral morphine per day. Other patients, with pain that progresses slowly over time allowing for tolerance to the sedating effects of high-dose opiates, may require up to 1,000 mg oral morphine per day or even higher. The much-feared sedation and respiratory depression rarely, if ever, happen to cancer patients being titrated up on their opiate medication. The dose-limiting toxicities with prolonged use of high doses of opiate are myoclonus and delirium, signs of opiate-induced hyperalgesia. Ultimately, opiate-induced hyperalgesia, if unrecognized, leads to an upward spiral of pain, more medication, and still more pain.

Routes of Administration

The correct route of administration is the one that the patient prefers and/or is able to utilize. While oral administration is the most straightforward, transdermal, sublingual, or subcutaneous IV administration will be more appropriate in many cases.

■ MANAGEMENT OF BOWEL OBSTRUCTION

Nausea and vomiting are perhaps the most distressing symptoms that patients with advancing gynecological cancers will experience. Patients with ovarian cancer, in particular, are prone to carcinomatosis and partial or complete bowel obstruction (8). Complete bowel obstruction is unlikely to be misdiagnosed, with its hallmarks of feculent emesis and air-fluid levels on radiographic examination. Partial small bowel obstruction will be more difficult to discern. These patients will have waxing and waning symptoms, and frequently will be able to keep down some amount of food. Radiographs are often unrevealing. Telltale symptoms include early satiety and the vomiting up of food eaten many hours before.

Nausea and vomiting are not the same. Nausea is a subjective symptom, characterized by a feeling of distress in the abdomen. Vomiting is the forcible ejection of stomach contents. In general, nausea is far more distressing than vomiting, in that nausea may be constant and unrelenting, while vomiting is brief and transitory, and often leads to at least temporary relief of nausea.

Treatment

Pharmacological treatment of nausea depends on the underlying cause of the nausea. For intraabdominal disease, the antidopaminergic drugs such as prochlorperazine (Compazine) or haloperidol (Haldol) are useful. The combined antidopaminergic/antihistaminic agent promethazine (Phenergan) is also effective though somewhat more sedating. These medications are best given as scheduled, to prevent nausea, rather than as rescue medications. The serotonin 5-HT3 receptor antagonists such as ondansetron (Zofran) are extraordinarily effective at preventing the vomiting of chemotherapy. They have little effectiveness in treatment the chronic nausea of patients with advancing intraabdominal disease.

While partial small bowel obstruction often can be managed by limiting oral intake and pharmacological control of nausea, complete bowel obstruction usually requires some intervention to manage the gastric and intestinal secretion that back up from the obstruction. Options include placement of a nasogastric tube, insertion of a draining percutaneous gastric tube (9), or medical treatment with octreotide to markedly diminish the production of gastric, pancreatic, and biliary fluids (10). Patient preference and prognosis should guide which of these interventions is chosen. Having the option of stomach drainage allows the patient to take in some amount of liquid, as long as the drainage tube is successful in promptly removing the liquid from the stomach.

IV Fluids Versus Total Parenteral Nutrition (TPN) Versus Limited Oral Intake

For patients with bowel obstruction, the question will arise of whether, and with which fluids, to provide hydration and nutrition. Prognosis and, to a lesser extent, patient preference should guide this decision. For a few select patients with a slowly progressive cancer and a good performance status, TPN may be indicated (11). These patients may not yet be in the anorexia/cachexia phase of their cancer, and may still be able to make use of the calories and nutrients provided by TPN. For patients with a prognosis of many weeks, IV fluids will help prolong life and probably help maintain quality of life. For these patients, TPN is contraindicated and will typically lead to fluid overload, encephalopathy, and risk of infection without providing any benefit. When patients are expected to live only days to a few weeks, the provision of fluids of any type will be unlikely to change the time to dying and will be associated with a substantial logistical burden for families and caregivers and a risk of causing symptomatic edema or ascites.

■ DEPRESSION

There is the common misperception that patients dying of advancing disease must be depressed. This confuses the normal and almost universal sadness and grief experienced by the dying patient with depression. Depression is characterized by a loss of self-worth and an inability to find any hope or meaning in one's last days. In one study, the single question, "Are you depressed?" was as accurate a tool for diagnosing depression as much more extensive instruments. Depression in the terminally ill can respond to pharmacologic interventions. Successful treatment can markedly improve the quality of life for a dying patient. The psychostimulant methylphenidate (Ritalin) at doses between 5 and 20 mg per day can have an effect within days (12).

■ DELIRIUM/AGITATION

Delirium is perhaps the most challenging symptom for families to manage when caring for a loved one at home. In particular, the patient who is still strong enough to get out of bed, yet without the judgment to keep herself safe, will require nearly constant attention. Delirium can have many causes, including medications and infections. At times, a search for reversible causes of delirium will be

indicated. More often, the delirium results from a generalized, irreversible "brain failure" that heralds the nearness of dying.

Reversible Delirium. When delirium is thought to be reversible, then treatment with antidopaminergic agents such as haloperidol (Haldol) or chlorpromazine (Thorazine) and removal of offending agents is indicated.

Irreversible Delirium. Terminal delirium near the end of life is best treated with benzodiazepines, which will provide a desirable level of sedation that will be welcomed by family caregivers. Occasionally, benzodiazepines will produce a paradoxical excitation and be ineffective as sedatives. In this circumstance, higher doses of haloperidol or barbiturates may be necessary.

■ HOSPICE

Palliative care refers to a body of knowledge and a set of skills available to any practitioner for any patient with advancing disease. Hospice refers to a very specific program of services, constrained by very specific eligibility criteria and reimbursement models.

When to Refer

Hospice eligibility is commonly understood to be for patients in the last 6 months of life. However, most hospice patients are referred in the last few weeks of life. This reflects the reality that the 6-month prognosis is not the most important criterion for determining if a patient is eligible for hospice care. The more important criteria for hospice eligibility are that patients must let go of all life-prolonging treatments and the expectation of returning to the hospital for further diagnostic testing to assess the progress for the disease. For many patients and their physicians, it is not until dying is quite near that they are willing to make that change in the direction of care. It is likely, however, that earlier discussion of the limited benefits of further diagnostic studies, treatments, and hospitalizations will lead to more timely referrals to hospice.

Where Is Hospice Provided?

Most hospice care is provided in a patient's home, though this can be a private residence, adult foster care home or long-term care facility. Hospice also provides short-term, 5-day admission to nursing facilities as a respite for caregivers. Short-term acute hospice care can also be provided in a hospital or hospice facility when symptoms are beyond what can be controlled at home.

How to Refer

Unfortunately, discussion of hospice often is used to provide the first hint from the physician that treatment is no longer effective and that dying is near. Thus, hospice gets unfairly associated with the emotional distress of that news. Instead, hospice probably should be one of the last topics discussed in a conversation with patients and families about next steps. Only when patients and families have come to the acceptance that further treatment will not be effective and have chosen the goal of being at home for their remaining time should hospice be presented as a tool to accomplish that goal.

Scope of Service

Hospice provides guidance and support for the family and caregivers (or for the staff in long-term care facilities) of patients whose primary goal is remaining at home for their last days, weeks, or months of life. Hospice provides multidisciplinary care, including home visits by nurses, social workers, chaplains, bath aides, and volunteers. Moreover, all medications and equipment needs related to the terminal diagnosis are provided by hospice. Hospice programs also offer short-term inpatient stays for acute symptom management and 5-day respite stays in care facilities to provide caregivers with needed relief.

■ CARE IN THE LAST HOURS OF LIFE

Historically, death was a common, familiar occurrence that took place in a person's home. In the last century, death was transformed into a medical event occurring in a hospital. Due to this change, death is now unfamiliar to most families. Thus, there is a need to share with families what to expect in the last hours. Families should be told that most patients have a very peaceful end, that their body gradually weakens, and eventually even the strength to breathe is lost, leading to life's end.

■ ETHICS

Requests for Hastened Death

Requests for hastened death remain an area of controversy. Physician assisted death (PAD) refers to the practice in which the terminally ill patient is prescribed a lethal dose of a sedative, usually a barbiturate, which they must self-administer. This option is now legal in 4 states: Oregon, Washington, Montana, and Vermont. Euthanasia, in which the physician delivers a lethal injection of medication, remains illegal in all states. Data from the now 15-year history of legal PAD in Oregon indicate that while many patients may contemplate the option of

PAD, few make a specific request for PAD to their physician and yet fewer (less than 1% of all deaths) end their lives with this method. Data indicate that for these few patients the dominant motivations are a desire to control the time and manner of dying or a desire to avoid the inevitable loss of independence that accompanies dying (13). Conversely, those patients who pursue PAD out of fears of uncontrolled physical suffering at the end of life are nearly universally reassured by the provision of excellent palliative care and hospice, and thus never further pursue the request (14).

Suffering

A final word about suffering. Pain and suffering are not the same. As eloquently described by Eric Cassell, MD (15), pain is an experience of the body, and suffering is an experience of the person. As such, a person can experience great pain and yet have almost no suffering. Conversely, terrible suffering can and will occur even in the absence of any physical symptoms.

Cassell further elucidates that suffering occurs when there is any threat to the integrity of the person, in any or all the realms in which a person defines themselves—as a woman, a parent, a spouse, a professional, and so on. There is no more fundamental threat to the integrity of the person than the threat of dying. How is it, then, that most dying patients do not report suffering? Cassell suggests that it is through transcendence, a sense of greater purpose or meaning beyond one's self, that one overcomes the suffering of impending death. The job of good palliative care is to be in service of helping patients achieve that sense of transcendence, through accurate and compassionate discussion of prognosis and the lack of treatment options, through excellent symptom control, and through skillful referral to hospice care to allow patients to live out the remainder of their days in a location of their choosing.

■ REFERENCES

1. Weissman D. Consultation in palliative medicine. *Arch Int Med.* 1997;157(7):733–737.
2. von Gruenigen V, Daly B, Gibbons H, et al. Indicators of survival duration in ovarian cancer and implications for aggressiveness of care. *Cancer.* 2008;112 (10),2221–2227.
3. Christakis NA, Lamont EB. Extent and determinants of error in doctors' prognoses in terminally ill patients: prospective cohort study. *BMJ.* 2000;320:469–473.
4. Fromme EK, Smith MD, Bascom PB, Kenworthy-Heinige T, Lyons KS, Tolle SW. Incorporating routine survival prediction in a U.S. hospital-based palliative care service. *J Palliat Med.* 2010;13:1439–1444.
5. Kolomainen DF, Daponte A, Barton DPJ, et al. Outcomes of surgical management of bowel obstruction in relapsed epithelial ovarian cancer (EOC). *Gyn Onc.* 2012;125(1):31–36.
6. Back AL, Trinidad SB, Hopley EK, et al. What patients value when oncologists give news of cancer recurrence: commentary on

specific moments in audio-recorded conversations. *Oncologist.* 2011;16:342–350.

7. Temel JS, Greer JA, Muzikansky A, et al. Early palliative care for patients with metastatic non-small-cell lung cancer. *N Engl J Med.* 2010;363(8):733–742.

8. Herrinton LJ, Neslund-Dudas C, Rolnick SJ. Complications at the end of life in ovarian cancer. *J Pain Sym Manag.* 2007;34 (3):237–243.

9. Campagnutta E, Cannizzaro R, Gallo A, et al. Palliative treatment of upper intestinal obstruction by gynecological malignancy: the usefulness of percutaneous endoscopic gastrostomy. *Gynecol Oncol.* 1996;62(1):103–105.

10. Laval G, Rousselot H, Toussaint-Martel S, et al. SALTO: a randomized, multicenter study assessing octreotide LAR in inoperable bowel obstruction. *Bull Cancer.* 2012;99(2):1–9.

11. Madhok BM, Yeluri S, Haigh K, et al. Parenteral nutrition for patients with advanced ovarian malignancy. *J Hum Nutr Diet.* 2011;24(2):187–191.

12. Kerr CW, Drake J, Milch RA, et al. Effects of methylphenidate on fatigue and depression: a randomized, double-blind, placebo-controlled trial. *J Pain Symptom Manage.* 2012;43(1): 68–77.

13. http://public.health.oregon.gov/ProviderPartnerResources/EvaluationResearch/DeathwithDignityAct/Pages/index.aspx

14. Bascom P, Tolle S. Responding to requests for physician-assisted suicide: "these are uncharted waters for both of us." *JAMA.* 2002;288:91–98.

15. Cassell EJ. The nature of suffering and the goals of medicine. New York, NY: Oxford University Press; 1991.

Index